"With the help of this book, any intelligent person can obtain the information necessary to make informed choices. This unique book will provide the tools and confidence you need to have the best possible birth experience."

—Don Creevy, M.D., FACOG Clinical Assistant Professor
in Gynecology and Obstetrics at
Stanford University School of Medicine

"In Henci Goer, thinking women have a champion, and maternity caregivers have a challenger. Henci has applied her impressive intellect, wisdom, writing skills, common sense, and wit to produce *The Thinking Woman's Guide to a Better Birth*."

—Penny Simkin,
coauthor of *Pregnancy, Childbirth, and the Newborn*
and author of *The Birth Partner*

"*The Thinking Woman's Guide to a Better Birth* puts the power of the latest scientific findings on childbirth into the hands of women to help them discern the facts from the myths and make informed decisions about their maternity care."

—Maureen P. Corry, MPH,
Executive Director, Maternity Center Association

THE
THINKING
WOMAN'S
GUIDE TO A
BETTER BIRTH

Henci Goer

A PERIGEE BOOK

A Perigee Book
Published by The Berkley Publishing Group
A division of Penguin Group (USA) Inc.
375 Hudson Street
New York, New York 10014

First edition: October 1999

Published simultaneously in Canada.

The Penguin Group (USA) Inc. World Wide Web site address is
http://www.penguin.com

Library of Congress Cataloging-in-Publication Data

Goer, Henci.
    The thinking woman's guide to a better birth / Henci Goer. —1st
ed.
        p. cm.
    Includes bibliographical references and index.
    ISBN 0-399-52517-3
    1. Pregnancy Popular works.   2. Childbirth Popular works.
    I. Title.
    RG525.G51375 1999
    618.4—dc21   99-12456
                                                                   CIP

Printed in the United States of America

19 18 17 16 15 14 13 12 11

To my three children, the birth of whom, among other joys, led me into my life's work. And to my beloved husband, who gave me those children.

I also want to acknowledge the inestimable contribution of my writers' critique group, Alexis Rubin and Cindy Tolliver, and my agent, Diana Finch, who made it all possible.

We can no longer say that a great deal of American obstetric practice goes forth without adequate research. It is now more accurate to say that many interventions are used routinely or frequently in spite of research that has clearly shown that the procedure is being used inappropriately in this country.

—Judith Pence Rooks,
Midwifery and Childbirth in America

If you don't know your options, you don't have any.

—Diana Korte and Roberta Scaer,
A Good Birth, A Safe Birth

Contents

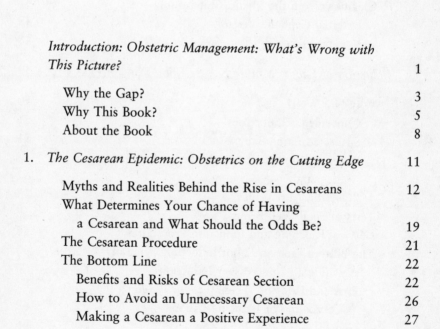

Contents

Contents

Contents

Contents

Contents

THE THINKING WOMAN'S GUIDE TO A BETTER BIRTH

Introduction

OBSTETRIC MANAGEMENT:
WHAT'S WRONG WITH THIS PICTURE?

Y OU'RE EXPECTING A baby or planning to become pregnant. Congratulations! You are embarking on a challenging and potentially highly rewarding journey. Without question, you want to have a safe and satisfying birth experience. I want that for you too, and I wrote this book because achieving that goal isn't as straightforward as it ought to be. Over the past thirty years, obstetric management has converted what should, in most cases, be a healthy, normal process into a high-tech event. Without anybody intending it to happen and with little recognition that it has happened, things have gone terribly wrong with maternity care in this country. Consider the following:

- Cesarean section is *the* most common major surgery performed in this country. Every year in the United States one in five—nearly one million—pregnant women have a cesarean section, despite the health risks, pain, recovery time, and expense. The consensus of the medical literature is that half of these operations were not needed.

1

- Doctors now use electronic fetal monitoring, a machine that records the baby's heart rate in conjunction with the mother's contractions, on four out of five laboring women. The percentage has risen steadily in the face of a stream of studies showing that its use doesn't improve babies' health. In fact, its routine use threatens the mother's health by increasing the odds of forceps or vacuum extraction deliveries and cesarean section.
- At some hospitals, almost every laboring woman has an epidural. Doctors assure women they are safe. Meanwhile, studies document a host of epidural complications affecting mother, baby, or both.
- Nearly half of women giving birth vaginally still have an episiotomy, a snip at the bottom of the vaginal opening. The research proves up, down, and sideways that, with rare exceptions, this procedure does no good and often does harm— sometimes serious and permanent harm.
- Most women who have a cesarean section automatically have them for subsequent babies. Reams of data show that vaginal birth after cesarean is safer for mothers, has advantages for babies, and will work for nearly three-quarters of women.
- Few women in this country give birth attended by a midwife. Yet studies consistently find that mothers and babies cared for by midwives experience fewer complications and have fewer tests and procedures compared with similar women managed by obstetricians. Midwives in several large studies have cesarean rates as low as 4 percent.
- Virtually no pregnant women managed within the conventional medical system escape without having tests, drugs, procedures, or restrictions that studies show offer little or no benefit when used indiscriminately but which introduce risks.

In short, there is a gap between how the typical obstetrician practices and what the medical literature supports. This gap goes largely unrecognized by obstetricians themselves. The obvious question becomes: "How can this be?"

WHY THE GAP?

OBSTETRIC PRACTICE DOES not reflect the research evidence because obstetricians actually base their practices on a set of predetermined beliefs. If you start from this premise, everything about obstetrics, including the inconsistencies between research and practice, makes sense.

There is nothing unique in shaping the care of childbearing women according to what one believes. Every culture does it. The problem is that obstetric beliefs don't fit the realities of pregnancy and childbirth. Obstetrician-gynecologists are surgical specialists in the pathology of women's reproductive organs. The typical obstetrician is trained to view pregnant and laboring women as a series of potential problems, despite the fact that pregnancy and childbirth are normal physiological processes that are no more likely to go seriously wrong than, say, digestion. Obstetric belief tends to become a self-fulfilling prophecy. It has been said that a healthy person is someone who hasn't undergone enough testing by specialists.

Obstetricians work within the medical model, a model that says drugs and procedures are the answer to whatever goes wrong. However, labor difficulties usually resolve themselves with tincture of time or simple remedies. Sterner, riskier measures are rarely required.

Obstetricians are also influenced by the broader culture in that it is believed that technology is superior to nature and machines are more reliable than people. This explains why they will not back off from technologies that have proven to be failures except to replace them with the next new and untested expensive technology that comes down the road. It also explains why *not* intervening has the burden of proving itself rather than the other way around.

Finally, until recently nearly all obstetricians were male, and even today, female obstetricians train in curricula devised by and mostly supervised by men. This means that gender bias permeates the system—as indeed it permeates all of medicine, only here all the patients are women, which intensifies its effects. One tenet of gender bias is that women's bodies are weak and defective and cannot be trusted to do what they are supposed to do. Little wonder, then, that the foundation of obstetrics is that obstetricians are needed to rescue babies from their mothers' bodies. Little wonder too that obstetric remedies rarely involve the mother's actions but are things done to her. If you see the mother as the problem, you don't see her as the solution. Gender bias also values the "masculine" qualities of control, efficiency, and predictability. This explains why obstetricians define "normal" within ever tighter limits around "average," although as with any bodily process, "normal" covers a wide range. It values action over inaction, hence the obstetric inclination to do something—anything—rather than nothing, even when "nothing" is the best thing to do. And it values top-down relationships, which explains why many obstetricians treat any questioning of their actions as a challenge to their authority and why they will not learn from any other source—midwives or nurses, for example—besides each other.

Returning to the question, "Why the gap?," one characteristic of beliefs is that they unconsciously color what those who hold them think and do. Believers "know" that their way of thinking and doing is the only right way. This means that obstetrics lacks a self-correcting mechanism. Research doesn't change practice, because a primary characteristic of belief is that evidence to the contrary makes no difference: "My mind is made up; don't confuse me with the facts." For this reason, anything that doesn't fit with the obstetric belief system will be denied or explained away, while anything that fits will be accepted without question. This prevents the recognition that obstetric management frequently doesn't work, that alternative strategies do, and most important, that obstetric management can cause harm. In other words, science and logic can have no effect unless obstetricians first change their beliefs, which is unlikely because those beliefs are the underpinnings of obstetrics.

WHY THIS BOOK?

THIS BRINGS ME back to my reasons for writing *The Thinking Woman's Guide to a Better Birth*. There is another model of care that, unlike obstetric management, fits the realities of pregnancy and childbirth. The midwifery model of care is founded on the belief that pregnancy and labor can be trusted to go right most of the time and that, as renowned French physician Dr. Michel Odent has said, "One cannot help an involuntary process. The point is not to disturb it." These terms indicate a philosophy, not a practitioner, although, of course, more obstetricians practice obstetric management and midwives offer midwifery care than vice versa. Emphasizing supportive rather than interventive care, the midwifery model demonstrably produces equally good and often better outcomes, a point I hope to prove to you in this book.

I also hope to give you the knowledge to make informed choices for yourself and your unborn baby. Unless you have medical background and a lot of free time, this knowledge is hard to come by. As we have just seen, what your caregivers tell you may be biased. And it is only human for caregivers to tell you only as much as will get you to do what they think best; the very concept of "informed consent" implies that once you are informed, you will consent. Without medical background, you have no way to evaluate the quality of your care, pick caregivers who practice according to the best research, or question your treatment. Like *Consumer Reports,* I will present the data you need to choose wisely and to practice "informed refusal" as well as "informed consent."

Finally, I will give you strategies that will enable you to avoid unnecessary medical intervention. An editor for whom I once wrote told me there isn't a lot of point in giving information unless your readers can do something with it. You have to give them some "take-home pay." Consider the strategies your "take-home pay."

You have no doubt gathered that this book will not be neutral. I don't profess to be any more objective than anyone else about what I think makes for optimal care. Yes, I will be trying to convert you to my way of thinking, but with a couple of differences. First, I will play fair. I will lay out the research data behind my thinking so that you can make up your own mind. You don't have to agree with me. Second, I want to give you the ability to decide what is right for you, not necessarily what I think would be right for me. To that end, I will offer a broad range of options and compare and contrast them.

I should add as well that I hold my opinions in good company. *A Guide to Effective Care in Pregnancy and Childbirth,* the summary of the conclusions of the *Cochrane Database of Systematic Reviews,* and *Pursuing the Birth Machine,* an analysis of the recommendations of the World Health Organization's consensus conferences on appropriate technology for care before, during, and after birth, agree with me pretty much on all points.

The problems with the medicalized, high-tech approach are well known to many people involved with maternity care in this country. A number of these organizations and individuals, including me, have come together to form the Coalition for Improving Maternity Services (CIMS, pronounced "kims"). Over a series of meetings, CIMS developed a consensus statement entitled the "Mother-Friendly Childbirth Initiative." Twenty-six organizations representing thousands of childbirth professionals ratified this document, including the professional associations of nurse-midwives, direct-entry midwives, maternity nurses, childbirth educators, labor support professionals, and lactation consultants. Twenty-seven prominent writers, researchers, and childbirth reform activists also ratified it. I was proud to be one of them. Since publication, many additional organizations and individuals have endorsed the document. The premises and conclusions of this book agree completely with the "Mother-Friendly Childbirth Initiative," reproduced at the back of this book.

Still, because I have biases (although I hope I am not prejudiced), I think you should know up front what those biases are. Here is my "full disclosure" statement.

I believe that the unconscious principles and resultant conscious practices of obstetric management fail to meet the needs of women and babies and cause many of the problems they claim to prevent or cure.

I am not antitechnology, but I am opposed to the routine use of intervention. I have attended labors in which the judicious use of technology probably saved the baby, and even in a case or two, possibly the mother, but the key word is *judicious*. I believe the injudicious use of technology is doing considerable physical and psychological harm to mothers and babies.

I am not antiobstetrician. I know personally and by reputation many fine obstetricians. I also believe that most doctors want to do well by their patients, although I have seen, experienced, and read about enough instances of arrogance, indifference, ignorance, and even cruelty to have no illusions. Still, the main problem is differing definitions of "doing well." Here is what I think defines good care. Good obstetricians, family practitioners, and midwives:

- Believe childbearing to be a fundamentally healthy and normal part of a woman's life.
- Treat women holistically, taking into consideration their thoughts, feelings, concerns, and priorities.

- Respect the right of women to make informed decisions for themselves and their babies.
- Respect labor as an experience with its own lessons and rewards.
- Offer supportive rather than interventive care.
- Evaluate individually and do not treat by rule.
- Start small when intervention becomes necessary.
- Keep abreast of the medical literature.

ABOUT THE BOOK

HERE ARE THE hows and whys of the book's organization.

Chapter 1 looks at the most pressing issue in maternity care: the cesarean epidemic. It serves as an overview and introduction to the rest of the book. The chapters that follow it discuss various issues of obstetric management in chronological order as you would encounter them during late pregnancy and labor. These prepare you for the last chapters, which give practical advice on how to choose someone who does professional labor support (a *doula* or *monitrice*), a caregiver, and a birth site.

The chapters all follow the same pattern. Each one begins with an overview that critiques mainstream belief and practices, followed by descriptions of any procedures, if relevant. Next comes "The Bottom Line." Here is where you will find summaries of the trade-offs of various approaches and strategies for avoiding unnecessary intervention. Every chapter other than chapter 1, "The Cesarean Epidemic," closes with "Gleanings from the Medical Literature." This section lists the conclusions I think can be drawn from the research data. I have keyed the statements within this section to chapter appendices that contain summaries of the evidence supporting each conclusion. The summaries include footnotes and reference lists. I chose this arrangement so you can look up what interests you without being distracted by the mini-reviews of the literature. Other appendices give the full text of the "Mother-Friendly Childbirth Initiative" and a list of organizations and resources related to pregnancy and childbirth.

I have tried to make this book responsive to many different needs. I wrote each chapter so that it can be read independently of any other chapter. This means you don't have to read sequentially and can skip around to whatever interests you. In particular, don't get bogged down in the research summaries if they aren't your cup of tea. I put them in for those of you who want to make your own evaluation and don't like taking anybody's word for it. You may also find them useful to show your doctor or midwife.

I have had to be selective in the data I presented, but I think I have included enough to make my case. For most chapters, I read two to three times the number of papers as appear in the bibliography and appendix reference lists. One tactic for dismissing a work like mine is to say that you can find a study to support any position, but that does not apply here. *The data uniformly failed to support common obstetric practice for most of the topics I researched.* (I should also point out that although studies will, of course, continue to be published after I complete this book, once there is a body of well-done studies that reach the same conclusion, future studies rarely reverse that conclusion.) Where there was surface agreement in the literature with what obstetricians typically do—pregnancies that go past their due date comes to mind—I think that agreement can be challenged by digging deeper and looking at the quality of the evidence on which it is based. By contrast, while it was almost always clear that current practice should be abandoned, what ought to be done instead was often less clear. I incorporated the pros and cons in these cases into "The Bottom Line."

You may be wondering about my credentials to write this book since I am not a doctor—either M.D. or Ph.D.—a midwife, or a nurse. I am a certified childbirth educator with a degree in biology from Brandeis University. Beyond that, I am self-taught. I am also the author of *Obstetric Myths Versus Research Realities: A Guide to the Medical Literature.* In that book, I organized and wrote hundreds of summaries of articles from the medical journals so that childbirth educators, midwives, and others could have at their fingertips the data supporting what most of them teach or practice. That book was well received. In fact, several midwifery schools have adopted *Obstetric Myths* as a textbook, and some childbirth education certification programs have made it required reading.

To those who would argue that you need more letters after your name in order to write a book like this one, let me respond with a story. Penny Simkin, a well-known educator, writer, speaker, and editor, was called on the carpet by an anesthesiologist, irate that she had written a handout listing the potential trade-offs of epidural anesthesia when she was not a doctor (although he did not dispute her accuracy). "What are your credentials?" he demanded. "I can read," she mildly replied. So can I.

One final point: The things you are about to read may well worry or distress you or even make you angry. I have not tried to be needlessly alarming, but I haven't pulled any punches either. This book was written on the same principle as sex education; namely, I would prefer you to be uncomfortable rather than ignorant. My goal is for you never to have cause to say "But I didn't know *that* was an option" or "I never would have agreed if I had known *that* could happen."

While my intent is to enlighten and offer strategies to meet a wide range of individual needs, you may also find yourself feeling overwhelmed by the many possibilities I present and their various trade-offs. Think of them merely as jumping-off points for discussions with your doctor or midwife—and, in fact, how he or she reacts to your raising these issues can tell you whether you have the right person. You can, of course, also leave all or most decisions up to your caregiver. That is a perfectly valid choice. The important thing is that it be a conscious *choice*, not one you felt constrained to make.

Chapter 1

THE CESAREAN EPIDEMIC:
OBSTETRICS ON THE CUTTING EDGE

IN 1970, THE U.S. cesarean rate was a stable 5 percent. By 1980, it had more than tripled. By 1983, one in five women was giving birth by major surgery, and the rate has yet to drop below that number. Some hospitals today perform cesareans on more than one-third of their obstetric patients, and a few surgically deliver as many as half. Cesarean section is *the* most common major surgical procedure performed in the United States.

No objective person could possibly believe that one in five women requires major surgery in order to be a healthy mother giving birth to a healthy baby. Experts estimate that the national rate could safely be halved, which means that at a minimum, nearly half a million women have unnecessary C-sections every year.

Compared with vaginal birth, cesarean section carries substantially increased risks of death and permanent injury. It takes a physical and emotional toll, and it casts a shadow over the rest of a woman's reproductive life. So the questions become:

What caused the rise, why hasn't it been reversed, and how can you protect yourself from an unnecessary cesarean?

MYTHS AND REALITIES BEHIND THE RISE IN CESAREANS

ALL OTHER FACTORS behind the rise in cesarean rate pale into insignificance beside obstetricians' beliefs about childbirth and cesarean section. Obstetrics (as opposed to midwifery) is based on the principle that the obstetrician's job is to use a full panoply of tests, drugs, and procedures to preserve mothers and babies from nature's "inept" process. Obstetricians believed this long before the rise in cesareans. What held the cesarean rate in check was that obstetricians viewed C-sections as even more dangerous than vaginal birth. Once improvements in surgical and anesthetic techniques changed that perception, the genie was out of the bottle.

Cesarean section has many things to recommend it from the obstetrician's point of view. By rescuing mother and baby from the supposed rigors and hazards of labor, it reinforces obstetric belief in the superiority of technology over nature, and the more cesareans, the stronger the illusion that such rescue is needed. C-sections enable obstetricians to do what they were trained to do. Obstetrics, despite all the rhetoric about being primary care or general women's-health practice, is a surgical specialty. It allows obstetricians to control what is otherwise an uncomfortably unpredictable process, while reinforcing the belief that their skills and knowledge are necessary and important.

The fit between cesarean section and obstetric belief leads obstetricians to hold positions that cannot be defended on any rational basis. Hard as it is to believe, more than one doctor has argued in print that all women should have cesareans. Recently, a group of obstetricians writing an editorial in the most prestigious U.S. medical journal, the *New England Journal of*

Medicine, argued against trying to lower the current one-woman-in-five cesarean rate.

It also leads obstetricians to exaggerate the problems of vaginal birth and minimize those of cesarean delivery. For example, the head of obstetrics and gynecology at the University Hospitals of Cleveland recently defended elective cesarean section (cesarean section for no other reason than that the mother wants one), saying, "In this day and age, the risks [of cesarean section] are manageable, and it's over in twenty minutes." A 1996 survey of obstetricians found that nearly one-third of the women and one-tenth of the men would choose a cesarean over a vaginal birth for themselves or their wives. It is no coincidence that in the countries with the highest cesarean and instrumental delivery rates in the world, obstetricians, rather than midwives, manage large numbers of normal pregnancies and births.

The reasons so many obstetricians in the survey favored elective C-section show obstetric prejudices at work. First, 80 percent of survey respondents believed that vaginal birth would injure the vagina, pelvic floor, or *perineum* (the block of tissue between the vagina and the anus). They thought cesarean section would prevent urinary incontinence, fecal incontinence, and sexual dysfunction. In reality, these injuries and their chronic effects arise almost exclusively from *episiotomies* (cutting the vaginal opening to enlarge it) and forceps and vacuum-extraction deliveries. Their belief that the natural process is always the problem and that drugs and procedures are always the cure effectively prevented them from seeing that obstetric management causes these problems, not childbirth per se. Second, 40 percent of respondents preferring elective cesarean feared that healthy babies could be damaged during vaginal birth, a belief that has no basis in fact. In fact elective cesarean is the greater hazard. It increases the incidence of babies born in poor condition, with breathing problems, admission to special-care nurseries, and jaundice compared with vaginal birth. Finally, more than one-quarter liked the idea of scheduling the delivery date. Only a major distortion of reality would allow someone to think that the convenience of scheduling the birth justifies major surgery.

Similarly, the main arguments against attempts to lower the cesarean rate in the *New England Journal of Medicine* editorial rested on the potential risks to the baby of laboring with a scarred uterus and the only recently appreciated dangers of vacuum extraction, a procedure the authors believed zealous physicians are substituting for cesarean section.* Bias blinds the authors to the obvious solution: Obstetricians should strive for spontaneous vaginal births, not complacency about the number of cesarean sections.

The strength of obstetric prejudices also explains why reversing the trend has proven so difficult. Beliefs do not respond to logic, science, or common sense. The fact that the cesarean rate is indefensible hasn't stopped obstetricians from defending it. Here are some excuses you may hear and why they are just that—excuses, not reasons or rationales.

- *We don't really know what the cesarean rate should be, and we should not try to lower it before we are certain that doing so will not compromise the health of mothers and babies.* This argument has gained prominence recently as a backlash to pressures to reduce the cesarean rate. It is disingenuous. Dozens of studies and statistical analyses, many of them cited or summarized in this book, document that the cesarean rate could safely be half to one-third of its current rate.
- *The rise in cesarean sections is responsible for the decline in perinatal mortality rates (the percentage of babies dying in the weeks before, during, or shortly after birth).* Just because two things happen at the same time doesn't mean one caused

---

*The rise in vacuum extraction is undoubtedly due to the increase in epidurals and the shift from forceps to vacuum extraction, not attempts to avoid cesarean.

the other. As one researcher pointed out, the rise in the British cesarean rate correlated equally well with, among other things, the rise in violent crime in the United States and the declining stork population in Holland. The two major causes of perinatal death are prematurity and congenital anomalies, neither of which can be fixed by cesarean section. The development of modern intensive care units and programs to fund prenatal care for low-income women have undoubtedly had more to do with falling perinatal mortality rates than did doing more C-sections. Medical research confirms that C-section rates and perinatal mortality rates are not connected. Comparisons of international cesarean rates versus perinatal mortality rates show no relation between the two. Studies at individual hospitals have shown equal declines in perinatal mortality rates at hospitals where cesarean rates remained low and at hospitals where they rose, no decline in death rates as cesarean rates went up, and that high cesarean rates can be slashed without adverse consequences.

- *Babies have gotten bigger.* Even if they have—and this is debatable—it shouldn't matter. The cesarean rate for babies weighing 8 lbs., 13 oz., or more (4,000 grams) was 3 percent in 1958 in Great Britain. Obstetricians currently may perform cesareans on as many as half of women with babies of this size, but this says something about obstetricians, not women's ability to birth big babies.

- *My cesarean rate is right on the national average.* A perennial favorite, this one amounts to "All the other kids are doing it."

- *Our hospital handles more high-risk cases.* Having a newborn intensive care unit (NICU) indicates that the hospital handles more high-risk cases. Public Citizen's Health Research Group periodically compiles data on over three thousand hospitals nationwide. In 1992, the average cesarean rate at hospitals with NICUs was 22.0 percent, versus 22.4 percent at hospitals that didn't have one. A perusal of individual hospital statistics also quickly reveals cesarean rates that are all over the map, regardless of the presence or absence of a NICU.

- *Women have the right to choose a cesarean even when it isn't medically indicated.* Until recently, this one mostly has had to do with the right to have a planned cesarean after having had a cesarean for a prior birth. I would be the first to champion making informed choices, but that is something else again. Offhandedly asking a woman who thinks her cesarean rescued her or her baby from a difficult labor if she wants to try labor again hardly constitutes informed choice. And that's the best most women get. By contrast, when doctors are enthusiastic and encouraging, and women get not only information but emotional support, few refuse labor. Simply by getting obstetricians to recommend vaginal birth after cesarean (VBAC, pronounced "vee-back") and offering VBAC classes or counseling to expectant mothers with prior C-sections, hospitals have been able to greatly increase the number of women willing to labor again.

    Popping up lately in the medical literature are arguments that women should be able to have first cesareans for the asking as well. Again, this is presented as a freedom-of-choice issue. But how much real freedom do women have in a culture that portrays labor as torture and C-sections as a "no muss, no fuss" option?

So if it isn't about women or achieving better outcomes, what is driving cesarean rates? The obstetric belief that choosing between a cesarean and a vaginal birth is like choosing between chocolate and vanilla opens the door to a number of other influences, all of which work subliminally but powerfully on the choices doctors and hospitals make.

- *Money.* Obstetricians often receive hundreds of dollars more for a cesarean. Hospitals make thousands of dollars more.

When a research project at a Chicago hospital lowered the cesarean rate from 18 percent to 12 percent between 1985 and 1987, the hospital involved lost $1 million in revenues. The need to fill hospital beds provides strong financial motives to perform cesareans. Public Citizen's Health Research Group points out other potential effects of that need: Because they bring in patients, hospital administrators may be reluctant to alienate obstetricians by interfering in their practices. I would add that profit may also motivate the use of other technologies that increase the cesarean rate as a by-product, such as epidural anesthesia and electronic fetal monitoring, which enables reduced staffing. Studies consistently show that for-profit hospitals have higher cesarean rates than non-profits, HMO-owned hospitals, or county hospitals. Private obstetricians also have higher cesarean rates compared with obstetricians caring for clinic patients, although low-income women have the higher medical risk.

- *Impatience.* About one-third of all cesareans are performed for reasons that amount to "she couldn't get the baby out." However, this is a purely subjective diagnosis, and the definition of how long is too long has shrunk considerably. Back in 1970, a British survey found that labor was considered "long" at eighteen hours, although that didn't necessarily demand action. By 1990, many obstetricians here and abroad had imposed a twelve-hour limit, a figure that may even be somewhat shorter than average, let alone abnormal, for first-time mothers. Experts and obstetric professional organizations also advise that cesareans for poor progress should not be done in early labor when progress in dilation is normally minimal, but doctors frequently ignore this caveat. As a result, between 1980 and 1989, the proportion of women deemed to have dysfunctional labor grew by 60 percent, and while not all of these women had cesareans, many did.
- *Convenience.* Studies have shown that obstetricians are less likely to perform cesareans late at night or on weekends.

Also, the cesarean rate is lower when obstetricians are in the hospital on-call with no other demands on their time.

- *Peer pressure and hospital culture.* Cesarean rates vary by region, by hospital, and according to rates at the institution where the obstetrician trained. In a glimpse into peer pressure and hospital culture at work, salaried doctors working for a new HMO had a 15 percent cesarean rate for low-risk first-time mothers during the first year of operation, compared with a 21 percent rate for private physicians at the same hospital. Leaving aside that both rates are too high, within a couple of years, the HMO doctors' rates approached that of their colleagues. Conversely, a new freestanding birth center reduced its cesarean rate from 18 percent to 7 percent over the first year as practitioners got the hang of out-of-hospital birth.

- *Defensive medicine.* This has actually played a smaller role than doctors and the media would lead you to think. The cesarean rate tripled before malpractice suits ever became an issue. Nonetheless, several analyses suggest that fear of being sued causes obstetricians to perform more cesareans and to use tests and technologies that increase the risk of cesarean without counterbalancing benefits. Currently, defensive medicine has been raising its ugly head in the matter of VBACs. Prominent obstetricians and the United States obstetricians' professional organization openly admit that malpractice suits are at the root of recommendations calculated to roll back twenty years of progress in VBAC rates (although they frequently couch the issue in terms of concern for women's and babies' health and women's freedom of choice (see page 166). Few challenge the ethics of the "defensive medicine" excuse. While I sympathize with the doctors' worry over unjustified malpractice suits, physicians have the obligation to use their skills to serve their patients, not themselves at their patients' expense. And when I consider the stakes involved, my sympathy for the doctors fades. The obstetrician may face the unpleasantness and distress of a court case; the woman could lose her uterus, a subsequent baby, or her life.

WHAT DETERMINES YOUR CHANCE OF HAVING A CESAREAN AND WHAT SHOULD THE ODDS BE?

WHETHER YOU HAVE a cesarean depends very little on your or your baby's state of health. When researchers selected a sample of 4,500 women who had no risk factors predisposing to cesarean and compared outcomes with women who had those factors, virtually identical numbers in both groups had cesareans. To give you an idea of the capricious nature of the cesarean decision, researchers asked five experts to review fifty cases of cesarean section for fetal distress. In nearly one-third of the cases, four of the five reviewers agreed the cesarean wasn't necessary. But that's not the worst of it. Three months later, given the same fifty cases, the experts changed their minds in 20 to 40 percent of the cases. Studies show that whether you have a cesarean depends on such factors as what part of the country you live in (the South is the worst, the West the best); whether the hospital is for-profit; the hospital culture and policies; which nurse you get; whether you have an obstetrician, family practitioner, or midwife; whether you plan to have your baby in a hospital, in a freestanding birth center, or at home; and most especially, your particular caregiver's cesarean rate. This last, in turn, depends on your caregiver's beliefs about birth.

Very few cesareans are done for reasons on which everyone agrees, such as when the placenta is covering the cervix (*placenta previa*). Most are done for reasons that depend on a judgment call or the individual caregiver's philosophy. Two-thirds of cesarean sections in this country are done for either insufficient progress or merely because the prior birth was a cesarean. Another 10 percent are for fetal distress. Breech presentation (when the baby is buttocks, knees, or feet down) accounts for another 10 percent or so. Premature babies and twins contribute another few percent. So all but about 10 percent of cesareans are done for reasons whose diagnosis and treatment vary enormously from place to place and practitioner to practitioner and for which the research shows that doing cesareans routinely doesn't improve outcomes.

What, then, is a reasonable rate? Over a decade ago, the World Health Organization concluded that since countries with some of the lowest perinatal mortality rates in the world had cesarean section rates of less than 10 percent, there was no justification for any region to have a cesarean rate more than 10 to 15 percent. Dr. Edward Quilligan, long-time editor of the *American Journal of Obstetrics and Gynecology,* estimated that based on occurrence rates of various complications of labor, cesarean section rates should range between about 8 percent and 17.5 percent, depending on the mix of low- to high-risk patients. However, several U.S. hospitals serving primarily high-risk, low-income women have been able to maintain cesarean rates in the 10 to 12 percent range without any detriment in newborn outcomes, which suggests that Quilligan's maximum is an overestimate. The authors of *A Guide to Effective Care in Pregnancy and Childbirth,* which summarizes the conclusions of ongoing analyses of the best medical research, observed that little improvement in outcomes occurs when cesarean rates rise above about 7 percent. A pair of British researchers performed an estimate similar to Dr. Quilligan's, and they also concluded that the national cesarean rate should be about 7 percent. Taking these opinions all together, the appropriate cesarean rate should lie within a few percentage points on either side of 10 percent.

Some years ago, faced with a cesarean rate approaching 25 percent, the U.S. government set the goal of achieving a 15 percent national cesarean rate by the year 2000. Ironically, in 1979, the National Institutes of Health viewed a 15 percent rate with such alarm that it convened a panel of experts to develop recommendations on how to lower it. Be that as it may, the likelihood of meeting the year 2000 target is nil. Even if we have turned the corner—and there are indications that the recent downturn is only temporary—we aren't likely to retreat to a 15 percent rate for years. A lot of mothers and babies will suffer before then. Some of them will die.

THE CESAREAN PROCEDURE

IN PREPARATION, NURSES will start an IV if there isn't one already in place. Most cesareans are performed under epidural anesthesia (see page 129 for the procedure). If you already have an epidural, the anesthesiologist will strengthen it so that you are numb up to your breastbone. Nurses will shave the pubic hair that shows when your legs are together, and insert a bladder catheter. Once you are on the operating table, your belly will be washed with antiseptic. Staff will place a screen across your chest that blocks your view of the operating field. If you are having general anesthesia, which is usually reserved for emergencies these days because of the increased risks, you will be put under by injecting a medication into your IV. Once you are unconscious, the anesthesiologist will put a tube down your throat to maintain an airway and deliver a gas anesthetic.

The operation generally takes about an hour. With rare exceptions, the roughly four-inch incision is made horizontally just above the pubic bone. A horizontal uterine incision is preferred because it produces a much stronger scar. However, in certain situations, such as when the placenta is covering the cervix, the incision is made vertically. You will feel pulling and tugging but no pain, similar to the experience of having a tooth pulled. The manipulations can make you queasy. The uterus and inner tissue layers are closed with stitches. The skin incision may be closed with conventional stitches, staples, or even tape strips.

THE BOTTOM LINE

BENEFITS AND RISKS OF CESAREAN SECTION

BENEFITS

A cesarean delivers the baby when vaginal birth would put mother or baby at risk or when the mother cannot deliver the baby vaginally.

RISKS

Intrinsic to cesareans are pain, debility, and a longer recovery period, all of which interfere with bonding with the baby and breastfeeding. In one study, one-quarter of the women reported pain when interviewed two weeks after their cesareans, and 15 percent still reported pain at eight weeks. More than 15 percent reported difficulties with normal activities such as getting out of bed, walking, bending, lifting, and tending the baby at two weeks. One in ten still reported problems at eight weeks.

Some cesarean complications relate strictly to the surgery and never occur with vaginal birth. Of those associated with both, all occur much more commonly with cesarean delivery.

During the operation, women with an epidural or spinal anesthetic may experience breathing difficulties if the anesthetic goes high enough to affect the breathing muscles. In some cases, women may have areas where there is no anesthesia. Hemorrhage and anesthesia complications may occur. According to one medical literature review, 1 to 6 percent of women lose enough blood to require a transfusion. Hemorrhage may sometimes require a hysterectomy. Accidental surgical injury to the bowel, bladder, uterus, or uterine blood vessels occurs in 2 percent of cases, although a ten-year review at one hospital reported that uterine injury occurred 10 percent of the time.

Postsurgical complications are also a problem. According to the same medical literature review, infection occurs 8 to 27 percent of the time after cesareans, 1 percent of women experience a paralyzed bowel (ileus), 6 to 18 women per 1,000 experience blood clots in their legs, and 1 to 2 per 1,000 experience clots that lodge in the lung (*pulmonary embolism*). The ten-year hospital review reported a 4.5 percent incidence of major complications—that is, severe hemorrhage, need for repeat surgery (generally to investigate bleeding), pelvic infection, blood clots, pneumonia, septicemia (blood poisoning), or clotting dysfunction (a result of severe hemorrhage). Nearly one-third of cesarean mothers experienced minor complications, including fever; hemorrhage; blood-filled swelling (*hematoma*); urinary tract, wound, or uterine infection; leg clots (*phlebitis*); or paralyzed bowel or bladder. In addition, long-term and chronic complications from scar tissue adhesions include pelvic pain, bowel problems, and pain during sexual intercourse.

Cesareans cause more maternal deaths than does vaginal birth. A 1989 analysis in Great Britain revealed that women were 550 percent more likely to die of an elective cesarean than a vaginal birth (9 versus 2 per 100,000). A Dutch study found that between 1983 and 1992, C-sections caused 700 percent more deaths than vaginal births did (28 versus 4 per 100,000). Obviously some factors that lead to C-section also threaten the mother's life. However, the British study compared elective cesarean, where there was no medical indication for the surgery, to vaginal birth to minimize that possibility, and the Dutch study investigated the exact cause of death. The numbers in the British study may also be low. Studies have found that data culled from vital statistics undercount cesarean death rates by 40 to 50 percent.

A cesarean poses risks to the baby as well. The baby may be cut, a complication that occurred in a little over 1 percent of head-down babies and 6 percent of breech babies in one hospital and in 1 percent of babies in the ten-year review. Cesarean-delivered babies are more likely to be in poor condition at birth. When researchers looked at 700 normal-weight babies born with low Apgar scores after healthy pregnancies, they found they were nearly half again as likely to be elective cesareans as vaginal births. Cesareans also increase the likelihood of breathing difficulties. Researchers compared outcomes for over 800 babies born by C-section for reasons unrelated to the baby's condition with 10,900 low-risk vaginal births. Babies born by cesarean were over three times as likely to be admitted to intermediate or intensive care (2.6 percent versus 8.7 percent) and five times more likely to need assistance with breathing (0.3 percent versus 1.5 percent). Another study compared elective cesareans—again, a situation where complications must be attributed to the cesarean, not the baby's condition—to women having trial of labor after a previous cesarean. It also documented more newborn breathing problems and more jaundice as well (see page 286).*

Women who have cesareans start motherhood behind a psychological eight ball. They face recovery from major surgery while trying to care for a newborn, and they must either cope with or suppress the host of negative feelings that swirl around both any experience of major surgery and the issues of needing an operation to have a baby. Beyond the natural feelings of disappointment, anger, frustration, or sadness at the loss of the expected birth experience, some women feel disfigured as well. Depression is more likely. Some women even experience post-traumatic stress reactions such as nightmares, flashbacks, or an overwhelming fear of pregnancy. A few women have difficulties forming an attachment to the baby. Psychological problems often lead to marital stress.

The trivialization of cesarean surgery compounds the situation. While it has long been recognized that major surgery has adverse psychological consequences, a recognition that enables

---

*Possible reasons are that the baby did not get the benefits of labor, which prepare her to breathe, or vaginal birth, which squeezes fluids out of her respiratory tract. The policy of giving a quart or more of IV fluid before surgery also plays a likely role. The resultant fluid overload causes fluid to collect in the lungs (see chapter 4).

medical staff to help surgical patients and their families expect and cope with those consequences, doctors and nurses rarely extend that acknowledgment to cesarean mothers. Every woman I interviewed for a magazine article on cesarean feelings said that medical staff and, as a result, their own families acted as if a cesarean were no big deal. Husbands, families, and friends expected the women to be "over it" physically and emotionally long before they really were. This left the women feeling inadequate as they struggled to recover from the operation while caring for a newborn. In addition, any expression of negative feelings was invariably met with "but the most important thing is a healthy baby," which left the women feeling guilty for experiencing feelings other than gratitude.

Finally, the scar tissue poses considerable risk to subsequent pregnancies and births. Cesarean section increases the risk of infertility and *ectopic pregnancy*, a life-threatening complication in which the embryo implants outside of the uterus, usually in the Fallopian tube leading to the ovary. Because the scar tissue interferes with placental attachment, cesareans increase the risk of the placenta detaching before the birth (*abruptio placentae*), growing over the cervix (*placenta previa*), or growing into or even through the muscular wall of the uterus (*placenta accreta* or *percreta*). The odds of placental complications soar with each succeeding cesarean, and the hemorrhage that results from placental attachment abnormalities or ectopic pregnancy can threaten the life and health of both mother and baby. The scar can also give way, causing massive bleeding and possibly expelling the baby into the abdominal cavity, an event that occurs in 4 per 1,000 women with horizontal scars and more often in women with vertical scars. In addition, pelvic scar tissue makes subsequent cesareans more technically difficult and injuries to other organs more likely.

HOW TO AVOID AN UNNECESSARY CESAREAN

- *Choose a caregiver with a low cesarean rate and a high vaginal birth after cesarean (VBAC) rate.* Based on the consensus that the cesarean rate should be around 10 percent, and allowing a generous margin, a doctor should have a cesarean rate of 15 percent or less, and a midwife's rate should be substantially less if she mostly cares for low-risk women, because twins, breeches, and serious health problems will be referred to an obstetrician. The VBAC rate should be at least 70 percent. It will be far easier to find midwives who fit those criteria than doctors.
- *Health permitting, have your baby at a freestanding birth center or at home.*
- *Have your baby in a hospital with a low cesarean rate and a high VBAC rate.* Again, look for a cesarean rate of 15 percent or less and a VBAC rate of 70 percent or more.
- *Choose a caregiver who deals with the emotional and psychological issues of pregnancy and childbirth.* This will almost certainly be a midwife. The mainstream medical model views labor strictly as a mechanical process and does not acknowledge the possibility that the mother's environment and her past experiences can influence labor progress.
- *Hire someone who does professional labor support (doula).*
- *Deal with psychological baggage.* If you don't, it can prevent you from making good choices and impede labor. Psychological baggage includes such issues as history of childhood sexual or physical abuse, prior traumatic birth experience, overwhelming fear of labor or birth, or overwhelming control issues such as might come from growing up with an alcoholic parent. Your midwife, doula, or childbirth educator may be able to help you. Mental health professionals may also be of assistance, although the research is relatively new, and many

counselors know little about the standard run of childbearing issues, let alone these problems. The following books may help you: *Creating a Joyful Birth Experience: Developing a Partnership with Your Unborn Child for Healthy Pregnancy, Labor, and Early Parenting* by L. Capacchione and S. Bardsley, *Courage to Heal: A Guide for Women Survivors of Sexual Abuse* by L. Davis and E. Bass, *Birthing from Within* by P. England and R. Horowitz, *I Can't Get Over It: A Handbook for Trauma Survivors* by A. Matsakis, *Banished Knowledge: Facing Childhood Injuries* by A. Miller, and *An Easier Childbirth: A Mother's Workbook for Health and Emotional Well-Being During Pregnancy and Delivery* by G. Peterson.

- *Don't plan a repeat cesarean.*
- *Refuse a planned cesarean for a big baby.*
- *Take steps to turn a breech baby head down.*
- *Consider vaginal breech birth.*
- *Consider refusing prenatal tests of fetal well-being. (See page 61.)*
- *Consider refusing induction of labor for going past your date or for rupture of membranes.*
- *Refuse routine continuous electronic fetal monitoring.*
- *Refuse routine breaking of the bag of waters (amniotomy).*
- *Refuse a cesarean for slow progress prior to 4 centimeters' dilation.*
- *Avoid an epidural.*
- *Stay active in labor.*

MAKING A CESAREAN A POSITIVE EXPERIENCE

- *Make an informed decision.* Barring an emergency, before you agree, make sure you understand the benefits and risks of the surgery and the benefits and risks of the alternatives to surgery, including doing nothing. Doctors tend to tell you just enough to get you to say yes.

- *Be awake during the operation.* You will not see the actual operation, and it permits you to be "present" when your child is born. Anything that makes the cesarean more like a birth is to your advantage.

- *Have your partner, doula, or other loved ones with you while being prepped for surgery and during the operation itself.* Having the support of familiar people can be comforting during this trying time—the anticipation of surgery can be more anxiety provoking than the actual operation. Partners sometimes have concerns about witnessing an operation. It may help to know that he or she will be seated at your head so that like you, your partner will be behind a screen and will not see the surgery. If your partner still cannot bring himself or herself to accompany you, or staff will not allow it, ask the nurse to help you through the experience.

- *Hold the baby and keep him with you in the operating room and during recovery.* Many hospitals automatically whisk the baby off to the nursery after the delivery, but most babies are born in good health. Ask that at least one arm be left free and that the screen be placed low enough on your chest to permit laying the baby on your breast. Your partner can also hold the baby.

- *Request that the anesthesiologist inject a narcotic into the epidural catheter at the end of the operation.* This provides hours of good pain control, which will enable you to (relatively) comfortably hold and breastfeed your baby.

- *Have patient-controlled analgesia.* This technique also improves pain control, which, again, enables you to care for and enjoy your baby. Basically, you push a button to get a dose of narcotic through the IV. A lockout mechanism prevents overdosing.

- *Get help with breastfeeding.* Ask a nurse or the hospital's lactation consultant, if they have one, to show you positions for holding the baby that don't put pressure on your incision. Get your family and friends to assist you with maneuvering the baby and taking care of other chores such as burping or diaper changing. Some hospitals allow your partner to stay with you overnight, which is ideal. *Note:* Many postsurgical patients run fevers; some develop infections. You should not be separated from your baby or advised not to breastfeed for these reasons.

- *Get help at home.* Your only responsibilities for the first few weeks should be looking after yourself and cuddling and breastfeeding the baby. This is true for all new mothers, but it is especially true after a cesarean.
- *Remember that you have had major surgery with all that entails in terms of recovery time and how you will feel physically.* Some women sail through their recovery, but most don't bounce back nearly as fast as they think they should. Don't get discouraged. You will feel like your old self again in time.
- *Remember that it is normal to feel disappointed, angry, frustrated, or sad about your cesarean.* You can feel relieved or grateful and have negative feelings as well. It's not an either-or proposition.

Chapter 2

THE FULL-TERM BREECH BABY:
Cesarean Section Is Not the Only Answer

At your eighth-month visit, ask your doctor or midwife whether your baby is *breech,* meaning the baby is presenting buttocks, knees, or feet to the birth canal. Many doctors don't see any point in telling women their babies are breech until the last few weeks of pregnancy, when it becomes likely that the baby will stay that way. All but about 3 percent to 4 percent will settle into a head-down position by this time. Either they don't perform *external cephalic versions* (ECV), an outpatient procedure for turning the baby head down by manipulating the mother's belly, or if they do, they don't know that there may be advantages in doing the procedure before the ninth month. Few doctors (as opposed to midwives) use alternative techniques that can be tried earlier. However, you may want to try one of these alternative techniques, schedule an ECV in your eighth month, or find a practitioner who does ECVs. Also, few U.S. caregivers will do a vaginal breech birth. This chapter will cover the pros and cons of vaginal breech birth versus planned cesarean. If you decide to go for a vaginal birth, you will need time to find a caregiver who does them and who can help you evaluate whether you are a good candidate.

WHAT'S THE PROBLEM WITH BREECH BIRTH?

MOST BREECH BABIES will do just fine. Nonetheless, breech babies are somewhat more likely to have problems than head-down babies. There are several reasons for this.

To begin with, the fact that full-term babies normally come out head first is no evolutionary accident. Coming head first allows the cervix to open to pass the largest part of the baby, and the contractions can gently shape the still-flexible skull to the mother's pelvis. In addition, the head fits neatly against the cervix like an egg in an egg cup. This prevents the umbilical cord from coming down ahead of the baby and getting pinched between the baby and the mother's pelvis. For these reasons, a very few breech babies will get into trouble. The mechanics of breech birth also increase the chance of injury to the baby during the birth.

Obstetricians have long known this, but up until about thirty years ago, U.S. obstetricians treated breech birth matter-of-factly. Part of their training was learning how to handle breech births. Then, in the 1970s, these concerns led obstetricians in this country to decide that all breech babies should be cesarean deliveries, this being the era when they decided that cesarean section was the panacea for all pregnancy and labor complications. They were wrong. Numerous studies since have shown that the changeover from mostly vaginal breech birth to nearly universal cesarean delivery didn't close the gap between breech and head-first outcomes. Here's why.

The main reason that breech babies overall don't fare as well as head-first babies is that babies born early are more likely to be breech. As the baby grows, gravity and the shape of the uterus together with the baby's normal movements eventually bring the baby head down and keep her that way. That process hasn't happened yet in babies who come early. Premature infants have more complications. Cesarean section won't fix them.

Another reason is that babies who have something wrong with them are also more likely to be breeches. Babies who are full term but severely undersized tend to be breech for the same reason as babies born early. Babies with inborn neuromuscular disabilities also tend to be breech because they don't engage in the active movements that help the baby end up head down. Certain physical abnormalities such as *hydrocephalus* (skull swollen with excess fluid) predispose to breech as well. Cesarean section won't help any but this last one.

Finally, panicked or unskilled doctors can cause deaths and injuries by hasty or forceful manipulations. C-section would seem to be the solution for this problem, at least, but it isn't. Maneuvering a baby through a cesarean incision poses the same hazards as a vaginal birth. More than one research obstetrician has observed that if you don't know how to do a vaginal breech birth, you don't know how to do a cesarean breech delivery either.

Despite these facts, most U.S. obstetricians today believe that the only safe breech delivery is an abdominal delivery, although as one author who recently reviewed the literature wrote, "The generally applied approach of cesarean to breech is not based on clinical facts." Authorities in other countries do not share this belief, and neither do a number of eminent American physicians, including the panel that produced the National Institutes of Health Consensus Development Statement on Cesarean Childbirth. These experts may debate who makes a good candidate for vaginal breech birth and how vaginal breech birth should be conducted, but they don't think every woman carrying a breech baby requires a cesarean.

Two other factors also come into play in the U.S. rise in cesareans for breech babies: defensive medicine and lack of training and experience. As I will repeat in almost every chapter, fear of being sued over a bad outcome should never be the reason behind medical care decisions. Training became a problem as doctors consigned more and more breeches to C-sections. As a result, fewer and fewer obstetric residents learned how to handle vaginal breech birth. But skills can be learned if you think you need them. And as for experience, Dr. Luis Cibils of the Department of Obstetrics and Gynecology at Chicago Lying-In Hospital writes, "The numbers are not as critical as good judgment, gentle hands, and a cool head."

All of these arguments against universal cesarean for breech notwithstanding, you are stuck in a system where the policy is likely to be planned cesarean section. For this reason, the first thing you want to do, if you can, is get the baby turned around.

TURNING THE BABY HEAD DOWN

THERE ARE SEVERAL ways of turning a baby head down. Let's begin with the technique that is simplest, costs nothing, and can be tried earliest in pregnancy, which is another point in its favor. The earlier in pregnancy you begin, the greater the odds of success because there is more amniotic fluid and the baby is smaller. Unless your caregiver objects, give one of these a try if your baby is still breech at six to eight weeks before your due date.

THE HOME VERSION

- The authors of *Pregnancy, Childbirth and the Newborn* recommend the following: Three times a day for ten to fifteen minutes, lie on your back with bent knees and your hips elevated about twelve inches on cushions, or lie on a propped ironing board. Pick times when the baby is active and your

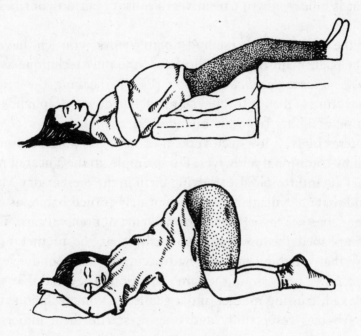

Home version positions

stomach and bladder are empty. Have someone help you get in and out of the tilt position. It helps if you concentrate on relaxing your trunk and visualizing what you want the baby to do. Placing personal stereo headphones playing classical music just above your pubic bone may coax the baby in the direction you want her to go. So may having your partner talk to the baby through a toilet paper roll placed in the same area. Keep the sound level at a volume that would be comfortable for you.

• The authors of *A Guide to Effective Care in Pregnancy and Childbirth* report that the knee-chest position may be effective. Kneel on a mattress with flexed hips and your upper body flat against the mattress. Your thighs should be apart so they do not press on your belly. Ideally, you do this every two waking hours for fifteen minutes for five days, which, to put it mildly, doesn't seem very realistic, but do your best.

If the do-it-yourself method doesn't work, you will have to get help. In mainstream medical care the only technique available is *external cephalic version* (ECV), meaning the practitioner turns the baby (version) head down (cephalic) by manipulating her from the outside (externally).

Interestingly, a low-tech version of ECV has long been practiced by traditional midwives. For example, in the Yucatan peninsula an anthropologist studying birth in the present-day Maya found that the village midwives routinely turned babies as part of the series of massages that formed part of prenatal care. They accomplished the procedure so easily that the mother never knew that anything unusual had occurred. Some midwives in this country carry on in the same tradition. They find that with a relaxed, trusting mother and a gentle, coaxing technique that treats babies respectfully and doesn't startle them into resistance, babies turn easily and without complications. Babies that don't want to turn should never be forced.

THE HIGH-TECH VERSION

Around week thirty-seven of pregnancy, you go to the hospital for an outpatient procedure. You have a preliminary ultrasound scan to evaluate the baby and the amount of amniotic fluid and to locate the placenta. You are given a drug through an IV to keep the uterus relaxed during the attempt; alternatively, the medication may simply be injected under the skin. Caregivers also begin external electronic fetal monitoring to keep track of the baby's heart rate. Once the medication has taken effect, the practitioner tries to flip the baby by manipulating your belly. The procedure may be uncomfortable, but it should rarely take more than five minutes; many ECVs take less than one. If the procedure fails or the baby turns back to breech, some practitioners will try again. Electronic fetal monitoring is continued for a while afterward to make sure the baby tolerated the procedure.

You do have some other options. Alternative-medicine techniques can be used as an adjunct to ECV or as something else to try.

ALTERNATIVE-MEDICINE VERSIONS

- One researcher hypnotized one hundred women carrying a term breech baby and made suggestions to induce relaxation and calm fears. Combining the numbers of women whose babies turned on their own with the number who had successful ECVs, 80 percent of babies in the hypnotized group were head down at the birth. Few conventional ECV studies have achieved this success rate. The secret may lie in relaxing a tense belly, a factor known to inhibit ECV.
- Chinese-medicine practitioners turn breeches with acupuncture or moxibustion. *Moxibustion* uses heat from a burning herb for stimulation instead of needles. The trigger points lie on the outside edge of the little toe's toenail at the base of the toenail. The treatment is done at or near full term because it may also trigger labor. A trial in which researchers randomly assigned women to moxibustion, or not, resulted in higher success rates with moxibustion than were achieved in most ECV trials.

THE BOTTOM LINE ON ECV

CONTROVERSIES AND TRADE-OFFS OF ECV

Obstetricians tend to fall into two camps depending on whether they think ECV is risky or safe.

ECV is risky—turn the baby once late in pregnancy. Almost all doctors wait until thirty-six or thirty-seven weeks' gestation, on the theory that ECV can cause fetal distress or hemorrhage, complications demanding immediate delivery. They reason that by waiting until the end of pregnancy, all babies who would have spontaneously converted to head down have turned. In addition, once the baby has been turned, it isn't likely to revert to breech, and should an emergency occur, the baby is mature. Most also think that the few babies who turn back to breech should be left alone.

ECV is safe—turn the baby early and often. Other doctors argue that if ECV is done gently, the risks are nil, so there is no reason to wait or not to try again if the baby flips back. Waiting reduces the odds of success because the baby is bigger and there is less amniotic fluid. Some women will miss their opportunity to have ECV because membranes will rupture or labor will begin. Of course, most breech babies turned earlier in pregnancy would have turned on their own, but you don't know which ones would and which ones wouldn't.

Studies agree that ECV is safe and effective when practiced as directed, but that overly forceful manipulations can be extremely dangerous.

STRATEGIES FOR IMPROVING THE ODDS OF SUCCESS OF ECV

Some of these suggestions may seem aimed more at medical professionals. I list them so that you know about them and can discuss them ahead of time with your doctor or midwife, who probably won't know about them unless he or she has recently researched ECV. The "Literature Summaries" appendix for this chapter may come in handy for your discussion.

- *Problem:* Success rates vary from practitioner to practitioner.
  Solution: If more than one practitioner in your community does ECV, shop around.
- *Problem:* Your practitioner says ECV will probably fail in your case, and he or she does not want to try.
  Solution: While the odds of success vary according to many factors, the fact that ECV is safe and cesareans aren't means you have nothing to lose and a lot to gain by trying.
- *Problem:* Your medical condition (high blood pressure, diabetes, heart disease) precludes the use of uterine relaxant medication (*tocolytics*).
  Solution: ECV can be done without it.
- *Problem:* Your caregiver is reluctant because you have had a prior cesarean or other uterine surgery.
  Solution: Uterine scar may not be a contraindication.
- *Problem:* A tense belly can inhibit the baby from turning.
  Solution: ECV provides an opportunity for you to practice your newly learned relaxation skills for what may be a trying couple of minutes. Deep breathing, consciously releasing the muscles of your torso, and other techniques learned in your childbirth class may help here just as they do in labor.
- *Problem:* The baby is facing your belly instead of your back, which makes a successful ECV less likely.
  Solution: Assume the hands-and-knees position for ten minutes before the attempt so that gravity can swing the baby's back against your belly.
- *Problem:* The baby's spine is in line with yours, which also inhibits ECV.
  Solution: If the baby is startled with a buzzer, a technique used in evaluating fetal well-being, she will almost always move off to the side.

- *Problem:* Labor has started. Some obstetricians consider labor a contraindication to attempting ECV.
  Solution: Provided the bag of waters hasn't broken, a tocolytic drug can be given to temporarily stop contractions, and ECV can be tried in labor. (Once membranes have ruptured, the umbilical cord could slip down into the birth canal during the procedure.)

THE BOTTOM LINE ON BREECH BIRTH

UNLIKE "FLIP THE baby and the problem goes away," there are no easy answers if your baby persists as a breech. Each choice presents advantages and disadvantages, and no choice guarantees that everything will be fine. Part of this can't be helped, but part of it, as you will see in a moment, relates to how obstetricians tend to manage vaginal breech birth. The best I can do for you is lay out the arguments and give you the conclusions I drew from the literature. This will give you a jumping-off point for discussions with your doctor or midwife.

TRADE-OFFS OF CESAREAN VS. VAGINAL BREECH BIRTH

CESAREAN BIRTH
Planned cesarean section may have a slight edge on reducing the percentage of babies born in distress. It may reduce the possibility of birth injury, and it may also just possibly reduce deaths. On the downside, cesarean section does not completely protect the baby from the risks of breech birth, but it markedly increases maternal risks in both the short and long term over vaginal birth. This increased risk is more than theoretical. Sprinkled here and there among the studies of breech birth are reports of women whose cesareans led to severe infections causing

prolonged hospital stays, hysterectomy for uncontrollable hemorrhage, and even maternal death.

However, the issue is more complex than it looks. Typical hospital vaginal breech protocols call for a large *episiotomy* (cutting the bottom of the vaginal opening) and forceps delivery of the head. Both episiotomy and forceps deliveries can cause maternal complications, some of which may result in long-term or chronic problems. In addition, women who labor still have a substantial probability of having a cesarean—the bulk of studies range from 25 percent to over 60 percent—and women having in-labor cesareans are more likely to develop infections than women having planned cesareans.

VAGINAL BIRTH

Many studies have concluded that the shift to planned cesarean delivery has not improved breech outcomes in either the short or long term. In addition, many centers reporting on selecting women for labor have not found that vaginal birth posed undue risk. The jury is still out, though, and likely to remain so. The authors of *A Guide to Effective Care in Pregnancy and Childbirth,* which represents the analysis and distillation of hundreds of studies, classify routine planned cesarean for breech under "Forms of Care of Unknown Effectiveness." They point out that complications occur so rarely among healthy, full-term breeches that it would take many thousands of cases to establish whether routine cesarean benefits breech babies, far more than have been studied to date.

Vaginal birth appears to increase the risk of birth injury compared with C-section, but differences in birth injury rates are also not as straightforward as they seem. Birth injuries such as broken collarbone and injuries to a complex of nerves and blood vessels controlling the arm muscles (*brachial plexus* injury, also called *Erb's palsy*) may be more common, but almost all babies recover. And babies born by cesarean are hardly home free. The same kinds of injuries also occur during cesarean delivery, as well as one new one: cuts severe enough to require suturing.

To sum up, the balance sheet looks like this: Even with optimal care, a baby may occasionally die or suffer permanent injury who would have been OK had the mother had a planned cesarean. To put this risk in perspective, fetal loss rates from amniocentesis, another situation where the mother's interest counterbalances the baby's, fall in the same range. More babies born vaginally will have birth injuries from which almost all of them will recover.

Similarly, even with optimal care, a mother may occasionally die or suffer permanent injury who would have been OK had she had a vaginal birth. More women having planned cesareans will have complications, such as postpartum infections, from which they will recover. Women having cesareans will have a scarred uterus, which increases their risk of the uterine scar giving way and certain placental complications in subsequent pregnancies. While rare, all pose life-threatening risks to mothers and babies.

Given these trade-offs, the situation is not nearly as clear-cut as obstetricians would make it seem. Depending on the individual case, vaginal birth is as much a reasonable, responsible choice as is planned cesarean section.

CONTROVERSIES OF VAGINAL BREECH BIRTH

- *Who should be eligible for labor?* The ideal vaginal breech birth candidate is a woman carrying a full-term or near full-term baby of average size in *frank breech* position, that is, buttocks down and with legs in pike position, hips flexed and knees straight (see drawing on page 43). Frank breech is by far the most common type of breech. With a frank breech, the buttocks are about the size of the head, which minimizes

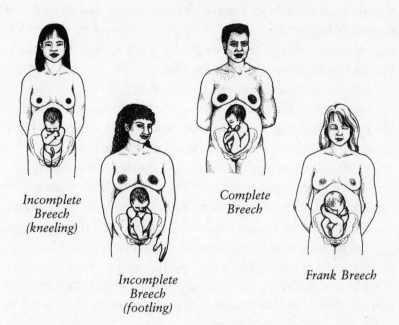

*Incomplete
Breech
(kneeling)*

*Complete
Breech*

*Incomplete
Breech
(footling)*

Frank Breech

the possibility that the cervix will dilate enough to pass the
body but not the head, and the chance of the umbilical cord
coming down ahead of the baby (*prolapsing*) is the same as
in head-down babies. Average size means the baby is neither
growth retarded, which could mean the baby has problems,
nor large enough to increase concern about birth injury or
worry that the mother's pelvis may be too small for the head.
The mother should have normal to ample pelvic measurements for these same two reasons.

Everyone agrees that "stargazers," that is, babies with
heads tipped back (*hyperextended neck*), should be planned
cesarean sections. These babies can be gravely injured during
vaginal birth, although cesarean delivery offers no guarantees. Everyone also agrees that babies with physical abnormalities should be cesarean deliveries unless the baby has
such severe problems that the baby will not be able to survive
regardless of what is done. There agreement ends. The major
controversies are:

- *Should complete breeches (babies presenting buttocks down with legs bent at knees and hips) or incomplete breeches (babies presenting feet or knees to the birth canal, most commonly footling breech) be cesareans?*
  - ➤ *Pros:* Complete breeches can convert to incomplete breeches at any time. Incomplete breeches have a higher risk of umbilical cord prolapse and of having the body slip through an incompletely dilated cervix.
  - ➤ *Cons:* With complete breeches, the buttocks fill up the lower uterus just like the frank breech. With incomplete breeches, electronic fetal monitoring will permit a timely cesarean, and unlike cord prolapse in head-down babies, the infant's soft legs protect the umbilical cord from compression. Vaginal birth avoids the risks of C-section.
- *Should X ray, CT scan, or other imaging techniques be used to take pelvic measurements? Should ultrasound be used to make fetal weight estimates?*
  - ➤ *Pros:* These evaluations rule out overly large babies and overly small mothers.
  - ➤ *Cons:* X-ray measurements of pelvic size (*pelvimetry*) expose the baby to radiation. In head-down babies, X-ray measurements have never been shown to improve the ability to predict who will give birth vaginally compared with physical examination, so there is no reason to think they will do better for breech babies. X-ray measurements also provide no information as to the degree to which soft tissues may help or hinder the birth, and they take static measurements when, in fact, the pregnant woman's pelvis can flex. Finally, decisions based on pelvic measurements assume incorrectly that no other factors such as positioning or epidural anesthesia affect the ability of a woman to push out her baby. Newer imagining techniques reduce radiation exposure, but all of the preceding objections still apply. Ultrasound weight estimates are inaccurate especially at the extremes of the scale. Where to

set the thresholds for qualifying or disqualifying women for vaginal breech birth is another problem. Ultrasonography can be used to rule out "stargazers," check for fetal abnormalities, and make sure the placenta isn't covering the cervix, the key points in deciding who should labor.

The data resolve neither dispute. Several things are clear, though.

- *Having a first baby should not disqualify a woman for vaginal breech birth.* The theory is that first-time mothers have an "untried pelvis," but studies have not found poorer outcomes in first-time mothers.
- *If the only contraindication to labor is that the baby is a stargazer, wait until labor begins and do a sonogram.* The baby may have moved.
- *Before planning a cesarean, have an ultrasound scan to rule out congenital anomalies incompatible with life.*
- *If having pelvimetry, do it via CT scan or some other technique that exposes the baby to less radiation than X rays.*

Once you and your caregiver decide to plan a vaginal birth, another set of controversies comes into play.

- *Should epidurals be given routinely?*
  - ➤ *Pros:* Epidurals prevent premature urge to push, which helps ensure full dilation, and allow obstetricians to apply forceps and manipulate the baby without causing pain.
  - ➤ *Cons:* Epidurals interfere with pushing, the last thing you want when a woman must rapidly and effectively push out a head that hasn't been shaped to the mother's pelvis by the pushing contractions. An epidural and the flat-on-the-back-with-legs-in-stirrups position would seem to be a recipe for birth injury—if not worse. Epidurals also introduce their own list of potential complications.

- *Should all or almost all breech babies born vaginally be forceps deliveries?*
  - ➤ *Pros:* Because of the risks of birth injury, using forceps to entirely deliver the baby should be reserved for emergencies, but once the baby's buttocks and legs emerge on their own, applying a specially designed forceps allows a controlled delivery of the head.
  - ➤ *Cons:* Forceps should rarely be needed with a mother who can push effectively and a pushing position that works for rather than against the birth forces. Forceps deliveries also are usually done in conjunction with a large episiotomy. Episiotomies and forceps can cause complications.

The medical literature does not support these practices:

- *Forbidding the use of oxytocin (trade name: Pitocin or "Pit"):* Some obstetricians believe that poor progress in labor warns of potential difficulties at the birth and indicates the need for cesarean. However, no data support this contention, and the careful use of oxytocin may spare a woman a cesarean section.
- *Performing episiotomy routinely:* As a routine practice, enlarging the vaginal outlet offers no benefits. Head entrapment, a rare life-threatening complication, is a problem of the bones or of the lower part of the uterus. Forceps deliveries do not routinely require episiotomies, and not doing an episiotomy reduces the chances of an anal tear. Some obstetricians do an episiotomy off to the side instead of straight down to prevent anal tears during forceps deliveries, but this has its own drawbacks.

SAFETY FACTORS IN VAGINAL BREECH BIRTH

- *Have a skilled, gentle birth attendant.* Interview potential birth attendants. Ask about their complication rates. Find out what they recommend to minimize the chance of problems. *Note:* You may find that your insurance plan does not include anyone who does vaginal breech births. However, most plans have a provision for going outside the plan for services not offered by covered providers. Expect to have to fight for your rights, though.
- *Monitor fetal heart tones closely.*
- *Delay pushing until full dilation.* Especially with a breech, you may experience the urge to push before full dilation, but you must resist. You want a straight shot through the birth canal with nothing constricting the way.

GLEANINGS FROM THE MEDICAL LITERATURE

EXTERNAL CEPHALIC VERSION (PAGES 219–220)

- Moxibustion is effective.
- ECV is safe.
- ECV is effective.
- Attempting ECV earlier in the last trimester and repeating it if necessary can also be safe and may have a higher success rate.
- Strategies to increase the odds of success include turning a *posterior* baby (the baby is facing your belly) to *anterior* (the baby is facing your back) by getting on your hands and knees and "buzzing" a baby that is lying in the midline so that it startles and moves off the midline.
- Medication to relax the uterus (tocolytics) is not essential.

- Uterine scar may not be a contraindication to ECV.
- ECV can be attempted in labor.

VAGINAL BREECH BIRTH (PAGES 220–223)

- Most of the poor outcomes in breech babies have nothing to do with birth route.
- Vaginal breech birth is a reasonable choice.
- Cesarean section does not remove the risks of breech birth, including birth injury, and it increases maternal risk.
- First-time mothers, women carrying nonfrank breeches, and women with a prior cesarean section need not be automatically disqualified from vaginal breech birth.
- Ultrasound estimates of fetal weight aren't very accurate.
- Forceps may not always be required at vaginal delivery.

Chapter 3

⌒

INDUCTION OF LABOR:
MOTHER NATURE KNOWS BEST

INDUCING LABOR IS intrinsically ironic. It works best when least needed and often fails when needed most. It also causes the very problems it was intended to prevent.

Despite common perception, obstetricians can't just switch labor on at will. Starting and intensifying labor involves a complex cascade of feedback mechanisms that mutually reinforce and limit each other. It is an elegant and delicate interplay of hormones and other substances between the baby, who initiates and controls the process, and the mother. You can't simply dump in any of the substances involved and expect it to work unless labor was on the verge of starting on its own. Inducing labor when the mother isn't ready to labor often ends in a C-section. So why not wait?

WHY NOT WAIT?

ONE ANSWER IS that doctors wrongly believe that the development of agents to ripen the cervix has done away with the problem of induction failures. However, while undeniably effective at softening and effacing the cervix, these agents do little to reduce the cesarean rate. The gap in cesarean rates between induced and spontaneous labor has closed, mainly because cesarean rates have soared in spontaneous labors. For example, in one large trial, women one week past their due date were randomly assigned to await labor or to induction. Despite using a cervical ripening agent, 29 percent of first-time mothers in the induction group had cesareans, versus 33 percent—one-third—of the "await labor" group. Cervical ripening may have offered some slight benefit, but *both* percentages are appalling, especially considering that these women lacked almost every risk factor for cesarean in that they were healthy, their babies were mature, the babies weren't breech, and they weren't carrying twins.

A second answer is that doctors induce labor when they are concerned about the baby's condition, which brings us to the other irony: Induction causes the problems it was intended to prevent. Induced labors are much harder on the baby than natural labor. For one thing, it takes greater contraction pressures over a longer time to get a labor going and keep it going than generally are needed for spontaneous labor.* For another, all of the conventional compounds used in labor inductions—namely, oxytocin (trade name Pitocin or "Pit"), prostaglandin E2 (also called dinoprostone, trade names Prepidil and Cervidil), misoprostol (also called prostaglandin E1, trade name Cytotec)—are

---

*This is why oxytocin causes complications more often when used to start labor than when used to strengthen labor. You need higher doses, which increases the likelihood of problems.

notorious for causing contractions that are overly long, strong, and close together (*uterine hyperstimulation*). In addition, breaking the bag of waters, a usual practice with inductions, removes the cushioning effect of amniotic fluid, allowing contractions to squeeze the umbilical cord. In other words, a baby who has enough reserves to withstand the stresses of a natural labor might not be able to tolerate the rigors of an induced one.

A third answer, the one I will address in this chapter, is that even if the baby is fine, doctors believe the risks of continuing the pregnancy outweigh the risks of induction. Unfortunately, because obstetric philosophy emphasizes the perils of the natural process and minimizes the dangers of intervening in it, what obstetricians think justifies induction and what the research evidence supports are two different things. Here are some common rationales for inducing labor in healthy women carrying healthy babies and what's wrong with them.

CONVENIENCE INDUCTIONS

When you're feeling huge and uncomfortable and anxious, or worse yet, your doctor or midwife announces that he or she is leaving town, inducing labor can seem like a good idea. It isn't. When there is no reason to induce, you run the risks of induction—and those risks are not inconsequential—without any balancing benefit. Inducing merely for reasons of convenience has been disapproved by the FDA.

SUSPECTED LARGE BABY

The theory goes that if you are carrying a baby believed to weigh 8 lbs., 13 oz. (4,000 grams) or more (*macrosomia*) or believed to weigh in the upper 10 percent of babies for that week of pregnancy ("large for gestational age"), inducing labor before the baby gets even bigger can spare you a cesarean section and the baby the possibility of *shoulder dystocia* (when the shoulders get stuck). The facts, however, are otherwise. To begin with, ultrasound weight estimates are so inaccurate that if your caregiver suspects a large baby, he or she could equally well flip a coin as order a sonogram. Moreover, studies comparing induced women with women allowed to begin labor on their own all show that induced women have more cesareans and equal numbers of shoulder dystocias. (Just so you know, planned cesarean is an even worse idea than induction.) It turns out that shoulder dystocia isn't very tightly tied to weight, and while it's a dangerous situation, handled properly it rarely results in permanent injury.

PRELABOR RUPTURE OF MEMBRANES IN FULL-TERM PREGNANCY

In the 1960s, a flurry of papers on the danger of infection with prolonged rupture of the fetal membranes resulted in the twenty-four hour rule: Once membranes rupture, the baby must be born within twenty-four hours. This policy means inducing any woman who does not begin labor on her own within a few hours of membrane rupture, stimulating slowly progressing labors with oxytocin, and performing cesarean sections on women who aren't close to giving birth by the twenty-four hour limit. In addition, it means babies born after or close to the limit are likely to be subjected to a series of tests for infection called a *septic workup*. Septic workups include drawing blood and often include a spinal tap. Many pediatricians confine the baby to the nursery and prescribe IV antibiotics until the baby's cultures come back negative. Even at the time the twenty-four hour rule was created, obstetricians expressed concern about raising cesarean section rates and observed that infections were rare when no vaginal exams were done. These hesitations were brushed aside on the grounds that high cesarean rates for failed induction or fetal distress were preferable to the deadly infections that would surely result from doing nothing. By the early 1970s, the twenty-four hour rule had become the standard of practice in full-term pregnancies.

The studies that sparked the rule had serious weaknesses. For example, many of them combined prelabor rupture of the membranes at full term with those occurring preterm. In many preterm cases, infection causes membrane rupture, not vice versa. Doctors also ignored the role they themselves played in precipitating infections. Studies show a clear connection between ruptured membranes, number of vaginal exams, use of internal monitoring devices, time, and infection. When membranes rupture, fluids wash out of the vagina, which means infective bacteria must migrate upstream, against the current, to enter the uterus. But, during a vaginal exam, the caregiver slides his or her fingers in, giving any organisms present a free ride up to and even into the cervix. Worse, internal electronic fetal monitoring and internal contraction-pressure monitoring create a pathway into the uterus itself. Waiting twenty-four hours or even more before inducing labor is safe as long as caregivers keep their fingers and internal monitoring devices out of the vagina—with one possible exception: women who are vaginally colonized by group B streptococci, also called *group B strep* or *GBS*.

GROUP B STREPTOCOCCUS (GBS)

To give you some background, between one and three in every ten healthy women have GBS living in their vaginas (*colonized*). Before the widespread use of preventative antibiotics during labor, two to three of every hundred colonized women would have a baby who developed a serious infection. About 4 percent of infected babies died, making the odds of a colonized mother losing a child to GBS 4 to 8 per 10,000. A few survivors suffered permanent neurological damage. However, since 1 in 4 newborn infections are in premature babies, and 1 in 5 are not early-onset disease, the odds of preventable disease are reduced in full-term pregnancies. Also, prolonged ruptured membranes is a risk factor, which suggests that obstetric management plays a role.

The solution would seem to be to test for GBS early in pregnancy and give antibiotics when it is present, but this doesn't work. Once the course of antibiotics ends, GBS often reappears. For these reasons, the Centers for Disease Control recommend the following:

Screen all pregnant women at thirty-five to thirty-seven weeks of pregnancy. Give all colonized women IV antibiotics in labor. When GBS status at onset of labor is unknown, give IV antibiotics when risk factors are present, namely, preterm labor, ruptured membranes for eighteen hours or more, fever during labor, or prior baby with a GBS infection. Women testing negative for GBS do not need IV antibiotics even if they have risk factors except for those with a previous infected baby.

The baby of a GBS-positive mother needs no evaluation or antibiotic therapy provided the baby shows no signs of infection, is at least 35 weeks of gestational age, and the mother began antibiotic treatment at least four hours before birth. If the baby is younger than 35 weeks or was born less than four hours after antibiotic treatment, the baby should have blood cultures. If the mother received antibiotics because of suspected uterine infection or the baby shows signs of infection, the baby should have a full septic work-up, including a spinal tap, and antibiotic therapy.

Cases of newborn infection declined with the introduction of routine testing and treatment in the 1990s and currently stands at 0.5 cases per 1,000 births. There is, however, a downside. Cases of severe maternal allergic reactions have occurred, and while penicillin-resistant GBS strains have not yet appeared,

GBS resistance to other antibiotics has. Even more concerning, the fall in GBS infections in preterm infants has been more than offset by a rise in deadly, penicillin-resistant E. coli infections.

"Overdue" Pregnancy

A better term than *overdue* would be the medically correct *post-dates*. "Overdue" implies that going past your due date is a problem, rather like overbaking a cake. On the contrary, inducing for exceeding your due date is a textbook case of how mainstream obstetric care keeps narrowing the definition of normal until practically no one fits, which then creates the "need" for intervention. True, a small percentage of women don't begin labor when they are supposed to. And, yes, placentas are not made to last forever. Still, mainstream postdates management has little scientific basis.

Up to the late 1980s, conventional obstetric wisdom held that if pregnancy continued two weeks past the forty-week due date, either labor should be induced or some sort of periodic testing of fetal well-being should be done. Nonetheless, induction became the norm. This sounds reasonable, but as with so much of obstetric management, nothing is as it seems.

To begin with, there are problems with the due date itself. You may be surprised to learn that the conventional forty-week pregnancy length is completely arbitrary. It was established by a German obstetrician in the early 1800s. He simply declared that a pregnancy should last ten moon months, that is, ten months of four weeks each. However, when researchers in a 1990 study followed a group of healthy, white women, they discovered that pregnancy in first-time mothers averaged eight days longer than this, and the average was three days longer in women with prior births.

In addition, ultrasonography, the current standard for assigning due dates, does not reliably establish due dates. Even in the first trimester, the date is plus or minus five days. This means the actual due date falls within a ten-day window. Sonograms done later in pregnancy are even less accurate.

It gets worse. While even the forty-two-week limit isn't sound, in recent years, the "time's up" date has backed up to forty-one weeks, with some researchers recommending forty weeks. Based on the above study, first-time mothers are not only not "late" at forty-one weeks, they haven't even reached the average pregnancy length.

The earlier and earlier time limit has come about mainly through tests intended to evaluate the baby's well-being. All these tests have poor positive predictive values, meaning that when the test says the baby of a healthy mother is in jeopardy, it is probably wrong. However, faced with a worrisome test result, obstetricians quite properly induce labor or perform a cesarean. The baby turns out to be fine—it always was—but now the obstetric belief system takes over. Most obstetricians have an unfounded faith in the accuracy of tests. A healthy baby only reinforces the erroneous idea that timely intervention saved him. The policy of beginning routine testing at forty-two weeks resulted in many babies seeming to be at risk. Obstetricians concluded from this that if so many babies were in trouble at forty-two weeks, they should begin testing earlier. Again, because of the high false-positive rates, many babies looked as if they had problems earlier, and the vicious cycle continued.

Ironically, inducing labor also reinforces the belief that allowing pregnancy to continue is dangerous. Inductions increase the risk of fetal distress and the incidence of cesarean section, problems that are then attributed to the baby's condition rather than to their real cause—the induction. For example, one researcher found huge jumps in complication rates (6 to 20 percent) and cesarean rates (7 percent to more than 25 percent) at forty weeks, the women's due dates, at his hospital. Forty weeks was when women were automatically transferred to the high-risk clinic. The researcher concluded that risk increased earlier in pregnancy than previously thought, but any unbiased person would see the obvious culprit: management in the high-risk clinic.

Still, postdates pregnancy isn't a "one size fits all" issue. Routinely inducing at some arbitrary date is not the solution mainstream obstetricians believe it to be. Testing in order to determine which babies would benefit from induction runs the risk of acting on false-positive results. Letting nature take its course is generally best, although that is not risk-free either. No course of action (or inaction) guarantees good outcome.

TESTS OF FETAL WELL-BEING

- *Fetal movement counts.* Starting the last few weeks before your due date, you pick a time every day when the baby is awake and count how long it takes for the baby to make ten distinct movements. If the time lengthens over successive days or there is a marked drop in the number of movements on a particular day, you report this to your caregiver, who should follow up with one of the following tests.
- *Nonstress test.* Your caregiver uses external fetal monitoring to track the baby's heart rate when the baby moves or when you have a prelabor (*Braxton-Hicks*) contraction. (See page 90 for a description of how external fetal monitoring is done.) The heart rate should speed up. However, the most common reason it doesn't is that the baby is asleep.
- *Vibroacoustic stimulation.* In this variation of the nonstress test, a buzzer is sounded against your belly. The baby's heart rate should speed up when he startles.
- *Contraction stress test or oxytocin challenge test.* You are hooked up to an electronic fetal monitor and caregivers start an IV containing oxytocin to see how the baby's heart rate responds to simulated labor contractions. Alternatively, and noninvasively, nipple stimulation can be done manually or

with an electric breast pump. Nipple stimulation causes natural release of oxytocin.

- *Biophysical profile.* In addition to a nonstress test, caregivers do an ultrasound scan to evaluate the placenta, the baby's movements, and how often the baby takes a practice breath (to conserve energy, babies in trouble stop moving around and stop practicing breathing). Caregivers give the baby an overall score on a scale of zero (worst) to ten (best).
- *Amniotic fluid volume measurement.* Caregivers use ultrasound to estimate the amount of amniotic fluid. Too little fluid increases the probability of fetal distress in labor.

CERVICAL RIPENING AND INDUCTION PROCEDURES

- *Nipple stimulation.* Stimulating the nipples causes oxytocin release. Low-tech stimulation can be through the application of warm, wet cloths, manual stimulation, or suckling by a baby or partner. To minimize the chance of overly strong contractions, begin by stimulating one nipple only. Stop the stimulation during contractions. If stimulating one nipple does not produce contractions, then stimulate both. High-tech techniques include stimulating the nipples with an electric breast pump or a TENS (transcutaneous electronic nerve stimulation) unit, a physical therapy device that painlessly delivers a low electric current through pads applied to the skin.
- *Sexual intercourse.* If you didn't know how to do this, you wouldn't be reading this book.
- *Castor oil.* Folk wisdom has long held that stimulating the digestive tract also stimulates labor contractions. Castor oil is often given with orange juice to disguise the taste and sometimes with vodka to reduce cramping.
- *Enema.* Enemas, running liquid into the rectum, have been given on the same principle as castor oil.

- *Acupuncture or TENS.* The acupuncturist places thin needles in particular points of the body and runs a low electric current through them to stimulate those points. Evidence in one study suggests that the same stimulation could effectively and non-invasively be given with a TENS unit.
- *Herbs.* Several herbs are reputed to stimulate labor, but I could find no studies in the mainstream research literature. Herbs are usually drunk as teas.
- *Stripping/sweeping the membranes.* During a vaginal exam, the caregiver inserts a finger into the cervix and lifts the amniotic sac off the cervix. This minor irritation triggers the local release of prostaglandins, compounds that ripen the cervix and stimulate contractions.
- *Mechanical dilators.* Inserted into the cervix, these materials absorb moisture and dilate the cervix as they gradually swell.
- *Prostaglandin E2 (PGE2).* This is currently the most popular technique for cervical ripening. The caregiver inserts a gel containing PGE2 (Prepidil) into the cervix. A newer formulation, Cervidil, packages PGE2 in an insert with a string, which allows it to be withdrawn should overly strong contractions occur and at the end of the ripening period. Contractions and the baby's heart rate must be carefully monitored for an hour or two because uterine hyperstimulation is a common side effect. Sometimes PGE2 is enough to start labor on its own, but usually IV oxytocin is needed as well.
- *Misoprostol (PGE1).* Misoprostol (trade name Cytotec), like PGE2, is inserted vaginally. Contractions and the baby's heart rate must be carefully monitored because misoprostol is even more likely than PGE2 to cause uterine hyperstimulation and fetal distress.
- *Rupturing membranes (amniotomy).* During a vaginal exam, the doctor or midwife snags the membranes with an *amnihook*, which looks like a flat, plastic crochet hook except that it has a small, sharp tooth under the curled-over tip. There

will be a gush of warm liquid. The procedure can be uncomfortable for you but doesn't hurt the baby because there are no nerves in the membranes.

- *Oxytocin*. The nurse starts an IV. The tubing is connected to two bags, one containing oxytocin (trade name: Pitocin, also called "Pit") and the other plain IV fluid. The medicated fluid is routed through a special machine that administers an adjustable number of drops per minute. The machine permits tight control over the dosage, a critical safety factor in administering this powerful drug. If contractions become too strong, the medication can be stopped while the plain IV is left running to keep the line open.

THE BOTTOM LINE ON LABOR INDUCTION GENERALLY

AVOIDING AN UNNECESSARY INDUCTION

Note: If this is your first baby, be especially leery of induction. You are at much greater risk of a cesarean. Induction may also pose a slightly greater risk of symptomatic scar separation in women with a prior cesarean.

- *Choose a caregiver who:*
  - ➤ has a low induction rate.
  - ➤ doesn't induce for suspected large baby.
  - ➤ at a minimum and in the absence of signs of infection, allows you twenty-four hours to begin labor on your own if membranes rupture.
  - ➤ doesn't consider you overdue until at least forty-two weeks of pregnancy.
- *Refuse an elective induction, that is, induction for convenience.*
- *Refuse an ultrasound to estimate fetal weight.* In a case of "what your doctor knows can hurt you," studies show that

when an obstetrician *thinks*, based on a sonogram, that the baby will weigh over 8 lbs., 13 oz., the mother is more likely to have a cesarean than if the baby *actually* weighs this much or more, but the doctor doesn't suspect.

- *Refuse an induction for suspected large baby.*
- *Don't permit your due date to be changed based on an ultrasound scan (sonogram) unless it was done within the first thirteen weeks and the result is more than ten days earlier than your current due date.* On the other hand, if you get a due date later than your current date, consider taking it. It may spare you hassle later over whether you should be induced for being postdates.
- *If you know when you got pregnant—for example, if you did an early pregnancy test—refuse a sonogram for the purpose of estimating your due date.*
- *Consider refusing routine tests of fetal well-being.* The American College of Obstetricians and Gynecologists (ACOG), the U.S. obstetricians' professional organization, acknowledges that there is no evidence that routine tests of well-being improve outcomes in postdates pregnancies. ACOG says to do them anyway because there is no evidence that testing has adverse effects, but there they are wrong. Because these tests have such high false-positive rates—30 percent or more—and because healthy women carrying full-term babies aren't very likely to have babies that are having difficulties, a positive result ("positive" means the test found a problem) is hugely more likely to be wrong than right. The consequences of a false-positive test are not trivial. For example, one study of amniotic fluid volume showed that having this test routinely done doubled the cesarean rate for fetal distress without improving newborn outcomes. Another study found that using one technique for estimating amniotic fluid volume (*amniotic fluid index*) resulted in much higher rates of abnormal findings than a different technique (*maximum pool depth*). The amniotic fluid index led to more inductions and C-sections

with no improvement in newborn outcomes. Moreover, a negative result doesn't guarantee the baby is fine. While a negative test is generally reassuring, there can be false negatives, cases where either the baby's problem did not show up or something happened between tests.

- *Make sure you have been drinking plenty of fluids in the hours before you have an ultrasound measurement of amniotic fluid volume.* Drinking increases amniotic fluid volume, and even mild dehydration reduces it.
- *If a test of fetal well-being is positive, insist on repeating the test or doing a different test before agreeing to an induction or cesarean section.* Having two positive tests mathematically reduces the odds that the results are falsely positive.

PROS AND CONS OF TECHNIQUES FOR RIPENING THE CERVIX AND/OR INDUCING LABOR

MANUAL NIPPLE STIMULATION TO RIPEN THE CERVIX
> *Pros:* A natural and painless means of increasing circulating oxytocin levels, which ripens the cervix and can induce labor. It is noninvasive, costs nothing, and can be done at home.
>
> *Cons:* May require prolonged application to be effective— three one-hour sessions per day for three consecutive days in one study. May cause overly strong contractions.

NIPPLE STIMULATION BY BREAST PUMP OR TENS TO INDUCE LABOR
> *Pros:* Safe and effective. Studies are few and small, but because stimulation is readily controlled, it is unlikely to impose any more hazard than prostaglandins or oxytocin and probably imposes less.
>
> *Cons:* Some women induced with a breast pump complained of sore nipples.

SEXUAL INTERCOURSE

Because of the risk of infection, *never* engage in sexual intercourse with ruptured membranes.

Pros: Natural and pleasurable means of increasing prostaglandin levels. It costs nothing and can be done at home.
Cons: Effectiveness unknown.

CASTOR OIL

Pros: Reduces the need for oxytocin. Does not require hospitalization.
Cons: Causes diarrhea. Its effects cannot be halted once administered. Not enough data to determine whether there are adverse effects.

ENEMA

No data on either effectiveness or adverse effects.

ACUPUNCTURE OR TENS

Pros: Small studies have shown acupuncture to be effective at inducing labor, and TENS used at acupuncture points has been shown to increase the frequency of labor-strength contractions. Both acupuncture and TENS can be stopped should there be adverse effects. TENS is noninvasive and painless.
Cons: No adverse effects known of either, but studies have been small. The TENS study only looked at use over a few hours. While this caused contractions, it isn't known whether longer use would induce progressive labor.

HERBS

Pros: Anecdotal data suggests that herbs may be effective and freer of adverse effects than conventional treatments. Inexpensive, painless, home-based treatment.

Cons: No rigorous research into effectiveness or possible adverse effects. Cannot be stopped once administered.

STRIPPING/SWEEPING THE MEMBRANES

Pros: Slightly decreases the number of oxytocin inductions by reducing the number of postdates pregnancies. However, routine induction for postdates pregnancy has questionable value.

Cons: Potential of rupturing membranes, instigating infection, or causing hemorrhage if the placenta is overlaying the cervix (placenta previa). Does not decrease C-section rates.

MECHANICAL DILATORS

Pros: Cheaper than prostaglandins.

Cons: They may increase the odds of infection.

PROSTAGLANDIN E2 (PGE2; Cervidil or Prepidil)

Pros: Somewhat reduces the cesarean rate compared with straight oxytocin inductions with an unripe cervix. Cervidil can be removed if it causes problems.

Cons: Can cause uterine hyperstimulation and fetal distress. In some cases, fetal distress can lead to cesarean section. Prepidil cannot be removed once administered.

MISOPROSTOL (Cytotec)

Pros: It may be more effective at ripening the cervix and inducing labor than PGE2 or oxytocin alone. Some studies show that its use reduces the cesarean rate compared with other induction methods. Much cheaper than PGE2.

Cons: It increases the odds of both uterine hyperstimulation compared with PGE2 and abnormal fetal heart rate resulting from uterine hyperstimulation. Uterine rupture has been reported. Once administered, its effects cannot be stopped. Studies have not established a safe, effective dose.

Misoprostol was not formulated for use in inducing labor, and has not been approved by the FDA for this purpose.

RUPTURING MEMBRANES (Amniotomy)

Pros: In a woman on the verge of beginning labor, rupturing membranes may be enough to trigger labor.

Cons: Can precipitate umbilical cord prolapse. Increases the odds of episodes of abnormal fetal heart rate and cesarean section for fetal distress. Since the interval between rupture and birth may be long with an induction, it increases the risk of infection in women who subsequently have vaginal exams and women colonized with group B strep.

OXYTOCIN

Pros: Effective agent for inducing labor. Can be stopped if it is producing adverse effects.

Cons: Labor is more painful. Requires an IV and electronic fetal monitoring, which have their own potential adverse effects. Often causes uterine hyperstimulation, which can lead to fetal distress. Doubles the odds of the baby being born in poor condition. Also causes increased postpartum blood loss and newborn jaundice. Blood loss and jaundice may relate to direct effects of oxytocin; increased use of IV fluids, especially IV fluids that don't contain salts; or both. Increases the risk of C-section, which also has grave potential adverse effects.

RUPTURING MEMBRANES AND OXYTOCIN

Pros: One study where women were assigned to oxytocin alone or oxytocin with amniotomy concluded that doing both was the more effective option. However, a statistical analysis of that study concluded that participating obstetricians had almost certainly sabotaged the random assignment process because of their preconceived belief that amniotomy was also needed.

Cons: Another trial that randomly assigned women to induction with early or late amniotomy found that early amniotomy was associated with increased likelihood of fetal distress and maternal infection but had no effect on cesarean rate. Three-fourths of the early-amniotomy cesareans for fetal distress were for abnormal heart rate patterns typical of umbilical cord compression due to lack of amniotic fluid.

GENERAL ADVICE ON INDUCTION

- *If cervical ripening is necessary, ask for Cervidil because it comes enclosed in a net and attached to a string.* Unlike the gel formulation, it can be removed should uterine hyperstimulation occur.
- *You can go home during the ripening process.* The American College of Obstetricians and Gynecologists recommends an observation period between thirty minutes and two hours before going home to make sure uterine hyperstimulation is not occurring.
- *Start oxytocin at night.* Although there are no data on timing of induction, the uterus is most sensitive to oxytocin at night, which is why labor usually starts at night.
- *Although this should be standard practice, make sure the IV fluid contains salts.* Salt-free fluids, especially in combination with oxytocin, one of whose effects is fluid retention, can cause serious blood-chemistry imbalances.
- *Have continuous electronic fetal monitoring.* It reduces the risk of newborn seizures. (See page 245.)
- *Insist on a low-dose oxytocin regimen that allows at least thirty minutes between dose increases, because high-dose regimens increase the risk of adverse effects.* The chance of developing adverse effects goes up with the total amount of oxytocin given and the peak dose. High-dose regimens greatly increase both.

- *Once you are actively dilating, try turning off the oxytocin.* Sometimes, once labor kicks in, it will continue on its own without extra oxytocin. This will be much more comfortable for you and easier on your baby. As long as the IV line is kept open, the nurse can always restart the oxytocin if needed. Low-dose, long-interval protocols increase the odds of being able to turn the oxytocin drip down or off in active labor.
- *Avoid or at least hold off on an epidural.* Epidurals slow labor and, with prolonged use, cause fevers. A fever in labor indicates a possible infection in mother or baby, and you and the baby will be treated accordingly.
- *Refuse rupture of membranes until 5 centimeters' dilation or more.* For one thing, you can back out if the induction doesn't work. For another, you eliminate the risk of infection and avoid IV antibiotics and septic workups should labor be slow to start.
- *Limit vaginal exams once membranes are ruptured.* There is a clear relationship between length of time since rupture, number of vaginal exams, and infection.
- *Refuse internal contraction-pressure monitoring.* It requires rupture of membranes, increases the odds of infection, introduces risks of its own (see page 93), and doesn't improve outcomes.

THE BOTTOM LINE ON LABOR WITH A LARGE BABY

STRATEGIES TO AVOID UNNECESSARY INTERVENTION

- *Have a caregiver with a low cesarean rate.* Obstetricians with low cesarean rates are less likely to opt for C-sections when they suspect a large baby.
- *Avoid an epidural.* Epidurals interfere with effective pushing and prevent you from doing the activities and assuming the positions that will maximize your chances of birthing a large baby. Avoiding an epidural will also help you . . .

- *Avoid a low or outlet forceps delivery.* These are deliveries done when the baby's head has passed through the pelvis, which means they are mostly unnecessary except in cases of sudden fetal distress. Evidence suggests that low and outlet forceps deliveries are more likely to injure a large baby than spontaneous delivery.
- *Preplan with your caregiver to use the all-fours maneuver should there be problems birthing the baby's shoulders.* Assuming an all-fours position seems to be the best and safest technique for releasing the shoulders (see page 234). The potential need for this maneuver is another reason to avoid an epidural, although with coordinated assistance, even a mother with an epidural could be quickly helped into this position.

THE BOTTOM LINE ON INDUCTION FOR PRELABOR RUPTURE OF MEMBRANES

GENERAL ADVICE

- *If membranes rupture, have someone listen to the baby's heart.* It should tick along at two beats per second or more (120–160 beats per minute). If it is much slower than this, or if you are having contractions and it slows down drastically during a contraction, go to a hospital immediately. The umbilical cord may have slipped down ahead of the baby, which can pinch it between the baby's head and your pelvis.
- *Refuse vaginal exams before active labor.* The main reason to do one is to determine whether the umbilical cord has come down into the vagina, but this can be ruled out simply by listening to the baby's heartbeat.
- *Limit vaginal exams even after labor kicks in.*
- *If you and your caregiver aren't sure membranes actually ruptured, consider refusing induction.* The common tests for

membrane rupture will incorrectly diagnose ruptured membranes in equivocal cases in one-quarter or more women.

- *Refuse internal contraction-pressure monitoring.* It increases the risk of infection and it does no better than external contraction monitoring for determining oxytocin dose.
- *Avoid having an epidural early in labor.* Epidurals cause fevers, especially with prolonged use. Epidural-induced fever can lead caregivers to mistakenly conclude that you have an infection. (See page 269.)

COMPARE AND CONTRAST THREE APPROACHES TO PRELABOR RUPTURE OF MEMBRANES

WAIT AT LEAST 24 HOURS BEFORE INDUCING LABOR UNLESS YOU SHOW SYMPTOMS OF INFECTION	INDUCE LABOR IMMEDIATELY OR SHORTLY WITH PROSTAGLANDIN E2 (PGE2) FOLLOWED BY OXYTOCIN	INDUCE LABOR IMMEDIATELY OR SHORTLY WITH OXYTOCIN
Have to wait. This can be nerve-wracking if you are confined to bed in a hospital.	No waiting.	No waiting.
Allows time for natural cervical ripening.	Ripens an unripe cervix.	Potential failure with unripe cervix.
Allows most women to begin labor on their own. One study showed that waiting 24 hours didn't increase the time from membrane rupture to birth but greatly reduced the need for oxytocin.	————	————
Probably a more pleasant labor because most women will start labor spontaneously.	Labor probably more painful and difficult than spontaneous labor if oxytocin also needed.	Labor probably more painful and difficult than spontaneous labor.

(continued)

WAIT AT LEAST 24 HOURS BEFORE INDUCING LABOR UNLESS YOU SHOW SYMPTOMS OF INFECTION	INDUCE LABOR IMMEDIATELY OR SHORTLY WITH PROSTAGLANDIN E2 (PGE2) FOLLOWED BY OXYTOCIN	INDUCE LABOR IMMEDIATELY OR SHORTLY WITH OXYTOCIN
Spontaneous labor easiest on baby.	Increased likelihood of episodes of abnormal fetal heart rate.	Greatest likelihood of episodes of abnormal fetal heart rate and fetal distress.
Infection rate low, provided no vaginal exams and mother not colonized with group B strep.	According to one large, multicenter study, infection may be a risk for group B strep carriers. See page 71.	Infection rate low.
IV antibiotics may be needed to keep infection rates low in group B strep carriers if labor does not begin shortly.	IV antibiotics may solve the problem of the association between PGE2 and infection in group B strep carriers.	IV antibiotics less likely to be needed in group B strep carriers.
The (likely) longer time period from membrane rupture to birth may lead to pressure to give you and/or your baby IV antibiotics and to do a septic workup on the baby regardless of group B strep status.	May reduce pressures to treat you and/or your baby with IV antibiotics or to do a septic workup on baby.	May reduce pressures to treat you and/or your baby with IV antibiotics or to do a septic workup on baby.
When there is thick *meconium* (the baby's first stool) in the amniotic fluid, the pros and cons of awaiting labor are unknown.	When there is thick meconium in the amniotic fluid, the pros and cons of using PGE2 are unknown. However, thick meconium sometimes indicates a compromised baby. A baby with problems may have a harder time tolerating an induced labor.	If there is thick meconium in the amniotic fluid, oxytocin may increase the likelihood of inhaling it. (Inhaling meconium can cause a life-threatening pneumonia after birth.)

Note: Many doctors want you in the hospital once membranes rupture, but you can just as well and much more comfortably await labor at home. A large study that randomly assigned women to induction versus awaiting labor found that women preferred induction. However, this preference applied only to women admitted to the hospital while awaiting labor. Women allowed to go home like expectant management just fine.

POINTS FOR GBS-POSITIVE WOMEN TO CONSIDER

GBS migrates to the vaginal outlet from the colon. It is rarely found in the upper vagina, but almost all newborn GBS infections arise from the bacterium invading the uterus. This suggests that conventional obstetric management could cause infection by transferring GBS to the cervix or opening a pathway into the uterus via prenatal cervical checks, vaginal exams in labor—*especially* after membranes rupture, rupturing membranes, and internal fetal heart rate or contraction monitoring. The effect cannot be measured because we have no unexposed GBS-positive comparison group. Still, infection in general is associated with ruptured membranes, number of vaginal exams, use of internal monitoring devices, and time. You may wish to refuse potentially contributory practices since none of them have offsetting benefits. Wiping from front to back might also keep GBS from getting into the vagina.

You should know that inducing labor for ruptured membranes is not a Centers for Disease Control recommendation. If you agree to induction, know that using prostaglandin E2 quadrupled the incidence of infection in GBS-positive women compared with oxytocin alone. None of the women, though, had IV antibiotics in labor. Know too that the CDC guidelines specifically state that colonization is not a reason for scheduled cesarean section. Finally, GBS positive status doesn't rule out home birth. IV antibiotics could be administered and the baby observed or a blood sample taken if warranted.

INDUCTION FOR
POSTDATES PREGNANCY

COMPARE AND CONTRAST THREE POSTDATES OPTIONS

INDUCE AT 41–42 WEEKS	DO PERIODIC TESTS TO ASSESS THE BABY'S WELL-BEING AND INDUCE ONLY IF THERE SEEMS TO BE A PROBLEM	AWAIT LABOR
Ends uncertainty.	Uncertainty continues. If the test says the baby is fine, the baby is almost certainly fine (low false-negative rate).	Uncertainty continues.
According to one large multicenter trial, inducing may slightly reduce the chance of cesarean with a typical obstetrician. However, induction has usually been shown to increase the odds of cesarean even with PGE2 to ripen the cervix.	Tests of fetal well-being all have high false-positive rates, which means there is a good probability of having an induction or a C-section for a perfectly healthy baby.	Very rarely, a normally formed baby suddenly dies in the womb. If it happens after the mother's due date, it appears that a routine induction would have prevented the tragedy. However, hindsight doesn't take into account the risks of induction. Because of these risks, while a routine induction policy would save some babies, other babies and even mothers would be lost.
Induced labors usually more painful and prolonged.	Fewer inductions.	Fewest inductions.
Induced labors harder on baby. May be enough to distress or harm a baby who would have tolerated natural labor.	Even with a true positive, the baby may tolerate natural labor better than induced labor.	Fewest inductions.

INDUCE AT 41–42 WEEKS	DO PERIODIC TESTS TO ASSESS THE BABY'S WELL-BEING AND INDUCE ONLY IF THERE SEEMS TO BE A PROBLEM	AWAIT LABOR
Baby may be born premature, although not by enough to endanger him.	Less likelihood of caregiver-caused prematurity because fewer inductions.	Least likelihood of caregiver-caused prematurity because fewer inductions.
Less likelihood of passing meconium into the amniotic fluid because the probability increases with age. Occasionally the baby inhales it into the lungs (*meconium aspiration*), causing a kind of pneumonia.	More likelihood of passing meconium. This increases the odds both of meconium aspiration and of inappropriate treatment (aggressive suctioning, putting a tube down the baby's throat) for harmless amounts of meconium (light meconium or *tea-staining*).	More likelihood of passing meconium. This increases the odds both of meconium aspiration and of inappropriate treatment (aggressive suctioning, putting a tube down the baby's throat) for harmless amounts of meconium (light meconium or *tea-staining*).

GLEANINGS FROM THE MEDICAL LITERATURE
(PAGES 227–234)

- Nipple stimulation, castor oil, acupuncture, and TENS stimulation have all been found effective at ripening the cervix and/or inducing contractions, and sexual intercourse increases the local concentration of prostaglandins involved in initiating labor.
- Oxytocin, especially in the quantities required for induction of labor, has risks.
- Physiological oxytocin-induction regimens offer advantages over high-dose regimens.

- Prostaglandins have not solved the problem of induction leading to more cesareans.
- Inducing labor for reasons of convenience or other nonmedical reasons (elective induction) increases the risk of cesarean and fetal distress.
- Ultrasound weight estimates followed by induction for suspected large baby increases the risk of cesarean without improving outcomes.
- Waiting for labor onset for at least twenty-four hours after membrane rupture is safe, provided there are no symptoms of infection, the mother tests negative for group B strep, and no vaginal exams are done.
- Inducing with oxytocin shortly after membrane rupture may greatly increase the odds of C-section compared with awaiting labor.
- Inducing with PGE2 shortly after membrane rupture results in similar cesarean rates to those for awaiting labor, but it doesn't decrease infection rates.
- The obstetric powers that be have decided that labor should be routinely induced at forty-one weeks, but the situation is not nearly as clear-cut as it seems.
- The all-fours maneuver is a rapid, safe, and effective technique for relieving stuck shoulders.

Chapter 4

⌒

IVs:
"WATER, WATER EVERYWHERE, NOR ANY DROP TO DRINK"

IN THE 1940S, back in the days when general anesthetics were administered through opaque face masks, doctors began forbidding food to patients undergoing surgery because they realized that vomiting and inhaling food particles into the lungs (*aspiration*) was a grave and often fatal complication of surgery. Since laboring women during this time were usually heavily drugged and often had general anesthesia even for vaginal births, doctors extended the policy to childbirth. On no grounds whatever, and despite knowing that clear liquids empty rapidly from the stomach, the ban included drinking too. Thus, "nothing by mouth," or NPO for the Latin *non per os*, became standard practice before surgery and during labor.

Today, changes in anesthetic and obstetric practice have made aspiration a vanishingly rare event. Less than 2 per 1,000,000 pregnant women in the United States between 1988 and 1990 died of *any* anesthesia-related complication—not just aspiration—during delivery. Better training of anesthesiologists and the modern anesthetic practice of *intubation*, putting a tube down the throat to protect the airway, are largely responsible for the improvement. The virtual disappearance of general anesthesia for vaginal birth and its replacement with epidural and spinal (*regional*) anesthesia for most C-sections has also contributed. Nonetheless, NPO in labor remains the norm at many hospitals because many doctors erroneously believe that eating and drinking in labor is risky and that IV fluids are a risk-free replacement for oral intake.

THE ILLOGIC OF "NOTHING BY MOUTH"

TO BEGIN WITH, eating and drinking in labor are safe. In three large U.S. studies totalling seventy-eight thousand women in labor who ate and drank freely, there was not one case of aspiration. The anesthesia-related maternal mortality rate in England and Wales, where oral intake in labor is usual, is identical to the rate in the United States, where it is not. Nor is aspiration a problem in other countries that permit eating and drinking in labor, such as Japan and the Netherlands.

The real problem is the occasional incompetent anesthesiologist. Experts agree that poor technique is *the* major cause of airway-related anesthesia deaths, including aspiration. Doris Haire, long-time childbirth activist and writer on maternity care issues, says, "I have searched back through twenty years of the medical literature, and there is not a single documented case of aspiration in an individual [not just pregnant women] who was properly anesthetized by today's standards of anesthesia."

Secondly, medical research does not support NPO or routine IV policies. The authors of *A Guide to Effective Care in Pregnancy and Childbirth,* the bible of evidence-based obstetric care, place both under "Forms of Care Unlikely to Be Beneficial."

Why, then, the strenuous objections to oral intake and the insistence on routine IVs? What we have, once again, is an obstetric belief system that defines childbirth as a medical-surgical event. Eating and drinking do not fit this model. IVs do.

Consider the following: Doctors know that "nothing by mouth" is a futile exercise. The threshold of risk should aspiration occur is generally agreed to be about two tablespoons (25 ml) of stomach fluid. However, as studies attest, no time interval since the last oral intake guarantees a stomach volume below this amount in a pregnant woman. In fact, no time interval guarantees a volume of less than 100 ml. Prudence dictates that anesthesiologists always assume laboring women have full stomachs and treat them accordingly. Nonetheless, NPO is the rule before surgery, so doctors impose it in labor too. Doctors also know that narcotics slow stomach emptying, cause nausea and vomiting, and relax the esophageal sphincter. Narcotics confer at least as much risk of aspiration as do eating and drinking, but no doctor suggests limiting narcotic use in labor. Narcotic medication, unlike eating and drinking, fits the medical-surgical model. Doctors know, too, that water rapidly absorbs directly through the stomach walls. Whatever possible argument could be made against food, none can be made against water. Yet many hospital policies continue to limit women to the meager ice chips. Finally, what other reason besides fervently and irrationally held beliefs could explain how an American Society of Anesthesiologists brochure educating pregnant women about epidurals can gloss over the very real risks of epidurals but warn in oversized capital letters against eating or drinking in labor?

These same beliefs also explain why doctors find IVs an acceptable substitute. IVs are problematic by nature. Hunger and thirst and our natural responses to them invoke complex feedback loops that maintain delicate chemical balances in both mother and unborn child. These balances are disrupted when they are bypassed by dumping huge amounts of fluids, often over a short period of time, directly into the bloodstream. Pregnancy renders women particularly vulnerable because the physiological changes (increased amounts of fluids in the tissues, for example) cut down on the margin for error. As you can see in the appendix for this chapter, complications believed to be "just one of those things" or intrinsic to pregnant women, difficult labor, or cesarean surgery can be linked to IVs. However, none of this stops doctors from writing articles that describe the numerous and sometimes serious potential complications of IVs but that then fail to arrive at the obvious solution: Let laboring women do as thirst and hunger dictate. On the contrary, a study that found a blood-chemistry disturbance emblematic of fluid overload in women with IVs but not in women allowed to drink clear liquids does not recommend abandoning routine IVs. Instead, the authors admire "the resiliency" of the pregnant women's circulatory systems and kidneys when "confronted with iatrogenic [doctor-caused] stresses" because none of the women actually developed fluid in the lungs. Two articles conclude that a glucose IV should be given despite the hazards. The authors of yet another pair of articles, no doubt proceeding on the basis that if you can't solve the problem, simply deny it's a problem, decide that an IV isn't necessary; prolonged fasting in labor won't hurt. A sports-medicine physician would be horrified at the suggestion that an athlete engage in an endurance event with no food, nourishing drinks, or even water, but obstetricians and anesthesiologists are too wedded to their beliefs about labor to see it in these terms.

Routine IVs and NPO make no sense in modern-day obstetrics. These days, the odds are minuscule that a laboring woman will require general anesthesia. Until such time as we require "nothing by mouth" and IVs for downhill skiers, football players, and drivers entering the freeway—all activities where surgery under general anesthesia might also suddenly become necessary—we should not require it of laboring women.

THE BOTTOM LINE

Pros and Cons of Forbidding Food and Drink in Labor

Pros: None. Some caregivers tell women that what goes down in labor will only come back up, so there is no use in attempting oral intake, but this is not true. Few women allowed to eat and drink as they wish will vomit.

Cons: Hunger and especially thirst cause considerable discomfort. Midwives observe that dehydration may cause fever. Dehydration and starvation are associated with longer labors, increased use of oxytocin (trade name: Pitocin or "Pit") to stimulate stronger contractions, and instrumental delivery. In addition, during pregnancy, starvation causes a faster, sharper drop-off in blood sugar levels and an earlier switch to metabolizing body fat. Vigorous exercise—in this case, labor—accelerates this process. This is a problem when women fast in labor because metabolizing fat produces *ketones*. In animal studies, ketones have been shown to cross into fetal circulation, making the fetal blood more acidic (*acidosis*). Acidosis is a symptom of fetal distress. Also, undiluted stomach acid poses a severe hazard to lung tissue should it be aspirated.

Pros and Cons of Routine IVs

Pros: None.

Cons: IVs inhibit mobility; painful inflammation can occur at the site with time; and the punctured blood vessel may leak, causing a painful, long-lasting bruise.

The main problem with IV fluids is fluid overload, which is all too common especially with rapid administration of large (*bolus*) amounts (one or more liters), as is done before administering an epidural or beginning a cesarean section under epidural or spinal anesthesia.* This can lead to fluid in both mother's lungs (*pulmonary edema*) and baby's lungs (*neonatal tachypnea*). More than one author thinks bolus administration explains why babies born by cesarean section are more likely to have breathing difficulties due to fluid in the lungs. Bolus IV-fluid administration also dilutes the blood, which decreases the concentration of red blood cells (*anemia*). Lower red blood cell concentration means fewer oxygen-carrying cells per unit volume for the baby and the uterine muscle cells. Another problem with anemia in childbirth is that it predisposes to bleeding.

Glucose-containing IV fluids, also called "dextrose" IVs, can raise maternal and fetal blood glucose levels to diabetic levels (*hyperglycemia*). Hyperglycemia in the baby increases the production of lactic acid, a metabolic by-product when there is insufficient oxygen. This additional source of lactic acid can add to the stress of a baby already experiencing difficulties; in fact, animal studies show that excess glucose renders the fetal brain more vulnerable to injury during periods of oxygen deprivation. Excess glucose in the baby's circulation causes the baby to pour out insulin in response. After the birth, the baby is abruptly cut off from the source of glucose. The excess insulin can then cause a precipitous and sometimes dangerous drop in the baby's blood sugar levels (*hypoglycemia*). Monitoring a newborn's blood glucose levels means one or more painful heel sticks and possibly a bottle feeding with sugar water or formula, which can interfere with establishing breastfeeding.

---

*The standard recommendation for fluid intake has long been eight cups of liquid per day. This is equivalent to two liters (bags) of IV fluid. You can see that giving one or more liters of IV fluid in less than an hour is grossly unphysiological—even over two or three hours is excessive.

Although this can happen with any type of IV, glucose infusions, because they typically lack salts (*electrolytes*), greatly increase the probability and danger of fluid overload. They can cause newborn jaundice,* a type of transient pneumonia called "wet-lung syndrome" (*transient neonatal tachypnea*), and low blood sodium (*hyponatremia*), which puts the newborn at risk for such neurological problems as pauses in breathing (*apnea*) and seizures. They also result in a transfer of water into the baby's tissues. This extra fluid inflates the baby's birth weight and the subsequent weight loss after birth. Doctors and others often gauge breastfeeding adequacy by how fast the baby regains her birth weight, so this misleading weight loss may lead a doctor or mother to mistakenly conclude that breastfeeding is inadequate.

Finally, any problem that requires treating the newborn will result in separation from the mother, interfere with bonding and breastfeeding, and cause worry and expense.

What Should You Eat or Drink During Labor?

Fat delays digestion. Solids must be broken down into tiny bits to pass into the intestines. High concentrations of sugar and acid and either low or high concentrations of salt also slow digestion. Heavily sweetened drinks can also cause nausea and acid in the stomach, which, as we have seen, should be avoided. Icy liquids empty more slowly as well. Given these criteria, choose food and drink that you know you tolerate well, the kind you would consume if you were recovering from the stomach flu. Examples might be soft, nonacid fruits; nonfat yogurt;

---

*Severe fluid overload causes jaundice because the excess fluid swells and bursts red blood cells. Jaundice results from excess circulating levels of bilirubin, a yellow pigment and a breakdown product of red blood cells.

cooked cereal; eggs; graham crackers; toast and jam; puddings; custard; fruit smoothies made with nonacid fruits; sweetened, noncaffeinated teas; nonfat milk; or noncreamy soup with noodles or rice. Eat or drink small quantities frequently rather than large quantities infrequently. One midwife recommends carbohydrates early in labor, moving to at least four ounces of calorie- and electrolyte-containing fluids per hour in late labor. If you vomit, cut back to sips of clear, nonacid liquids.

WAYS TO MINIMIZE THE CHANCE OF ASPIRATION

Note that when doctors abide by these recommendations, the problem of aspiration disappears whether you eat or drink or not.

Doctors should:

- *Do fewer cesareans.* Fewer cesareans means fewer opportunities for anesthesia complications.
- *Perform cesareans using epidural or spinal (regional) anesthesia.* This has become the norm in most hospitals, but it wouldn't hurt to ask if this is the case at yours. Aspiration can't happen when you are conscious.
- *Ensure that anesthesiologists use proper techniques.*
- *Avoid IV-fluid overload.* The excess fluid causes tissue swelling and makes it hard to intubate for general anesthesia.

You should:

- *Maintain some form of oral intake.* The most dangerous form of aspiration is aspiration of undiluted stomach acid because it chemically burns the airways. Presurgical antacid treatment is not completely preventative.
- *If you are having a narcotic, including a narcotic epidural, limit oral intake to small, frequent amounts of clear, nonacid,*

moderately sweetened or salted liquids. Narcotics cause nausea and vomiting as well as relax the esophageal sphincter.

If there is a high probability that general anesthesia may be needed, you should:

- *Limit oral intake to small, frequent amounts of clear, nonacid, moderately sweetened or salted liquids.*
- *Avoid narcotics.*

GLEANINGS FROM THE MEDICAL LITERATURE
(PAGES 239–242)

Note: We do not know what the normal biochemistry of laboring women and newborns is like because, almost universally, all control groups were kept NPO and usually had an IV, too. The few cases where oral intake was permitted give tantalizing glimpses as to how much NPO policies and routine IVs derail normal physiology. Also, there are no studies of nutrition during labor other than one published study of the effects of eating and drinking on nausea and vomiting and a small unpublished study of their effects on labor.

- Fasting during labor causes a rise in maternal ketone levels, which may have adverse effects on the labor.
- Fasting does not guarantee an empty stomach.
- Hunger and especially thirst are a source of considerable discomfort in laboring women.
- Eating and drinking in labor does not increase the risk of vomiting, avoids the hazards of IV-fluid overload, and may have beneficial effects on labor progress.
- IVs can cause pain and inflammation at the IV site.
- Caregivers may commonly overdose IV fluids.
- IV fluids can cause problems related to fluid overload, prob-

lems that are greatly exacerbated by giving large amounts of IV fluids rapidly or fluids that don't contain salts.

- Glucose IVs can cause high blood sugar in the baby before birth and low blood sugar after the birth, both of which can cause problems.

Chapter 5

⌒

ELECTRONIC FETAL MONITORING AND CESAREAN FOR FETAL DISTRESS:
THE MACHINE THAT GOES *PING!*

THE OPENING SEQUENCE of the Monty Python movie *The Meaning of Life* shows obstetricians preparing for a birth. "More apparatus!" the doctors command. "Get the machine that goes *ping!*" They especially want this machine because it is extremely expensive and will impress the hospital administrator should he drop by. The delivery room fills with equipment. All seems in readiness until one of the doctors notices that something is missing—the patient. Amused at their oversight, they retrieve her gurney from behind the equipment and shift her onto the delivery table. "The administrator is coming," warns the nurse. Hurriedly the doctors order her to switch everything on. The administrator enters. "Ah," he says, suitably impressed, "I see you have the machine that goes *ping!* Carry on." With a great show of busy self-importance and barking out of orders, the doctors deliver the baby and clap it into an isolette. Everybody rushes out with the equipment and the baby, leaving the bewildered mother behind.

Electronic fetal monitors are the machines that go *"ping!"*

Lights blink, sounds thump, a tracing crawls across an oscillo-scope, reams of data transcribe onto graph paper. It's mesmer-izing. Nobody pays attention to the mother who's attached to one—not her partner, not the medical staff. Everything centers around the machine. You would think *it* was having the baby. Fathers sit intently gazing at . . . the machine. "You're starting a contraction," they say, as if she wouldn't know this on her own. Nurses and doctors come in to tend and scrutinize the machine. One study analyzing medical staff behavior during the pushing phase of labor records that during one arbitrarily cho-sen five-minute segment of videotape, the nurse looked at the monitor nineteen times.

Despite all we know about the benefits of supportive care in labor, a supposed *advantage* of electronic fetal monitoring (EFM) systems is that one nurse can monitor an entire labor ward of women by watching screens at a central station. Ig-noring the mother wouldn't be so bad if the machine did what everybody thinks it does: tell doctors the baby is in trouble and allow them to rescue her from harm, but it doesn't do that.

As a medical journal editorial commented, "When the req-uisite randomized controlled trials were finally done, the con-sensus was striking: routine electronic fetal monitoring confers no demonstrable benefit to the fetus, yet poses a significantly increased risk of operative delivery (e.g., cesarean delivery or forceps) for the woman. Even for high-risk fetuses, evidence of the benefit of electronic monitoring . . . is lacking. After two de-cades of use, electronic fetal monitoring has not been shown to be superior to intermittent [listening]."

HOW DID WE GET INTO THIS MESS?

H. L. MENCKEN SAID, "For every complex problem there is a solution that is simple, neat—and wrong." EFM exemplifies that truism. The basic premise behind EFM is that insufficient oxygen (*hypoxia, asphyxia*) in labor is a common cause of severe mental retardation, death, and especially cerebral palsy, and that changes in the fetal heart rate precede brain damage. Based on that premise, obstetricians reasoned that intermittent listening had been unable to prevent brain injuries because it provided too little information too late. The solution, then, became a machine that made a continuous tracing of the fetal heart rate and how it reacted to contractions. Unfortunately, however, the premise was wrong on both points.

To begin with, less than 10 percent of cases of cerebral palsy or mental retardation during or shortly after birth result from oxygen deprivation during labor. Even when doctors suspect that lack of oxygen played a role, often other factors did too.* Consider the following: The number of cases of oxygen deprivation in labor has declined steeply since 1979. If birth asphyxia were largely responsible for cerebral palsy, the cerebral palsy rate should have declined too. It hasn't. Moreover, continuous EFM has become nearly universal since the 1980s. If it worked, it should have affected the cerebral palsy rate by now, but the rate remains unchanged. An editorial in the journal *Lancet* states, "In light of the evidence . . . , the continued willingness of doctors to reinforce the fable that [labor] care is an important determinant of cerebral palsy can only be regarded as shooting the specialty of obstetrics in the foot."

Second, there really isn't much connection between what the baby's heart rate does during labor and measures of the baby's condition at birth, such as the pH of the baby's blood or the baby's Apgar score. Few babies diagnosed with fetal distress are born in poor condition. A bedrock truth of EFM is that if the monitor says the baby is fine, the baby is almost certainly

---

*In fact, data suggest that many so-called cases of birth asphyxia are actually due to a silent infection during pregnancy. The misattribution occurs because the symptoms of infection mimic those of oxygen deprivation.

fine, but if the monitor says the baby is not fine—that is, that she has *nonreassuring* heart rate patterns—the baby is also probably fine. There is even less connection between poor condition at birth and eventual handicap. If heart rate patterns don't predict condition at birth very well, and poor condition at birth doesn't predict long-term outcome very well, then EFM couldn't possibly have much effect on long-term outcomes.

Basically the situation looks like this: When the monitor says the baby is in trouble, it is usually wrong (false positive), and even when it is right (true positive), often you can't do much about it. Cesarean delivery will make no difference. But there's more. Although almost all babies who look good during labor are born healthy, some babies with low blood pH or Apgar scores at birth show no signs of distress during labor (false negative). And with certain rare emergencies, such as *umbilical cord prolapse* (the umbilical cord comes down into the birth canal ahead of the baby) or *placental abruption* (the placenta detaches from the uterus before birth), the monitor picks up the problem all right, but the event can be so catastrophic that even a prompt cesarean may not be fast enough to avert disaster. On the other hand, as studies document, sometimes caregivers don't respond to a baby who is clearly in trouble, in which case it doesn't matter how they monitored the baby.

Finally, machines don't always work right. For example, it is possible for the electronics of the monitor to double or halve the baby's heart rate. It is also possible for the monitor to pick up the mother's pulse instead, which can lead to an erroneous diagnosis of abnormally slow fetal heart rate (*bradycardia*).

Even as studies failed to find EFM beneficial, usage steadily rose. As of 1995, 81 percent of all U.S. women having live births had EFM. When you consider the percentage of women who had scheduled cesareans or arrived at the hospital on the point of giving birth, this means practically everybody else had EFM. If EFM doesn't work, why haven't obstetricians abandoned it?

First and foremost, EFM fits so neatly with obstetric biases that doctors and researchers refuse to let go of it. It also fits with the broader cultural fascination with high-tech equipment. Obstetricians and hospital administrators can be as susceptible to slick marketing and as interested in having the latest equipment in their field as any other enthusiast. For this reason, EFM swept the marketplace and became the norm before research ever established whether it had value. EFM is expensive, scientific, and complicated. It simply *had* to be better than putting a stethoscope or even a Doptone—the little hand-held ultrasonic device—to the tummy. This is also why many researchers cannot seem to understand that the problems with EFM are intrinsic. They assume they just need to try harder. Lately, for example, studies of computer analyses of EFM tracings and studies looking to see whether some subtle aspect of the baby's heartbeat correlates with outcomes pepper the obstetric literature.

EFM's high false-positive rate also reinforces belief that it works. "Fetal distress" appears, the obstetrician performs a cesarean or forceps delivery, the baby is born healthy, and everybody thinks that EFM saved the baby—only, of course, the baby was fine all along.

Another excuse for not abandoning EFM is the liability issue. Doctors and administrators argue that EFM monitor strips provide documentation that will protect them in a lawsuit. Not only are we once again confronted by "our interests before our patients' interests," but ironically, doctors are hanging themselves. Litigators can always find an "expert" to point to some squiggle on the strip and claim there was fetal distress. Along these same lines, obstetricians argue that EFM is the "standard of care," so not using it lays them open to accusations of substandard care. But intermittent listening is equally acceptable. The American College of Obstetricians and Gynecologists officially holds the position that intermittent listening performed according to appropriate guidelines "is equivalent to continuous electronic monitoring." The Society of Obstetricians and Gynecologists of Canada goes even further, stating, "The preferred method of fetal health surveillance for low risk women during labour is [to listen intermittently] with a hand-held ultrasound Doppler." An American legal review of EFM similarly states that failure to use EFM does not render a doctor liable, because abundant evidence from the medical research shows intermittent listening to be equally good. In fact, the reviewer adds that the doctrine of "informed consent" may demand that obstetricians inform women that EFM does not improve outcomes but increases cesarean and vaginal instrumental delivery rates.

Finally, obstetricians say they can't switch back to intermittent listening because hospitals don't have enough nurses to listen to the baby as often as it needs to be done. This is another way of saying that hospitals don't have enough staff to properly watch over laboring women. The legal reviewer thinks doctors may be obliged to inform women of that too. Moreover, when the staff of a big, busy labor and delivery unit looked to see whether intermittent listening was feasible, they found that it was. Nurses had to use EFM because of lack of staff only 3 percent of the time.

None of this is to say that doctors should ignore the baby's heart rate. It says that most of the time, intermittent listening can tell medical caregivers when the baby is fine and when to worry. EFM usually just clouds the issue, although in its place, EFM can occasionally help. The task is to make EFM the servant, not the master.

HOW EFM IS DONE

THE ELECTRONIC MONITOR is a bread box–sized instrument that displays the baby's heart rate in parallel with uterine pressure as tracings on an oscilloscope screen. The heart rate and contraction patterns are also traced onto a long strip of graph paper that is calibrated so that medical caregivers can see how the baby's heart responds to contractions, how it varies over time, and how long, strong, and close together the contractions are. The strip provides a permanent record. The monitor collects data basically in one of two ways: externally and internally.

External EFM

Nurses put two belts snugly around your belly, each with its own sensor, or the sensors are held in place by a wide elastic mesh band. The lower belt's sensor picks up your baby's heart rate via ultrasound. It uses the same technology as the hand-held Doppler devices used by most doctors and midwives during prenatal visits. If the baby moves or you do, the sensor may lose the signal, which can be alarming to parents but means nothing except that the nurse has to reposition the sensor. The upper belt picks up contractions. When you have a contraction, your uterus lifts up and forward, pushing in a button on the sensor. The monitor plots this as a series of hills as the contractions come and go. External contraction monitoring does not measure contraction intensity in any rigorous way, although as time passes, the peaks tend to get higher. If the sensor is not positioned just right or you are on the heavy side, strong contractions may barely register. Conversely, mild, nondilating contractions (*Braxton-Hicks contractions*) may register strongly. This can confuse you and sometimes misleads nurses.

Internal EFM

With internal heart rate monitoring, the lower belt is replaced by a wire that plugs into a small box strapped to your thigh. Leads from the box then go into the monitor. The wire ends in a thin, stiff, sharply pointed spiral needle. The medical caregiver catches the needle under the baby's scalp (or buttocks if the baby is breech) and twists to anchor it and keep it from coming loose, although they sometimes come loose anyway and have to be replaced. The contraction sensor belt can also be replaced by a thin tube filled with water that is vaginally inserted into the uterus. The tube acts as a pressure gauge. It permits reasonably accurate measurements of contraction strength.

THE BOTTOM LINE

COMPARING EXTERNAL AND INTERNAL MONITORING

EXTERNAL EFM	INTERNAL EFM
Less accurate, sometimes loses the baby's heartbeat, but good enough for most situations.	More accurate, less likely to lose the baby's heartbeat, which may be important when there is concern.
When you or your baby moves, the signal may be lost.	Not affected by you or your baby moving.
Often attached via a snug belt around your belly, which can be uncomfortable, although some hospitals use a broad mesh band.	No belt.
Noninvasive—nothing goes inside you.	Invasive procedure. A spiral needle catches under the baby's scalp, and wires extend from the scalp, through the vagina, and to the outside. This increases the risk of infection.
Does not require that membranes be ruptured.	Requires that membranes be ruptured. Breaking the bag of waters increases the risk of fetal distress and, in rare cases, may cause umbilical cord prolapse if the head is still high in the pelvis when it is done.

EXTERNAL EFM	INTERNAL EFM
Readjusting the sensing device is painless.	If the monitor lead comes off the baby's head, it must be replaced, which is uncomfortable for the mother and makes another small scalp wound in the baby.

EXTERNAL CONTRACTION MONITORING	INTERNAL CONTRACTION MONITORING
Doesn't measure actual contraction pressures, but knowing when contractions begin and end is almost always good enough.	Measures actual contraction pressures, but studies have not established the usefulness of this in making decisions about treatment.
Often attached via a snug belt around your belly, which can be uncomfortable, although some hospitals use a broad mesh band.	No belt.
Noninvasive—nothing goes inside of you.	Invasive procedure in which a catheter is inserted into the uterus. This increases the risk of infection. Other reported complications include piercing the uterus, rupturing blood vessels on the inner surface of the placenta, and becoming entangled with the umbilical cord and causing fetal distress.
Not sensitive to your changing position.	For the most common type of sensor used, changing levels will throw off the measurement. This pretty much confines you to lying in bed. There is another type that doesn't have this problem, but it is less popular in the United States.

SITUATIONS WHEN THE MEDICAL LITERATURE SUPPORTS THE USE OF CONTINUOUS EFM*

- *Oxytocin use.* EFM appears to have an advantage over intermittent listening in women receiving oxytocin, a hormone that stimulates contractions and can cause fetal distress.
- *When intermittent listening indicates there may be a problem.* When caregivers suspect or know that the baby is having a problem, EFM can be useful in tracking it, determining whether it is getting worse, and evaluating whether treatment is helping.
- *Vaginal birth after cesarean (VBAC).* (See page 173 for the arguments for and against EFM in VBAC labors.)

WAYS TO AVOID THE DRAWBACKS OF EFM

- *Don't have your baby in a hospital.* Few freestanding birth centers have electronic monitors, and, of course, home birth practitioners don't use them.
- *Avoid its use.* Insist on intermittent listening. If that won't wash or seems likely to provoke more conflict than you want to deal with, fall back on intermittent EFM—say, fifteen minutes per hour—going to continuous monitoring during pushing. (Once you begin pushing, you are likely to be in or near the bed anyway.) Many hospitals insist on at least having an initial "test strip" when you are admitted. Sometimes the test period can drag on. One nonconfrontational solution is to ask the nurse how long she wants to run the test strip. If she doesn't come in within a few minutes of that time, call her in and ask how the baby is doing. If she says, "Fine," ask to be disconnected.

*One trial concluded that routine EFM had important benefits, but there are serious problems with how it was conducted. (See page 246.)

- *Refuse routine internal EFM.* The key questions are "What is the problem?" and "What information will you get that could change my care that you are not getting from the way you are monitoring the baby now?"
- *Refuse routine internal contraction monitoring.* Ask the same questions as for internal EFM.
- *Don't have an epidural.* If you have an epidural, you will almost certainly have EFM because of the potential side effects of the epidural and the likelihood of needing oxytocin to stimulate stronger contractions.
- *Barring an emergency, make sure suspected fetal distress is confirmed by a follow-up test.* This reduces your chances of a cesarean section for an erroneous diagnosis. The classic means of confirming fetal distress is to take a blood sample from the baby's scalp and analyze it. This procedure is uncomfortable, tricky to do, takes time, and makes a wound in the baby's head. Studies show that it can be almost if not entirely replaced by rubbing the baby's head and observing whether her heart rate reacts.
- *Don't allow EFM to keep you from moving around and changing positions.* You will be more comfortable and it may promote labor progress.
- *Request a telemetry monitor.* A telemetry monitor enables you to be up and around because it uses wireless technology. Few hospitals have them.
- *Turn the monitor away or cover it with a towel and turn off the sound.* You should be the center of your partner's attention—and your own attention, for that matter—not a machine.
- *If the hospital uses belts and not the mesh band and you have more than one person with you, ask that someone be allowed to hand-hold the device that picks up the baby's heart rate while another person marks the beginning and end of contractions on the graph paper.* Tight belts can add considerably to your discomfort in active labor.

WAYS TO AVOID PROBLEMS WITH THE BABY

- *Avoid epidurals.* I put epidurals first because they can not only cause problems for the baby on their own but can lead to a cascade of other interventions that can also cause problems, namely:

  Oxytocin. Oxytocin, especially high-dose oxytocin regimens and when it is used to induce labor, can cause fetal distress due to overly long, overly strong contractions (*tetanic contractions, uterine hyperstimulation*). Uterine hyperstimulation can lead to . . .

  Medications to suppress contractions (tocolytics). However, tocolytics can also cause abnormal fetal heart rate patterns.

- *Avoid narcotics.* Narcotics can cause loss of normal variability of the fetal heart rate. Although this can also happen when the baby is sleeping, it is mildly concerning.
- *Avoid having the membranes routinely ruptured (amniotomy).* Because a liquid cannot be compressed, as long as the bag of waters is intact, the fluid protects the umbilical cord from the pressure of contractions. Once membranes are ruptured, contractions can impede blood flow through the cord, which can compromise the baby's oxygen supply. In rare cases, rupturing the membranes when the head is high can cause the umbilical cord to come down ahead of the baby and get pinched between the baby's head and the mother's pelvis. This is an emergency requiring immediate cesarean delivery.
- *Avoid lying on your back.* Lying on your back compresses the large blood vessels that serve the uterus and placenta.
- *Avoid prolonged breath holding during pushing.* Women pushing spontaneously rarely hold their breaths for more than six seconds, and most will groan or grunt while they push, which relieves the strain on their hearts and circula-

tions. Prolonged breath holding has been shown to compromise the baby's oxygenation. Despite this fact, nearly all women giving birth in hospitals will be told to bear down for ten or more seconds at a time and not to make any noise. (See page 281.)

It amazes me how many elements of typical obstetric management can cause nonreassuring heart tones, fetal distress, or both, and how little attention is paid to this. Doctors don't seem to worry that they might jump in unnecessarily or that they might dismiss true distress as an artifact of medication or that their practices might put a baby who was just able to handle normal labor over the edge. One obstetrician defended EFM on the basis that half the admissions to newborn intensive care come from healthy women who started labor with healthy babies. What a powerful, though unintended, indictment of obstetric management!

GLEANINGS FROM THE MEDICAL LITERATURE
(PAGES 244–247)

- Few cases of cerebral palsy arise from events in labor.
- The baby's heart rate during labor correlates poorly with measures of the baby's condition at birth.
- Measures of the baby's condition after birth correlate poorly with long-term outcomes.
- The baby's heart rate during labor correlates poorly with the incidence of cerebral palsy.
- Comparisons of EFM and intermittent listening show that EFM offers no long-term benefits in either low- or high-risk pregnancies, although it may have short-term benefits especially when oxytocin is used.
- Comparisons of EFM and intermittent listening show that EFM increases the likelihood of cesarean and vaginal instru-

mental delivery, infection, and cerebral palsy in premature babies.
- Selective EFM produces equally good outcomes as routine EFM.
- Intermittent EFM produces equally good outcomes as continuous EFM.
- Stimulating the baby's scalp can usually replace fetal scalp blood sampling as a follow-up test.

Chapter 6

WHEN DOCTORS BREAK THE MEMBRANES:
IF IT AIN'T BROKE, DON'T BREAK IT

Ask a typical obstetrician about routinely breaking the bag of waters, called *amniotomy* or *artificial rupture of membranes*, and he or she will tell you that it's a harmless way to shorten labor, to "get the show on the road," so to speak. Although at the time that this belief arose, no one had studied whether amniotomy actually did this, it turned out that obstetricians were right. Trials of early amniotomy versus conservation of membranes have since shown that early amniotomy shortens labor by an hour or two. However, we need to look at why obstetricians think shortening labor is beneficial, whether they are right, and whether amniotomy really is harmless.

To begin with, obstetricians believe that amniotomy circumvents the need for riskier remedies for poor progress: IV oxytocin (trade name: Pitocin or "Pit") to stimulate stronger contractions and cesarean section. It doesn't reduce cesarean sections, though. All nine trials that randomly assigned women to early amniotomy versus "conserve membranes" groups have shown an *increase* in cesarean sections—in particular, an increase in cesareans for fetal distress in the early-amniotomy group. The odds of that happening by chance are the same as the odds of flipping a coin and getting "heads" nine times in a row—in other words, very small. As for avoiding oxytocin, while amniotomy seems to reduce the use of oxytocin, that virtue derives from a circular argument. Obstetricians generally have unrealistic expectations of how fast labor should progress. So because of their unrealistic expectations, amniotomy, an invasive and potentially hazardous intervention, averts the use of a yet more risky and invasive intervention: IV oxytocin. With a little patience on the part of obstetricians, the "need" for amniotomy, oxytocin, and, for that matter, C-section for poor progress disappears in most cases. Meanwhile, getting out of bed and walking—which some obstetricians won't let women do with ruptured membranes—and pushing in an upright position do more to shorten labor than does amniotomy, and they pose no risks whatever (see pages 258 and 281).

Some obstetricians also believe that normal labor stresses the baby. They see labor as a race between the clock and the development of fetal distress. If this characterization is accurate, it is far more likely to result from labor management practices than from labor itself. Many components of standard obstetric management are known to have adverse effects on the baby, including laboring flat on the back, being directed to push as long and hard as you can (see page 281), epidurals, narcotics, oxytocin, and—last but not least—amniotomy.

The possibility that early amniotomy can cause complications in the baby shouldn't be news to obstetricians. They have long known that lack of amniotic fluid associates with fetal heart rate abnormalities. As long as membranes remain intact, the baby and the umbilical cord, which carries blood between the baby and the placenta, float inside a water balloon. The fluid protects umbilical cord blood vessels from the pressure of uterine contractions because liquids cannot be compressed. Remove the fluid, however, and that protection is gone, and uterine contractions can impede blood flow through the cord. In some babies, this leads to abnormal heart rate patterns. In fact, the past few years have seen a series of studies exploring the value of putting fluid back by running a catheter through the vagina into the uterus and infusing sterile saline (*amnioinfusion*). Obstetricians on the one hand act as if releasing the amniotic fluid never causes problems, while on the other hand they treat women for not having enough of it.

If your labor starts with spontaneous rupture of membranes, though, don't worry. Healthy, full-term babies can compensate. Nonetheless, the fact remains that if left alone, two-thirds of laboring women reach full cervical dilation with membranes intact, and there are advantages to this.

Another danger with early amniotomy is precipitating umbilical cord prolapse—that is, the umbilical cord coming down into the birth canal ahead of the baby. This is an obstetric emergency demanding immediate cesarean section because the cord will be pinched between the baby's head and the mother's pelvis during contractions. While rare, this problem is more likely in early labor when the head is still high. Once the head moves down into the pelvis, it fits against the cervix like an egg in an egg cup, and prolapse cannot occur. This is why some obstetricians want women with ruptured membranes to be flat in bed; they think it will prevent prolapse. In point of fact no studies have been done, and common sense says women would be better off upright. In upright positions, gravity brings the head lower in the pelvis.

Finally, several studies that evaluated infection rates found that early amniotomy increased the likelihood of maternal infection. One study suggested a possible mechanism: Early amniotomy increased the number of vaginal exams performed after membrane rupture.

So much for routine early amniotomy. What about amniotomy for a specific reason?

One reason doctors and midwives perform amniotomies is to

get a labor that has gotten stuck going again. The theory is that amniotomy will bring the head directly against the cervix, where it can do a better job of helping to open it. However, some studies have not found amniotomy beneficial. Still, done late in labor, at least, amniotomy would not violate the natural timing of membrane rupture and would be unlikely to cause the potential complications of early amniotomy.

The other reason for performing an amniotomy, which is accepted without question even by opponents of routine amniotomy, is to evaluate a baby who has symptoms of fetal distress. The amniotomy may be performed to insert a fetal scalp electrode for internal electronic fetal monitoring or to inspect the fluid to see whether the baby has passed *meconium,* the baby's first stool, into it. (Meconium in the amniotic fluid may signal current or previous fetal distress and may cause pneumonia if it gets into the baby's lungs.) This provides another paradoxical image. Replacing amniotic fluid has two purposes: relieving umbilical cord compression, thereby relieving fetal distress, and diluting thick meconium, thereby reducing the chances of the baby developing inhalation pneumonia. I can imagine a labor ward where in one room an obstetrician is rupturing membranes to verify fetal distress or the presence of meconium, while next door another obstetrician is putting fluid back in hopes of alleviating distress or diluting meconium.

In summary, there are trade-offs to rupturing membranes even for a specific indication. Meanwhile, routine amniotomy has little value and potential risks. For example, what if *this* baby cannot tolerate labor with ruptured membranes? Let's turn the tables on those who defend routine intervention "just in case." Shouldn't caregivers refrain from routine amniotomy— just in case?

THE AMNIOTOMY PROCEDURE

DURING A VAGINAL exam, the doctor or midwife snags the membranes with an *amnihook*, which looks like a flat, plastic crochet hook with a small, sharp tooth under the curled-over tip. The procedure can be uncomfortable for you but doesn't hurt the baby, because there are no nerves in the membranes. After the membranes are broken, there is usually a gush of warm liquid. You may get little gushes with every contraction thereafter until the head gets down into the pelvis far enough to plug the cervix. You will probably experience an increase in contraction intensity after membrane rupture, but you'll adapt within a few contractions.

THE BOTTOM LINE

PROS AND CONS OF ROUTINE AMNIOTOMY

Pros: Routine early amniotomy shortens labor by an hour or two. It appears to reduce the incidence of five-minute Apgar scores below 7 but has no other effects on the infant's condition at birth. It may reduce the use of oxytocin and the number of women who report the most intense degree of labor pain. However, the use of oxytocin, which makes labor more painful, and pain medication, especially epidurals, makes it difficult to determine the relationship between amniotomy and labor pain.

Cons: Amniotomy increases the incidence of abnormal fetal heart rate patterns. Studies may underestimate this risk because women not having early amniotomy are more likely to receive oxytocin, which also increases the odds of abnormal fetal heart rate patterns. Routine early amniotomy consistently increases the cesarean rate. When data from seven trials in which women were randomly assigned or not assigned to early amniotomy were analyzed (*meta-analysis*), women in the early-amniotomy group were 20 percent more likely to have a cesarean. An additional two studies not included in the meta-analysis also reported more cesareans in the early-amniotomy group. The percentage found in the meta-analysis may be low because caregivers in several trials were not able to stop doing amniotomies in the "conserve membranes" group. Specifically, half or more of women in the "conserve membranes" group in the two biggest trials had amniotomies, albeit somewhat later in labor. If amniotomy does, in fact, lead to C-section, this would tend to minimize the differences in cesarean rates between the two groups. Early amniotomy may also increase the risk of infection.

PROS AND CONS OF AMNIOTOMY FOR INDICATION

Pros: Rupturing membranes may help labor progress, allow closer monitoring when there is concern about the baby, and permit caregivers to determine whether the baby has passed meconium into the amniotic fluid.

Cons: Studies suggest that early amniotomy may not benefit slowly progressing labors and that late amniotomy may have unpredictable effects. Valerie El Halta, a prominent home birth midwife, suggests one reason why: If the baby is *posterior*—that is, facing the mother's belly instead of her back—labor often progresses slowly until the baby turns into the anterior position. With membrane rupture, the head may surge downward into the pelvis and get stuck. As for permitting closer monitoring for suspected fetal distress, releasing the amniotic fluid adds to the baby's stress by exposing the umbilical cord to compression during contractions. In addition, one potential cause of fetal distress is that the umbilical cord has slipped between the head and the cervix. Rupturing membranes could then cause prolapse.

AVOIDING AMNIOTOMY

AVOIDING ROUTINE AMNIOTOMY

Many caregivers consider amniotomy so trivial that they may not think to advise you that they are about to do one. For this reason, you must tell your caregiver that you do not want one done as a matter of course. Even so, your partner should pay attention when you have vaginal exams during labor. If a doctor or midwife plans an amniotomy, he or she will take an amnihook (described earlier) out of a long, slim paper tube. This is your cue to initiate a discussion. You should also know that internal electronic fetal monitoring, which uses an electrode that catches under the baby's scalp, requires an amniotomy if membranes have not yet broken.

AVOIDING AMNIOTOMY FOR INDICATION

The decision to perform an amniotomy should be made as part of a discussion with your caregiver in which you have the ultimate say-so. Under the doctrine of "informed consent," any time an intervention is suggested, you have the legal right to know what is being recommended—meaning that you must be told this in language you can understand—why it is being recommended, its potential problems and side effects, alternative ways to handle the problem, and the pros and cons of the alternatives, including doing nothing. Obviously you wouldn't take the time to go through this process in an emergency, but performing an amniotomy is never an emergency.

GLEANINGS FROM THE MEDICAL LITERATURE
(PAGES 250–253)

- Amniotomy shortens labor by only a modest amount and is a minor variable in determining the length of labor.
- Early amniotomy may not prevent or correct poor progress.
- Amniotomy can cause fetal heart rate patterns indicative of fetal distress.
- Amniotomy increases the risk of cesarean section, especially for fetal distress.
- Early amniotomy may increase the risk of maternal infection.
- Amniotomy may precipitate umbilical cord prolapse.

Chapter 7

~~~~~~

SLOW LABOR:
Patience Is a Virtue

Obstetricians treat women who are laboring slowly the way Peter Pan treated the Lost Boys. Peter expected everyone to adapt to his ideas of the way things should be. If they didn't, he saw to it that they did. For example, the boys entered the Neverland underground home through hollow trees. If a boy didn't fit his tree, James Barrie writes, Peter "did something" to the boy. So too with obstetric management. Obstetricians have inflexible ideas of how labor ought to go. If your labor doesn't conform to that pattern, typical doctors "do something" to you to make you fit. There are, as you may gather, a number of drawbacks to this myopic approach.

The first is that the standard for labor progress doesn't give you nearly enough time before you are declared over the line. Doctors base their standard on studies from the 1950s and 1960s, supposedly of normal labors—but many women had interventions that could shorten labor, such as oxytocin (trade name: Pitocin or "Pit") or forceps delivery. A recent study evaluating healthy women who had no interventions that would affect labor length got very different results. For example, the standard says that starting from 4 centimeters' cervical dilation, the average first-time mother will take 6 hours to achieve full dilation of 10 centimeters. Doctors set the cutoff defining "abnormal" progress in dilation at 12 hours for first-time mothers and 6 hours for women with previous births because, according to the standard-setting studies, only 5 percent of women will take longer than this. However, the new study found that average duration in first-time mothers was 7½ hours, not 6, the threshold for abnormal fell at 19½ hours, not 12, in first-time mothers and over 13½ hours, not 6, in women with prior births. The standard also stipulates smooth, linear progress. More than a relatively brief halt is thought to require action. However, averaging many labors together evens out the variations. Individual labors often don't work this way.

A second drawback is that obstetric management can obstruct progress. Epidural anesthesia is a notable example of this. Confinement to bed and pushing while lying on one's back may also interfere. Refraining from these things would seem obvious, but mainstream obstetricians rarely recognize their management as the problem. Within the obstetric mindset, all labor difficulties originate with the woman or her body. Doctors are always the "fixers," never the "breakers."

Finally, doctors have few ideas about what to do. They can rupture membranes, which is supposed to speed things up, although that is debatable (see page 250). They can strengthen contractions by giving IV oxytocin, or they can deliver the baby via vacuum extraction, forceps, or cesarean section. This limited repertoire has its own drawbacks.

To begin with, weak contractions are only one of several reasons why labor progress may be slow or come to what is in most cases a temporary halt. To cite three:

- The baby may be in the *occiput posterior* position, a hidden factor in as many as half of all cesareans for poor progress.

In the posterior position, the back of the baby's head (*occiput*) is toward the mother's back. During labor with a baby in the favorable anterior position, contractions push the rounded crown of the baby's head downward against the cervix, which helps open it. However, the posterior baby can't help because the cervix lies against the broad middle of the baby's head. (Think of it like trying to pull on a tight turtleneck sweater.) In addition, most posterior babies cannot fit through their mother's pelvis without swiveling to anterior.

- Sometimes in early labor the cervix, the neck-like opening of the womb, impedes progress. During pregnancy, the cervix's job is to keep the baby in against the pull of gravity. In preparation for labor and during early labor, the firm connective tissue in the cervix softens like a dry sponge absorbing water, shifts forward so as to be in line with the force of contractions, and *effaces*, meaning it draws up into the body of the uterus (see drawing on page 110). If the cervix has not finished this process, dilation will proceed slowly if at all.
- Fear, anxiety, and other psychological issues can also hold up labor.

If weak contractions aren't the problem, oxytocin isn't the answer. In addition, rupturing membranes, IV oxytocin, vacuum extraction, forceps delivery, and cesarean section can pose serious risks to baby or mother. These interventions should be the last, not the first—let alone the only—resorts, but, unlike most midwives, many doctors don't know any alternatives.

As a result of obstetric impatience and injudicious management, in 1995, about 1 in 5 U.S. women who began labor on their own had oxytocin stimulation, and nearly 176,000 women had cesareans for failure to progress, prolonged labor, dysfunctional labor, or *cephalopelvic disproportion* (the baby didn't fit). These diagnoses are all ways of saying the baby didn't come out within somebody's idea of a reasonable time, but "reasonable" is primarily a matter of philosophy, not physiology, as

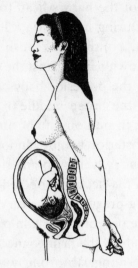 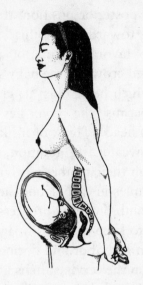

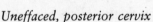

Uneffaced, posterior cervix   *Effaced, anterior cervix*

the enormous variation in cesarean rates among caregivers attests. As one editorialist all too aptly put it, "Unfortunately, we have spent the last 25 years managing labor *without knowing what we do.*"

ACTIVE MANAGEMENT OF LABOR

DOCTORS THINK THEY have at last found a way to make labor adhere to their pattern. In recent years active management of labor has swept the English-speaking obstetric world. From the obstetric viewpoint, it has everything to recommend it. Its rigid, precise protocol sounds reassuringly scientific. It is supposed to eliminate cesareans for poor progress even in the face of epidurals, which slow labor down. And best of all, it allows doctors to orchestrate every contraction. However, nothing about active management is as it seems except the control.

Active management of labor came out of the Dublin, Ireland,

National Maternity Hospital in the 1970s. According to its developers, it was intended to benefit first-time mothers by preventing prolonged labor. Obstetricians guaranteed that women would not labor for more than twelve hours, that is, ten hours to dilate and two to push out the baby—this being the maximal labor length they thought women could tolerate without pain medication. (They never asked women what they thought, though. Several studies have shown that women don't like oxytocin because it makes contractions hurt more.) Whatever the Dublin doctors believed their reasons for active management were, their book, *Active Management of Labor,* reveals who active management really benefits: It spares *obstetricians* the "tedious hours" of waiting until full cervical dilation, and it transforms "the previously haphazard approach" to planning for staffing.

Active management attracted attention outside Ireland because in an era where cesarean rates in many countries—including the United States—were skyrocketing, the National Maternity Hospital cesarean rate remained stable at about 5 percent without any apparent disadvantage in maternal and newborn outcomes. Active management was not responsible, however. The cesarean rate was even lower before its introduction.

The cornerstone of active management is to rupture membranes once labor is established and give IV oxytocin to any first-time mother who fails to dilate at 1 centimeter or more per hour. It begins at dosages considerably above blood levels produced naturally and ends with dosages that are twice the amount that are permitted in protocols that attempt to mimic normal oxytocin levels. The active-management oxytocin regimen may seem scientifically precise, but it was not based on any experimental data, and its rationales had nothing to do with science. For example, the Dublin doctors linked the drip rate strictly to contraction frequency to prevent soft-hearted midwives from turning down the drip rate when women complained of the pain. Indeed, the doctors of the National Maternity Hospital state in their book that the laboring woman's job in this scheme of "military efficiency" with a "human face" is to take orders and not to disturb the labor unit by making "the degrading scenes that occasionally result from the failure of a woman to fulfill her part of the contract."

Does active management work? Yes and no. It does tend to shorten labor compared with lower-dose oxytocin regimens, and a few studies have shown that it reduces the cesarean rate, although others do not. All this means, though, is that if more women can be forced to fit their doctors' unrealistic expectations of labor duration—forced to "fit their Neverland tree," so to speak—their doctors may operate less often.

Also, some of the components that almost certainly contribute to reducing the odds of cesarean for poor progress didn't make the transatlantic crossing. The Dublin protocol mandates a trained woman who never leaves the laboring woman's side. A body of research attests to the benefits of this practice. According to the protocol, women will not be admitted to the labor unit unless they are in progressive labor with effaced cervixes. By contrast, U.S. hospitals frequently admit women who are in very early labor or are having prelabor contractions.* Because progress is normally slow in early labor and nil if the mother isn't in labor, early admission plus impatience often equal unnecessary intervention. As originally conceived, active management assumed a minimal use of epidurals. The Dublin obstetricians believed that the promise of a twelve-hour-or-less labor length would enable women to get through labor without pain medication. Epidurals increase the cesarean rate for poor progress even when doctors practice active management.

---

*Penny Simkin, noted educator and author, uses "prelabor contractions" instead of "false labor" because there is nothing false about these very real and sometimes painful contractions, and they do eventually lead to progressive labor.

Active management also has serious drawbacks. First-time mothers are given oxytocin if they don't steadily progress at the *average* rate—a rate that is probably an underestimate. At one stroke, deviation from the average has been defined as "abnormal." Studies have shown that with active management, 40 percent or more of first-time mothers will receive oxytocin. Telling nearly half of first-time mothers their bodies are incapable of birthing a baby without help could have significant psychological consequences. For example, the use of labor interventions, not surprisingly, links to postpartum depression. And high-dose oxytocin increases the chances of overly long, overly strong contractions, which, by depriving the baby of oxygen, can cause fetal distress and worse. Setting arbitrary time limits on the pushing phase of labor can also lead to unnecessary and potentially risky procedures. In a study of thirteen thousand labors at the Dublin National Maternity Hospital, the authors reported that three babies delivered by forceps for prolonged pushing phase died of forceps injuries. In this country, doctors generally don't use forceps unless the head is low enough to make forceps relatively safe. However, faced with a "time's up" situation, they would do a cesarean instead—not exactly an improvement!

The sad thing about these disadvantages is that active management isn't necessary. Numerous studies have demonstrated that other, less aggressive regimens work just as well. This, however, brings up the real question, which is, "Do you need universal amniotomy and liberal use of oxytocin at all?" All studies have compared active management with standard management. This is like comparing the frying pan to the fire. If active management does better—and it doesn't always—it's still the frying pan. Midwives, especially those attending births in freestanding birth centers and homes, have achieved equally low cesarean rates and equally good, if not better, maternal and newborn outcomes with much less use of oxytocin, instrumental delivery, or C-section. In fact, active management makes a good litmus test of whether a practitioner works from the obstetric or midwifery model. If your doctor or midwife thinks it's great, head for the door.

PROCEDURES

- *Rupturing membranes* (amniotomy). See page 103.
- *Oxytocin IV.* For details of the procedure, see page 60. There are several schools of thought behind the various oxytocin regimens for strengthening (*augmenting*) labor. Doctors began using IV oxytocin years before researchers had the technology to study its metabolic properties. Older regimens were based on uterine response: Start the drip slowly; turn it up every fifteen minutes or so until the mother had what seemed to be three adequate contractions in ten minutes (the average rate in normal, progressive labor); and turn the drip down if contractions got too strong, long, or close together. This is probably still the most common method in the United States today. Low-dose regimens evolved out of research that determined blood levels during functional labor, how long oxytocin took to metabolize, what dosage rate maintained a steady blood level of oxytocin, and how long it took to produce a maximal response when the dose was increased. Low-dose regimens attempt to imitate the natural process, the goal being to reduce the frequency of adverse effects by minimizing the amount of oxytocin used to bring contractions up to par. Proponents of high-dose regimens such as active management think that giving more oxytocin faster will reduce the number of augmentation failures. High-dose regimens start where low-dose regimens typically end. In addition, the interval for judging response and deciding whether to turn up the drip is much shorter than the time actually required for uterine muscle to fully respond.
- *Vacuum extraction.* The apparatus consists of a flexible plas-

tic cap attached to a handle, tubing, and a vacuum source. The doctor uses the vacuum to hold the cap to the baby's head. The doctor then pulls while the mother pushes. Vacuum extraction can be used to swivel the baby from facing the mother's stomach (*posterior*) or her side (*transverse*), which are unfavorable for birth, to facing her back (*anterior*).

- *Forceps delivery.* For safe forceps delivery, the head must be at least partially through the mother's pelvis. The doctor inserts the curved blades on either side of the baby's head, locks them together, and pulls. Forceps can also be used to turn the baby from posterior or transverse to anterior.
- *Cesarean section.* See page 21.

THE BOTTOM LINE

BENEFITS AND RISKS OF TECHNIQUES FOR COPING
WITH POOR PROGRESS

NONMEDICAL TECHNIQUES
These include activities such as pelvic rocking or walking, assuming positions such as all fours or squatting, eating and drinking, massage and acupressure, warm tub baths or showers, and talking.

Benefits: Studies suggest that activity and positioning can intensify contractions, bring the baby down, expand the pelvis,* and turn the baby to the favorable anterior position. Eating and drinking can help the mother avoid fatigue and dehydration, which may slow labor. Massage, acupressure, and warm tub baths or showers can ease pain and induce relaxation, which may enhance progress. Warm-water im-

---

*The hormones of pregnancy soften the joints of the normally rigid pelvis.

mersion has been called the "midwives' epidural." Talk can provide comfort, reassurance, and encouragement; relieve anxiety; and explore what psychological or emotional issues or adverse environmental elements might be affecting labor. Using these strategies as the primary approach avoids unnecessary use of oxytocin, instrumental delivery, and C-section along with their attendant risks.

Risks: A full squat may be inadvisable in women with varicose veins or knee joint problems. Women may develop a fever if submerged too deeply for too long in warm water, but this can be alleviated by lifting more of the body out of the water or getting out of the tub, and infection is *not* a risk with ruptured membranes. As an experiment using a starch-impregnated tampon and iodine in the water proved, bath water does not enter the vagina. Exploration of possible underlying psychological factors may lead a woman to think that slow progress results from not thinking the "right" thoughts, which could lead to self-blame. Contrary to common obstetric belief, eating and drinking in labor pose *no* risks.

NIPPLE STIMULATION

Benefits: Causes secretion of additional oxytocin. Unlike intravenous oxytocin, oxytocin naturally secreted within the brain elevates mood and has amnesiac properties. IV oxytocin cannot cross the blood-brain barrier. Avoids unnecessary use of oxytocin, instrumental delivery, and C-section along with their attendant risks.

Risks: May produce overly long, overly strong contractions. Stopping or reducing the stimulation will rapidly normalize contractions.

AMNIOTOMY
See page 103.

IV OXYTOCIN

Benefits: Strengthens contractions by increasing circulating oxytocin levels. May avoid the need for instrumental delivery or C-section.

Risks: Increases pain. Especially when given in high-dose regimens, oxytocin can produce overly long, overly strong contractions and abnormally high resting uterine-muscle tension, which may deprive the baby of sufficient oxygen. If this is not addressed, it may result in fetal distress (abnormal heart rate patterns), brain damage, or death. Treatments include reducing or turning off the drip, giving medication to suppress contractions (*tocolytics*), or, if distress continues unabated, cesarean section. With prolonged use, oxytocin increases the risk of postpartum hemorrhage. It may also increase the risk of newborn jaundice. The authors of a recent review of research into oxytocin commented, "If oxytocin had been discovered in the 1990s we would not sanction its widespread routine use and would conduct further clinical trials."

VACUUM EXTRACTION

Benefits: Adds to maternal pushing efforts and can be used to turn the baby from posterior to anterior. Less likely to injure maternal tissues than forceps and may avoid the need for C-section.

Risks: Doctors may be more likely to perform an episiotomy, although it is not necessary for this procedure. Episiotomy introduces several risks (see page 155). The vacuum cup may cut the baby's scalp, although plastic cups are less likely to do this. Vacuum extraction can cause a blood-filled swelling (*cephalohematoma*) beneath the cup, which increases the likelihood of developing jaundice. Occasionally, profuse bleeding occurs beneath the scalp (*subgaleal* or *subaponeurotic* hemorrhage). Unlike the relatively benign cephalohematoma, this bleeding poses a grave risk. Bleeding within the brain is another rare, serious complication. The growing number of reports on serious complications and deaths resulting from vacuum extractions has caused the FDA to issue a warning advisory about this procedure.

FORCEPS DELIVERY

Benefits: Delivers the baby when the mother cannot accomplish the birth on her own. Forceps can also be used to turn the baby into the favorable anterior position. May avoid the need for C-section.

Risks: As typically practiced in the United States, forceps poses little risk of life-threatening injury to the baby. However, the baby's face may be cut or bruised, the collarbone may be broken, or there may be injury, usually temporary, to a nerve complex that controls the arm (*brachial plexus injury* or *Erb's palsy*) or to the nerve that controls the facial muscles. Forceps sometimes also cause cephalohematomas. Forceps delivery increases the risk of *shoulder dystocia* (the shoulders hang up during the birth), which can be life-threatening, but is almost always resolved without incident. Using forceps to rotate the baby 90 degrees or more can cause spinal cord injury. Doctors will almost certainly perform an episiotomy, although it is not always needed, which introduces several maternal risks. Forceps delivery with episiotomy greatly increases the risk of anal tears, which, even though repaired, may permanently weaken the anal sphincter. The forceps may also cut or bruise the vaginal wall. For these reasons, forceps also increase the probability of severe pain in the days after birth.

CESAREAN SECTION

Benefits: Delivers the baby when no lesser means will serve and the baby will be endangered by continuing labor.

Risks: While relatively safe as major surgeries go, cesarean section poses considerable short-term and long-term risks to the mother and to any future pregnancies.

STRATEGIES TO AVOID THE NEED FOR IV OXYTOCIN, INSTRUMENTAL DELIVERY, OR CESAREAN SECTION

- *Have a patient caregiver who sees his or her role as attending your birth, not delivering your baby.* Sheila Kitzinger, world-famous British author and founder of Britain's National Childbirth Trust, says that the most invasive and potentially dangerous technology—because from it proceeds all others— is the clock.
- *Have your baby at a freestanding birth center or at home.* Oxytocin-use rates and instrumental and cesarean delivery rates are much lower for out-of-hospital births.
- *Hire a professional labor support person.* She will know non-medical techniques to help keep or get your labor back on track. She will also provide continuous support, encouragement, and reassurance to you and your partner.
- *Have confidence in yourself and your body.* Doctors tend to instill doubt. The fact that cesarean section is so common these days does the same: If you don't think you can birth your child, it may become a self-fulfilling prophecy.
- *Have realistic expectations of labor length and difficulty.* Impatience and frustration are your worst enemy. They can lead you to make choices you may regret.
- *Address emotional issues that may be problematic in labor.* For example, women who experienced sexual abuse in childhood or have prior traumatic birth experiences or have strong control issues may sometimes have difficulty surrendering to the labor. If this is true for you, consciousness of this can help you and those with you work out strategies to prevent

or cope with their potential effects on labor. Please, though, do *not* blame yourself if labor is slow and you can't "fix" it.

- *Avoid induction of labor.* See chapter 3.
- *Unless there are medical reasons to go to the hospital early in labor, stay home until labor becomes active.* If you aren't sure, during the day you can go into your caregiver's office to be checked, and at night, they can check you at the hospital. Don't stay, though, if not much is happening. Studies show that women who are admitted in prelabor or very early labor are more likely to have oxytocin, instrumental vaginal delivery, and C-sections.
- *Refuse a cesarean for poor progress prior to active-phase labor.* This means at least 3 to 4 centimeters' dilation if you have had children before and 4 to 5 centimeters' dilation if you haven't. Both the U.S. and Canadian obstetricians' professional organizations state that cesareans for this reason should not be done in early labor.
- *Avoid frequent vaginal exams, but when you have them, get information on more than just dilation.* Avoid frequent exams, because finding that there is little or no change in dilation can be intensely disappointing. Find out about the state of the cervix, how far down the baby is, and, if possible, the baby's position. You may be making important progress even though you are not dilating, and often, advances in these areas may be necessary before dilation continues.
- *In labor, stay active, change positions frequently, maintain liquid and calorie intake, use warm tub baths or showers, and avoid flat-on-the-back or nearly flat-on-the-back pushing positions.* These strategies promote good progress. You can bathe or shower with an IV, as it can be covered with plastic and taped. You can bathe with ruptured membranes.
- *Take steps to rotate a posterior baby.* Don't wait until you are dilated enough for someone to tell the baby's position by feeling her head vaginally. Assume a posterior baby if contractions are strong but produce little progress. None of these

recommendations will hurt if the baby isn't posterior. Activities such as climbing stairs, crawling, pelvic rocks, and hip swivels help jiggle the baby around. Assuming an all-fours position or an open lunge during the cervical dilation phase and all-fours or squatting during pushing uses gravity to swing the baby's back into your belly or the leverage of your legs to expand the pelvis. Likewise, the double-hip squeeze opens the pelvis. Assuming a knee-chest position in early labor (this may be too uncomfortable in active labor) disengages the head from the pelvis, and the dangle during pushing elongates the torso, both of which give the baby more room to come around (see page 122). Some midwives may offer to turn the baby manually early on during a vaginal exam. This will be painful but can transform the labor according to midwives who do it. However, there are no formal data on the efficacy or safety of this procedure.

- *Avoid epidural anesthesia.* Epidurals slow labor, cause persistent posterior babies, and increase the risk of cesarean for poor progress.

- *Nipple stimulation can intensify weak contractions and can avoid the need for IV oxytocin.* Stimulating the nipples causes the release of additional oxytocin. Stimulation can be manually, by electric breast pump, or via a TENS (transcutaneous electronic nerve stimulation) unit, a physical therapy device that painlessly delivers a low electric current through pads applied to the skin.

- *If you require oxytocin, make sure it is given a fair trial.* A study of a protocol mandating at least four hours of adequate contractions on oxytocin in women with arrested labor progress and longer if contractions could not be brought up to par achieved an 8 percent cesarean rate. This was despite nearly all woman having epidurals (epidurals slow labor). If, as is not uncommon, cesareans had been done after two hours on oxytocin with inadequate progress, the cesarean rate would have been 23 percent.

ROTATING A POSTERIOR BABY

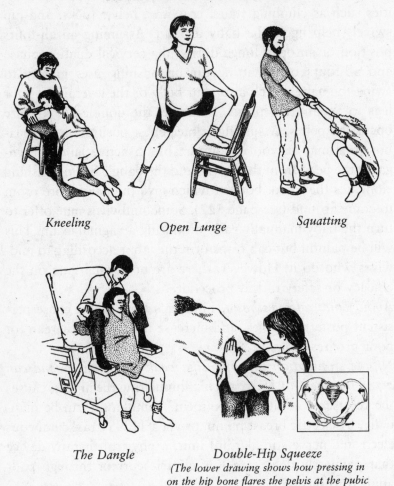

Kneeling   *Open Lunge*   *Squatting*

The Dangle   *Double-Hip Squeeze*
(The lower drawing shows how pressing in
on the hip bone flares the pelvis at the pubic
joint, making more room for the baby.)

- *Refuse an instrumental delivery or cesarean section recommended solely on an arbitrary time limit.* Both the Canadian and U.S. obstetricians' professional organizations state that there is no need to deliver the baby provided some progress is being made and the baby is doing well.

GLEANINGS FROM THE MEDICAL LITERATURE
(PAGES 254–261)

- Nonmedical factors often determine the diagnosis and treatment of slow labor.
- High-dose oxytocin regimens pose risks.
- Active management is at worst ineffective, and at best unnecessary.
- Active management does not eliminate the adverse effects of epidurals.
- Simple, noninvasive strategies may safely and effectively enhance labor progress during the dilation and pushing phases of labor as well as make for a more pleasant labor.
- Women admitted to the hospital in early labor or prelabor may be more likely to have labor interventions.

Chapter 8

EPIDURALS AND NARCOTICS:
A SHOT IN THE DARK

IF YOU HAVE reached the point in pregnancy when labor looms even larger than you do, you have almost certainly considered pain relief medication for labor. Obstetric management offers only two options: injected narcotics and epidurals. While you can usually get a balanced picture of the trade-offs of narcotics, epidurals are another matter. Your friends, most mainstream medical caregivers, and even some childbirth educators will tell you that epidurals are anesthesia's gift to women and you would be crazy to go through labor without one. While epidurals are, as advertised, the Cadillac of anesthesia, I recommend looking under the hood before deciding to purchase. You should know what kind of trouble you may be buying before deciding to drive this particular model off the lot. The same goes for narcotics.

WHY YOU DON'T HEAR ABOUT THE
DOWNSIDE OF EPIDURALS

THERE ARE SEVERAL reasons why friends and medical caregivers don't tell you about the problems of epidurals or why, if you bring them up, medical caregivers often brush them aside. To begin with, your friends may not have experienced any side effects—or maybe they did, but no one told them their epidural was the culprit. I attended a labor some years ago where within five minutes of injecting the epidural medication, the baby's heart rate took a nose dive. When it didn't recover within a few minutes, the staff rushed my client off for an emergency cesarean. Everyone told my client that sometimes this happens even with healthy babies. "It was just one of those things," they said. But it wasn't. Epidurals can cause profound, prolonged drops in babies' heart rates.

Your medical caregivers have likely been silent for one or a combination of the following reasons: mindset, money, or ignorance. First, many anesthesiologists, doctors, nurses, and even some midwives tend to live in a black-and-white world. They believe that labor pain has no value, mastering labor pain has no value, epidurals have no defects. These beliefs color perception in ways that are obvious to those who don't share them but invisible to those who do. For example, two studies that concluded that epidurals significantly increased the likelihood of having a cesarean for poor progress went on to say that this was acceptable because epidurals are so good at relieving pain. Recovering from a cesarean doesn't hurt? Another article recommended epidurals for high-risk babies on the theory that the mother's stress reaction to pain can reduce blood supply to the placenta and further increase the baby's risk. The same article stated that a fall in maternal blood pressure is the most common epidural side effect, and a high-risk baby may not be able to tolerate even a modest drop.

The belief that epidurals protect babies from fetal distress, a belief not uncommon among anesthesiologists and obstetricians, typifies how a mindset works. There isn't a shred of evidence to support it. I have never seen a study where babies whose mothers had epidurals were less likely to experience fetal distress. In fact, the reverse is true. But those who think that labor pain is bad and epidurals are good don't need evidence. All that is required is that the theory fits beliefs, and this one does. It even carries a bonus, lifting epidurals out of the realm of personal choice and providing a rationale for advocacy: "Well, you can choose to martyr yourself, but think about your baby."

Differing definitions of safety also play a part. Doctors often feel unconcerned about side effects—even life-threatening side effects—provided they know what they will do to treat them and that the life-threatening ones occur reasonably rarely. So, two doctors writing for their colleagues can say reassuringly: "These [epidural] complications should not cause fatalities if trained personnel and adequate resuscitation facilities are available." Loose translation: If a laboring woman develops a life-threatening complication from an epidural, she or her baby won't die of it provided hospital staff are on the ball.

Medical professionals can hardly be blamed for their attitudes. As I explained in the Introduction, these attitudes arise from deep-seated beliefs that go to the heart of what our culture believes about women, labor, pain in general, labor pain in particular, medicine, and technology. Unfortunately, they can lead to an astonishing amount of denial. The American Society of Anesthesiologists put out a 1995 press release recommending that women have epidurals because a study showed they reduced stress and anxiety in husbands. Consider their nonchalance in the face of what *A Guide to Effective Care in Pregnancy and Childbirth,* also published in 1995, has to say about epidurals. It begins, "Well-established complications include . . ." and goes on to list low blood pressure with associated nausea and vomiting, prolonged labor, and increased use of forceps, vacuum extraction, and cesarean section. Rare complications, it continues, include nerve damage, toxic drug reactions, breathing difficulties, and maternal death. "Possible, but as yet unproven complications" include problems with urinating, chronic headache, long-term backache, and numbness.

The second reason caregivers may be silent about the dark side of epidurals is that they generate big bucks for anesthesiologists and hospitals. Epidural charges range from $500 to $2500. A hospital consultant explained to me that hospitals have to maintain staff anesthesiologists around the clock to handle obstetric emergencies. In order for these doctors to make what they consider an adequate income, the hospital has to maintain something like an 80 percent epidural rate. Given this, how strongly do you think medical staff would resist the notion that epidurals are not always a good thing and most women can cope without them?

Consider the brochure put out by the American Society of Anesthesiologists entitled, "Anesthesia & You . . . Planning Your Childbirth." It never lies outright, but it skates circles around the truth. Among its evasions, obfuscations, and inversions is the statement that epidural anesthesia "can be safe." The brochure was published in 1992, the same year the authors of a review of the medical literature were dismayed to find only nine reasonably well-designed studies of epidurals conducted over a twenty-year period. The studies totaled less than six hundred women and documented serious complications. The authors concluded that remarkably little was known about the short-term and long-term effects of epidurals.

Finally, caregivers themselves may be misinformed, generally because they are passing on what they have been told. Nurses are particularly prone to this because they tend to get their information about epidurals from obstetricians and, of course, anesthesiologists.

Even your childbirth educator may not tell you about the risks. This may be because she doesn't know them or possibly because she has been gagged. I keep meeting hospital educators who have been forbidden to discuss epidurals in class. Anesthesiologists and obstetricians, they were told, would take care of telling women all they needed to know. In a couple of cases the stated reason was that listing the drawbacks of epidurals might give women second thoughts about having one. In fact, an article in *Ob. Gyn. News* about the 1998 annual meeting of the Society for Obstetric Anesthesia and Perinatology reports that speakers explicitly expressed concern that controversy around the safety of epidurals might scare women away. They blamed "biased" studies for "misleading patients" and childbirth educators for making data from those studies available to their couples. ("Biased," in this case, meant any study concluding that epidurals could cause problems.)

So, for a lot of reasons, you probably won't get objective information about epidurals from the people you would ordinarily trust to give it to you. I will try to give you a more balanced picture of epidurals (and narcotics as well). As with any other medical intervention, such as cesarean sections or IVs, epidurals and narcotics have their place. Certainly, though, the wise woman will not make the decision to have pain medication lightly, because when it comes to pain medication—and especially when it comes to epidurals—there is no free lunch.

THE EPIDURAL PROCEDURE

To prepare you for an epidural, nurses will start an IV and run in about a quart of fluid in an attempt to prevent a fall in blood pressure. They will attach electronic fetal monitor belts in order to pick up any epidural-caused problems with the baby's heart rate. They also place a blood pressure cuff so that your blood pressure can be closely monitored. In some hospitals the cuff periodically inflates and records your pulse and blood pressure automatically. Finally, you will be asked to either sit

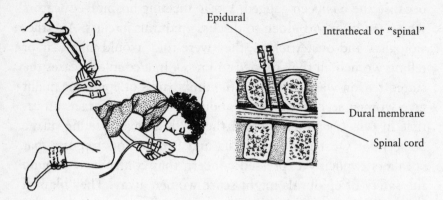

Injection sites

up on the side of the bed or lie on your side while your back
is washed with antiseptic and covered with a sterile drape.

For the actual procedure, you will be asked to arch your back
like a "mad cat" or a rainbow. The anesthesiologist will numb
the skin with local anesthetic and then will push a large needle
between two of the spinal vertebrae a little above the level of
your waist. You must hold absolutely still while the needle is
in your back even if you have a contraction, and you will probably have one or two before this part of the procedure is over.
The anesthesiologist will guide the needle in slowly and carefully, feeling for the loss of resistance that indicates that the
needle is in the epidural space. An epidural is placed outward
of the two membranes that cover the spinal cord (see drawings,
above). The anesthesiologist will perform one or more tests to
check that the needle has neither pierced a blood vessel nor gone
below the epidural space, which can cause life-threatening complications. These precautions may include pulling back on the
plunger of the syringe to see if blood flows in, injecting a small
dose of anesthetic and asking if you experience certain symptoms such as a bitter taste, or injecting a dose of adrenaline
(epinephrine), which is supposed to warn that the needle is in
a blood vessel by increasing the pulse rate. If all seems well, the

anesthesiologist will thread a tiny flexible plastic catheter through the needle and withdraw the needle. Then he or she will inject the full dose of anesthetic, and the catheter will be looped and taped to your back to keep it from shifting position. None of these precautions is fail-safe.

The anesthesiologist will evaluate the quality of anesthesia. If it is inadequate, you may be asked to shift position to redistribute the dose, or the anesthesiologist may inject more. The anesthesiologist will also test the extent of the anesthetized area with pinpricks or ice, which, as with the test dose, may warn that the anesthetic has been delivered into the wrong space.

In order to maintain anesthesia, the anesthesiologist may connect the catheter to a syringe and place the syringe in a pump that slowly depresses the plunger (*continuous infusion*). This delivers a continuous dose. Alternatively, the anesthesiologist may cap the catheter and return to inject more anesthetic (*periodic top-ups*) when you complain of returning pain.

Ideally you will feel no pain but will have some control over your legs. However, about 5 to 10 percent of women will experience "windows" of no anesthesia, or the anesthetic will not take on one side despite the anesthesiologist's best efforts. Anesthesiologists may reduce the anesthetic concentration when you approach full cervical dilation so that again, ideally, you remain comfortable but have enough sensation to push effectively.

The procedure can easily take close to an hour if you start from inserting the IV and end when the anesthetic has taken full effect. It can take much longer if the anesthesiologist is not readily available when you request an epidural. The period during which you must hold still generally lasts five to ten minutes.

Most centers use bupivacaine (trade name: Marcaine), but some use lidocaine (trade name: Xylocaine). Anesthesiologists vary considerably as to the amount and concentration of anesthetic they use, but the trend is to use lighter doses in an attempt to minimize side effects. At many hospitals, anesthesiologists have reduced the anesthetic concentration and added a narcotic (*narcotic epidural*). Some anesthesiologists perform a *combined spinal-epidural*. The anesthesiologist injects an initial dose of anesthetic or narcotic beneath the outermost membrane covering the spinal cord (see drawing, page 130) and inward of the epidural space (*intrathecally*). He or she then threads a catheter through the needle and withdraws the needle, leaving the catheter in the epidural space.

THE BOTTOM LINE

WHAT AN EPIDURAL DOES

An epidural stops pain by injecting an anesthetic of the same type that dentists use. An epidural also interferes with the ability to move your legs and with certain functions of the autonomic nervous system such as sweating.

THE TRADE-OFFS OF EPIDURALS

Pros: Epidurals almost always completely eliminate pain while leaving you awake and alert. This allows you to rest or sleep. In a difficult labor, epidurals can transform what otherwise would be a harrowing experience into a positive one. In some cases, epidurals seem to promote progress in labors that have gotten "stuck."

Cons: Epidurals slow labor, which results in increased use of IV oxytocin (trade name: Pitocin or "Pit") to stimulate stronger contractions, and usually leads to higher episiotomy rates, forceps or vacuum-extraction rates, and cesarean rates, especially in first-time mothers. Epidurals require electronic fetal monitoring and a precautionary IV. You are also more likely to need bladder catheterization.

Body temperature rises over time, so you are more likely to develop a fever.

These procedures, problems, and cures have secondary consequences. Electronic fetal monitoring increases the odds of cesarean section. IVs, especially when given in large amounts over a short time, as they are when administering an epidural, can cause fluid overload. Fluid overload leads to fluid in mother's and baby's lungs, maternal anemia, and blood chemistry disturbances in mother and baby. Bladder catheterizations can cause urinary tract infections. Oxytocin can lead to overly forceful contractions and fetal distress. Forceps delivery and episiotomy increase the probability of anal tears, which can have long-term effects on sexual satisfaction and fecal continence. Cesarean section has both short- and long-term risks. Maternal fever may stress the baby during labor. And because fever may signal uterine infection, the baby is more likely to be separated from you after birth for observation and subjected to blood tests, a spinal tap, and other diagnostic procedures to rule out this alarming possibility. Some data suggest that epidurals increase the probability of actual infection in the baby.

The procedure itself, apart from the drugs involved, can cause problems. An epinephrine test dose can cause fetal distress. Using air to locate the epidural space can cause neurological and other complications. The catheter can injure blood vessels and irritate nerves.

Potential postpartum complications include temporary urinary incontinence, nerve injury causing temporary muscle weakness or abnormal sensation, a blood-filled swelling (*hematoma*), and an excruciating, incapacitating headache (*spinal headache*), which can last for days. In the newborn, epidurals may cause adverse physical and behavioral effects.

Epidurals also cause potentially life-threatening complications. Some women will experience a considerable drop in blood pressure, despite the IV fluid given to prevent it. This may endanger the baby if it is not promptly recognized and countermeasures taken, up to and including an emergency cesarean section if lesser measures fail. Although the anesthetic is delivered into the cerebrospinal fluid and not the bloodstream, it readily passes into maternal blood vessels and crosses the placenta into the baby's circulation. Here, it may act directly to slow the fetal heart, which again may endanger the baby depending on the degree of the effect and whether it is recognized and promptly treated. If the needle or catheter pierces a blood vessel, which is easy to do in pregnancy because blood vessels are enlarged, or the needle goes deeper than the epidural space, or the catheter migrates inward, convulsions, respiratory paralysis, and/or cardiac arrest can occur. These latter two complications have been reported to occur as commonly as 1 in 3,000 cases. To give you some perspective, drugs causing serious adverse reactions in this range have been withdrawn from the market or forced into restricted use. Allergic shock is also a possibility. On rare occasions, women have died from epidural anesthesia. Doctors take precautions to prevent these complications, but they still occur.

Epidurals have adverse psychological effects as well. By the time you are hooked up to an IV, an oxytocin delivery pump, a fetal monitor, an automated blood pressure cuff, an epidural pump, and have a bladder catheter, what was a perfectly normal labor has been transformed into a high-tech event. This has profound consequences for how you view yourself and your labor and how your partner, other support people, and medical caregivers perceive you and your labor as well.

Recent innovations in technique have not reduced the incidence of problems, including lowering the anesthetic concentration (*low-dose epidural*), using a pump to provide continuous anesthetic, replacing some of the anesthetic with narcotic (*narcotic epidural*), and using a combined spinal-epidural technique. Moreover, combined spinal epidurals markedly increase the odds of spinal headache; spinally and epidurally injected narcotics cause nausea and itching; and spinally injected narcotics can cause life-threatening episodes of respiratory depression.

WHAT AN INJECTED NARCOTIC DOES

Nurses inject narcotics into your hip muscle or into a port on the IV tube, which delivers the medication into a vein. Narcotics dull, but don't abolish, pain. They can also make you feel drowsy or drunk. In the doses given today, they won't usually put you out unless you are very tired. The drugs work because they are chemically similar to endorphins, the body's own natural pain relievers. The medication takes effect almost instantly when it goes into a vein, but it doesn't last as long as when injected into a muscle.

Narcotics in common use include Nubain, butorphanol (trade name: Stadol), and fentanyl (trade name: Sublimaze). Unlike Demerol of old, the newer narcotics last only an hour or two, which is good because the baby is less likely to be born before you metabolize them. A study comparing Stadol and fentanyl concluded that Stadol gave better pain relief. This agrees with my observations of my labor support clients.

THE TRADE-OFFS OF INJECTED NARCOTICS

Pros: Compared with epidurals, injected narcotics don't involve a needle in the back or tie you up to monitoring equipment, an IV, or a bladder catheter. The delay between asking for pain relief and getting it is brief. Narcotics don't slow labor or interfere with pushing. They allow you to experience labor and feel in control of your body. Narcotics can be especially helpful in back labors where there is pain in between contractions because they will eliminate this pain and give you a break. You may get better pain relief than with nonmedication strategies, but the difference is smaller than you might think.

Cons: Narcotics depress your breathing. This is not a problem for you, but it could be for your baby in situations where the baby is already having difficulties. Narcotics adversely affect fetal heart rate (see page 96), and babies are more likely to be born with low blood pH, an indicator of inadequate oxygenation. Babies whose mothers have narcotics can have trouble breathing. If this happens, doctors will inject a drug that counteracts the narcotic and provide temporary breathing support if necessary. Research shows that Demerol interferes with newborn behavior, including the ability to suckle. No one has studied the neurological effects of the newer narcotics. As far as drawbacks for you, narcotics can make you nauseated. This happens so commonly that they are often given along with an antinausea medication. Some women don't like the fuzzy-headed feeling. And, of course, narcotics don't eliminate pain.

THE TRADE-OFFS OF NATURAL CHILDBIRTH

In the interest of full disclosure, I am a proponent of natural childbirth. I think labor offers an unparalleled opportunity to discover inner resources, capacities, and strengths you never knew you possessed, and I know personally and from hearing from others that there can be great value in such an experience. However, I also understand that women bring to labor widely differing beliefs, goals, and past experiences. Many women do not want to pursue natural childbirth, and wanting a narcotic or an epidural says nothing about strength of character. Nor does it follow that women who want natural childbirth and change their minds in labor have somehow "failed." No one can predict how long or hard a labor will be, and everyone has a point at which they say "enough." Still, keep in mind that many hospitals are hostile to natural childbirth. Many women who desired natural childbirth end up with pain medication because they didn't get emotional support or practical help from hospital staff and sometimes, too, from their nearest-and-dearest who were too uncomfortable seeing their loved one's pain.

Pros: As for the virtues of avoiding drugs, in 1981 the author of a review of the medical literature on the neurologic effects of pain medication in labor on the newborn wrote, "All the widely used [pain relieving medications] pass to the baby so that it is rare today for the baby's progress of adaptation to extra-uterine life to begin without a drug being present in the bloodstream. When drugs are used as widely as this, it is reasonable to demand very high standards of safety. However, given our ignorance of the physiological and behavioral effects of these drugs, safety (or otherwise) is much more a matter of luck than judgment." With the proliferation of designer narcotics and the various permutations of drug combinations since that time, we know even less today.

Natural childbirth has positive effects too. The pain and stress of normal labor have value for both you and your baby. For you, nerves in the cervix, and later the pelvic floor muscles and vagina, transmit stretching sensations as well as pain. These stretch receptors signal the pituitary gland within the brain to secrete more oxytocin. Secreting more oxytocin intensifies the labor, causing further cervical dilation. Once the cervix is completely open and the head stretches the pelvic floor and vagina, surges of oxytocin create the urge to push. Because they numb the nerves, epidurals wipe out the positive feedback mechanism.

Pain guides you. Usually, the positions and activities you find most comfortable are also those that promote good labor progress or help shift the baby into the best position for birth.

Your body responds to labor pain by secreting adrenalines and endorphins. Adrenalines give you stamina. Endorphins relieve pain and elevate mood. They are responsible, for example, for "runner's high." By the time of the birth, endorphins are found at levels thirty times higher than in nonpregnant women, and levels can be twenty times higher in women with prolonged or difficult labors than in women with uncomplicated labors. The natural oxytocin secreted within the brain has mood-elevating and amnesiac properties too. (IV oxytocin does not because it cannot cross the blood-brain barrier.)

The normal pain and stress of labor also benefit your unborn baby. The stress hormones produced in response to labor trigger the final preparation of your baby's lungs to breathe air, mobilize glucose for energy, and, by shunting your baby's blood away from the limbs and to the brain and heart (exactly opposite of the effect in adults), protect your baby against lack of oxygen (*hypoxia*) during labor. Extreme anxiety or fear may, indeed, compromise the baby's oxygen supply, a point used in arguments for epidurals. However, according to one study, epidurals do not relieve emotional distress. This is probably because it often arises from the typical features of hospital birth— lack of privacy, discomforts and deprivations, painful and invasive procedures, and lack of emotional and physical support from caregivers—rather than from pain.

Nondrug pain management strategies also have advantages. They tend to promote labor progress rather than inhibit it, and unlike drugs, any adverse effects can instantly be reversed by discontinuing the technique. Natural childbirth strategies facilitate labor both physiologically and psychologically. They raise endorphin levels, whereas epidurals reduce them and narcotics substitute for them. You gain knowledge, skills, and self-confidence from learning and using nondrug techniques. Studies show that a key to a positive labor experience is mastery—a sense of control over events. With epidurals in particular, control is completely given over to medical staff. As sociologist Barbara Katz Rothman wrote, "[O]ne mother, awake, but unable to feel the birth because of an epidural block, said, 'It's like seeing a rabbit pulled out of a hat.' Being the hat is a far cry from being the magician."

Cons: Labor will hurt. Probably a lot. But whether this is negative is another matter. Pain and suffering differ, as anyone who engages in activities demanding strength and endurance can tell you. A laboring woman can be in a great deal of pain, yet feel loved and supported and exhilarated by the power of the creative forces flowing through her body and her ability to meet labor's challenges. Conversely, a woman with an epidural may experience no pain, yet feel intensely distressed because she feels ignored or helpless. Of course, pain and suffering may coincide, as many women who have labored would hasten to tell you. Still, the key seems to be who controls the pain medication decision. Pain becomes a drawback only when pain medication is being withheld or a woman is not getting the support and help she needs to master it.

You may also not hurt as long as you think. A childbirth educator used a father's detailed recording of his wife's contractions to calculate how much of the time she was actually in pain during a twenty-four-hour labor. All told, it amounted to 3½ hours, not all of which would have been spent in intense pain.

Moreover, labor pain differs from other severely painful experiences in ways that make coping with it easier. It is self-limiting, rarely lasting more than twenty-four hours. Contractions usually last no longer than a minute, are rhythmical in pattern, and the pain stops in between (back labor can be the exception).* This means that periods of pain are brief, you have breaks in which to recover, and you can predict and prepare for the next episode. Both individual contractions and the labor itself usually start off mildly, then grow stronger, which provides a chance to adapt. This makes labor like getting into a hot tub: If you jump in, it seems unbearably hot, but if you ease in, you can tolerate it. Finally, the pain and effort are gloriously rewarded, making labor more like running a marathon or climbing a mountain than experiencing an injury or illness.

STRATEGIES TO AVOID PAIN MEDICATION

- *Consider not having your baby in a hospital.* Few freestanding birth centers offer epidurals, and they are never used at home births. What the eye doesn't see, the heart doesn't grieve after. Many freestanding birth centers but few home birth practitioners offer narcotic injections.
- *Consider using a midwife or family practitioner.* Women attended by midwives or family practitioners are less likely to have epidurals because the philosophy of care differs, although individual caregivers may prove to be exceptions to

---

*Back labor is when you feel the contractions in your lower back. It is commonly caused by a baby in the posterior position, that is, head down but looking toward your belly instead of your back. In this position, the bony back of the baby's skull presses on your lower back, adding to the pain of contractions and sometimes causing pain between contractions as well.

the rule. In hospitals, at least, caregiver type doesn't seem to affect narcotic use.

- *Consider hiring a professional labor support companion or have a loving, supportive female relative or friend accompany you throughout labor.* Fewer women who are accompanied throughout labor by a caring woman have pain medication.

- *Learn nondrug methods of coping with labor pain.* These include warm baths or showers, massage, acupressure, application of heat or cold, structured breathing, visualization, hypnosis, transcutaneous electronic nerve stimulation (TENS), walking, and many others.

- *Request that nurses not suggest pain relief medication.* This should be at the top of your birth plan, and your partner should remind nurses at each change of shift. Telling a laboring woman that pain medication is available is like waving a box of doughnuts under the nose of someone on a diet. If you want it, you can always ask for it.

- *Preplan on sterile water injections to relieve intense back pain.* Midwives increasingly know about this option, but few doctors do. With this technique, a tiny amount of sterile water is injected just under the skin at four points on the lower back. The injections sting but then produce profound relief of back pain that lasts an hour or more. The procedure can be repeated, and there are no known adverse effects (see page 273).

- *Have a code word or phrase.* Most laboring women will reach a point where they doubt their ability to continue without pain medication. A code word or phrase can help your support team distinguish between "give me reassurance" or "come up with something else" and "get me pain medication."

- *Prearrange a set amount of time between requesting pain medication and calling the nurse.* This should be some reasonable amount of time—say, five contractions or thirty minutes—for your support people to try to make you more comfortable. One of three things will happen: Something you try will work, you will get over the hump, or you will still want pain medication, in which case you will know that you've used up your other options and can feel at peace with your decision to go ahead with medication.

- *Have a vaginal exam before going ahead with the medication.* Sometimes labor progresses rapidly, and a woman who found contractions unbearable because she thought she was still in early labor will be okay with them once she realizes she is more advanced than she thought she was. Especially with an epidural, it may take considerable time to locate the anesthesiologist and get set up. Some women have gotten an epidural just in time to prevent them from pushing effectively.

QUESTIONS TO ASK WHEN HELPING A LABORING WOMAN DECIDE WHETHER TO HAVE PAIN MEDICATION

This section is for those who will accompany and support you during labor. If you reach the "should I or shouldn't I?" point, the answers to these questions can help your labor support team guide you to a decision you will be happy with long-term.

- *How strongly did she feel before labor about avoiding pain medication?* The stronger she felt about avoiding pain medication, the stronger your efforts should be to discourage her and vice versa.
- *Do events in her past make natural childbirth more problematic?* For example, for some women who had a prior traumatic labor or who have a history of physical or sexual abuse, the knowledge that an epidural is available on request may be the thing that makes labor possible.
- *How far dilated is she?* Epidurals should be discouraged in

early labor because they greatly increase the odds of cesarean, and late in labor because the hardest part of labor is likely to be almost over, and epidurals interfere with pushing. Narcotics should be discouraged late in labor because they can cause respiratory depression in the baby.

- *How long has she been in labor?* A woman who got six hours' sleep before beginning labor and is progressing nicely differs from a woman who has taken two days to get to 4 centimeters' dilation.
- *Has she just had discouraging news?* Requesting pain medication may sometimes be part of an urge to throw in the towel—an urge that will soon pass.
- *What other pain-coping techniques have you tried?* Is your bag of tricks empty or can you still shake out a few more ideas?

STRATEGIES TO MINIMIZE THE RISKS AND SIDE EFFECTS OF AN EPIDURAL OR SPINAL-EPIDURAL

- *Make sure your hospital has the ability to perform an emergency cesarean and that trained staff and equipment are available to perform resuscitation of mother or baby at any time of day.* This will ensure optimum care in case you are one of the rare women who develops a life-threatening reaction. Many small community hospitals do not have this capability around the clock.
- *If you have an epidural and develop trouble breathing or you have a spinal narcotic and become very drowsy and nonresponsive, your partner should get medical help immediately.* In the first case, the epidural may be affecting your breathing muscles. In the second case, when a narcotic is the "spinal" part of the combined spinal-epidural, it can cause life-threatening respiratory depression on rare occasions.
- *Choose a doctor or midwife with a low cesarean rate.* Epi-

durals slow labor, but whether you have a cesarean as a result depends on your caregiver's philosophy.

- *Delay an epidural until 5 centimeters' dilation or later, especially if this is your first baby, your prior birth or births were cesarean sections, or labor progress is slow.* Women having their first baby who have an epidural are much more likely to have a cesarean for lack of progress, and the earlier in labor the epidural is given, the greater the odds. The risk is highest of all with an early epidural in a slowly progressing labor. Epidural anesthesia also increases the cesarean rate for poor progress in women who have given birth vaginally before, but the numbers are low because poor progress occurs so rarely in women with prior vaginal births. Finally, while I have no data specifically on women with prior cesareans, studies show that they tend to have labor patterns more like those of first-time mothers. If labor progress is slow, take measures to help enhance progress and rotate a posterior baby (head down, facing the mother's belly) into the favorable anterior position (facing her back) (see the drawing on page 122).

- *Stay off your back after having an epidural.* The research shows that epidurals inhibit fetal rotation from posterior to anterior. When you lie on your back, even semi-reclining, gravity keeps the baby from shifting to the favorable anterior position. Lie on your side or sit up instead, or if you have the strength and control of your legs, as you may with a low-dose epidural, try hands and knees, the optimal position for rotating a posterior baby, for a few contractions.

- *Keep cool by having someone fan or sponge you or by lowering the temperature in the room.* No guarantees, but it may help keep you from developing an epidural-caused fever and the consequent newborn diagnostic tests and treatments and separation from your baby while medical staff rule out infection.

- *Make sure you don't get into awkward positions and that*

you change positions from time to time. This is thought to be the reason why women with epidurals may be more likely to develop chronic backache after giving birth.

- *Refuse an instrumental delivery or cesarean section based solely on arbitrary time limits.*
- *Delay pushing until the head begins to show or you feel an urge to push.* Many noninterventionist practitioners believe this practice increases the number of spontaneous births. One small study found delaying pushing reduced forceps deliveries because it allowed more posterior babies to rotate. Another study found delaying pushing reduced the need for instrumental rotations, although this didn't significantly reduce the instrumental delivery rate overall.
- *Let the epidural wear off for pushing.* This is a last resort because it will be difficult to take back the pain of labor after being pain-free. Still, it can be done, and it is worth trying if the next stop is a cesarean. Letting the epidural wear off allows you to feel what you are doing when you push and also enables you to try helpful positions such as squatting.
- *If natural childbirth was your goal and you have had to abandon it, a review of the measures you tried, praise for what you accomplished, and sympathy for your disappointment can help you accept this change of plans in the most positive manner.* Opting for pain medication seems to cause more problems for women who have an epidural than for women who have a narcotic, probably because the labor experience doesn't change so much with a narcotic. Medical staff can unintentionally make things worse by making remarks like "Now we'll see some smiles again," or "Natural childbirth makes about as much sense as natural dentistry." They think they are helping women feel good about choosing to have an epidural, but the hidden message is that natural childbirth was not a worthwhile goal and you never should have tried it.

GLEANINGS FROM THE MEDICAL LITERATURE
(PAGES 264–273)

Note: Keep in mind as you review the studies that virtually all comparison women also had drugs (oxytocin, narcotics, a different type of epidural), procedures (IVs, rupture of membranes), or restrictions (confinement to bed, nothing by mouth) that could also affect labor progress, the baby's condition, and so on. Also keep in mind that every variation in epidural procedure and anesthetic dose and each of the various designer narcotics could affect mothers and babies differently, but *none* have undergone scrutiny before becoming widely used.

- Epidurals slow labor.
- Epidurals increase the use of oxytocin.
- Epidurals increase the likelihood of vaginal instrumental delivery.
- Epidurals can increase the likelihood of cesarean delivery, especially in first-time mothers.
- Having an epidural early in labor, when dilating slowly, or when the head is still high in the pelvis increases the risk of cesarean for poor progress, probably at least partly because epidurals inhibit rotation of the baby from posterior to anterior.
- Whether an epidural increases the odds of cesarean depends on the caregiver's philosophy.
- Epidurals cause complications, including life-threatening complications, even with experienced anesthetists using correct procedures and despite taking proper precautions.
- Epidurals cause fevers, increasing the likelihood that the baby will be kept in the nursery, subjected to diagnostic tests (septic workup), and given preventative intravenous antibiotic treatment.
- Epidurals may cause long-term, even chronic problems.

- Epidural anesthetics "get" to the baby, as does the narcotic component of narcotic epidurals.
- Far from protecting babies from fetal distress, epidurals can cause profound disturbances of the fetal heart rate.
- Epidurals may have adverse effects in the newborn.
- Lower dosages and newer techniques have not reduced the adverse effects of epidurals.
- Narcotics adversely affect the baby's oxygenation before birth, can cause breathing problems at birth, and interfere with early breastfeeding.
- Sterile water injections are a safe, effective means of relieving intense back pain.

Chapter 9

EPISIOTOMY:
The Unkindest Cut

In a branch of medicine rife with paradoxes, contradictions, inconsistencies, and illogic, episiotomy crowns them all. Routine episiotomy—snipping or cutting the *perineum,* the block of tissue between the bottom of the vagina and the anus, shortly before birth—is the quintessential example of an obstetric procedure that persists despite a complete lack of evidence for it and a huge body of evidence against it.

Here is what routine episiotomy is supposed to do for you. Obstetricians claim that episiotomies protect the muscles of your pelvic floor from tears during vaginal birth and prevent them from overstretching, which in turn is supposed to prevent urinary incontinence, vaginal or uterine prolapse, and loss of sexual sensation for both partners during intercourse. Obstetric lore says that by shortening the time period from full cervical dilation until birth, episiotomy prevents brain damage. Episiotomies are also supposed to be less painful, easier to repair, and heal better than spontaneous tears, or as doctors say, "a nice clean cut is better than a jagged tear."

Even before reviewing the data, anybody can see that the major reputed benefits are absurd on their face. How do you prevent injury to a muscle by cutting into it? Specifically, episiotomies are supposed to prevent deep tears into or through the anal sphincter muscles. Anyone who has ever snipped a piece of fabric in order to tear off a length knows that the *last* thing you would want to do if you wanted to prevent the perineum giving way is cut into it. As for the second so-called advantage, how do you prevent overstretching when episiotomy is not done until the baby's head is at the vaginal outlet (*crowning*), at which point, as one research reviewer observes, the pelvic floor is already at full stretch? And if episiotomy prevents urinary incontinence and vaginal and uterine prolapse, how come all the older women having repair surgery for these problems—and their name is legion—all had generous episiotomies? We know they did because until fairly recently, virtually every U.S. woman who gave birth vaginally in a hospital had one. Finally, the rationale behind shortening the second stage of labor is that it cuts short the time the baby's head spends "pounding on the perineum" and prevents damage from the accumulating effects of oxygen deprivation during pushing. The perineum is a hammock of soft stretchy muscle. "Pounding" on it is about as harmful as bouncing on a trampoline. And episiotomies aren't done until the very end. They couldn't possibly cut more than a few contractions off the labor.

The research fails to support any of the claims made for routine episiotomy. Going back as far as 1983, every review of the medical literature has concluded that episiotomies do not perform as advertised and that they introduce considerable risks.

First and foremost, episiotomies don't prevent deep tears; they cause them. Without exception, the medical literature shows that anal injuries almost never occur except as extensions of an episiotomy. This is a major problem because tears into or through the anal sphincter often have serious short- and long-term consequences.

Vaginal birth may lead to a certain amount of pelvic floor relaxation, but no one has shown that episiotomy prevents that or that episiotomy has any effect on urinary incontinence or genital prolapse. In fact, data suggest the opposite. Women with the strongest pelvic floors after childbirth are those with intact perineums.

As for the baby, no one has shown that routine episiotomy protects even the most fragile of premature babies from brain hemorrhage. How, then, could it help a healthy, full-term newborn? Trials in which women were randomly assigned to "perform episiotomy liberally" versus "restrict episiotomy" groups also show that full-term newborns are none the worse for wear when born without episiotomies.

Finally, episiotomies do not appear to be less painful or heal better than spontaneous tears. They are certainly more painful for women whose episiotomies extend into the anus! They are also certainly harder to repair in these cases. And, as one medical reviewer points out, even if the standard episiotomy is easier to repair—and we have no evidence that it is—"ease of repair" would be an acceptable reason for episiotomy only "if it were definitively shown not to harm the patient in the process." A glance at the "cons" of episiotomy that follow will show you that episiotomy fails that test.

It is also unclear to what extent obstetric practitioners cause some of the problems believed to be inevitable or frequent results of childbirth by the way they manage the pushing phase of labor and the birth itself. Obstetricians decided that shortening second-stage labor by performing an episiotomy was good because they observed that the longer the time women spent pushing, the worse the baby's condition at birth. No wonder. Lying flat on the back, the standard pushing position until recently—and probably still the standard in some hospitals—puts about ten pounds' worth of baby and uterus on top of the major maternal blood vessels serving the uterus and placenta. Add to that how women were—and still are—typically instructed to push. Studies show that the usual instructions to hold the breath and push "as long and hard as you can" and not to take more than a quick breath between pushes cause symptoms of fetal distress. Left to their own devices, women don't push like that. They grunt and groan, and when they hold their breaths, they hold it for no longer than six seconds. They usually take several breaths between pushes. Studies show that spontaneous pushing does not adversely affect the baby. It may take a little longer to push out the baby, but despite this, babies are born better oxygenated. Data also suggest that giving birth in an upright position, which is how women in every traditional culture do it, preserves the perineum from tears and reduces the need for episiotomy. As for birth overstretching the pelvic floor, nurses normally tell women to begin pushing at full cervical dilation whether they feel like it or not. Prolonged straining in defiance of the natural urge exhausts the mother and would seem to be a recipe for overstressing pelvic floor muscles and connective tissue.

WHY ARE DOCTORS STILL DOING ROUTINE EPISIOTOMIES?

LIKE ALL TRUE believers, obstetricians who believe in episiotomy don't let clear-cut evidence get in their way. Episiotomy fits with the obstetric premise that childbirth is a dangerous and difficult business and that the obstetrician's role is to rescue the baby from the clutches of its mother's untrustworthy body. It also fits with the obstetrician's role as a surgeon.

By contrast, midwives generally have lower episiotomy rates because they work from a model that trusts the natural process. Hospital-based midwives, however, may be infected with the obstetrical mindset. Midwives' episiotomy rates in some hospital studies rival those of doctors.

You can see obstetric beliefs at work in a large trial of midline episiotomy in which women were randomly assigned to liberal or restrictive use-of-episiotomy groups. The researchers found that some doctors couldn't stop doing episiotomies in the "restrictive" group even though they had agreed to try. Doctors who usually did episiotomies were more likely to exclude their patients from the study and to diagnose fetal distress and "impending tear" (although tears occur or not; they don't impend) in the ones they allowed in. When the researchers grouped doctors by their opinion of episiotomy and compared those holding a high opinion with those holding a low opinion, they found that doctors who viewed episiotomy favorably were also more likely to distrust labor and women's bodies in other respects. They stimulated more labors with oxytocin (trade name: Pitocin or "Pit"), delivered more women on their backs with legs in stirrups (*lithotomy* position), diagnosed fetal distress more frequently, and performed more cesarean sections.

Still, episiotomy is such an egregious example of the chasm between evidence and practice that the realization is slowly having an effect. In 1987 the U.S. episiotomy rate was 62 percent. As of 1993, it was 50 percent of all vaginal births. This is hardly cause for celebration, though. Excluding newborns, episiotomy was *the* most common surgical procedure performed in the United States in that year. In 1996, the episiotomy rate had declined to 43 percent. However, two literature reviews have recommended 20 percent and 30 percent as maximum rates, and noninterventionist practitioners commonly have rates under 20 percent.

Not long ago you could use episiotomy rates as a touchstone for practice philosophy. Nowadays, even some interventive doctors are abandoning routine episiotomy, which means that having a low episiotomy rate may or may not be good news, although a caregiver who does them routinely is definitely bad news. I would think twice about staying with a doctor or midwife who gives you any of the standard justifications for routine episiotomy, who tells you most first-time mothers need one, or whose episiotomy rate exceeds 30 percent, the higher of the

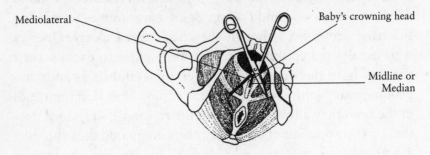

Mediolateral

Baby's crowning head

Midline or
Median

The Two Types of Episiotomy

recommended maximums. It is a clear and unequivocal sign that he or she does not practice evidence-based medicine.

WHAT IS AN EPISIOTOMY?

AN EPISIOTOMY IS a cut made at the base of the vaginal opening to enlarge it for birth. The cut may go straight down (*median* or *midline* episiotomy) or down and off to one side (*mediolateral* episiotomy) (see drawing above). Doctors and midwives in the United States and Canada usually perform midline episiotomies, although some caregivers may routinely do mediolateral episiotomies or do them under certain circumstances, such as for forceps deliveries. European practitioners prefer the mediolateral type. According to *Williams Obstetrics*, the classic obstetrics textbook, compared with mediolateral episiotomies, midline episiotomies are easier to repair, hurt less afterward, cause less blood loss, cause fewer complications during healing, give better anatomical results, and are less likely to cause pain during intercourse. However, midline episiotomies are much more likely to extend into or through the anal sphincter.

Perineal wounds, injuries to the block of tissue between the base of the vagina and the anus, are graded according to depth. *First-degree* injuries include the skin and connective tissue;

second-degree injuries go into the underlying perineal muscle; *third-degree* injuries extend into but not through the anal sphincter; and *fourth-degree* injuries go completely through the anal sphincter. Some researchers lump all anal injuries into third-degree injuries. An episiotomy makes a second-degree wound.

THE BOTTOM LINE

PROS AND CONS OF ROUTINE EPISIOTOMY

Pros: None.

Cons: Episiotomies increase the number of women with perineal injuries; cause considerable pain, sometimes for weeks or months; and increase blood loss. Because episiotomies predispose to tears into or through the anal sphincter, they increase the likelihood of developing stool incontinence in the short or long term, pain with intercourse, infection, wound breakdown, and the formation of openings between the vagina and the rectum (*rectovaginal fistulas*).

TRADITIONAL INDICATIONS FOR EPISIOTOMY

- *Fetal distress.* If the baby is in trouble, your doctor or midwife may not want to wait the few minutes it may take for the birth without an episiotomy.
- *Shoulder dystocia (the head is born, but the shoulders are hung up behind the pubic bone).* Because shoulder dystocia is not a soft-tissue problem, cutting the perineum will not relieve it, and shoulder dystocia can usually be resolved without maneuvers that require making room for the practitioner's hands. Nonetheless, shoulder dystocia is an emergency, so whether you have an episiotomy will probably not be up for debate.

- *Forceps delivery.* Several studies have shown that doing forceps deliveries without an episiotomy reduces the incidence of deep perineal tears. Not doing an episiotomy may increase the incidence of vaginal tears, but unlike tears involving the anus, vaginal tears do not seem to cause long-term complications.
- *Vacuum extraction.* Vacuum extractions don't require routine episiotomies any more than spontaneous births do.
- *Inelastic perineum.* The problem here is judgment. If your birth attendant has a low episiotomy rate—say 10 percent—you can trust his or her judgment, but if the rate is high—say 50 percent—you can't.
- *Maternal exhaustion.* This should be your call. Keep in mind, though, that you are only saving yourself a few contractions.

Strategies to Protect the Perineum

- *Have a caregiver with a low episiotomy rate.* Yes, you can refuse an episiotomy, but caregivers who routinely do episiotomies don't know how to prevent tears, and they tend to find excuses to do them.
- *Refuse routine episiotomy.* If you have a caregiver who you know does episiotomies routinely or you don't know the policy of the person who turns up at the birth, tell him or her that you don't want an episiotomy unless the baby is in trouble. Tell him or her that you accept the fact that you may tear. If you are dealing with someone who you don't think knows how to prevent tears, do what you can yourself— namely, relax your bottom, insist on having your legs no more than comfortably apart for the birth, and don't push forcefully as the head emerges. A recent trial shows that you may do just as well if your caregiver keeps hands off than if he or she uses techniques to protect the perineum.

Note: If your caregiver usually does episiotomies but seems open to change, recommend Thompson's "No Episiotomy?!" (see the chapter bibliography). The author, an obstetrician, describes his technique. Using it, he reduced his episiotomy rate from 78 percent to 7 percent and increased his intact perineum rate from 16 percent to 68 percent.

- *Do pelvic-floor contractions.* These are also known as "Kegels," after the doctor who first prescribed them as a treatment for urinary incontinence. Instructions for doing these contractions can be found in any pregnancy and childbirth "how-to" book. Exercising your pelvic floor will make it stronger and more elastic. Learning how to contract and release the muscles around the vagina will also help you consciously relax those muscles for the birth.

- *Engage in regular exercise.* Women who exercise regularly are less likely to have episiotomy extensions. Women whose lifestyle includes regular exercise recover stronger pelvic muscles after birth.

- *Do prenatal perineal massage.* Gentle stretching of the perineum in the last weeks of pregnancy reduces the odds of episiotomies and tears, provided that your caregiver doesn't usually do episiotomies. Women in the massage group were instructed as follows. Once a day for five to ten minutes, they or their partner should massage vegetable oil such as olive oil into the perineum and lower vaginal wall. Then they or their partner should massage using a U or "sling" movement, stretching just enough to produce a slight burning sensation. (The massager must have impeccably clean hands and short nails.)

- *Avoid an epidural.* Epidurals increase the odds of episiotomy, instrumental vaginal delivery, and of a baby that persists in the posterior position (facing your belly instead of your back).

- *If the baby is facing your belly (posterior) or directly to one side (transverse), try strategies to rotate him into the anterior position (facing your back).* Posterior babies associate with a higher incidence of perineal injury, probably because they increase the odds of episiotomy and instrumental delivery. (See page 120 for strategies.)

- *Push with the natural urges, breathing as your body directs you.* This should minimize the chance of becoming exhausted or developing fetal distress. Expect to have to fight off the troops on this one. Despite the complete lack of evidence for pushing on command or beginning to push at full dilation without an urge, most hospital staff members are convinced that no baby can be born without such pushing. You want to avoid confrontation, so your best bet is to explain that this is what you want to do, and if there is concern about the baby's condition or no progress in two hours, you will certainly be open to a change in pushing technique.

- *Give birth upright, or at least avoid giving birth in a position that stretches the legs wide apart.* If your perineum is already under tension, it has nowhere to go. Upright positions reduce the incidence of tears and the need for episiotomy and instrumental delivery.

- *Think in terms of breathing rather than pushing the baby out.* A slow, controlled birth of the head and shoulders allows tissues to fan out.

- *Don't allow injection of a local anesthetic into the perineum on a "just in case" basis.* The liquid swells the local tissues, reducing elasticity. Your partner should watch for the birth attendant picking up a syringe.

- *Refuse a forceps or vacuum extraction delivery recommended only because some arbitrary time limit has passed.* Both the Canadian and U.S. obstetricians' professional organizations state that as long as you are making progress and the baby is fine, there is no need to curtail labor. This is especially important if you have had an epidural.

- *If you must have an instrumental vaginal delivery, have a vacuum extraction rather than forceps delivery.* Studies show much less incidence of deep tears with vacuum extraction than with forceps. (Both procedures can cause trivial or major complications in the baby.)

- *Don't have an episiotomy with an instrumental delivery.* You reduce the odds of deep perineal tears.

While many midwives and doctors use one or more of these last three strategies to help avoid tears, we have little formal data and only one random-assignment trial on their effectiveness or possible adverse effects.

- *Apply warm compresses to the perineum.*
- *Apply oil and massage the perineum during the birth.*
- *Keep the head flexed and support the perineum as the head is born.* A random-assignment trial comparing routine versus selective use of these techniques resulted in similar outcomes in both groups.

GLEANINGS FROM THE MEDICAL LITERATURE (PAGES 276–282)

- Episiotomies don't prevent tears into or through the anal sphincter.
- Episiotomies don't prevent relaxation of the pelvic floor muscles, urinary incontinence, herniations of the bladder into the vagina (cystocele), or vaginal or uterine prolapse, or preserve sexual satisfaction during intercourse.
- Episiotomies don't prevent brain damage.
- Episiotomies don't cause less pain than do tears.
- Episiotomies don't appreciably shorten second-stage labor.
- Primarily, but not entirely because they predispose to anal tears, episiotomies increase the risk of infection, delayed healing, wound breakdown, the formation of an opening between

the vagina and the rectum (*rectovaginal fistula*), and gas or stool incontinence.

- Episiotomies increase blood loss.
- Forceps deliveries greatly increase the risk of tears into or through the anal sphincter compared with vacuum extractions.
- Selective episiotomy reduces perineal injury rates during instrumental vaginal deliveries.
- Breathing and pushing according to the mother's natural inclinations and giving birth in an upright position, or at least not on one's back or with legs spread wide apart, produces the best perineal and infant outcomes.
- Women who exercise regularly have stronger pelvic floors and appear less likely to have anal tears when they have episiotomies.

Chapter 10

⌒

ELECTIVE REPEAT CESAREAN:
JUST SAY NO

IF YOU HAVE had a cesarean section, you may be wondering why you wouldn't want another one for your next baby. Perhaps labor was prolonged and difficult, and having fallen off that horse, you have no desire to try riding again. Perhaps your surgical recovery was so smooth and rapid that cesarean section seems much simpler and easier and more convenient. Perhaps you think your chances of vaginal birth are so small that laboring again is pointless. You may even think that vaginal birth after cesarean (VBAC, pronounced "vee-back") is risky—or at least riskier than elective repeat cesarean. Unfortunately, typical obstetricians are all too ready to grant requests for C-section without giving you the information you need to make an informed decision, much less helping you overcome the psychological obstacles that may prevent you from making the best choice for you and your baby.

Frankly, VBAC should be a nonissue by now. You should no more be choosing whether to labor this time than you did before you had a cesarean. Based on two decades of studies to-

161

taling many thousands of women, the consensus of the experts—including the official guidelines of the American College of Obstetricians and Gynecologists (ACOG) and the Society of Obstetricians and Gynaecologists of Canada—is that in the absence of a specific reason for cesarean section, the routine policy for women with prior cesareans should be labor. (ACOG has recently backtracked on VBAC, but not for valid reasons, as I will explain shortly.)

VBAC has become the norm in other countries, but not in the United States. With nearly half a million U.S. women per year becoming pregnant after having a cesarean, such a policy would soon spare hundreds of thousands of women unnecessary major surgery and the risks that surgery entails. Yet while the VBAC rate is rising—it reached 28 percent in the United States in 1995—the most common reason for cesarean section remains that the woman has had one before.

SO WHY HASN'T VBAC BECOME ROUTINE?

NORTH AMERICAN OBSTETRICIANS have had to be dragged into doing VBACs. Research had produced rock-solid evidence that VBAC was safe and effective, and ACOG had begun recommending VBAC years before the annual VBAC rate in this country rose above single digits. Similarly, in Canada, a concerted effort to persuade obstetricians to follow their own professional organization's VBAC guidelines had only slight effect. What finally put on the pressure in this country was this: Not doing repeat cesarean sections is the quickest and simplest way of reducing the cesarean rate. Insurance companies and health maintenance organizations began refusing to pay for elective repeats. Hospital quality-control committees began insisting on VBACs. However, on the principle that you can always find a reason for not doing something you don't want to do, the next line of defense for reluctant obstetricians was to argue that it wasn't their fault. Women preferred repeat cesareans, and their preference should be respected. But as the evidence shows, patient preference has nothing to do with it.

A 1990 survey of ACOG members reported that over 90 percent of obstetricians "encouraged" VBAC, but over 40 percent of women refused. Several studies that looked at women's decision making concerning VBAC got similar results, but let's look closer. In these studies, negotiating with obstetricians *always* meant negotiating to have an elective cesarean, *never* a vaginal birth. The doctors who believed in "once a cesarean, always a cesarean" wouldn't negotiate. How much freedom of choice do you really have if all you can say is "yes" to a cesarean but never "no"? Women chose repeat cesarean for such reasons as wanting the convenience of scheduling the delivery, knowing what to expect, fearing the pain of labor, or believing that VBAC is riskier for women. The first three reasons are hardly indications for major abdominal surgery, and the last isn't true. VBAC is safer for the mother. How much accurate information—let alone encouragement—does this imply doctors are really giving women about VBAC?

Reluctant doctors like to believe that they haven't much influence over their patients, but that is clearly not the case. Several studies have found that when doctors genuinely encouraged women to have VBACs, most of them did, and when they said nothing or acted neutral, most women didn't. Finally, when obstetricians discouraged VBAC in women who wanted to try it, *none* of them did.

A study of interactions between women and obstetricians offers an explanation. It described three levels of increasing power imbalance: In the first, you fight and lose; in the second you don't fight because you know you can't win. However, in the highest level of power differential, your preferences are so manipulated that you act against your own interests, but you are content. Elective repeat cesarean exemplifies that highest level.

Doctors also find excuses not to do VBACs. Half of planned

repeat cesareans in one study were done for specious reasons such as high head or unfavorable cervix at term.

In recent years, pressure on obstetricians to do VBACs has resulted in a growing VBAC-lash. It began in 1996 with a study published in the prestigious *New England Journal of Medicine*. The study concluded that "major maternal complications" were twice as likely in women laboring compared with women having elective cesareans. VBAC opponents latched on to this as proving that VBAC was riskier than previously thought. However, preeminent VBAC researcher Dr. Bruce Flamm points out that the authors coded wound infections and hemorrhage requiring transfusion as "minor complications," both of which occurred more often in the planned cesarean group. If you classify these as major complications, the difference between the two groups disappears. Dr. Flamm adds that even without doing this, major complication rates were quite low—a bit less than 1 percent in the planned cesarean group, a bit more than 1 percent in the labor group—hardly unimpeachable evidence favoring planned cesarean.

That same year, news of malpractice suits—justified or not—over VBAC labors spread throughout the obstetric community. This led to the development of a so-called "informed consent" form for VBAC. It details all the horrible things that could potentially happen should the scar give way during a VBAC. But this form is not really about informed consent because it says nothing about all the equally horrible things that could potentially result from an elective cesarean. In fact, the obstetrician editor of *OBG Management,* who devised its prototype and promotes use of such forms, openly admits that the motivation behind them is forestalling lawsuits and that using them will "send your C/S rate soaring."

VBAC-lash culminated in ACOG's new VBAC guidelines, issued late in 1998. Taking a giant step backward, the new guidelines state, "It is reasonable for women to undergo a trial of labor in a safe setting, but the potential complications should be discussed thoroughly." The 1995 version said, "Neither repeat cesarean delivery nor a trial of labor is risk free," and "VBAC is not associated with an increase in maternal and perinatal morbidity and mortality rates." The new wording substitutes a one-sentence acknowledgement that vaginal birth has fewer complications than repeat cesarean followed by two paragraphs dwelling on the risks of VBAC. Nothing is said about the hazards of repeat cesareans. Gone too are statements that trial of labor in women suspected of carrying large babies or who have more than one prior cesarean "should not be discouraged." These factors have been relegated to the "iffy" category. Postdates pregnancies have been added to that same category. New on the list of reasons not to allow VBAC is "Inability to perform immediate emergency cesarean delivery because of unavailable surgeon, anesthesia, sufficient staff, or facility." Now while I will argue in chapter 13 that this capacity is the only reason for a healthy woman to have her baby in a hospital and recommend that VBAC moms choose such a facility, this caveat tells you that obstetricians are thinking about their welfare—not yours. The general population has about the same potential for an emergency in labor as the potential for the uterine scar giving way. If it isn't safe for VBAC labors in hospitals that cannot meet these criteria, then it isn't safe for anyone to labor there.

Based on ACOG's new guidelines, the only women having VBACs in future will be women no more than a week past their due dates, carrying average-weight babies, whose previous cesarean was for some reason other than lack of progress, who have no more than one prior cesarean, and who plan to have their babies at a major medical center with an obstetric residency program and in-house anesthesia. They will also have to demand a VBAC and persist in that demand in the face of consent forms that detail the risks of VBAC but say little about the risks of cesareans. Few women will fit through that narrow doorway.

Most recently, VBAC-lash has taken an uglier turn. The 1998 VBAC guidelines and a 1999 *New England Journal of Medicine* editorial widely reported in the popular press position obstetricians as defenders of maternal and child health and safety and protectors of a woman's right to make medical decisions with her physician and without outside pressure, which in this case means her right to choose a cesarean. They imply that the only proponents of VBAC are government agencies, HMOs, and the like, whose sole interest in promoting VBAC is to save money. That the "right" to elective cesarean is the only instance in which obstetricians have ever championed a woman's right to determine any aspect of her care should raise extreme suspicion of the motive. And to impugn the well-established safety and effectiveness of VBAC at reducing unnecessary cesareans is, to say the least, disingenuous.

Let me call a spade a spade. The VBAC-lash is a particularly glaring instance of doctors abandoning their duty to their patients and opting to look out for themselves at their patients' expense. Worse yet, they are putting the onus on their victims in the bargain. The VBAC debate is not about the safety of VBAC versus elective repeat cesarean or about whether VBAC works. Those points have been established. And it isn't about women's rights to determine their care, although I think many doctors honestly believe it is. It is about doctors ducking their professional responsibilities and leaving women holding the bag.

THE BOTTOM LINE

PROS AND CONS OF VBAC VS. ELECTIVE REPEAT CESAREAN

VBAC
  Pros: The consensus of the research is that:
  ➤ VBAC is safe.

➤ Elective repeat cesarean poses greater risks to the mother's life and health than does vaginal birth. It poses hazards to the baby as well, especially with succeeding pregnancies and more than one cesarean.

➤ Most women, including women whose prior cesarean was for lack of progress or who are believed to be carrying a big baby, will birth vaginally if allowed to labor.

Cons: The healed uterine scar is tough. Still, in a few women, the scar will open up enough for the umbilical cord or the baby to pass through the opening or for bleeding to occur. The number usually quoted for women with one prior cesarean is less than 1 percent, based on the fact that several big studies found rates of symptomatic scar separation in 7 or 8 per 1,000 labors. However, based on calculations made on all twenty-nine studies I've found, the number is about half that, or 4 per 1,000.* Even should this rare event occur, few babies will be harmed if a cesarean is promptly performed. In fact, the perinatal mortality rate (deaths around the time of birth) in those twenty-nine studies was 3 out of 10,000 for both VBAC labors and planned cesareans.

Note: Medical professionals use loaded language when speaking of VBAC. The expression "successful VBAC" implies that a labor that ends in repeat cesarean is a "failure." "Attempted VBAC" suggests that labor is not the norm and vaginal birth is doubtful, as does "trial of labor." Worst of all, they speak of "uterine rupture," a term that creates so vivid an image that it's a wonder any woman tries VBAC after hearing it. I tell you

---

*The reason for the difference is that the large studies are from Los Angeles. Many women in them are Mexican immigrants, which means more of them have the higher-risk vertical uterine scar. Also, policies at the study hospitals may increase the risk of scar separation (see pages 285 and 288).

this so that you will not be subliminally affected by the terminology.

ELECTIVE REPEAT CESAREAN

Pros: Since there is no labor, there is no chance of symptomatic scar separation, at least not during labor. Prelabor cesareans have lower infection and other complication rates than cesareans done in labor, although infections, at least, could be at least partly avoidable. Women who labor are likely to have membranes ruptured, multiple vaginal exams, and internal monitoring, all of which associate strongly with infection.

Cons: Compared with vaginal birth, cesarean section substantially increases the risk of infection, injury to other organs, hemorrhage, and anesthesia complications. These complications, in turn, increase the risk of prolonged hospitalization, hysterectomy, and maternal death. Repeat cesarean sections are more technically difficult to perform because of scar tissue. For this reason, injury to other organs is more common. Scar tissue formation (*adhesions*) can cause chronic pain and bowel problems. Elective cesarean also increases the baby's risk for poor condition at birth, breathing difficulties, and jaundice. Each successive cesarean greatly increases the risk of developing *placenta previa* (in which the placenta grows over the cervix) and/ or *placenta accreta* (in which the placenta grows into and sometimes through the uterine muscular wall, sometimes invading other organs) in subsequent pregnancies. Both of these complications pose life-threatening risks to mother and baby. Cesareans also increase the odds of infertility and ectopic pregnancy, another life-threatening danger, in subsequent pregnancies. Women with multiple prior cesareans have a slightly increased risk of symptomatic scar separation during VBAC.

Note: Jaundice and breathing difficulties at birth are almost certainly due to large amounts of IV fluid being given preoperatively in an attempt to prevent low blood pressure from spinal or epidural anesthesia. (See pages 241 and 288.) You may wish to refuse this since studies, including a random-assignment trial to preload IV fluid or not, show it doesn't work anyway.

THE ODDS OF VBAC

Among thirty-four studies reporting VBAC rates, all but one reported rates above 60 percent. Half the studies reported rates between 70 percent and 79 percent. Therefore, your odds of having a vaginal birth should be about three out of four, and you would be well advised to seek another caregiver should your doctor or midwife have a VBAC rate of less than 70 percent. If your prior cesarean was for poor progress, your odds of VBAC are somewhat less, but not markedly so. I have eighteen studies reporting VBAC rates when the prior cesarean was done for this reason. All but two report half or more of woman with this previous diagnosis giving birth vaginally. Half the studies report rates between 60 percent and 69 percent, so your odds in the hands of a supportive practitioner should be about two out of three. The other situation that may lead women to doubt whether trying labor is worthwhile is having had more than one prior cesarean. However, four studies reporting VBAC rates for women with more than one previous cesarean all report rates between 60 percent and 79 percent or better than three out of five.

FACTORS THAT EXCLUDE VBAC

- *Vertical (classical) uterine scar or extensive prior uterine surgery.* In almost all countries, low transverse uterine incisions are the norm. Reasons for a classical incision include *placenta previa* (in which the placenta is growing over the cervix), occasionally *breeches* (when the baby presents buttocks, knees, or feet down), and sometimes emergency cesareans.

FACTORS THAT DON'T EXCLUDE VBAC

The following are often cited as reasons for not trying labor, but they are not valid.

- *Prior cesarean for poor progress (also known as "failure to progress," "labor dystocia," "cephalopelvic disproportion").* Studies have shown that the odds of vaginal birth are 2 out of 3.
- *Suspected large baby.* Ultrasound doesn't accurately predict birth weight (see page 230). Even when babies weighed over 8 lbs., 13 oz. (4,000 grams), the VBAC rate in three studies ranged from over half to nearly three-quarters.
- *Type of uterine scar not known.* Unless the prior cesarean was done in Latin America or certain other countries or for the reasons listed previously, the odds are 99 to 1 the scar is transverse.
- *Low vertical uterine scar.* This incision is done when the baby is premature because the lower part of the uterus isn't well enough developed for a transverse incision. Data suggest this scar is as strong as a transverse scar.
- *More than one prior cesarean.* The odds of symptomatic scar separation may increase slightly, but not enough to mandate planned cesarean. The odds of vaginal birth are still excellent (see page 169).
- *Twins.* We lack sufficient data on twins, but what data we have do not suggest that VBAC poses undue risk.
- *Breeches.* We also lack data on breeches, but if you are oth-

erwise qualified for vaginal birth, there is no reason to think a prior cesarean should be an obstacle. What little data we have on *external cephalic version* (turning breech babies head down from the outside) after prior cesarean suggests that the procedure is safe.

Factors That Promote Safe Vaginal Birth

WARNING! If you experience continuous abdominal pain or vaginal bleeding that is more than streaking or spotting (bleeding that looks like the start of your period), get to a hospital immediately for further evaluation.

- *Have a confident caregiver with a high VBAC rate.* Almost all complications occur in women who have repeat cesareans, so the better your odds of vaginal birth, the lower your chances of experiencing one of them. You want an encouraging caregiver who performs only medically indicated repeat cesareans and who has a VBAC rate of 70 percent or more.
- *Commit yourself to vaginal birth.* It isn't uncommon for women in the heat of labor to decide they want the baby out and they don't care how—except that if you have a prior cesarean, doctors are much more likely to grant your request. See pages 173–175 for better solutions to pain, fear, and emotional distress than major surgery.
- *Give birth in or near a facility capable of performing a cesarean within twenty minutes of making the decision and that can care for a distressed baby.* Surprisingly, considering that the major argument for hospital birth is faster response in an emergency, many hospitals don't have these capabilities. To meet these requirements, the hospital must have round-the-clock, in-house obstetricians and anesthesiologists and twenty-four-hour blood banking. They must also have at least a Level II nursery, which means they can take care of

babies with moderate problems and can stabilize sicker babies for transport to a facility with a Level III, or newborn intensive care, nursery. The hospital should also have at least a 1-to-1 nurse (RN)-to-patient ratio for women in active labor as well. Find out whether your hospital meets these qualifications. This recommendation does not preclude out-of-hospital birth, provided you are being closely monitored and the birth center or your home is close enough to such a hospital.

- *Avoid induction of labor.* One large study found an increased rate of the scar giving way in women who were given oxytocin (trade name: Pitocin or "Pit") before 2 centimeters' dilation. Even though these women were already having some ineffective contractions on their own, physiologically, these were inductions.
- *Refuse oxytocin to strengthen labor before active labor (3 to 5 centimeters' dilation and painful, regular contractions).*
- *Avoid an epidural.* Epidurals not only reduce your odds of vaginal birth, but also cause episodes of abnormally slow fetal heart rate in about 10 percent of laboring women. The most reliable sign that the scar has opened and is causing the baby problems is abnormally slow fetal heart rate, which means that an epidural puts you at greater risk of an emergency cesarean for suspected scar separation.
- *While it is best to avoid these, know that prostaglandin gel to ripen the cervix for induction, oxytocin to induce or strengthen labor, and epidural anesthesia can be used in VBAC labors.* A good case can be made that mainstream practitioners grossly overuse these procedures to the detriment of mothers and babies, but that isn't likely to change any time soon. Meanwhile, in the real world, your doctor's unwillingness to use the first two when he or she thinks they are indicated means you end up with an avoidable cesarean, and refusal to allow epidurals may keep you from trying labor.

- *No arbitrary time limits should be set on labor.* There is no evidence that length of labor has any effect on scar integrity if you haven't been induced. At the very least, caregivers should give you as much time as if you had never had a baby. Studies show that women with a prior cesarean have labor lengths more like those of first-time mothers than of women who have given birth before.

- *Consider having continuous electronic fetal monitoring (EFM).* Abnormal fetal heart rate is the most common indication of uterine scar problems requiring intervention. Dr. Bruce Flamm, a preeminent VBAC researcher, has argued that periodic listening may miss the change because it may be sudden, and time is of the essence if it occurs. Others have responded that symptomatic scar separations are no more common than other unpredictable obstetric emergencies. If women generally have not been shown to benefit, we should be cautious about subjecting women with prior cesareans to the disadvantages of EFM. The American College of Obstetricians and Gynecologists' 1995 VBAC practice guidelines mandate close monitoring but do not prescribe EFM. The 1998 VBAC practice guidelines recommend continuous EFM. If you agree to continuous EFM, see page 94 for how to minimize its drawbacks.

- *Limit vaginal exams and avoid having membranes ruptured (amniotomy) and internal fetal monitoring.* These procedures increase the likelihood of infection. They may be one reason, if not the main reason, why in-labor cesareans have higher infection rates than nonlabor cesareans.

FACTORS THAT PROMOTE A POSITIVE BIRTH EXPERIENCE

- *Use a midwife.* Midwives are more likely to be sensitive to and willing to help with the fears, anxieties, and doubts that may assail women before or during VBACs.

- *Take care of emotional issues and fears surrounding labor.* Consider what worries or distresses you when you think about laboring again. What can you do to address those concerns? What will you need to feel safe? What will you need to feel taken care of in labor? (See page 27 for suggested reading.)

- *Hire professional labor support.* In labor, it helps to have someone with you continuously to whom you can express doubts or anxieties and who will encourage and reassure you. This is often not your partner, who may be experiencing doubts and anxieties of his or her own. A professional will also know techniques to help you relax and to ease pain and promote progress.

- *Plan on having an epidural.* For some women, planning to have an epidural makes VBAC possible. (See page 143 for tips on how to minimize the risks of epidurals.) In the past, doctors refused epidurals for VBAC labors on the grounds that the epidural might mask pain from the scar giving way, but pain isn't a reliable symptom, and experts agree that epidurals should not be withheld in VBAC labors.

- *Have realistic expectations.* If things don't go as you hoped, you may wish you had planned a cesarean, but you don't know what might have happened had you made this choice. It might have gone smoothly, but then again, maybe not. As with many things in life, with VBAC, you plan the best you can, but you get no guarantees.

- *Take an active role in planning a VBAC that will meet your emotional and physical needs and, barring an emergency, in making decisions during the labor and birth.* One of the difficult issues for cesarean mothers can be feelings of loss of control. Ironically, many women give "wanting to feel in control" as a reason for planned cesarean, although, of course, you are never in less control than you are during surgery. When you take charge of the childbirth experience, even another cesarean can be empowering.

- *Refuse the routine use of an intrauterine pressure catheter or manual exploration of the scar after birth.* These procedures have not been shown to increase the safety of VBAC, and they add to your discomfort.
- *Refuse a routine IV and insist on being allowed to drink clear liquids.* With the possible exception of continuous electronic fetal monitoring, you should not be treated any differently than any other laboring woman. If it seems too hard to refuse an IV, compromise on a *heparin lock*. With a heparin lock, the IV catheter is inserted, but rather than connecting to an IV bottle, it connects to a short rubber tube that is taped to your hand or arm. It frees you from an IV pole, but an IV can be started simply by plugging into the rubber tube.

GLEANINGS FROM THE MEDICAL LITERATURE
(PAGES 284–288)

- VBAC is safe provided the baby is closely monitored and caregivers can respond promptly to the rare problem with the scar.
- Elective repeat cesarean increases the mother's risk of hysterectomy and death and baby's risk of death in subsequent pregnancies.
- Elective cesarean increases the baby's risk of poor condition at birth, breathing difficulties, and jaundice.
- Women should not be disqualified from VBAC because they have an unknown uterine scar type.
- Women should not be disqualified from VBAC because they have more than one prior cesarean.
- Women should not be disqualified from VBAC because they have a low vertical incision.
- Women should not be disqualified from VBAC because of twins.

- Using intrauterine pressure catheters does not increase the safety of VBAC.
- Manual exploration of the scar after birth does not increase the safety of VBAC.
- Prostaglandin gel to ripen the cervix for induction may be used in VBACs.
- Oxytocin to start labor or stimulate stronger contractions may be used in VBACs; however, induction or oxytocin before active labor may increase the risk of symptomatic uterine scar separation.

Chapter 11

PROFESSIONAL LABOR SUPPORT:
Mothering the Mother

IF YOU ARE a first-time mom planning a hospital birth, you're probably assuming that your nurse will shepherd you and your partner through labor. Ever-present, she will comfort and tend you. I suppose it happens occasionally, but not often. Studies show that the average labor and delivery nurse spends fifteen minutes of her eight-hour shift offering physical comfort measures, providing emotional support, or advocating for her patients. Another study showed that time with laboring women didn't increase even with a group of nurses who acknowledged the importance of labor support and when that was the study's intent. Meanwhile, with staff cutbacks the order of the day, even the best-intentioned nurse has no time to labor-sit. More than one nurse who tried has told me she was criticized during her review for "spending too much time with patients." As for doctors, unless there are complications, they normally have nothing to do with labor support. Your odds are better with midwives, but they too may have time constraints, particularly hospital-based midwives. If you want an expert to help you and your partner meet one of life's greatest and most rewarding challenges, you will have to bring her with you. Known by many names, she is the first line of labor support for the soon-to-be mom.

Perhaps the most complicated thing about this new profession is the terminology. Dana Raphael first popularized the term *doula,* a Greek word meaning "woman caregiver," in her 1973 book, *The Tender Gift.* She used it to describe women who provided help and support to women after childbirth. Drs. Marshall Klaus and John Kennell adopted the term in the first of their studies, but they meant a labor support companion. Today, women who offer postpartum home-care services and women who do labor support both call themselves doulas, and some women do both. Polly Perez and Cheryl Snedecker, authors of *Special Women,* first published in 1990, distinguished between a *monitrice* and a doula. A monitrice has medical skills to monitor mother and baby and assess labor progress. *Birth assistant, childbirth assistant*, and *labor assistant* have all been used as synonyms for *doula* but may also be used to describe a midwife's assistant. I will use the term *doula.*

DO YOU REALLY NEED PROFESSIONAL LABOR SUPPORT?

YOUR MEMORIES OF labor stay with you the rest of your life, including the full intensity of the attached emotions. In particular, you will remember whether you felt loved, supported, encouraged, and cherished, or the reverse. That alone is a good reason to try to ensure that the memories will be positive ones. But there's more.

Randomized controlled trials produce the strongest kind of research evidence because researchers randomly assign participants to have the treatment or not, which eliminates all kinds of biases. We now have more than a dozen randomized controlled trials. Various trials have shown that the continuous presence of a caring, experienced woman can reduce the length of labor, the use of pain medication, the need for intravenous oxytocin (trade name: Pitocin or "Pit") to stimulate stronger contractions, the likelihood of having an episiotomy (snipping or cutting the vaginal opening), the percentage of instrumental vaginal deliveries, and the C-section rate. Doulas can reduce the number of babies born in poor condition and the number who are admitted to special-care nurseries, have prolonged hospital stays, or have evaluations for infection. These studies also show that women who have a doula experience less pain and anxiety in labor, express greater satisfaction with the labor, feel that they coped better, have a heightened appreciation of their bodies' strength and performance and themselves as women, breastfeed longer, and experience less difficulty in mothering. They can have more positive feelings toward the baby, better self-esteem, a better relationship with the father, and less postpartum depression. The fact that these studies took place in different countries with different populations of women under different circumstances and consistently found benefits further strengthens confidence in the validity of their results. The author of an analysis of the random-assignment doula trials concluded, "Given the clear benefits and no known risks, . . . every effort should be made to ensure that all labouring women receive support, not only from those close to them but also from specially trained caregivers. This support should include continuous presence, the provision of hands-on comfort, and encouragement."

Here's what doulas do that differs from what others do, at least at hospital births.* Doulas stay with mothers throughout labor and are in close proximity if not actual physical contact virtually all of the time. They offer physical comfort measures

---

*All doula studies have been in hospitals. Both medical professionals and loved ones are likely to behave quite differently at free-standing birth centers and home births.

such as cool cloths, massage, and hand-holding; emotional support, including praise, reassurance, and encouragement; and information or instruction, such as explanations of what is happening, what the doctor said, or how to push. They also provide advocacy in that they help the woman communicate her needs to hospital staff, act on her behalf, and support her decisions. In short, they "mother the mother."

However, we don't know why doulas have the effect they do, although we have some ideas. I think the reduction in medical procedures and drug use and the improvements in outcomes partly stem from the reduction in the use of pain medication, especially epidurals. Epidurals in particular are associated with nearly every one of the medical interventions and problems researchers report that doulas reduce. In proof of this, some studies with high epidural rates in the doula group found no effect on medical intervention and complication rates. Drs. Klaus and Kennell explain that doulas reduce stress and anxiety, factors that can inhibit labor, and that a doula's close contact and massage stimulates oxytocin production. Unlike intravenous oxytocin, in addition to strengthening contractions, naturally secreted oxytocin produces drowsiness, feelings of well-being, and a raised pain threshold. All of these things help the mother relax, which also fosters progress.*

Dr. Klaus and Dr. G. Justus Hofmeyr and his group, who also conduct research on doulas, speculate that having a doula produces short- and long-term psychological benefits because the qualities of labor render the mother particularly open and vulnerable. What happens to her during that time makes an especially deep impression. If she emerges from the labor feeling strong, confident, and nurtured, she will be in a much better

---

*The pituitary, located within the brain, secretes oxytocin both into the bloodstream, where it causes uterine contractions, and into the brain, where it has the effects just mentioned. Intravenous oxytocin cannot cross the blood-brain barrier. It produces more painful contractions without compensating psychological effects.

position to nurture her baby in turn and to cope with stresses and strains that inevitably accompany the early weeks of life with a newborn. Klaus and colleagues cite a survey of birth customs in various cultures. In 126 out of 127 cultures, laboring women had one or more experienced women with them continuously throughout labor. Anything that universal almost certainly serves an important purpose.

WHAT ABOUT THE FATHER'S ROLE?

YOU ARE PROBABLY thinking, "Don't childbirth preparation classes teach my partner how to do labor support?" A study that observed fathers with their partners in labor found that most fathers did not act as "coaches." Of the men that didn't, some wanted to play an active role, but needed guidance from someone else. That can be you in early labor, but not as labor advances, and as we have seen, the guidance isn't likely to come from the nurse. The rest wanted to be present for the birth of their child but did not do much in the way of labor support. Studies also show that labor support from fathers, friends, and family members has not shown the beneficial effects that are associated with doula care. This, of course, is not to say that fathers (or family members or friends, for that matter) shouldn't be there. It only says that we have created a role for fathers that doesn't really suit most of them.

You needn't worry that a doula will replace your partner. A good doula enhances rather than detracts from the father's participation. One study found that fathers in the doula group were more likely to offer physical comfort measures, equally likely to offer emotional support, and only slightly less likely to advocate for their partners compared with fathers in the control group. Fathers lost ground only when it came to giving information or instruction, which you would expect with the more knowledgeable doula on the scene. Interviewed afterward, fathers uniformly liked having a doula and did not feel that she interfered with their role. Fathers reported that not only did doulas help them help the moms, but many of the doula's support actions were directed personally at them. I tell couples who want to know what I do at a birth that, really, I am the father's hired handmaiden.

THE BOTTOM LINE

IF YOU ARE planning to have a midwife attend your birth, you may not need a doula. Traditionally, midwives stay with you, providing comfort and support as well as medical supervision and care. However, midwives attending hospital births may not do this. This may sometimes be true as well at freestanding birth centers and for midwives with home birth practices, although one-on-one continuous labor support is certainly usual. Even when your midwife or her assistant provides labor support outside of the hospital, they may not come with you should you transfer into the hospital. Finally, you may want a doula outside of the hospital in any case if you need someone to handle household tasks during the birth such as preparing food, cleaning up after meals, changing bed linens, and doing laundry.

PROS AND CONS OF PROFESSIONAL LABOR SUPPORT

Pros:
> *Continuity of care.* Most doulas meet with you one or more times before the birth, stay with you throughout labor, and make one or more postpartum visits. Because of this, they know your concerns and priorities regarding labor, they can help you debrief and digest the labor experience, and they can help with breastfeeding and parenting concerns.

➤ *Support for the father or partner.* Fathers or partners can participate to the extent that they feel comfortable. Fathers especially need nurturing and care during this major life transition.

➤ *Accessible resource.* You and your partner do not have to worry about forgetting what you learned in childbirth preparation classes.

➤ *Another pair of hands.* During long labors, the partner and the doula can spell each other. During intense periods, more than one person may be needed to help you.

➤ *Credibility.* You know that unlike the father, the doula knows how hard labor can be. You will trust that what the doula asks can be done because you know the doula is experienced with labor support and, in most cases, has labored herself.

➤ *Advocacy.* Accountable only to the couple, the doula has no conflict of interest with the hospital or doctor. She is ideally situated to facilitate communication between you and medical staff and to help ensure that you make informed decisions.

➤ *Reduced rates of medical procedures and complications.* Doulas are not magic, though. If your obstetrician has a high cesarean rate or you are planning an early epidural, a doula may not be able to overcome that.

Cons:

➤ *Hiring the wrong person.* This would be someone who imposes her ideas of the "right" way to do things or who pushes your partner aside.

➤ *Hospital staff hostility.* This may be the doula's fault, but more likely it arises from doctors or nurses seeing the doula as an intruder into their territory or as a competitor. Hospital staff may also feel threatened if the doula's presence leads you to ask questions or resist procedures. In their view, the doula has made you a "difficult patient."

Comparison Between Labor Support from a Female Relative or Friend and a Doula

FEMALE RELATIVE OR FRIEND	DOULA
She knows you and your partner well. Ties of affection make you comfortable with her in the intimacy of labor and birth.	She knows you, but the fact that you have no ongoing relationship means you don't have to perform for her or worry about what she might think of you.
She may have beliefs and experiences with labor that may color her behavior and bias her advice.	While caring, she is likely to be more objective.
She has no special training or experience, but she may not need it. The most effective and important component of doula care is loving touch.	She knows about labor, techniques to promote good progress, and comfort measures. She can help facilitate communication between you and your caregivers. She, too, provides a loving touch.
She costs nothing, but you have no authority over her.	She charges for her services, but her responsibility is to please you.

Comparison Between a Doula and a Monitrice

DOULA	MONITRICE
She offers only nonmedical labor support skills.	She combines labor support skills with nursing skills such as taking blood pressures, listening to the fetal heart tones, and performing pelvic examinations to assess progress.

DOULA	MONITRICE
Her only role and focus is labor support. If complications and problems arise, she will be the only one whose duties begin and end with your emotional needs.	Her perspective may be different because she wears two hats: labor support and medical caregiver. However, she can help you decide such things as when to leave for the hospital.
	Because she offers additional skills, her services may cost more.

Choosing a Professional Labor Support Companion

Talk to more than one person if at all possible. The comparison can be instructive. Although either you or your partner can do the preliminary screening, both of you should participate in the final face-to-face meeting because you must both be comfortable with her. The feelings you get during the give and take of the interview process will tell you more about whether you want to hire this person than will answers to specific questions. Here are some questions you may want to ask.

- *What is your background, training, and experience relevant to doing labor support? Are you certified by a doula training program?* Certification guarantees a minimal degree of knowledge and skill, which can be useful information. However, it does not guarantee that this person is competent, and many highly competent doulas are not certified.
- *What do you see as your strengths?*
- *How do you see your role at the birth?*
- *How do you feel about _____?* Fill in the blank with anything on which you have an opinion or that is part of your plans, such as pain medication, prayer during the labor, the presence of your other children, home birth, and so on.
- *What services do you offer?*

- *What do you charge? If relevant: Are you open to alternate financial arrangements, such as time payments or barter?*
- *What are your backup arrrangements? May I meet or speak with your backup?*
- *How many clients do you take a month? Do you have anyone else due close to my due date?*
- *Do you work with any particular hospitals, doctors, or mid-wives?* Working with certain practitioners or in certain hospitals can be positive in that this person will be known and respected. It may be a disadvantage in that it may create a conflict of interest between pleasing you and pleasing her source of referrals.
- *Do you have any limitations on where you will go or which caregivers you work with?*
- *Will you provide references?*

GLEANINGS FROM THE MEDICAL LITERATURE
(PAGES 291–294)

- Whether a mother experiences her labor as positive or negative depends on how well supported she feels.
- Doulas can decrease the use of medical procedures and treatments for both mother and baby.
- For reasons beyond their control, doulas don't always reduce intervention rates.
- Doulas improve psychological and social outcomes.
- Fathers don't do what doulas do.
- Doulas complement and enhance the father's care.
- Labor and delivery nurses don't generally offer supportive care.

Chapter 12

OBSTETRICIANS, MIDWIVES, AND
FAMILY PRACTITIONERS:
SOMEONE TO WATCH OVER YOU

As I HAVE documented in the rest of this book, whether you have a C-section or any other procedure or medication in labor has little to do with your or your baby's condition. What happens to you depends almost entirely on your caregiver's practice style and philosophy.

This is vital information because all procedures and medications introduce risks. For this reason, you will want to choose a caregiver who avoids using them on a routine or frequent basis. You want someone who knows an array of no-risk strategies to facilitate labor progress, maintain labor normality, and put errant labors back on track. You want someone who individualizes care rather than treats by rule and who knows when to sit on his or her hands. You want someone who understands that childbirth is more than a mechanical process, that it involves the head and the body, that the two affect each other, and that childbirth is a powerful emotional, psychological, and spiritual event. Finally you want a practitioner who, when more aggressive intervention is justified, intervenes judiciously. In short, you want someone who provides midwifery-style care, not obstetric management. Now, while individual caregivers vary widely within professions, you will not be surprised to hear that midwives mostly practice midwifery, obstetricians tend toward obstetric management, and family practitioners, who are, after all, doctors, although not surgeons like their obstetrician colleagues, usually fall in between. In other words, the dice are loaded in your favor with midwives, somewhat less so with family practitioners, and against you with obstetricians. Or, as the obstetrician said to the pregnant woman, "You're in labor? I'm in management!"

Typical obstetricians, of course, would tell you differently. They would say, "Why would you want a midwife or family practitioner when you can have the superior skills and knowledge of a specialist?" At best, they would acknowledge that midwives have a place, but that place is firmly under the control and direction of an obstetrician. Typical obstetricians see no reason why family physicians should do maternity care at all. Typical obstetricians dismiss studies showing that midwives and family practitioners achieve excellent outcomes, saying that their statistics look good only because midwives and family physicians care only for low-risk women. Furthermore, they would add, why disturb the status quo? Studies show that most women are satisfied with their care under the current system.

Let me take these objections one by one.

To begin with, the obstetrician's special skills hurt, not help, most pregnant women. The rest of this book establishes that the routine or indiscriminate use of medical tests, procedures, drugs, and restrictions—the hallmarks of obstetric management—does far more harm than good. It could not be otherwise. As I stated before, obstetric interventions introduce risks as well as benefits. If they are used on women who do not have a problem or who have a problem that could be resolved by lesser means, then they expose those women and babies to the risks of the intervention without any possible benefit. Case in point: When researchers compared outcomes for all U.S. women cared for by nurse midwives in 1991 with outcomes of similar women managed by doctors, they found, among other benefits of midwifery care, that one-third fewer babies died during the first week of life. As the authors of an analysis comparing birth outcomes of midwives and obstetricians comment, "In all economically developed countries except Holland, maternity care has come to be organised so as to give full effect to the theory that childbirth is always safer if it takes place under the management of obstetricians in a hospital. . . . It is a remarkable fact that obstetricians have never at any time had valid evidence to support the theory they have so successfully propagated."

Second, because midwifery care is superior to medical management for low- and moderate-risk pregnant women, obstetricians should not control midwives or labor and delivery policies. In a maternity-care system that makes sense, such as Holland's, midwives and family physicians would care for pregnant women, and at their discretion they would consult with or refer to obstetricians those women who developed complications. This, of course, is the arrangement in all other instances of generalists and specialists.

Third, research disproves the argument that the fact that obstetricians handle high-risk cases accounts for differences in procedure and medication rates. For one thing, midwives don't just take care of low-risk women. Hospital-based midwives, at least, care for women with risk profiles comparable to—and for some factors worse than—the national average. For another, when you compare low-risk women managed by obstetricians with low-risk women cared for by midwives or family practitioners, the midwives and family practitioners consistently come out behind on intervention rates. Moreover, the percentage of high-risk women in obstetricians' practices doesn't begin to explain some of the huge gaps in intervention rates. For example, Public Citizen's Health Research Group surveyed 419 hospital-based nurse-midwifery practices. The cesarean rate in the

127,300 women cared for by the midwives between 1991 and 1993 was 12 percent, roughly half the national cesarean rate of 23 percent.

Finally, yes, it is true that when women are surveyed, they almost all express satisfaction with their maternity care, but the issue is not that clear-cut. Joy in the birth of a baby creates a halo effect around the whole experience, particularly if the survey is done shortly thereafter. Even so, studies where women were randomly assigned to midwifery versus obstetric care found that while almost all the women liked their care, the ones assigned to midwifery care liked it better. We also have research that shows that satisfaction with birth depends on feeling a sense of mastery over events. Conversely, experiencing lack of support and respect and having many medical procedures during pregnancy and labor increase the probability of developing postpartum depression. So regardless of whether women express satisfaction, they may be suffering the fallout of obstetric management. Why would women generally say they were happy with care that by all objective standards has hurt them? Perhaps the explanation lies in an old Jewish saying about the worm who was perfectly happy in a horseradish—because it had never known a nice, juicy apple.

THE BOTTOM LINE

A GUIDE TO THE QUALIFICATIONS OF BIRTH ATTENDANTS

OBSTETRICIANS

Obstetricians are physicians who have completed a residency specializing in obstetrics and gynecology. They may be *board certified* in obstetrics, meaning they have passed a national qualifying exam.

FAMILY PRACTITIONERS

Also known as *family physicians* or *general practitioners*, family practitioners are physicians who have completed a residency in family practice. They, too, may be board certified in family practice. About 30 percent of family physicians currently practice obstetrics.

MIDWIVES

Midwives come in several varieties. The best accepted in mainstream maternity care is the *certified nurse-midwife*. Nurse-midwives have an RN and have completed additional postgraduate training at an institution accredited by the American College of Nurse-Midwives (ACNM). *Direct-entry midwives* have trained as midwives but without obtaining an RN, as is the norm in Europe. The Midwifery Education Accreditation Council (MEAC) has begun accrediting direct-entry midwifery training programs. Two organizations offer certification to direct-entry midwives: the ACNM and the North American Registry of Midwives (NARM). The ACNM certifies only midwives who have graduated from ACNM-accredited education programs and who have a bachelor's degree either before entering or by the time they graduate. NARM will certify any applicant who demonstrates the requisite skills and knowledge, regardless of background or source of training. Not all midwives are certified.

PROS AND CONS OF VARIOUS CLASSES OF BIRTH ATTENDANTS

Note: The rest of this section will focus on selecting hospital-based caregivers, which excludes direct-entry midwives. Questions for out-of-hospital caregivers, that is, those practicing at freestanding birth centers or with home birth practices, and the trade-offs between certified nurse-midwives and direct-entry midwives will be addressed in chapter 13.

OBSTETRICIANS

Pros: Obstetricians have the knowledge and skills to diagnose and treat serious complications of pregnancy and childbirth. Rarely would you require transfer to someone else's care.

Cons: Obstetricians are surgical specialists in the pathology of women's reproductive organs. This high-risk mentality often spills over onto the care of low-risk women, where it does no good and considerable harm. Unlike most midwives, typical obstetricians have a limited repertoire, and all their options carry considerable risks, or, as one wit put it, "If you don't want to get cut, don't go to a surgeon." Typical obstetricians think of pregnancy, childbirth, women, and the role of the obstetrician in ways that are adverse to healthy physical and psychological outcomes. Few obstetricians attend births at freestanding birth centers and virtually none attend home births.

FAMILY PRACTITIONERS

Pros: Family practitioners tend to be less interventive than obstetricians. Instead of shuttling among an internist, pediatrician, and obstetrician-gynecologist, all members of the family can see one person. This fosters building a relationship and increases convenience. For example, it allows one-stop doctoring when everybody has the same illness, or you can get information or advice about your postpartum concerns during well-baby visits.

Cons: Pregnancy or labor complications may mean transferring care to an obstetrician. Although the average family practitioner is less interventive than the typical obstetrician, typical family practitioners still tend to intervene more than typical midwives. Few family practitioners attend births at freestanding birth centers, and virtually none attend home births.

MIDWIVES

> *Pros:* As a class, midwives offer care that is flexible, individualized, supportive rather than interventive, and attentive to emotional issues. Midwives apply a broad array of low-risk strategies for correcting problems arising in pregnancy or labor. The typical midwife's practices, and in particular, the midwife's use of tests and procedures, come closer to guidelines recommended by official physicians' organizations than those of the typical obstetrician. Many midwives offer well-woman gynecological care, which allows you to continue your care with someone more likely to be sensitive and knowledgeable about such issues as postpartum depression, sexuality, and eventually menopause. Some midwives attend births at freestanding birth centers, and, with rare exceptions, only midwives attend home births.
>
> *Cons:* Pregnancy or labor complications may mean transferring care to an obstetrician. Many midwives only have hospital-based practices.

INTERVIEWING A CAREGIVER

GENERAL PRINCIPLES

- *Don't make assumptions about practice style or philosophy based on sex or type of practitioner.* You cannot assume that a woman will be sensitive, flexible, and noninterventive and a man will not. You cannot assume that all midwives and family physicians work from the midwifery model and all obstetricians follow the obstetric model. There are obstetricians who are excellent "midwives" and midwives who are obstetricians in midwives' clothing.
- *Interview several caregivers.* If the name is based on a personal recommendation, ask what the recommender liked about this practitioner because you may feel differently.

Childbirth educators, professional labor support providers, and La Leche League or other breastfeeding counselors often know which local doctors and midwives work from the midwifery model.

- *Ask open-ended questions.* Don't give away your own opinions, which you will surely have if you have read this book. Examples of open-ended phrasing include "What is your approach to . . . ," "When do you recommend . . . ," "Why is it important to . . . ," and "What is your opinion of. . . ."
- *Follow up on vague answers.* Responses such as "I only do that when it is necessary" or "We'll have to see at the time" tell you nothing. Continue with "How often do you find it necessary?" or "Under what circumstances would _____ be inadvisable?"
- *Ask yourself, "Am I getting facts or feelings?"* For example, if you asked about episiotomy and were told, "Which would you rather have: a nice clean cut or a jagged tear?" you got feelings. Compare that answer with "I do them about 15 percent of the time in first-time mothers, and I don't remember the last time I did one in a mother who had already had a baby. I do them when the baby is in trouble right at the end, or I may suggest one if I feel you aren't stretching well. Sometimes, but not always, I do them as part of a forceps delivery."
- *Ask yourself, "Would I feel comfortable asking this person a 'dumb' question?"* Look elsewhere if the answer is no.
- *If this book or your interview leads you to think you have chosen the wrong caregiver, remember that it is never too late to switch.* And it is almost always better to switch than fight.

SPECIFIC QUESTIONS
- *Are you board certified?* (physicians only—nurse-midwives are certified by definition) Board certification does not guarantee you somebody wonderful, nor does lack of certification

necessarily mean lesser qualifications, but it is a benchmark of achievement.

- *Under what circumstances would you transfer my care to an obstetrician (midwives and family physicians only)?* You may also wish to meet or at least talk with that person.
- *Do the midwives attend births?* (if you are choosing a practice of obstetricians and midwives) In some practices, midwives only do prenatal and postpartum care.
- *What is the likelihood that you will attend my birth?* Many caregivers practice in groups and rotate call among the members. They won't necessarily share the same philosophy toward birth, so you need to speak with all of them. Caregivers also take vacations.
- *What are your dietary recommendations? How much weight should I gain?* Prenatal care should include help in planning a nutritious, varied diet that takes into account your food preferences and addresses such problems as allergies, morning sickness, or history of an eating disorder. You should be told to gain a minimum of twenty-five pounds if you are of average weight, more if you are underweight, and less if you are overweight, but you should not be told to lose weight or hold the line once you reach a certain weight. You should not be told to restrict salt.
- *What is your policy on sonograms (ultrasound imaging)?* Be wary of caregivers who routinely do more than one sonogram in a normal pregnancy or who promote them as a means of "bonding" with your unborn baby. Medical tests should be done only if there's concern about the baby or to gather information that will help determine your care. Studies have not shown any value to routine sonograms. A caregiver who treats this technology lightly may have the same attitude toward more invasive and risky procedures.
- *Under what circumstances do you recommend inducing labor?* (See chapter 3.)

- *How do you handle slowly progressing labors?* (See chapter 7.)
- *What are your policies regarding monitoring the baby's heart rate in labor, IVs, drinking or eating in labor, breaking the bag of waters (amniotomy), epidurals, episiotomies?* (See chapter 4, 5, 6, 8, and 9.)
- *What are your reasons to do a cesarean? How often do you find it necessary? How do you try to avoid the need for cesarean?* (See page 20 for a reasonable cesarean rate.)

RED FLAG RESPONSES

These behaviors will tell you that you have the wrong person, someone who wants to coerce rather than convince you. All the examples are real statements made by real doctors. I don't want to stereotype caregivers, but the fact is that these tactics are common among obstetricians, occasionally found in family practitioners, and almost unheard-of in midwives.

- *Scare tactics.* "We can do that—if you don't care what happens to the baby." "Which would you rather have: a nice experience or a healthy baby?" You can have both. In fact, the things that make a nice experience also make for a healthy baby. "I can't be responsible if you insist on/won't do _____." "This is a premium baby; we don't want to take any chances." This one is used on older women expecting a first and perhaps only child. The hidden assumption is that vaginal birth carries more risk for the baby than cesarean section, but in fact the opposite is true (see page 286).
- *Anger.* "And where did *you* go to medical school?" "I can't take care of you if you don't trust me." Of *course* you should trust your caregiver, but that trust must be earned.
- *Ridiculing your concerns, desires, opinions, or competency to participate in decisions about your care.* "I see you've been reading those women's magazines." "You want natural child-

birth? I think that makes about as much sense as natural dentistry."

- *Patronizing you.* "Don't worry about a thing; just leave everything to me."
- *Vagueness.* It's a bad sign when you can't pin a caregiver down enough to get at least ballpark estimates of personal statistics such as cesarean rates or percentages of women who give birth vaginally after a prior cesarean. It's also bad when the caregiver says you can do anything you want during labor and won't specify what situations might preclude that.
- *Attempts to co-opt your partner.* This may occur with male doctors and male partners. You'll know it is happening if the doctor addresses himself to your male partner and ignores you. The hidden message amounts to "You and I together will take care of the Little Woman," and it can be seductive to caring, protective, expectant fathers. This bodes ill for the labor, as the following story illustrates. A friend of mine doing labor support wandered out into the hall in time to overhear her client's obstetrician trying to talk her client's husband into persuading her client to agree to the episiotomy that she had refused. If not for my friend's pointing out that it was his wife's vagina and she had the right to decide whether it was cut, the obstetrician might have succeeded. Imagine how you would feel to suddenly find your husband and doctor in league against you. Conversely, acting as if your partner is a fifth wheel isn't good either.

WHEN CHOICE IS LIMITED

WHEN THE PROBLEM IS MEDICAL COVERAGE
- *Talk to the prospective caregiver about your problem.* He or she might have suggestions.
- *Switch insurance plans.* You may be able to switch to a dif-

ferent plan during open enrollment or to your husband's or partner's plan.

- *Go outside the plan.* Your insurance plan may allow you to use caregivers outside the plan by paying a premium, usually 20 percent of costs. If your plan doesn't include midwives, here is some leverage: As of 1998, thirty-one states had mandated third-party reimbursement for nurse-midwifery services, which means private insurance companies and managed-care plans must pay for nurse-midwifery services, although, as just mentioned, they may charge a co-payment for nonmember providers. Medicare now stipulates that women be allowed direct access to women's health care specialists, including nurse-midwives. Medicare policies often become templates for employers and private insurers. If you start early enough and can get to someone in a position to authorize exceptions, you may be able to get coverage by convincing that person that you are opting for more cost-effective care than is provided in the standard plan. A friend of mine got her home birth with a midwife covered by doing this. Finally, as of 1995, nine states have mandated that managed care organizations include any licensed nurse-midwife who is willing to particpate. This could be a wedge to get your birth covered as well.

- *Pay for the birth out-of-pocket.* This may amount to several thousand dollars, but it may be cheap at the price when you consider the potential costs of an unnecessary cesarean to you and your subsequent children. Midwives in independent practice (as opposed to employees of a physician practice) are more likely to be able and willing to negotiate fees and terms or to make alternate payment arrangements, such as barter. If you do not have medical problems, you can substantially reduce your costs without compromising safety by having your baby at a freestanding birth center or—provided you have a trained birth attendant—at home.

WHEN THE PROBLEM IS NOT INSURANCE RELATED

Suppose the problem is that your medical condition limits options or there are no acceptable caregivers within reasonable distance of your home.

- *Except in an emergency, politely refuse any procedure or drug until you understand its advantages and disadvantages as well as the pros and cons of any alternatives, including doing nothing.* Your partner must be prepared to assist you in this. This includes scheduled cesarean section, induction of labor, an IV, electronic fetal monitoring, internal electronic fetal monitoring, rupture of membranes, oxytocin augmentation of labor, episiotomy, vacuum extraction or forceps delivery, and in-labor cesarean section. Unless you are given a good reason to do otherwise—and this book will help you determine what's a "good" reason—politely insist on being allowed freedom of activity and position and freedom to drink unrestricted amounts of clear, calorie-containing liquids.
- *Don't have an epidural.* All too often epidurals lead to other interventions, including C-sections. You and your partner must be well prepared to cope with the pain of labor without an epidural.
- *Hire a professional labor support companion.* She can help you get the information you need to make informed decisions. She can also help you avoid an epidural by offering alternative pain management techniques and strategies.
- *Go to the hospital as late as your circumstances allow and go home as early as you can.* The less time you spend in the hospital, the less time staff members have to do things to you or your baby. A professional labor support person with medical skills (*monitrice*) can be especially helpful in determining when to go to the hospital because she can monitor you and the baby and determine labor progress by vaginal exams.

- *Have an unattended home birth.* Do not take this option lightly. While rare, there are life-threatening problems that can arise during labor or at birth in a previously healthy mother carrying a healthy baby. Studies show that the safety of out-of-hospital birth depends on having a trained attendant. A knowledgeable and skilled birth attendant can spot complications coming in time to transfer into the hospital or can treat or stabilize them. However, birth in the hospital with a highly interventive caregiver also poses risks. You have the right to decide whether the risks of hospital birth outweigh the risks of unattended home birth.

GLEANINGS FROM THE MEDICAL LITERATURE
(PAGES 295–304)

- The midwifery model of care differs from the obstetric model in ways that are beneficial to mothers and babies.
- What medications and procedures you have depends mainly on your caregiver's philosophy, not your medical condition.
- Midwifery care produces equally good or better maternal and infant outcomes as does obstetric management, with much lower procedure and medication rates.
- Family practitioners tend to be less interventive than obstetricians, but may intervene more than midwives.
- Midwifery-style care may be distorted or limited by a high-tech environment or one where obstetricians dictate policy.
- Female physicians have practice styles and philosophies similar to those of their male counterparts.

Chapter 13

 ⁓

THE PLACE OF BIRTH:
Location, Location, Location

ODDS ARE, YOU are planning a hospital birth as a matter of course. You've probably never considered birth at home or at a freestanding birth center. If asked why not, you would almost certainly respond with some variation of "Because it's safer," the usual one being, "What if something goes wrong?" This is an unexamined assumption well worth examining.

The obstetric tale goes like this: Birth is a risky business. Up to the early 1900s, many women and babies died in childbirth. Then doctors took over maternity care from ill-trained and ignorant midwives, and childbirth moved into the hospital. As a result, maternal and infant death rates plummeted, and today almost everybody lives healthily and happily ever after thanks to the skills of obstetricians and the superior resources available in hospitals.

The only problem with this story is it isn't true.

HISTORY REEXAMINED AND A FEW CURRENT FACTS

FIRST, DEATH RATES did not decline as birth began to move into the hospital and under the control of physicians. They rose. In the 1920s in the United States, middle-class women began having babies in hospitals with physician attendants. By the mid-1920s, half of urban births took place there, and by 1939, half of all women and three-quarters of urban women gave birth in hospitals. In 1915, prior to the major changeover, 60 mothers died per 10,000 births. Despite the shift, the 1932 U.S. maternal mortality rate reached 63 deaths per 10,000 births, and in cities, where hospitalization for birth was more common, it stood at 74 deaths per 10,000 births, substantially worse than the overall rate. Meanwhile, between 1915 and 1929, as the shift in birth site and attendant occurred, infant deaths from birth injuries increased by 40 to 50 percent.

Maternal mortality in the United States did not begin to fall until the late 1930s, when sulfa drugs and antibiotics to treat infection were introduced and—this is worth emphasizing—*more stringent controls were placed on obstetric training and practices*. Many factors contributed to reducing maternal deaths, including better living conditions and nutrition, child spacing, and the development of blood transfusions, but moving birth into the hospital and under doctor control was not one of them.

In fact, several studies suggest that the doctor takeover and institutionalization of birth actually retarded improvements in mortality rates. One analyst looked at British data from the Isle of Man. The maternal mortality rate there dropped from about 70 per 10,000 births to less than 30 per 10,000 in the early years of the twentieth century as public health improved, only to climb right back up to 70 per 10,000 by 1929. The only change on the island during the climb was the replacement of midwives by physicians and the opening of a maternity hospital. Another statistician projected that had the British campaign to move birth into the hospital failed, the 1981 stillbirth rate would have been lower. In the 1960s, in a rural, impoverished California county, introducing midwives into the county hospital more than halved the newborn death rate. When doctor opposition to midwives blocked renewal of the program, the newborn death rate promptly tripled.

As late as 1970, the picture hadn't changed. This can be seen from an analysis of British data, where, unlike in the United States, home birth and birth in maternity homes had not yet disappeared. A 1970 survey assigned pregnant women risk scores ranging from "very low" to "very high." Hospital *perinatal mortality rates* (deaths of babies in the weeks before, during, or within a week after birth) exceeded out-of-hospital mortality rates at every level of risk except the highest. In fact, the perinatal mortality rate for *high*-risk births *outside* of the hospital (16 per 1,000) was lower than that for *low*-risk *in-hospital* births (18 per 1,000). In addition, the perinatal mortality rates for the categories "very low," "low," and "moderate" risk births at home or in maternity homes held steady at 4 to 5 per 1,000. By contrast, hospital perinatal mortality rates doubled with each increase in risk level, rising from 8 per 1,000 to 32 per 1,000. This suggests that hospital management actually intensified the risks!

Think that hospital birth must at least have the edge these days? Think again. No study has ever shown that out-of-hospital birth resulted in worse outcomes provided women were prescreened for risk factors and had a planned out-of-hospital birth with a trained attendant. And while individual studies may be too small to show significant differences in the occurrence of adverse outcomes because such outcomes are exceedingly rare in healthy women, collectively they affirm the safety of out-of-hospital birth. Moreover, the Netherlands, where home birth never disappeared and nearly one-third of women continue to have their babies at home today, has excellent outcome statistics for mothers and babies. The British, at least, have recognized this fact. In 1992, the House of Commons Health Select Committee published a report that concluded, "The policy of encouraging all woman to give birth in hospitals cannot be justified on grounds of safety. . . . Women should be given . . . an opportunity for choice, . . . including the option, previously denied to them, of having their babies at home, or in small maternity units."

How can women and babies do just as well without the benefits of modern hospitals? To begin with, in the more relaxed, physically and emotionally supportive out-of-hospital setting, problems may be less likely to develop. Feeling helpless or threatened can inhibit labor. Furthermore, animal studies suggest that these emotions may cause fetal distress. Second, when problems do arise, most are resolved with "tincture of time" or such no-risk strategies as walking, changes of position, oral fluids, warm baths, or investigating what might be causing the mother to feel fearful or anxious. As for the "What if something goes wrong?" argument, the things that go wrong in labor tend to go wrong slowly, such as a labor that doesn't progress or a baby who gradually becomes less able to tolerate labor. Provided the mother is under close observation, which is a major advantage of out-of-hospital birth, the caregiver can see problems coming and either fix them or move into the hospital before the situation becomes urgent. Unpredictable emergencies do occur, of course, but they are rare, and the most common ones—a baby whose head is born but whose shoulders are stuck, a baby that requires resuscitation, heavy bleeding after the birth—can be resolved or stabilized for hospital transport by a skilled pair of hands and readily portable medication and equipment.

Besides equivalent safety, out-of-hospital birth also has some advantages. Some studies report fewer maternal and newborn complications. Most studies show less use of drugs such as oxytocin to stimulate labor and procedures such as cesarean section and greater use of comfort measures such as baths and food and drink. And women just plain like the care better.

THE SAFETY OF HOSPITAL BIRTHS

ACTUALLY, WE COULD well turn the tables and ask, "Are hospital births safe?" A good case can be made that for low-risk women, at least, the answer is "No."

The main reason is the injudicious use of drugs and procedures so typical in hospitals. Every intervention into the normal process introduces risks as well as benefits. As indications for use broaden beyond a few limited cases, the balance between risks and benefits begins to tip toward risks. When intervening becomes routine, meaning there is no reason for it, only risks remain. Moreover, because one intervention tends to lead to another, it produces a "cascade effect." So, for example, electronic fetal monitoring confines women to bed, which may slow labor. Doctors may then give oxytocin, which increases pain, causing women to want an epidural. The epidural may slow labor or cause abnormal heart rate patterns, ending the cascade in a cesarean section for poor progress or fetal distress.

Ironically, authors of studies purporting to show that things go wrong in labor too often to make out-of-hospital birth safe actually unwittingly document the dangers of hospital birth. One study reviewed the hospital records of the 1,300 women out of 32,400 that reviewers felt were low enough risk to qualify for birth out of the hospital. The reviewers were alarmed to find that sixty-five (5 percent) of the babies needed assistance with breathing. However, eleven of these babies received naloxone (Narcan) during resuscitation. Naloxone is a drug given to reverse the respiratory depressant effects of narcotics given in labor. The authors of another study attribute a 10 percent cesarean rate, 13 percent forceps rate, and a greater than 20 percent use of oxytocin to strengthen contractions in a group of ultra-low-risk women to the inherently unpredictable difficulties of labor. They see nothing strange in so many healthy women with normal pregnancies having these interventions. Yet studies of out-of-hospital births report half or less of these rates with equally good or better outcomes. To repeat my quote from the Introduction, as renowned French physician Michel Odent has said, "One cannot help an involuntary process. The point is not to disturb it."

Then, too, many hospitals are not really better prepared to handle obstetric emergencies. To respond promptly to an emergency, a hospital must have twenty-four-hour in-house obstetric, anesthetic, and pediatric coverage and blood banking and a nursery capable of handling babies with moderate problems and stabilizing sicker babies for transport to an intensive care unit. Many hospitals lack these qualifications.

Cost-cutting measures have also taken their toll. Many hospitals have cut back on the number of registered nurses or replaced them with staff members with lesser training or both. This means fewer skilled caregivers monitoring women and babies. And when there is a mix of high- and low-risk cases and skilled care is at a premium, low-risk women and babies will surely get the short end of the stick. Even where nurse-to-patient ratios are adequate, nurses are often kept too busy monitoring and adjusting equipment, performing procedures, setting up for and assisting physicians as they perform procedures, and record keeping to pay proper attention to what is going on with their patients.

Clearly, women with complicated pregnancies should have their babies in hospitals. But for most women, it comes down to a matter of choice. The real question about safety is not, "Do you want a pleasant birth outside the hospital or a safe birth in the hospital?" It is, "Do you want to give birth outside a hospital and run the minuscule risk of an emergency that might (but not necessarily would) be handled better in the hospital, or do you want to give birth in the hospital and run the considerably increased risk of infection, the certainty of additional stress, and the near certainty of having unnecessary (and potentially risky) interventions?"

A (RELATIVELY) NEW OUT-OF-HOSPITAL OPTION

HOME BIRTH, OF course, has been the norm throughout humanity's history up to the beginning of the twentieth century and still prevails in regions of the world today. However, in 1974, the Maternity Center Association in New York introduced a new option: a birth center separate from, but close to, an acute-care hospital. In the birth center, as in their own homes, low-risk women could have whomever and however many people they wished with them, including children. They could eat and drink, move around freely, take showers and baths, and labor and give birth in positions of their choice. The idea was to offer home birth–style care with the added advantages of the staffing, protocols, and equipment of an institution, to create, as the authors of one journal article put it, a "maxi-home," not a "mini-hospital."

The ideal would be an in-hospital birth center, but the entrenched obstetric model, in which childbirth is viewed as a medical crisis, does not permit homelike care in a hospital setting. This can be seen in the rise and fall of "alternative birth centers" and "family birth rooms" in the 1970s and early 1980s. Most women never found out they existed; many who did were discouraged from using them; those who persisted were often disqualified; and intervention rates for the few who managed to give birth there were mostly unchanged. They vanished only to be reincarnated on cost-cutting and marketing grounds as "single-room maternity care." Still, while laboring, giving birth, and recovering in the same room is an improvement, nobody even pretends any more that reducing medication and procedure rates is a goal.

The freestanding birth center concept spread rapidly. By 1981, some 125 to 150 centers had been established in twenty-seven states. Freestanding birth centers represent a major challenge to the obstetric model of care, so obstetricians mostly opposed them despite their excellent track records. As early as 1983, based on four studies, the American Public Health Association stated, "Births to healthy mothers can occur safely in birth centers outside of an acute-care hospital." By 1995, additional studies, including a study of nearly 12,000 women giving birth in 84 U.S. birth centers, led a reviewer of the medical literature to state, "Comprehensive data have clearly demonstrated that birth centers are as safe as hospitals for low-risk births." Yet, as of the end of 1997, the American College of Obstetricians and Gynecologists continues to oppose freestanding birth centers on the grounds of insufficient data.

Obstetrician opposition has hampered development, which, together with the usual economic vicissitudes of any new business, has forced the subsequent closure of many birth centers. These obstacles, though, have not managed to kill them off. In 1983, the National Association of Childbearing Centers (NACC) was founded. One of NACC's earliest efforts was to develop national accreditation criteria. As of winter 1998, there were forty-seven accredited freestanding birth centers and four more working on accreditation in twenty-two states. An additional twenty-two centers in an additional twelve states, Canada, and the Bahamas maintain membership in NACC but are not currently accredited. Because they offer superb care at half the cost of conventional hospital birth, in these days of managed care, freestanding birth centers may be a concept whose time has come.

COMPARING BIRTH SITES

	HOSPITAL	FREESTANDING BIRTH CENTER	HOME
Philosophy:	Doctors deliver babies. Birth is a medical crisis and is normal only in retrospect. Difficulties should be resolved with medications and high-tech procedures.	Women give birth. Birth is a normal, healthy event, albeit one needing supervision and care. Most difficulties will resolve on their own in time or by using low-tech, no-risk strategies and techniques. However, risk-out and hospital transfer rates in labor are generally higher than with home birth.	Women give birth. Birth is a normal, healthy event, albeit one needing supervision and care. Most difficulties will resolve on their own in time or by using low-tech, no-risk strategies and techniques.
Safety:	Safe, provided caregivers are trained and competent.	Safe, provided caregivers are trained and competent.	Safe, provided caregivers are trained and competent.
If problems arise:	All diagnostic and treatment equipment is available on-site. However, proximity often breeds overuse. Many hospitals cannot perform a cesarean at all times within thirty minutes of making the decision, as recommended by the American College of Obstetricians and Gynecologists (ACOG).	Most, though not all, problems can be resolved on-site. Medications and equipment to treat or stabilize emergencies are kept on-site. Accreditation criteria require emergency protocols, drills, and formal hospital backup arrangements. Most birth centers can meet ACOG's thirty-minute "decision to incision" recommendation.	Most, though not all, problems can be resolved on-site. Home birth practitioners should carry medications and equipment to treat or stabilize emergencies. Some homes may be too far from a hospital to meet ACOG's thirty-minute "decision to incision" recommendation.

(continued)

	HOSPITAL	FREESTANDING BIRTH CENTER	HOME
Infection:	Infection with antibiotic-resistant organisms is an ineradicable risk because of the mix of numerous staff, sick patients, surgical patients, and central nurseries.	Infection, especially with antibiotic-resistant organisms, is extremely unlikely because freestanding birth centers lack the characteristics that foster infections.	Safest of all environments with regard to infection.
Social dynamic:	Institutional and bureaucratic. It's their territory and their rules. Policies are "one size fits all" and designed to process diverse people as efficiently and economically as possible.	It's their territory, but the hallmark of freestanding birth centers is individualized, supportive care.	It's your territory and everyone present is your invited guest. You and your needs are the sole focus of attention.
Hassle factor:	May be high if you want a midwifery-style childbirth in an obstetric-management hospital.	Birth centers are more accepted than home birth, so there is less hassle for planning a birth there. Birth centers should have standing arrangements with a hospital, so hassle is less likely for transferees than for home birthers.	May be high in pregnancy because society deems home birth irresponsible. May be very high if you or your baby require hospital admission during labor or after the birth.

(continued)

	HOSPITAL	FREESTANDING BIRTH CENTER	HOME
Staffing patterns:	May be understaffed or using staff with low-level training in place of RNs. Often difficult to get what you need when you want it. You will be alone most of the time. If the birth attendant is an M.D., he or she is usually not on-site until the time of the birth.	Accreditation criteria stipulate that no mother should be left by herself.	One-on-one care from your birth attendant. May be more than one attendant, especially around the time of birth.
Ambience:	Varies. Often noisy, impersonal, lack of privacy, intrusions by strangers. Homelike hospital birth is an oxymoron.	Varies. Usually peaceful, intimate, homelike, and without the need to worry about cleaning up or what neighbors might hear.	All the comforts and familiarity of home and no strangers. However, someone must take care of housekeeping, cooking, and laundry.
Pain control:	Drugs available and used as the primary modality. Some nondrug techniques such as showers or whirlpool baths may be available.	Narcotics rarely available, epidurals never. A wide variety of nondrug techniques are used. May have equipment such as whirlpool baths not found in the typical home.	Drugs not available. A wide variety of nondrug techniques used. In addition, the comfort and familiarity of home reduce stress and anxiety, important sources of labor distress.

(continued)

	HOSPITAL	FREESTANDING BIRTH CENTER	HOME
Breastfeeding friendliness:	Baby is usually separated from you at least some of the time. Rooming-in rules can be a problem, as can staff giving newborns pacifiers and bottles of water or formula. Nurses may not know how to assist breastfeeding mothers. Some hospitals have trained lactation consultants available.	Baby is never separated from you. Bottles and pacifiers are not an issue.	Baby is never separated from you. Bottles and pacifiers are not an issue.
Convenience:	You have to pack up and go elsewhere in labor.	You have to pack up and go elsewhere in labor.	Barring complications, everything comes to you.

COMPARING DIRECT-ENTRY MIDWIVES AND NURSE-MIDWIVES

A few obstetricians and family practitioners attend births at freestanding birth centers, but virtually none attend home births, which makes out-of-hospital birth almost exclusively midwife territory. Nurse-midwives predominate at freestanding birth centers, and direct-entry midwives predominate at home births. (See page 191 for the differences between the two.)

You cannot make any hard-and-fast rules about this, but because nurse-midwives have had to go through nursing training, they are more likely to have assimilated the medical model of childbirth. And as nurse-midwifery has become more accepted, more nurses have trained as midwives simply as a career move, not because they have a commitment to a particular philosophy of birth. As a result, some nurse-midwives have medication and procedure rates that rival those of typical obstetricians. On the other hand, direct-entry midwives tend to be more "counter-culture," which at its extreme can make them unsafe practitioners. There has been a movement in recent years to meet in the middle. The American College of Nurse-Midwives has begun giving more support and validation to home birth, while the North American Registry of Midwives has developed certification criteria to verify competency among direct-entry midwives. Also, the Midwifery Education Accreditation Council accredits direct-entry midwifery training programs. (See also chapter 12.)

INTERVIEW QUESTIONS

HOSPITAL

These questions will help you choose a hospital that can handle emergencies and that has family-friendly policies.

- *Do you have twenty-four-hour in-house obstetrician, anesthesiologist, and pediatric coverage and twenty-four-hour blood bank availability?* The major advantage of the hospital is its ability to respond rapidly in an emergency. If the hospital does not have these things, it does not have this ability.
- *What is your RN-to-patient ratio? How many women are admitted to the unit at present and how many RNs are currently on duty?* It should be one-to-one for women in active labor. If no one—or, at least, no one competent to spot trouble—is keeping an eye on you, all the technology in the world won't make a difference if something goes wrong. The second question will help you determine if there is a gap between policy and reality.

- *What level nursery do you have?* A Level III nursery is an intensive care unit capable of caring for the sickest and smallest babies. A Level II nursery can care for newborns with moderate problems and stabilize very sick babies for transport. You want at least a Level II nursery or you are not getting what you chose the hospital for.

- *What is your cesarean rate? What is your vaginal birth after cesarean (VBAC) rate?* These numbers tell you about the hospital's overall climate and birth philosophy. Refusal to give you these numbers is a red flag. The cesarean rate should lie within a few percentage points on either side of 10 percent, although you will be hard put to find a hospital with cesarean rates this low. The VBAC rate should be 70 percent or better. Don't buy the argument that the cesarean rate is high because the hospital handles high-risk cases or has a newborn intensive care unit. Data show that cesarean rates have little to do with these factors.

- *What are your routine policies for laboring women?* As discussed in earlier chapters, continuous routine electronic fetal monitoring, IVs, and forbidding oral intake are bad ideas.

- *What percentage of women have an epidural for labor?* You want epidurals to be available, of course, but if nearly all women have epidurals, it tells you a lot about the attitude toward natural childbirth.

- *Do you have showers, tubs, or whirlpool baths available for laboring women?* This is a touchstone for whether the hospital has a commitment to natural childbirth. Deep tub baths in particular have been called the "midwife's epidural."

- *Can I labor, give birth, recover, and spend my postpartum stay all in the same room? Under what circumstances would that not be possible?* Many hospitals have converted to single-room maternity care. Being moved at the point of giving birth is disruptive and distressing.

- *How many people may be with me and under what circumstances would I be separated from them?* Ideally, the answer should be "It's up to you" and "Never, unless they are caus-ing a problem," including during a C-section.

- *What is your rooming-in policy for babies, and under what circumstances would my baby be separated from me?* You should be able to keep a healthy baby with you at any and all times from the moment of birth, including after a C-section.

- *What are your routine newborn-care policies?* You should be able to delay putting ointment in the baby's eyes, and, al-though this is now generally the case, they should use anti-biotic cream, not silver nitrate, which is both extremely irritating and ineffective. A breastfed baby should not be given any bottles or pacifiers, as they can interfere with learn-ing to breastfeed.

- *What assistance is available for breastfeeding mothers? Is this hospital certified as "Baby Friendly"?* See page 349 for in-formation about the World Health Organization's "Baby-Friendly Initiative."

FREESTANDING BIRTH CENTER

The National Association of Childbearing Centers recommends that you ask the following questions:

- *Is the center licensed by the state?* This means it meets safety and health standards for medical facilities; for example, Cal-ifornia licensing regulations require gurney-accessible birth-ing rooms, which ensures that a woman can be readily moved under emergency conditions.

- *Is the center accredited by the Commission for the Accredi-tation of Birth Centers?* If the answer is yes, the center fol-lows the national standards for birth centers, which means, among other things, that the center is prepared to handle emergencies.

- *Are birth attendants licensed health care providers?* The state licenses health care providers. Some states do not license direct-entry midwives. Unfortunately, since one of the accreditation criteria is having licensed birth attendants, this means that accredited centers cannot use direct-entry midwives in states that do not license them.

- *What are the arrangements for care if complications arise that require care by an obstetrician or admission to a hospital?*
- *How long have your birth attendants been attending out-of-hospital births?* Studies show that transfer rates into the hospital drop as birth center practitioners become more confident and comfortable with out-of-hospital birth.
- *What percentage of your clients become ineligible for the birth center during pregnancy (antenatal transfer rate)? What percentage of women or babies are transferred to the hospital during labor or after the birth (intrapartum and postpartum maternal and infant transfer rates)?* Some birth centers are far more restrictive than they need to be. See page 315 for the range of transfer rates.
- *What pain management options are available?*

HOME BIRTH

- *What is your background and training? Are you certified?* Certification does not guarantee you somebody wonderful, nor does lack of certification necessarily mean lesser qualifications, but it is a benchmark of achievement. (See page 191.)
- *What equipment and medications do you carry to the birth?*
- *What problems are you prepared to deal with at home and which ones require hospital transfer?*
- *What are the arrangements for care if complications arise that require care by an obstetrician or admission to a hospital?*
- *What is your role once I transfer into the hospital?* Your caregiver may continue to participate in your care, may continue on as labor support only, or may withdraw.

ADVICE IF YOU DECIDE ON AN OUT-OF-HOSPITAL BIRTH

- *You must accept that your or your baby's condition may require a move into the hospital.* As many as one-third of the women who start off planning out-of-hospital birth in early pregnancy end up having their baby in the hospital or transferring there after birth. Most of these will be first-time mothers. Kitty Ernst, past director of the National Association of Childbearing Centers, says a transfer in labor is not necessarily a disadvantage. Many women choose a birth center because they want to avoid unnecessary intervention. (This is equally true of women choosing home birth.) When they are part of the decision-making process, the transfer becomes an acknowledgment that intervention is now appropriate and necessary.

- *You must be psychologically committed to natural childbirth and prepared to cope with labor without pain medication.* Few birth centers offer narcotics, and none offer epidurals because their potential complications demand the resources of a hospital. Neither would be available at a home birth. However, this is a case of "I think I can, I think I can." A study showed that the likelihood of unmedicated birth depended on the woman's confidence in her ability to cope with labor without drugs.

- *Consider having an ultrasound scan in the third trimester to rule out problems in the baby that may require hospital facilities at birth and breech presentation (the baby is buttocks, knees, or feet down instead of head down).*

GLEANINGS FROM THE MEDICAL LITERATURE
(PAGES 307–318)

- Planned home birth with a trained attendant is safe for low-risk women.

- Birth in a freestanding birth center is safe for low-risk women, provided the center has the staff and resources to handle an emergency.
- Studies show no differences in outcomes between direct-entry midwives and nurse-midwives.
- Out-of-hospital birth attendants achieve equally good outcomes with less use of potentially problem-causing drugs and procedures, especially cesarean section.
- In-hospital practitioners tend to see problems that aren't there.
- The superior outcomes achieved outside the hospital are not because those women are at lower risk or in any way special or different from women planning hospital births.
- Hospital management may increase fetal and newborn complication rates.
- Risk-out and transfer rates vary markedly among studies, but home birth rates generally are lower than freestanding birth center rates.
- Out-of-hospital birth attendants are more likely to use comfort measures.
- Women prefer midwifery-style, homelike care.

Appendices

⸻⸻

LITERATURE SUMMARIES

Chapter 2
The Full-Term Breech Baby:
Cesarean Section Is Not the Only Answer

EXTERNAL CEPHALIC VERSION

Moxibustion is effective.

Researchers randomly assigned 260 first-time mothers with breech babies at thirty-three weeks of pregnancy to daily or twice daily moxibustion treatment or not.[3] Two weeks later, three-quarters of babies had turned head down in the treated group versus half of the untreated group. Excluding women who subsequently had ECV, three-quarters of the treated group were still head down at birth versus just over 60 percent of the untreated group. Moxibustion is believed to work by increasing the baby's activity, and in fact, babies in the treatment group moved signficantly more often as recorded during a daily one-hour observation period.

ECV is safe.

I have twenty-six reports on ECV totalling 3,700 women.[2,4–5,7–8,10,13-14,17–34] There were only two reported instances of ECV complications leading to cesarean section.[17–18]

ECV is effective.

An analysis of data pooled from six trials in which women were randomly assigned to ECV or not found that ECV reduced the chance of having a breech baby at the birth by 60 percent and halved the cesarean rate.[15] Among twenty-six ECV studies, success rates ranged from 40 percent to 80 percent.

Attempting ECV earlier in the last trimester and repeating it if necessary can also be safe and may have a higher success rate.

Three studies in which women underwent ECV reported no complications in over 1,000 women having more than 1,450 ECV attempts, although, of course, not all of the attempts took place before thirty-five weeks. One study reported a 97 percent success rate overall.[28] The other two reported success rates in three-quarters or more of attempts made before thirty-seven weeks, dropping to half of attempts in one study and two-thirds of attempts in the other when done later.[17,30]

Strategies to increase the odds of success include turning a posterior baby (the baby is facing your belly) to anterior (the baby is facing your back) by getting on your hands and knees and "buzzing" a baby that is lying in the midline so that it startles and moves off the midline.

Three studies found associations between ECV failure and posterior baby.[6,9,12] "Posterior baby" can be fixed. Researchers randomly assigned eighty full-term pregnant women with posterior babies to assume the hands-and-knees position for ten minutes and twenty women, the control group, to upright in a chair.[1] In the control group no baby rotated to anterior versus three-quarters of the other hands-and-knees groups.

In sixteen women, two attempts at ECV failed apparently because their babies lay on the midline.[16] Researchers applied an electronic larynx to the women's bellies to startle the babies with a loud noise, a technique also used in tests of fetal well-being. All sixteen babies moved off to one side. A repeat ECV then succeeded in fifteen of the sixteen women.

Medication to relax the uterus (tocolytics) is not essential.

Of five trials of ECV without tocolytics, all concluded that they were not required for success, and two concluded that tocolytics offered no advantages.[4,10,21,29–30]

Uterine scar may not be a contraindication to ECV.

Two studies of external cephalic version in women with a uterine scar found no untoward effects, but they totaled only sixty-seven women.[11,31] A third included three women with prior cesareans, making the total seventy.[18] This isn't enough cases to draw a conclusion about safety, but common sense says that a gentle attempt to turn the baby shouldn't overstress a uterine cesarean scar.

ECV can be attempted in labor.

Several studies report attempting ECV in labor, although together they total only thirty-four women.[5,8,12,17]

VAGINAL BREECH BIRTH

Most of the poor outcomes in breech babies have nothing to do with birth route.

A recent study of the risk factors for breech presentation revealed that premature birth, low birth weight, *hydrocephalus* (skull swollen with excess fluid), and malformed infant were associated with increased risk of breech presentation.[53]

Raw statistics make cesarean look like the better bet because infants who die before birth or who are thought to be unlikely to survive birth are more likely to be born vaginally. For example, one study analyzed outcomes in 1,600 breech infants weighing more than 2lbs. at birth.[52] Mortality rates during labor and the first month afterward did not differ for vaginally born versus cesarean delivered infants. However, mortality rates in late pregnancy through the first week after birth (*perinatal mortality*) favored cesarean section because breech infants that died before labor were more likely to be born vaginally. Two analyses, of 400 and 850 breech births, respectively, concluded that cesarean section did not improve outcomes once birth weight, prematurity, and inborn abnormalities were taken into account.[37,54] Finally, three follow-up studies of infants eighteen months old or more all concluded that long-term handicap didn't relate to birth route either.[43–44,55]

Several studies have concluded that performing cesareans for breeches did not improve infant outcomes. One compared outcomes at the same hospital during an earlier period when less than one-quarter of breech babies were cesarean deliveries and a later one when nearly all breeches were cesareans.[48] The change did not affect death or injury rates in breech infants. A study of 102,000 births, of which 3,800 were breeches, found no correlation between deaths around the time of birth and cesarean rate.[35] A third study looked at outcomes in over 1,200 breech infants who weighed over 2 lbs. at birth, were normally formed, and lived until hospital discharge.[42] Complication rates did not differ between cesarean born and vaginally born infants. Finally, a fourth study found that in 57,800 infants, breech mortality exceeded head-down mortality at every gestational age, but cesarean section did not help.[58] Breech mortality was higher regardless of birth route.

Vaginal breech birth is a reasonable choice.

Because adverse breech outcomes among healthy, mature infants are so rare, it would take thousands of cases to show whether routine cesarean is better. Individual trials of vaginal breech haven't been large enough to draw conclusions. Two analyses pooled data from nine trials and twenty-four trials respectively in an attempt to settle the question.[39,46] Both concluded that cesareans have an edge over vaginal birth in protecting breech babies from deaths and complications.

However, these analyses have their own drawbacks. In the larger pooled data analysis, the overall death rate for planned vaginal births calculates as 1 baby per 1,000, but one of the trials reported a vaginal-birth infant mortality rate of 66 per 1,000, skewing the outcome. In the smaller pooled data study, the mortality rate was 4 babies per 1,000 planned vaginal births, but six of the seven deaths occurred in one trial. Are these striking variations due to chance or to how breech was managed at a particular site?

You also cannot tell from statistics alone whether the death was truly attributable to birth route. In an Israeli series of 850 breech births, two babies in the planned vaginal delivery group died.[57] One died of meconium aspiration (the baby passes stool into the amniotic fluid and inhales it at birth, causing a type of pneumonia) after an uneventful vaginal birth, and in the other case, a cesarean section was performed in early labor when a sonogram revealed the baby to be an undiagnosed "stargazer," a baby whose head is tipped back. The delivery was traumatic and the baby was born in poor condition, dying a month later. In neither instance does the labor seem responsible.

I also have a study of deaths during labor and shortly after birth among all 6,550 breech babies born at or near full term during 1991 and 1992 in Sweden.[51] After excluding congenital malformations, the death rate was 2 out of 2,250 or 1 per 1,000 in vaginally born babies, again, the same as in the pooled studies. However, neither baby had electronic fetal monitoring (EFM) and both babies were thought to be in distress during pushing. EFM might have allowed earlier diagnosis and a timely cesarean.

I have ten studies comprising 1,800 women who labored with a full-term breech baby.[36,40–41,45,47,49,56–57,59–60] Two babies died who might have lived had the mother had a cesarean, making a birth-route related mortality rate of 1 per 1,000 vaginal breech births.[47,56] However, one of these deaths occurred because a woman became hysterical during an otherwise uncomplicated birth, and the baby died before doctors could get her under general anesthesia. Fifteen babies in the planned vaginal birth group sustained a birth injury for a rate of 8 per 1,000 vaginal breech births. These injuries were damage to the complex of nerves and blood vessels in the neck that controls the arm (*brachial plexus* injury or *Erb's palsy*), broken bone, or cuts needing suturing. All babies with birth injuries recovered fully except one with a brachial plexus injury who was improving but was lost to follow up at one month. If you assume that baby did not regain full strength in its arm, the permanent injury rate falls to less than 1 per 1,000. While valuable, keep in mind that 1,800 women aren't enough women to show statistically significant differences, and the studies are all over the map when it comes to who got to labor, how labor was conducted, and what percentage of labors ended in a cesarean.

Cesarean section does not remove the risks of breech birth, including birth injury, and it increases maternal risk.

In the same ten studies, cited in the summary just above, no babies died among nearly 1,200 women having a planned cesarean. However, one baby died subsequent to a traumatic cesarean delivery in the "planned vaginal birth" group. Doctors discovered in early labor that the baby was a "star gazer" (head tipped back—*hyperextended* neck). The birth injury rate for babies born by planned cesarean was 8 per 1,000, the same as for vaginally born babies. All recovered.

As for mothers, 5 percent of women planning vaginal birth experienced serious complications (infection, hemorrhage, the need for transfusion, emergency hysterectomy to control hemorrhage, "hypertensive crisis," and extensive lacerations of the vagina and cervix), compared with 13 percent of women planning cesarean birth. One woman in the planned cesarean group died of an uncontrollable hemorrhage during the surgery. One woman in the planned vaginal birth group versus two women in the planned cesarean group had an emergency hysterectomy, which makes a permanent injury rate of about 1 per 1,000 versus 2 per 1,000. Most of the maternal complications in the planned vaginal birth group were in women who ended up with cesareans. Clearly, the more women giving birth vaginally, the better off they will be. However, the ideal cesarean rate from the baby's standpoint is open to debate.

First-time mothers, women carrying nonfrank breeches, and women with a prior cesarean section need not be automatically disqualified from vaginal breech birth.

Studies that include women falling into these categories do not have excessive death or complication rates.[45,47,49,56,57] However, in the case of nonfrank breeches, the numbers are too small to draw conclusions about safety.

Ultrasound estimates of fetal weight aren't very accurate.

One study concluded that fetal weight estimates in breech babies were less accurate than estimates in head-down babies.[38] Ultrasound weight estimates in head-down babies are notorious for wrongly predicting large babies (see page 230). Given this, the breech estimates must be truly dismal.

Forceps may not always be required at vaginal delivery.

Several studies have had spontaneous birth rates ranging from 18 percent to 100 percent in one small study where midwives attended the births.[45,49–50,56,59]

REFERENCES

EXTERNAL CEPHALIC VERSION

1. Andrews CM and Andrews EC. Nursing, maternal postures, and fetal position. *Nursing Res* 1983;32(6):336–341.
2. Brocks V, Philipsen T, and Secher NJ. A randomized trial of external cephalic version with tocolysis in late pregnancy. *Br J Obstet Gynaecol* 1984;91:653–656.
3. Cardini F and Weixin H. Moxibustion for correction of breech presentation: a randomized controlled trial. *JAMA* 1998;280(18):1580–1584.
4. Chung T et al. A randomized, double blind, controlled trial of tocolysis to assist external cephalic version in late pregnancy. *Acta Obstet Gynecol Scand* 1996;75(8):720–724.
5. Cook HA. Experience with external cephalic version and selective breech delivery in private practice. *Am J Obstet Gynecol* 1993;168(6 Pt 1): 1886–1890.
6. Donald WL and Barton JJ. Ultrasonography and external cephalic version at term. *Am J Obstet Gynecol* 1990;162(6):1542–1547.
7. Dyson DC, Ferguson JE, and Hensleigh P. Antepartum external cephalic version under tocolysis. *Obstet Gynecol* 1986;67(1):63–68.
8. Ferguson JE and Dyson DC. Intrapartum external cephalic version. *Am J Obstet Gynecol* 1985;152(3):297–298.

9. Ferguson JE, Armstrong MA, and Dyson DC. Maternal and fetal factors affecting success of antepartum external cephalic version. *Obstet Gynecol* 1987;70(5):722–725.

10. Fernandez CO et al. A randomized placebo-controlled evaluation of terbutaline for external cephalic version. *Obstet Gynecol* 1997;90(5):775–779.

11. Flamm BL et al. *Am J Obstet Gynecol* 1991;165(2):370–372.

12. Fortunato SJ, Mercer LJ, and Guzick DS. External cephalic version with tocolysis: factors associated with success. *Obstet Gynecol* 1988;72(1):59–62.

13. Hanss JW. The efficacy of external cephalic version and its impact on the breech experience. *Am J Obstet Gynecol* 1990;162(6):1459–1464.

14. Hofmeyr GJ. Effect of external cephalic version in late pregnancy on breech presentation and caesarean section rate: a controlled trial. *Br J Obstet Gynaecol* 1983;90:392–399.

15. Hofmeyr GJ. External cephalic version at term. In: Neilson JP, et al. (eds.) *Pregnancy and Childbirth Module of the Cochrane Database of Systematic Reviews*, updated July 1995.

16. Johnson RL et al. Fetal acoustic stimulation as an adjunct to external cephalic version. *J Reprod Med* 1995;40(10):696–698.

17. Kornman MT, Kimball KT, and Reeves KO. Preterm external cephalic version in an outpatient environment. *Am J Obstet Gynecol* 1995;172(6):1734–1741.

18. Lau TK, Kit KW, and Rogers M. Pregnancy outcome after external cephalic version for breech presentation at term. *Am J Obstet Gynecol* 1997;176(1 Pt 1):218–223.

19. Mahomed K, Seeras R, and Coulson R. External cephalic version at term. A randomized trial using tocolysis. *Br J Obstet Gynaecol* 1991;98:8–13.

20. Marchik R. Antepartum external cephalic version with tocolysis: a study of term singleton breech presentations. *Am J Obstet Gynecol* 1988;158(6 Pt 1):1339–1346.

21. Marquette GP et al. Does the use of a tocolytic agent affect the success rate of external cephalic version? *Am J Obstet Gynecol* 1996;175(4 Pt 1):859–861.

22. Mauldin JG et al. Determining the clinical efficacy and cost savings of successful external cephalic version. *Am J Obstet Gynecol* 1996;175(6):1639–1644.

23. Megory E et al. Mode of delivery following external cephalic version and induction of labor at term. *Am J Perinatol* 1995;12(6):404–406.

24. Morrison JC et al. External cephalic version of the breech presentation under tocolysis. *Am J Obstet Gynecol* 1986;154(4):900–903.

25. Newman RB et al. Predicting success of external cephalic version. *Am J Obstet Gynecol* 1993;169(2 Pt 1):245–250.

26. O'Grady JP et al. External cephalic version: a clinical experience. *J Perinat Med* 1986;14(3):189–196.

27. Rabinovici J et al. Impact of a protocol for external cephalic version under tocolysis at term. *Isr J Med Sci* 1986;22(1):34–40.

28. Ranney B. The gentle art of external cephalic version. *Am J Obstet Gynecol* 1973;116:239–248.
29. Robertson AW et al. External cephalic version at term: is a tocolytic necessary? *Obstet Gynecol* 1987;70(6):896–899.
30. Scaling ST. External cephalic version without tocolysis. *Am J Obstet Gynecol* 1988;158(6 Pt 1):1424–1430.
31. Schacter M, Kogan S, and Blickstein I. External cephalic version after previous cesarean section—a clinical dilemma. *Int J Gynaecolog Obstet* 1994;45(1):17–20.
32. Stine LE et al. Update on external cephalic version performed at term. *Obstet Gynecol* 1985;65(5):642–646.
33. Van Dorsten JP, Schifrin BS, and Wallace RL. Randomized control trial of external cephalic version with tocolysis in late pregnancy. *Am J Obstet Gynecol* 1981;141(N 4):417–424.
34. Van Veelen AJ et al. Effect of external cephalic version in late pregnancy on presentation at delivery: a randomized controlled trial. *Br J Obstet Gynaecol* 1989;96(8):916–921.

BREECH BIRTH

35. Acien P. Breech presentation in Spain, 1992: a collaborative study. *Eur J Obstet Gynecol Reprod Biol* 1995;62(1):19–24.
36. Bingham P, Hird V, and Lilford RJ. Management of the mature selected breech presentation: an analysis based on the intended method of delivery. *Br J Obstet Gynaecol* 1987;94(8):746–752.
37. Brown L, Karrison T, and Cibils LA. Mode of delivery and perinatal results in breech presentation. *Am J Obstet Gynecol* 1994;171(1):28–34.
38. Chauhan SP et al. Sonographic assessment of birth weight among breech presentations. *Ultrasound Obstet Gynecol* 1995;6(1):54–57.
39. Cheng M and Hannah M. Breech delivery at term: a critical review of the literature. *Obstet Gynecol* 1993;82(4 Pt 1):605–618.
40. Christian SS et al. Vaginal breech delivery: a five-year prospective evaluation of a protocol using computed tomographic pelvimetry. *Am J Obstet Gynecol* 1990;163(3):848–855.
41. Collea JV, Chein C, and Quilligan EJ. The randomized management of term frank breech presentation: a study of 208 cases. *Am J Obstet Gynecol* 1980;137(2):235–244.
42. Croughan-Minihane MS et al. Morbidity among breech infants according to method of delivery. *Obstet Gynecol* 1990;75(5):821–825.
43. Danielian PJ, Wang J, and Hall MH. Long-term outcome by method of delivery of fetuses in breech presentation at term: population based follow up. *BMJ* 1996;312(7044):1451–1453.
44. Faber-Nijholt R et al. Neurological follow-up of 281 children born in breech presentation: a controlled study. *Br Med J* 1983;286:9–12.
45. Flanagan TA et al. Management of term breech presentation. *Am J Obstet Gynecol* 1987;156(6):1492–1502.

46. Gifford DS et al. A meta-analysis of infant outcomes after breech delivery. *Obstet Gynecol* 1995;85(6):1047–1054.

47. Gimovsky ML et al. Randomized management of the nonfrank breech presentation at term. *Am J Obstet Gynecol* 1983;146(1):34–40.

48. Green JE et al. Has an increased cesarean rate for term breech delivery reduced the incidence of birth asphyxia, trauma, and death? *Am J Obstet Gynecol* 1982;142(6 Pt 1):643–648.

49. Laros RK, Flanagan TA, and Kilpatrick SJ. Management of term breech presentation: a protocol of external cephalic version and selective trial of labor. *Am J Obstet Gynecol* 1995;172(6):1916–1923.

50. Lieberman JR et al. Breech presentation and cesarean section in term nulliparous women. *Eur J Obstet Gynecol Reprod Biol* 1995;61(2): 1111–1115.

51. Lindqvist A, Norden-Lindeberg S, and Hanson U. Perinatal mortality and route of delivery in breech presentations. *Br J Obstet Gynaecol* 1997;104:1288–1291.

52. Petitti DB and Golditch, IM. Mortality in relation to method of delivery in breech infants. *Int J Gynaecol Obstet* 1984;22:189–193.

53. Rayl J, Gibson PJ, and Hickok DE. A population-based case-control study of risk factors for breech presentation. *Am J Obstet Gynecol* 1996; 174(1 Pt 1):28–32.

54. Rosen MG and Chik L. The effect of delivery route on outcome in breech presentation. *Am J Obstet Gynecol* 1984;148(7):909–914.

55. Rosen MG et al. Long-term neurological morbidity in breech and vertex births. *Am J Obstet Gynecol* 1985;151(6):718–720.

56. Roumen FJ and Luyben AG. Safety of term vaginal breech delivery. *Eur J Obstet Gynecol Reprod Biol* 1991;40(3):171–177.

57. Schiff E et al. Maternal and neonatal outcome of 846 term singleton breech deliveries: seven-year experience at a single center. *Am J Obstet Gynecol* 1996;175(1):18–23.

58. Schutte MF et al. Perinatal mortality in breech presentations as compared to vertex presentations in singleton pregnancies: an analysis based upon 57819 computer-registered pregnancies in the Netherlands. *Eur J Obstet Gynecol Reprod Biol* 1985;19(6):391–400.

59. Stein A. A cooperative nurse-midwifery medical management approach. *J Nurse-Midwifery* 1986;31(2):93–97.

60. Watson WJ and Benson WL. Vaginal delivery for the selected frank breech infant at term. *Obstet Gynecol* 1984;64(5):638–640.

Chapter 3
Induction of Labor:
Mother Nature Knows Best

Nipple stimulation, castor oil, acupuncture, and TENS stimulation have all been found effective at ripening the cervix and/or inducing contractions, and sexual intercourse increases the local concentration of prostaglandins involved in initiating labor.

Nipple Stimulation: Researchers in two studies, of 100 and 200 women, respectively, randomly assigned women to perform breast stimulation three times a day in 1-hour sessions or to avoid sexual intercourse and breast stimulation.[25,67] Both concluded that nipple stimulation could ripen the cervix and bring on labor. The smaller study used electronic fetal monitoring during the first stimulation session and found no uterine hyperstimulation.

A study randomly assigned sixty-two women to induction of labor using an electric breast pump or to oxytocin induction.[12] Nipple stimulation substantially reduced the times from onset of stimulation to having three contractions in ten minutes, achieving contraction pressures sufficient for dilation, and achieving active phase labor. Three women had induction failures in the breast pump group versus four in the oxytocin group; however, one of the three in the breast pump group had had breast reduction surgery. Nearly half the women in the oxytocin group had cesareans versus one-quarter of the breast pump group. Five women using the breast pump complained of soreness, which was relieved by turning down the pump suction. A sixth woman asked that the breast pump be discontinued. No woman using the breast pump experienced skin injury. An even more promising study used mild electrical (TENS) nipple stimulation to induce labor in twenty-one women.[76] Fifteen achieved progressive labor. The six who didn't had unripe cervixes. No woman experienced nipple discomfort. Uterine hyperstimulation in five women was easily corrected by adjusting the TENS unit.

Castor Oil: A researcher compared outcomes in 196 women with ruptured membranes, of whom 107 took castor oil and 89 simply waited for labor.[17] Seventy-five percent of first-time mothers taking castor oil began labor spontaneously, versus 60 percent of control first-time mothers. However, 75 percent of the women with prior births in both groups began labor spontaneously. More women whose labors started with castor oil subsequently needed oxytocin to strengthen labor than women whose labors began spontaneously (14 percent versus 2 percent). The cesarean rate was 6 percent in the castor oil group versus 16 percent in the await labor group.

Acupuncture and TENS: Labor induction with acupuncture using electrically stimulated needles succeeded in 85 percent of thirty-four women induced for postdates pregnancy.[79] Fourteen percent of the twenty-nine successful inductions ended in cesarean section. Researchers in another study delivered electrical stimulation to acupuncture points via the pads of a TENS unit.[22] The researchers compared results in ten women receiving TENS stimulation and ten in whom the unit was attached, but not turned on. After two hours of stimulation, nine of ten women receiving TENS showed an increase in contraction frequency versus three of the control women, and women receiving TENS were more likely to experience labor-strength contractions.

Sexual Intercourse: A study of prostaglandin concentrations in cervical mucus during pregnancy found that concentrations increased ten- to fifty-fold above baseline two to four hours after intercourse.[77] Prostaglandins ripen the cervix and can induce labor.

Oxytocin, especially in the quantities required for induction of labor, has risks.

Uterine hyperstimulation is a common and potentially serious problem with induction because hyperstimulation can cause fetal distress, which, if not promptly treated, can lead to brain damage and death. I have ten studies comparing oxytocin regimens that report hyperstimulation rates.[7,16,30,40,47,55,58–59,64,69] At the lower oxytocin dose, hyperstimulation rates ranged from 2 percent to 60 percent, and six of the studies reported rates of 15 percent or more. At the higher dose, hyperstimulation rates ranged from 13 percent to 63 percent, and half reported that one-quarter or more of the women experienced hyperstimulation. Four of these studies reported fetal distress rates.[40,47,55,68] One reported an 8 percent rate at the lower dose; the rest reported rates ranging from 15 percent to 54 percent. Another study looked at factors associated with low blood pH at birth, an indication of oxygen deprivation in labor, and found that having oxytocin doubled the odds.[37]

Increasing oxytocin dose also correlates with increasing postpartum blood loss, although some of this effect could be due to diluting the blood with IV fluid, which can interfere with clotting. A study of 111 women found that postpartum hematocrit values, a measure of anemia, declined with duration of oxytocin use and greater maximal dose.[28] Another study compared labor characteristics in 86 women who experienced postpartum hemorrhage with 351 women with normal blood loss.[27] One-quarter of the induced group had a postpartum hemorrhage versus 5 percent of women not induced. Researchers in a third study found that among ninety women with five or more previous pregnancies undergoing induction, nearly 25 percent hemorrhaged after birth on a regimen where the oxytocin dose was doubled every fifteen minutes versus less than 10 percent of those whose dose doubled every forty-five minutes.[60]

Two studies have shown oxytocin use was associated with newborn jaundice and that the more oxytocin used, the greater the chance of jaundice.[11,20] This could partly be due to using salt-free IV fluids to deliver oxytocin. Salt-free IV fluid increases fluid retention (see page 241). Fluid retention causes jaundice because excess water outside cells causes water to flow into red blood cells (*osmotic pressure*), making them stiffer and more liable to damage. The newborn cannot process the excess destroyed red blood cells, and one circulating breakdown product, *bilirubin*, makes the body look yellow or jaundiced. However, oxytocin also plays a role. A third study found that newborns of induced mothers had more red blood cell destruction than the infants of women laboring spontaneously or having planned C-sections (these women would have had IVs too), and also that the red blood cells were less flexible.[9] Finally, a study found that independent of amount of IV fluid, oxytocin increased the odds of symptoms of fluid overload but only when given in quantity such as would happen in an induction.[73]

Physiological oxytocin-induction regimens offer advantages over high-dose regimens.

I have ten studies comparing oxytocin regimens that report hyperstimulation rates.[7,16,30,40,47,55,58-59,64,69] They vary in design, but all have a group receiving a lower peak dose and/or less oxytocin overall. In every case but one, uterine hyperstimulation was less common in the lower-dose group. In that one case, the difference was trivial.[64]

Four studies report fetal distress rates.[40,47,55,68] In all four, fetal distress was less common in the lower-dose group. Still, the rates are all alarmingly high, ranging from 8 percent to 34 percent in the lower-dose group and 18 percent to 54 percent in the higher-dose group. While the reasons for inducing labor might explain some cases of fetal distress, it is unlikely that they could explain all or even most of the excess.

I also have eleven comparison studies reporting cesarean rates.[16,30,40,47,55,58-59,64,68-69,83] Cesarean rates range from 3 percent to 26 percent in the lower-dose group and from 4 percent to 24 percent in the higher-dose group. While cesarean rates do not favor the lower dose as consistently as hyperstimulation and fetal distress rates, more studies report lower cesarean rates in the lower-dose group (eight to three).

Prostaglandins have not solved the problem of induction leading to more cesareans.

Researchers studied 600 women undergoing labor induction, all of whom had prostaglandin E2 (PGE2) treatment if the cervix wasn't ripe.[85] Thirty-three percent of first-time mothers had a cesarean when the cervical ripeness score before beginning induction was three or less (on a scale of one to ten) versus 20 percent of first-time mothers with initial scores of three or more. However, the cesarean rate was only 12 percent for women beginning labor spontaneously. Similarly, among women with previous births, cesarean rates were 29 percent with a cervical score of three or less, 15 percent with a score of three or more, but only 8 percent among women starting labor naturally.

Three analyses of multiple studies agreed that applying PGE2 before labor induction had at best a modest effect on reducing cesarean rates. One analyzed data from eighteen trials totalling 1,800 women who were randomly assigned to PGE2 or not before induction.[61] Taken all together, they found no statistically significant difference in cesarean rates. Another analyzed data from four random assignment trials totalling over 500 women and found cesarean rates of 29 percent in the PGE2 group and 33 percent in the control group, again, a difference likely to be due to chance.[78] Finally, the third analyzed data from forty-four trials totalling 3,300 women and found that the potential reduction in cesarean rate could be as little as 1 percent or as much as 30 percent with the actual reduction probably roughly halfway between.[44]

Data conflict on prostaglandin E1 (misprostol). One researcher looked at twenty-six studies of misoprostol versus oxytocin or misoprostol versus PGE2.[39] Cesarean rates ranged from a large reduction with misoprostol to no advantage. On the downside, misoprostol substantially increased the odds of uterine hyperstimulation causing fetal distress. The author speculates that the variation in cesarean rates among studies may reflect to what degree doctors responded to fetal distress with cesarean section.

Inducing labor for reasons of convenience or other nonmedical reasons (elective induction) increases the risk of cesarean and fetal distress.

A hospital compared outcomes between 250 women having elective inductions with 250 similar women who began labor spontaneously.[49] One-third of first-time mothers having elective inductions had cesareans versus about one-fifth of first-time mothers having spontaneous labors. Among first-time mothers with unripe cervixes, *half* the induced population had cesareans. Another study looked at 8,600 women and found that women having elective inductions were half again as likely to have cesareans as women whose labors began spontaneously.[41] A third study found that 30 percent of babies testing normal on fetal well-being tests developed fetal distress when labor was electively induced, and the cesarean rate was 15 percent in induced women versus 2 percent for spontaneous labors.[19] (See also page 232 "The obstetric powers that be. . . .")

Ultrasound weight estimates followed by induction for suspected large baby increases the risk of cesarean without improving outcomes.

I have six studies of outcomes for large (*macrosomic*) babies.[14,18,26,29,46,82] In one, women suspected of carrying macrosomic babies were randomly assigned to induction or not, a study design that produces the strongest evidence.[29] Every study found that induced labors resulted in more cesareans and vaginal instrumental deliveries without any compensating benefit for the baby.

Ultrasound diagnosis of macrosomia also hurts rather than helps. Five studies found that ultrasound predictions that the baby would be macrosomic were wrong one-third to one-half the time.[13–14,18,48,62] In addition, two studies looked at the effect of ultrasound diagnosis of macrosomia on outcomes.[48,82] Both found that when the obstetrician believed, based on ultrasound, that women were carrying macrosomic babies, half had C-sections versus less than one-third of women not thought to have macrosomic babies but who actually did.

Waiting for labor onset for at least twenty-four hours after membrane rupture is safe provided there are no symptoms of infection, the mother tests negative for group B strep, and no vaginal exams are done.

A study of over three hundred women with ruptured membranes for longer than twenty-four hours found that a major factor in newborn infections was length of time between vaginal exam and the birth.[70] If no vaginal exams were done, it didn't matter how long membranes were ruptured. A trial in which over five thousand women with ruptured membranes were randomly assigned to induction with either oxytocin or prostaglandin E2 gel or to await labor for four days followed by induction with one or the other method confirms this result.[35] Having a vaginal exam (the study combined manual and speculum exams) increased the risk of newborn infection. However, infection was a problem primarily among women testing positive for group B strep. Eight to 10 percent of the newborns of mothers vaginally colonized with group B strep developed infections in the await labor groups while in the immediate oxytocin induction group, the rate was 3 percent, the same rate as among women testing negative for group B strep. It may be that vaginal exams are the key factor in starting newborn infections in group B strep carriers. They could do this by transporting the bacteria up to and even into the cervix.

Vaginal examinations also increased the odds of uterine infection in this same large study.[71] The odds of developing a uterine infection went up along with the number of vaginal exams. Women having more than eight vaginal exams have five times the odds of uterine infection compared with women having fewer than three. Multiple vaginal exams were a much more important risk factor in uterine infection than testing positive for group B strep. Another study also found strong associations between vaginal exams, ruptured membranes, and time.[74] When membranes were ruptured twelve hours or less before birth, the maternal infection rate was 3 percent in women having four or fewer vaginal exams versus 9 percent in the group having more than four. If membranes were ruptured longer than twelve hours, the infection rate in women having four or fewer vaginal exams was virtually unchanged at 4 percent, but among women having more than four, it jumped to 20 percent.

I have twelve studies comparing induction with oxytocin after a longer versus a shorter time that reported newborn infection rates.[1,21,31,34,50,52–53,63,66,72,80–81] Eleven of the twelve randomly assigned women to one group or the other, a strategy that provides the strongest evidence. In the large study mentioned above, over 2,500 women were assigned to the oxytocin induction versus await labor arm of the trial. Most studies found little or no difference in newborn infection rates, including this big one. Infection rates ranged from 0 percent to 5 percent in the groups allowed longer times before induction and from 0 percent to 4 percent among women induced shortly after membrane rupture, except for one study where the rate was 12 percent.

Finally, researchers analyzed data from twenty-three trials, totalling 7,500 women, in which women were randomly assigned to various strategies for management of prelabor rupture of membranes at term.[54] They concluded that newborn infections would be reduced from 2 per 100 to 1 per 100 with immediate induction of labor with oxytocin compared with awaiting labor, but that this would increase cesarean deliveries from about 9 per 100 to 11 per 100.

Inducing with oxytocin shortly after membrane rupture may greatly increase the odds of C-section compared with awaiting labor.

I have sixteen studies comparing induction with oxytocin after a longer versus a shorter time that report cesarean rates.[1, 21,31,34,38,42,45,50,52–53,56,63,66,72, 80–81] Fourteen of the sixteen studies randomly assigned women to one group or the other. Seven of them reported that early induction tripled or quadrupled the chances of C-section while the rest reported similar cesarean rates, including a comparison involving over 2,500 women.

Inducing with PGE2 shortly after membrane rupture results in similar cesarean rates to those for awaiting labor, but it doesn't decrease infection rates.

An analysis of pooled data from fifteen studies comparing awaiting labor with induction with PGE2 found no differences in cesarean rates or newborn infection rates.[32] Since PGE2 increases the incidence of uterine hyperstimulus, this means there are no advantages and a possible disadvantage to using PGE2 compared with awaiting the onset of labor.

The obstetric powers that be have decided that labor should be routinely induced at forty-one weeks, but the situation is not nearly as clear-cut as it seems.

The bible for evidence-based care is the *Cochrane Database of Systematic Reviews*, an ongoing series of analyses (*meta-analyses*) of data from multiple *randomized controlled trials*, that is, trials in which participants are randomly assigned to the treatment under study or to standard care (control group). The meta-analysis covering postdates management looks at nineteen trials comparing routine induction at a particular time with awaiting labor either indefinitely or for some longer period of time.[15] It concludes that when the due date is known, pregnancy should be routinely induced at forty-one weeks because such a policy would reduce the number of babies that die shortly before, during, or after birth (*perinatal mortality rate*) without increasing the cesarean rate. However, I think both parts of this statement can be challenged.

To begin with, closer examination reveals a narrower gap in perinatal mortality with routine induction at forty-one weeks than would appear at first glance. Among the nineteen studies, 9 babies among 3,800 women died shortly before, during, or after labor in the await labor group versus 1 baby among 4,125 women in the routine induction group, an impressive difference. However, two of the deaths in the await labor group occurred in a study of only 110 women published in 1969. This study and those deaths can be eliminated on the grounds that the obstetrics of that era and the perinatal death rates simply don't apply to modern-day care. That leaves 7 perinatal deaths in 3,750 women versus 1 in 4,050 women. This calculates to 1.9 per 1,000 babies versus 0.2 per 1,000. But two of the seven deaths occurred suddenly, prior to labor, and before forty-one weeks of pregnancy. A policy of routine induction at forty-one weeks wouldn't have prevented them. In addition, researchers in one trial attributed a death during a planned induction at forty-two weeks to ignoring fetal distress.[51] This death, then, had nothing to do with the labor occurring after forty-one weeks. In fact, given that oxytocin increases the incidence of fetal distress, the induction may have contributed to, if not caused, the death. Be that as it may, removing deaths unrelated to exceeding forty-one weeks of pregnancy reduces the number of perinatal deaths in the await labor group from seven to four. We now have a perinatal mortality rate of 1.1 per 1,000 in the await labor group versus 0.2 per 1,000 among planned inductions. A difference this small is almost surely due to chance.

As for not increasing cesarean rates, we know that labors induced with oxytocin generally have higher cesarean rates than spontaneous labors and ripening the cervix with PGE2 gel hasn't solved that problem (see page 229, "Prostaglandins have not solved the problem . . ." above). Why should postdates pregnancy be an exception to that rule?

First, the way randomized controlled trials are conducted flattened out potential differences in cesarean rates between groups. Properly done randomized trials keep participants with their assigned group regardless of what treatment they actually received. In many studies, substantial percentages of women in the await labor group were induced because the doctor or mother got tired of waiting, or a time limit was reached, or cervical ripeness score increased, or fetal tests of well-being indicated that the baby could be in trouble.[5–6,10,23–24,33,43,57,75,84] Percentages induced in the await labor groups typically exceeded 20 percent and ranged as high as 36 percent. Conversely, in several studies, substantial percentages of the women in the induction group began labor spontaneously. In four trials, including by far the largest randomized controlled trial (3,400 women when one other studied 700 women and the rest studied 400 or less), about one-third of women in the induced group began labor spontaneously before their scheduled induction.[10,23,33,84]

Several trials allow us to tease out the effect of planned induction on the cesarean rate. Of twenty women who had no medical reason for induction (*elective induction*) in one randomized trial of postdates management, nine—nearly half the inductions—ended in cesareans.[10] In another study, researchers compared cesarean rates in two hundred women who had routine inductions at forty-two weeks to two hundred women who had routine inductions at forty-three weeks.[3] After removing inductions for medical reasons, induced women were half again as likely (18 percent versus 12 percent) to have cesareans as women beginning labor spontaneously. Virtually the same difference was found in yet another study randomly assigning two hundred women to either routine induction at forty-two weeks or to await labor.[65] Cesarean rates were similar between the planned induction and await labor groups overall (16 percent versus 18 percent) but only because so many women went into labor spontaneously before their scheduled induction: seventeen out of ninety-six women, *none* of whom had cesareans. If you compare cesarean rates between all women who began labor spontaneously with all women who had planned inductions, 20 percent of those who had planned inductions had cesareans versus 13 percent of women who began labor spontaneously. (See also page 230, "Inducing labor for reasons of convenience. . . .")

The largest of the postdates management studies, the one comprising 3,400 women, doesn't allow me to separate elective from medically indicated inductions, but it provides some provocative data nonetheless. The authors did a follow-up analysis of cesarean rates within each group according to how labor actually began.[36] Among mothers in the await labor group, one in five had a cesarean if labor began spontaneously, already an indefensibly high percentage, but it rose to a whopping one in three if labor was induced. Among first-time mothers, who generally are at greater risk of cesarean section, cesarean rates went from one-fourth of women with spontaneous labors to nearly half of induced women. The cesarean rate for fetal distress was 7 percent in women induced as planned in the routine induction group, again, an appalling percentage for healthy women carrying full-term babies, but it was twice as high among women induced in the await labor group. It simply isn't credible that inherent problems of postdates in healthy women caused a doubling of cesareans for fetal distress.

This brings me to the second reason the meta-analysis didn't find more cesareans in the induction group. Obstetricians also caused an excess of cesareans in await labor groups by inducing women in response to worrisome results on tests of fetal well-being. These tests, you may recall, are much more likely to be wrong in healthy women than they are to be right, which means the baby was fine and an induction wasn't really needed in most cases. Induction in response to worrisome test results is the worst possible circumstance under which to be induced. An anxious doctor reluctant to back out if the induction doesn't work will perform a cesarean at the least little blip on the electronic fetal monitor. Even if the test was right and the baby isn't doing well, induction stresses the baby more than normal labor.

Data support my contention here too. Researchers in one study randomly assigned 145 women at forty-two weeks of pregnancy to one of two schemes of testing for fetal well-being.[2] One scheme was more likely to produce abnormal results. This more than tripled the odds of induction for this indication and doubled the odds of C-section without any improvement in newborn outcomes. And as mentioned in the induction chapter, a researcher found that complication rates at his hospital jumped from 6 percent to more than 20 percent and cesarean rates from 7 percent to more than 25 percent in week forty, the week that women reached their due date and were transferred to the high-risk clinic.[4]

The all-fours maneuver is a rapid, safe, and effective technique for relieving shoulder dystocia.

The authors report on a series of eighty-two cases of shoulder dystocia treated primarily with the all-fours maneuver and compare results with seven other series using other techniques.[8] With the all-fours maneuver, one woman experienced heavy bleeding but did not require a transfusion (1 percent complication rate), one infant had a broken arm, three infants (including the infant with the broken arm) had low 1-minute Apgar scores, a measure of condition at birth, and one infant had not fully recovered by five minutes after birth (5 percent complication rate). Sixty percent of women had no episiotomy and no tears. By contrast, in the other series, infant death rates ranged from 5 percent to 32 percent and infant complication rates ranged from 15 percent to 71 percent. In the four studies reporting maternal outcomes, complication rates ranged from 17 percent to 100 percent (all women were treated by replacing the head and performing a cesarean section in one study). One woman died and complications included transfusion and hysterectomy due to ruptured uterus.

REFERENCES

1. Alcalay M et al. Prelabour rupture of membranes at term: early induction of labour versus expectant management. *Eur J Obstet Gynecol Reprod Biol* 1996:70(2):129–133.
2. Alfirevic Z and Walkinshaw SA. A randomised controlled trial of simple compared with complex antenatal fetal monitoring after forty-two weeks of gestation. *Br J Obstet Gynaecol* 1995;102:638–643.

3. Almstrom H, Granstrom L, and Ekman G. Serial antenatal monitoring compared with labor induction in post-term pregnancies. *Acta Obstet Gynecol Scand* 1995;74:599–603.

4. Arias F. Predictability of complications associated with prolongation of pregnancy. *Obstet Gynecol* 1987;70(1):101–106.

5. Augensen K et al. Randomised comparison of early versus late induction of labour in post-term pregnancy. *Br Med J* 1987;294:1192–1195.

6. Bergsjo P et al. Comparison of induced versus non-induced labor in post-term pregnancy. A randomized prospective study. *Acta Obstet Gynecol Scand* 1989;68(8):683–687.

7. Blakemore KJ et al. A prospective comparison of hourly and quarter-hourly oxytocin dose increase intervals for the induction of labor at term. *Obstet Gynecol* 1990;75(5):757–761.

8. Bruner JP et al. All-fours maneuver for reducing shoulder dystocia during labor. *J Reprod Med* 1998;43(5):439–443.

9. Buchan PC. Pathogenesis of neonatal hyperbilirubinaemia after induction of labor with oxytocin. *Br Med J* 1979;2:1255–1257.

10. Cardozo L, Fysh J, and Pearce JM. Prolonged pregnancy: the management debate. *Br Med J* 1986;293:1059–1063.

11. Chalmers I, Campbell H, and Turnbul AC. Use of oxytocin and incidence of neonatal jaundice. *Br Med J* 1975;2:116–118.

12. Chayen B, Tejani N, and Verma U. Induction of labor with an electric breast pump. *J Reprod Med* 1986;31(2):116–118.

13. Chervenak JL et al. Macrosomia in the postdate pregnancy: is routine ultrasonographic screening indicated? *Am J Obstet Gynecol* 1989; 161(3)753–756.

14. Combs CA, Singh NB, and Khoury JC. Elective induction versus spontaneous labor after sonographic diagnosis of fetal macrosomia. *Obstet Gynecol* 1993;81(4):492–496.

15. Crowley P. Interventions to prevent, or improve outcome from, delivery at or beyond term. In: Neilson JP et al., eds. *Pregnancy and Childbirth Module of the Cochrane Database of Systematic Reviews*, updated December 1997.

16. Cummiskey KC and Dawood MY. Induction of labor with pulsatile oxytocin. *Am J Obstet Gynecol* 1990;163(6):1868–1874.

17. Davis L. The use of castor oil to stimulate labor in patients with premature rupture of membranes. *J Nurse Midwifery* 1984;29(6):366–370.

18. Delpapa EH and Mueller-Heubach E. Pregnancy outcome following ultrasound diagnosis of macrosomia. *Obstet Gynecol* 1991;78(3):340–343.

19. Devoe LD and Sholl JS. Postdates pregnancy. Assessment of fetal risk and obstetric management. *J Reprod Med* 1983;28(9):576–580.

20. D'Souza SW et al. The effect of oxytocin in induced labour on neonatal jaundice. *Br J Obstet Gynaecol* 1979;86:133–138.

21. Duff P, Huff RW, and Gibbs RS. Management of premature rupture of membranes and unfavorable cervix in term pregnancy. *Obstet Gynecol* 1984;63(5):697–701.

22. Dunn PA et al. Transcutaneous electrical nerve stimulation at acupunc-

ture points in the induction of uterine contractions. *Obstet Gynecol* 1989;73(2):286–290.

23. Dyson DC, Miller PD, and Armstrong MA. Management of prolonged pregnancy: induction of labor versus antepartum fetal testing. *Am J Obstet Gynecol* 1987;156(4):928–934.

24. Egarter C et al. Is induction of labor indicated in prolonged pregnancy?' Results of a prospective randomised trial. *Gynecol Obstet Invest* 1989; 27(1):6–9.

25. Elliott JP and Flaherty JF. The use of breast stimulation to prevent post-date pregnancy. *Am J Obstet Gynecol* 1984;149(6):628–632.

26. Friesen CD, Miller AM, and Rayburn WF. Influence of spontaneous or induced labor on delivering the macrosomic fetus. *Am J Perinatol* 1995; 12(1):63–66.

27. Gilbert L, Porter W, and Brown VA. Postpartum haemorrhage—a continuing problem. *Br J Obstet Gynaecol* 1987;94:67–71.

28. Goldberg CC et al. Effect of intrapartum use of oxytocin on estimated blood loss and hematocrit change at vaginal delivery. *Am J Perinatol* 1996;13(6):373–376.

29. Gonen O et al. Induction of labor versus expectant management in macrosomia: a randomized study. *Obstet Gynecol* 1997;89(6):913–917.

30. Goni S, Sawhney H, and Gopalan S. Oxytocin induction of labor: a comparison of 20- and 60-min dose increment levels. *Int J Gynaecol Obstet* 1995;48(1):31–36.

31. Grant JM et al. Management of prelabour rupture of the membranes in term primigravidae: a report of a randomized prospective trial. *Br J Obstet Gynaecol* 1992;99(7):557–562.

32. Hannah ME and Tan BP Prostaglandins for prelabour rupture of membranes at or near term. In: Neilson JP et al., eds. *Pregnancy and Childbirth Module of the Cochrane Database of Systematic Reviews,* updated December 1997.

33. Hannah ME et al. Induction of labor as compared with serial antenatal monitoring in post-term pregnancy. A randomized controlled trial. *N Engl J Med* 1992;326(24):1587–1592.

34. Hannah ME et al. Induction of labor compared with expectant management for prelabor rupture of the membranes at term. *N Engl J Med* 1996;334(16):1005–1010.

35. Hannah ME et al. Maternal colonization with group B streptococcus and prelabor rupture of membranes at term: the role of induction of labor. *Am J Obstet Gynecol* 1997;177(4):780–785.

36. Hannah ME et al. Postterm pregnancy: putting the merits of a policy of induction of labor into perspective. *Birth* 1996;23(1):13–19.

37. Herbst A, Wolner-Hanssen P, and Ingemarsson I. Risk factors for acidemia at birth. *Obstet Gynecol* 1997;90(1):125–130.

38. Hjertberg R et al. Premature rupture of the membranes (PROM) at term in nulliparous women with a ripe cervix. A randomized trial of 12 or 24 hours of expectant management. *Acta Obstet Gynecol Scand* 1996; 75(1):48–53.

39. Hofmeyr GJ. Misoprostol administered vaginally for cervical ripening and labour induction with a viable fetus. In: Neilson JP et al., eds. *Preg-*

nancy and Childbirth Module of the Cochrane Database of Systematic Reviews, updated December 1997.

40. Hourvitz A et al. A prospective study of high- versus low-dose oxytocin for induction of labor. *Acta Obstet Gynecol Scand* 1996;75(7):636–641.

41. Jarvelin MR, Hartikainen-Sorri AL, and Rantakallio P. Labour induction policy in hospitals of different levels of specialisation. *Br J Obstet Gynaecol* 1993;100(4):310–315.

42. Kappy KA et al. Premature rupture of the membranes at term. *J Reprod Med* 1982;27(1):29–33.

43. Katz Z et al. Non-aggressive management of post-date pregnancies. *Eur J Obstet Gynecol Reprod Biol* 1983;15:71–79.

44. Keirse MJNC. Prostaglandins in preinduction cervical ripening. Meta-analysis of worldwide clinical experience. *J Reprod Med* 1993;38(1 Suppl):89–100.

45. Ladfors L et al. A randomised trial of two expectant managements of prelabour rupture of the membranes at 34 to 42 weeks. *Br J Obstet Gynaecol* 1996;103(8):755–762.

46. Larsen JS, Pedersen OD, and Ipsen L. Induction of labor when a large fetus is suspected. *Ugeskr Laeger* 1991;153(3):181–183.

47. Lazor LZ et al. A randomized comparison of 15- and 40-minute dosing protocols for labor augmentation and induction. *Obstet Gynecol* 1993; 82(6):1009–1012.

48. Levine AB et al. Sonographic diagnosis of the large for gestational age fetus at term: does it make a difference? *Obstet Gynecol* 1992;79(1):55–58.

49. Macer JA et al. Elective induction versus spontaneous labor: a retrospective study of complications and outcome. *Am J Obstet Gynecol* 1992;166(6 Pt 1):1690–1697.

50. Marshall VA. Management of premature rupture membranes at or near term. *J Nurse Midwifery* 1993;38(3):140–145.

51. Martin DH, Thompson W, and Pinkerton JHM. A randomized controlled trial of selective planned delivery. *Br J Obstet Gynaecol* 1978; 85:109–113.

52. McCaul JF et al. Premature rupture membranes at term with an unfavorable cervix: comparison of expectant management, vaginal prostaglandin, and oxytocin induction. *South Med J* 1997;90(12):1229–1233.

53. Morales WJ and Lazar AJ. Expectant management of rupture of membranes at term. *South Med J* 1986;79(8):955–958.

54. Mozurkewich EL and Wolf FM. Premature rupture of membranes at term: a meta-analysis of three management schemes. *Obstet Gynecol* 1997;89(6):1035–1043.

55. Muller PR, Stubbs TM, and Laurent SL. A prospective randomized clinical trial comparing two oxytocin induction protocols. *Am J Obstet Gynecol* 1992;167(2):373–380.

56. Natale R et al. Management of premature rupture of membranes at term: randomized trial. *Am J Obstet Gynecol* 1994;171(4)936–939.

57. National Institute of Child Health. A clinical trial of induction of labor versus expectant management in postterm pregnancy. *Am J Obstet Gynecol* 1994;170(3):716–723.

58. Orhue AA. A randomized trial of 30-min and 15-min oxytocin infusion regimens for induction of labour at term in women of low parity. *Int J Gynaecol Obstet* 1993;40(3):219–225.

59. Orhue AAE. Incremental increases in oxytocin infusion regimens for induction of labor at term in primigravidas: a randomized controlled trial. *Obstet Gynecol* 1994;83(2):229–233.

60. Orhue AAE. A randomised trial of 45 minutes and 15 minutes incremental oxytocin infusion regimes for the induction of labour in women of high parity. *Br J Obstet Gynaecol* 1993;100:126–129.

61. Owen J et al. A randomized, double-blind trial of prostaglandin E2 gel for cervical ripening and meta-analysis. *Am J Obstet Gynecol* 1991; 165(4 Pt 1):991–996.

62. Pollack RN, Hauer-Pollack G, and Divon MY. Macrosomia in postdates pregnancies: the accuracy of routine ultrasonographic screening. *Am J Obstet Gynecol* 1992;167(1):7–11.

63. Ray DA and Garite TJ. Prostaglandin E2 for induction of labor in patients with premature rupture of membranes at term. *Am J Obstet Gynecol* 1992;166(3):836–843.

64. Reid GJ and Helewa ME. A trial of pulsatile versus continuous oxytocin administration for the induction of labor. *J Perinatol* 1995;15(5):364–366.

65. Roach VJ and Rogers MS. Pregnancy outcome beyond 41 weeks gestation. *Int J Gynaecol Obstet* 1997;59(1):19–24.

66. Rydhstrom H and Ingemarsson I. No benefit from conservative management in nulliparous women with premature rupture of the membranes (PROM) at term. A randomized study. *Acta Obstet Gynecol Scand* 1991;70(7–8):543–547.

67. Salmon YM et al. Cervical ripening by breast stimulation. *Obstet Gynecol* 1986;67(1):21–24.

68. Satin AJ et al. A prospective study of two dosing regimens of oxytocin for the induction of labor in patients with unfavorable cervices. *Am J Obstet Gynecol* 1991;165(4):980–984.

69. Satin AJ et al. High-dose oxytocin: 20- versus 40-minute dosage interval. *Obstet Gynecol* 1994;83(2):234–238.

70. Schutte MF et al. Management of premature rupture of membranes: the risk of vaginal examination to the infant. *Am J Obstet Gynecol* 1983; 146(4):395–400.

71. Seaward PG et al. International Multicentre Term Prelabor Rupture of Membranes Study: evaluation of predictors of clinical chorioamnionitis. *Am J Obstet Gynecol* 1997;177(5):1024–1029.

72. Shalev E et al. Comparison of 12- and 72-hour expectant management of premature rupture of membranes in term pregnancies. *Obstet Gynecol* 1995;85(5):766–768.

73. Singhi S et al. Iatrogenic neonatal and maternal hyponatraemia following oxytocin and aqueous glucose infusion during labor. *Br J Obstet Gynaecol* 1985;92:356–363.

74. Soper DE, Mayhall CG, and Froggatt JW. Characterization and control of intraamniotic infection in an urban teaching hospital. *Am J Obstet Gynecol* 1997;175(2):304–310.

75. Suikkari AM et al. Prolonged pregnancy: induction or observation. *Acta Obstet Gynecol Scand* 1983;116(Suppl):58.
76. Tal Z et al. Breast electrostimulation for the induction of labor. *Obstet Gynecol* 1988;72(4):671–673.
77. Toth M, Rehnstrom J, and Fuchs A-R. Prostaglandins E and F in cervical mucus of pregnant women. *Am J Perinatol* 1989;6(2):142–144.
78. Trofatter KF. Endocervical prostaglandin E2 gel for preinduction cervical ripening. Clinical trial results. *J Reprod Med* 1993;38(1 Suppl):78–82.
79. Tsuei JJ, Lai Y-F, and Sharma SD. The influence of acupuncture stimulation during pregnancy. 1977;50(4):479–488.
80. Van der Walt D and Venter PF. Management of term pregnancy with premature rupture of the membranes and unripe cervix. *S Afr Med J* 1989;75(2):54–56.
81. Wagner MV et al. A comparison of early and delayed induction of labor with spontaneous rupture of membranes at term. *Obstet Gynecol* 1989; 74(1):93–97.
82. Weeks JW, Pitman T, and Spinnato JA 2nd. Fetal macrosomia: does antenatal prediction affect delivery route and birth outcome? *Am J Obstet Gynecol* 1995;173(4):1215–1219.
83. Willcourt RJ et al. Induction of labor with pulsatile oxytocin by a computer-controlled pump. *Am J Obstet Gynecol* 1994;170(2):603–608.
84. Witter FR and Weitz CM. A randomized trial of induction at 42 weeks gestation versus expectant management for postdates pregnancies. *Am J Perinatol* 1987;4(3):206–211.
85. Xenakis, EM et al. Induction of labor in the nineties: conquering the unfavorable cervix. *Obstet Gynecol* 1997;90(2):235–239.

Chapter 4
IVs: "Water, Water Everywhere, Nor Any Drop to Drink"

Fasting during labor causes a rise in maternal ketone levels, which may have adverse effects on the labor.

Studies comparing the effects of glucose-containing IV fluids with nonglucose-containing fluids document that fasting, laboring women not given glucose have extremely low blood-sugar levels (*hypoglycemia*) and that their ketone levels, an indicator of starvation metabolism, rise over time.[6,18] Another study found ketones in the urine of 40 percent of laboring women.[4] The incidence rose from 10 percent in women laboring less than six hours to 66 percent of women laboring over twelve hours. The presence of ketones was strongly associated with the use of oxytocin to stimulate stronger contractions and with forceps delivery. The association remained after adjusting for length of labor. This means that fasting was still a factor even after accounting for the fact that longer labor led to oxytocin use and forceps deliveries. Conversely, feeding women may enhance labor as may be seen below, "Eating and drinking in labor. . . ."

Fasting does not guarantee an empty stomach.

Three studies that measured the amount of fluid in the stomach after an overnight fast in, respectively, women having an elective cesarean, women having a first-trimester abortion, and surgical patients (not pregnant women) got nearly identical results.[1,10,12] All found average fluid above the commonly agreed danger threshold of 25 ml. Some participants had volumes close to or exceeding 50 ml.

Hunger and especially thirst are a source of considerable discomfort in laboring women.

More than one-fourth of new mothers responding to a survey rated restriction of food "moderately" or "most" stressful while nearly half said the same of restriction of oral fluids.[19] Two studies of presurgical patients randomly assigned them to either continue an overnight fast or to have about half a cup of water (150 ml).[1,12] Predictably, the patients given water felt less thirsty.

Eating and drinking in labor does not increase the risk of vomiting, avoids the hazards of IV-fluid overload, and may have beneficial effects on labor progress. (See also page 241, "IV fluids can cause problems. . . .")

One study observed the effects of eating and drinking in labor on vomiting in 106 women.[16] Only 1 in 5 women vomited, of whom fewer than in 10 vomited more than once.

Researchers compared *colloid osmotic pressures* in blood samples taken after birth in 16 women having vaginal deliveries who were routinely given IV fluids with 12 similar women not having IVs who were allowed to drink clear liquids.[5] Colloid osmotic pressure is a measure of the factors keeping fluid from leaking out of capillaries into tissues such as the lungs. The "danger" threshold lies at 15.6 mm Hg. Average postpartum values were 16.4 mm Hg in the IV group versus 19.2 mm Hg in the oral intake group. No woman drinking clear fluids had values below 15.6 versus nearly one-third of the IV group. Another study reported that X rays showed that one-half to two-thirds of women had fluid in their lungs after birth, a problem that the authors attributed to the normal alterations of pregnancy physiology or the rigors of pushing, but the colloid osmotic pressure study shows that IVs were almost certainly responsible.[7]

As for symptoms of fluid overload in babies, a study randomly assigned 300 women to a glucose IV or sips of water.[22] Glucose IVs magnify the problems of fluid overload because they typically lack salts *(electrolytes)*. Fifteen percent of infants whose mothers had the IV experienced a type of short-term pneumonia *(transient neonatal tachypnea* or *wet lung syndrome)* versus 3 percent of infants whose mothers had sips of water. Similarly, researchers compared newborn outcomes between 106 women having glucose IVs and 97 women having oral fluids.[3] The newborns of mothers having IVs were much more likely to have abnormally low blood levels of sodium *(hyponatremia)* and greater newborn weight loss, both symptoms of severe fluid overload. Newborns in the IV group averaged a weight loss of 6 percent ranging up to 9 percent versus a weight loss of 4 percent ranging up to 6 percent in the oral water group. If we assume a birth weight of 7 lbs., a 2 percent to 3 percent difference in weight loss amounts to 2 oz. to more than 3 oz., no trivial difference. Low blood sodium can cause seizures, and indeed, the authors thought this might have been the reason for a seizure of otherwise unknown cause in one hyponatremic infant.

There are no studies of fed versus fasting women other than a small, unpublished study mentioned in a review article.[11] In this study, researchers compared labor outcomes in 44 women allowed food in labor versus 22 women allowed toast and tea in very early labor and sips of water thereafter. Women who ate used less pain relief medication, were less likely to have oxytocin to stimulate contractions, and had an average labor length ninety minutes shorter than women only allowed water.

IVs can cause pain and inflammation at the IV site.

Within eight hours of inserting an IV, three of twenty-seven patients had pain at the IV site.[8] By sixteen hours, the number had risen to ten. Nearly 60 percent of new mothers responding to a survey rated IV fluids "moderately" or "most" stressful.[19]

Caregivers may commonly overdose IV fluids.

Although orders were given for all patients to be given IV fluids at the rate of 125–150 ml per hour (1,000 ml or 1 liter equals roughly one quart), the actual average rate at one hospital was 360 ml per hour with some women receiving over 600 ml per hour.[2] During the birth, the average rate increased to 750 ml per hour with some women receiving over 1 liter per hour. This means the average woman laboring for five hours in this hospital before giving birth would have the equivalent of the contents of a 2-liter bottle of soda during that relatively brief time—more if she labored longer or was given IV fluids at greater than the average rate. In another study, women having both an epidural and oxytocin received IV fluids at an average rate of 200 ml per hour or 1 liter every five hours.[23] A few women received over 4 liters of IV fluid in total.

IV fluids can cause problems related to fluid overload, problems that are greatly exacerbated by giving large amounts of IV fluid rapidly or fluids that don't contain salts. (See also page 240 "Eating and drinking in labor. . . . ")

As can be seen in the cross-referenced section, IV fluids can lead to excess fluid in the tissues, which can cause water to accumulate in the lungs. Giving large amounts of IV fluids rapidly (*bolus*), as is done before giving an epidural or performing a cesarean under epidural or spinal anesthesia, aggravates this problem. One study measured *colloid osmotic pressure*, a measure of factors that keep fluids from leaking out of capillaries into tissues, after giving women one of three bolus amounts of fluids before planned cesarean.[17] By delivery, amounts of IV fluid averaged nearly 2 liters, 2½ liters, and 3 liters, respectively. All three groups experienced a marked fall in colloid osmotic pressure.

In addition, giving bolus IVs dilutes the blood. Two studies totalling fifty participants revealed that the dilution effect of 1½ to 2 liters of IV fluid prior to planned section rendered most women anemic and many women became severely anemic.[9,15]

Giving glucose IVs, which typically don't contain salts, can cause severe fluid overload. On page 240, "Eating and drinking in labor . . ." describes two studies. Besides these, three studies compared newborn outcomes between women having and not having glucose IVs. In the first, women in the IV groups were much more likely to have newborns with low blood-sodium levels.[23] Even including salts in the fluid did not completely prevent this problem. Newborns in the IV groups also lost more weight after birth, another symptom that can be attributed to excess fluids. In the second study, one-third of babies in the IV group versus one-tenth of the non-IV group had high bilirubin levels, and 15 percent versus 4 percent were considered to have newborn jaundice *(hyperbilirubinemia)*.[20] Fluid overload causes this complication by swelling red blood cells until they break. Bilirubin, a breakdown product, is a yellow pigment, and in sufficient amounts, circulating bilirubin makes the skin and eyes look yellow or "jaundiced." In the third study, only 6 percent of the infants whose mothers had no IV had hyponatremia versus nearly half of the oxytocin-glucose IV group and nearly one-third of the plain glucose group.[21] Hyponatremic babies were ten times more likely (19 percent versus 2 percent) to experience breathing problems due to fluid in the lungs *(transient neonatal tachypnea)*, and over half developed jaundice versus 20 percent of newborns with normal blood-sodium levels. Studies also find that babies born after planned cesarean experience more respiratory problems and jaundice than babies born after vaginal birth (see page 286).

Glucose IVs can cause high blood sugar in the baby before birth and low blood sugar after the birth, both of which can cause problems.

One study looked at the effect of glucose-containing IVs on women undergoing elective cesarean section and their newborns,[6] and three studies compared the effects of giving 1 liter of glucose-containing IV fluid with nonglucose-containing fluid.[14–15,19] All of them found that some women given IV glucose developed blood glucose levels in the diabetic range *(hyperglycemia)*. The babies of women given glucose IVs were more likely to develop blood sugar levels low enough to require treatment *(hypoglycemia)* compared with women given nonglucose IVs. The likelihood of newborn hypoglycemia rose with the mother's increasing blood sugar level.

REFERENCES

1. Agarwal A, Chari P, and Singh H. Fluid deprivation before operation: the effect of a small drink. *Anaesthesia* 1989;44:632–634.
2. Cotton DB et al. Intrapartum to postpartum changes in colloid osmotic pressure. *Am J Obstet Gynecol* 1984;149(2):174–177.
3. Dahlenburg GW, Burnell RH, and Braybrook R. The relation between cord serum sodium levels in newborn infants and maternal intravenous therapy during labour. *Br J Obstet Gynaecol* 1980;87:519–522.
4. Foulkes J and Dumoulin JG. The effects of ketonuria in labour. *Br J Clin Pract* 1985;39:59–62.

5. Gonik B and Cotton DB. Peripartum colloid osmotic pressure changes: influence of intravenous hydration. *Am J Obstet Gynecol* 1984;150(1): 99–100.

6. Grylack LJ, Chu SS, and Scanlon JW. Use of intravenous fluids before cesarean section: effects on perinatal glucose, insulin and sodium homeostasis. *Obstet Gynecol* 1984;63(5):654–658.

7. Hughson WG et al. Postpartum pleural effusion: a common radiologic finding. *Ann Intern Med* 1982;97(6):856–858.

8. Jones JJ and Koldjeski D. Clinical indicators of a developmental process in phlebitis. *NITA* 1984;7:279–285.

9. Kempen PM and Tick RC. Hemodilution, regional block and cesarean section. *Reg Anesth* 1990;15(1S):9.

10. Lewis M and Crawford JS. Can one risk fasting the obstetric patient for less than 4 hours? *Br J Anaesth* 1987;59:312–314.

11. Ludka LM and Roberts CC. Eating and drinking in labor. A literature review. *J Nurse Midwifery* 1993;38(4):199–207.

12. Maltby JR et al. Preoperative oral fluids: is a five-hour fast justified prior to elective surgery? *Anesth Analg* 1986;65:1112–1116.

13. Mendiola J, Grylack LJ, and Scanlon JW. Effects of intrapartum maternal glucose infusion on the normal fetus and newborn. *Anesth Analg* 1982;61(1):32–35.

14. Morton KE, Jackson MC, and Gillmer MDG. A comparison of the effects of four intravenous solutions for the treatment of ketonuria during labor. *Br J Obstet Gynaecol* 1985;92:473–479.

15. Murray AM, Morgan M, and Whitwam JG. Crystalloid versus colloid for circulatory preload for epidural caesarean section. *Anaesthesia* 1989; 44(6):463–466.

16. O'Reilly SA, Hoyer PJ, and Walsh E. Low-risk mothers. Oral intake and emesis in labor. *J Nurse Midwifery* 1992;38(4):228–235.

17. Park GE et al. The effects of varying volumes of crystalloid administration before cesarean delivery on maternal hemodynamics and colloid osmotic pressure. *Anesth Analg* 1996;83(2):299–303.

18. Philipson EH et al. Effects of maternal glucose infusion on fetal acid-base status in human pregnancy. *Am J Obstet Gynecol* 1987;157(4 Pt 1):866–873.

19. Simkin P. Stress, pain, and catecholamines in labor: Part 2. Stress associated with childbirth events: a pilot survey of new mothers. *Birth* 1986; 13(4):234–240.

20. Singhi S, Choo Kang E, and Hall J. Hazards of maternal hydration with 5% dextrose. *Lancet* 1982;2:335–336.

21. Singhi S et al. Iatrogenic neonatal and maternal hyponatraemia following oxytocin and acqueous glucose infusion during labor. *Br J Obstet Gynaecol* 1985;92:356–363.

22. Singhi SC and Choo Kang E. Maternal fluid overload during labour; transplacental hyponatraemia and risk of transient neonatal tachypnoea in term infants. *Arch Dis Child* 1984;59:1155–1158.

23. Tarnow-Mordi WO et al. Iatrogenic hyponatraemia of the newborn due to maternal fluid overload: a prospective study. *Br Med J* 1981;283:639–642.

Chapter 5
Electronic Fetal Monitoring and Cesarean for Fetal Distress: The Machine That Goes Ping!

Few cases of cerebral palsy arise from events in labor.

One study matched each of 183 cerebral palsy patients with three similar healthy children. In only 8 percent of cerebral palsy cases was it thought possible or likely that oxygen deprivation caused cerebral palsy.[1] Another study reviewed the records of 70 children with cerebral palsy and compared them with 591 healthy children.[23] Three-quarters of the cerebral palsy cases had no recorded evidence of distress. Nine percent of the cerebral palsy cases involved prolonged distress, but so did 3 percent of labors that resulted in healthy children. Eliminating all fetal distress would eliminate only 16 percent of cases of cerebral palsy. A third study looked at the records of 48 full-term babies with neurological impairments.[22] Seventy percent already had an abnormal heart rate at hospital admission for labor.

The baby's heart rate during labor correlates poorly with measures of the baby's condition at birth.

The baby's heart rate in labor predicts blood pH or Apgar scores poorly. In one study, three investigators who didn't know the outcomes reviewed the monitor tracings for 38 full-term infants believed to have experienced severe oxygen deprivation in labor and 120 healthy infants.[19] The investigators found no heart rate abnormalities in 5 oxygen deprived babies and found abnormalities in 35 healthy babies. They failed to predict poor condition at birth in 15 oxygen deprived babies and thought 11 healthy babies would be born in poor condition. If these proportions are extrapolated to all 3,700 babies born during the seventeen months the study covered, obstetricians would have been confronted with 338 tracings that at least two of three investigators predicted would result in a baby with low blood pH, but only twenty-three newborns would actually require admission to neonatal intensive care.

EFM and fetal scalp-blood testing in 2,660 women correctly identified less than two-thirds of babies born with low blood pH and low 1-minute Apgar scores.[31] The authors attribute this to misinterpretation of monitor tracings and delays between getting normal blood pH results on the scalp-blood sample and the birth instead of to EFM's intrinsic limitations. On the other hand, 95 percent of all babies predicted by EFM and/or scalp-blood testing to have low blood pH and 1-minute Apgar scores had neither. The authors attribute this to promptness in delivery instead of to EFM's propensity to misdiagnose healthy babies. The authors enthusiastically recommend EFM. Perhaps they, like the White Queen, start their days by believing six impossible things before breakfast.

When researchers compared 400 women who had continuous EFM with 450 women who had intermittent listening, 14 percent of the EFM women had forceps or cesarean deliveries for fetal distress but gave birth to healthy babies.[28] This never occurred in the listening group. EFM also offered no advantages in identifying babies in trouble. The same percentage of women in both groups gave spontaneous birth to a distressed baby.

Researchers correlated abnormal EFM tracings with low blood pH in 700 women and found that in one-third of cases with an abnormal tracing, the baby had normal blood pH.[27] I calculated that an abnormal tracing correctly predicted a baby with low blood pH less than 25 percent of the time.

Babies' heart patterns in labor also don't predict who will need resuscitation or have seizures. In a study of 6,800 labors, an abnormal fetal heart rate correctly identified only one-third of babies who needed breathing assistance at birth.[3] Thirty-two out of 56 infants who required a tube down their throats (*intubation*) as part of resuscitation efforts had normal EFM tracings.[16] An analysis of EFM tracings of 34 full-term newborns with seizures found that 15 of them had only mildly abnormal heart rate patterns.[13]

Measures of the baby's condition after birth correlate poorly with long-term outcomes.

Five studies correlated Apgar scores and blood pH at birth with neurological outcomes in time frames ranging from two weeks to ten years after birth.[4–5,17,24,33] All five found poor correlation between low blood pH and/or low Apgar scores and neurological status. To cite one example, one of these studies followed up 184 infants with 1-minute Apgar scores at birth of 3 or less (very poor condition) at age 5. Eighty-one percent had no impairment, including two-thirds of the children who also had low blood pH. Only 6.5 percent sustained serious impairment or died in the newborn period.

The baby's heart rate during labor correlates poorly with the incidence of cerebral palsy.

Researchers reviewed records of 95 children born at full term in four California counties over a three-year period who developed cerebral palsy and compared them with those of 378 healthy children.[20] Only 22 percent (twenty-one children) of cerebral palsy cases involved severe heart rate abnormalities as did 9 percent of labors that resulted in healthy children. If these results are extrapolated to all 155,600 children born in those counties over the same time period, then 9 percent of all healthy, full-term children experienced severe fetal heart rate abnormalities in labor as well as the 21 children who developed cerebral palsy. This calculates to a false positive rate, meaning EFM wrongly predicted the baby would have cerebral palsy, of 99.8 percent.

Comparisons of EFM and intermittent listening show that EFM offers no long-term benefits in either low- or high-risk pregnancies, although it may have short-term benefits especially when oxytocin is used.

The *Cochrane Database of Systematic Reviews,* a highly respected, ongoing series of analyses of randomized controlled trials (randomly assigning participants to one group or the other strengthens conclusions because it eliminates a major source of potential bias), has concluded that based on an analysis of data from nine such trials of EFM versus intermittent listening in both high- and low-risk women, the only significant benefit is a reduction in newborn seizures.[30] Even this may have no implications for long-term outcomes. One study followed up all newborns experiencing seizures in the largest (13,000 women) of these randomized controlled trials and found no differences between groups in cases of cerebral palsy at age four.[10] Premature babies, who are at higher risk during labor than full-term babies, would certainly seem more likely to benefit from routine EFM. However, one randomized controlled trial of EFM versus intermittent listening in women in premature labor found that at age 4, *more* children had developed cerebral palsy in the *EFM* group.[25]

EFM may, though, offer some protection from the risks of oxytocin. That same large trial reported a marked difference in seizure rates when oxytocin was given in the intermittent listening group compared with the EFM group: 12 per 1,000 versus 3.5 per 1,000.[18]

Note: You should know about a 1993 Greek trial because EFM defenders cite it as finally proving EFM's value.[32] Two renowned research analysts, Drs. Murray Enkin and Marc Kierse, both of whom are editors and authors associated with the *Cochrane Database*, have independently written scathing critiques discrediting the validity of this study.[8,14]

Comparisons of EFM and intermittent listening show that EFM increases the likelihood of cesarean and vaginal instrumental delivery, infection, and cerebral palsy in premature babies.

The *Cochrane Database of Systematic Reviews* has concluded that compared with intermittent listening, EFM increases the risk of cesarean section by one-third.[29] Using fetal scalp blood testing to confirm fetal distress narrows, but does not eliminate, that gap. The authors of the Cochrane review provide additional information in a medical journal article: high-risk women were half again as likely to have cesareans, and *low-risk* women were *twice* as likely to have them.[30] EFM also increased the risk of instrumental vaginal delivery by about 10 percent.

Second, if EFM increases the risk of cesarean section, you can take it as a given that it increases the rate of maternal infection because infection rates after cesareans considerably exceed infection rates after vaginal births. Nonetheless, only one trial comparing internal EFM with intermittent listening found a difference in infection rates. The authors reported that 13 percent of mothers in the EFM group developed postpartum infections versus less than 5 percent of the intermittent listening group.[11] Adjusting for the difference in cesarean rates did not completely eliminate the gap. Still, studies that look at factors associated with uterine infection have indicted internal monitoring. One found that more than 80 percent of uterine infections could be explained by duration of ruptured membranes and duration of internal monitoring alone.[21] Another found that internal monitoring doubled the odds of uterine infection.[26]

As for cerebral palsy, a follow-up study of a trial of EFM versus intermittent listening in 246 women having their babies prior to thirty-three weeks of pregnancy had these disturbing results: At eighteen months old, mental development scores and psychomotor scores were lower in the EFM group, and the children in the EFM group were nearly four times as likely to have developed cerebral palsy.[25] Even more disturbing, the average time between picking up an abnormal heart pattern and delivery was substantially longer in the EFM group: 104 versus 61 minutes, which suggests that EFM lulled staff into unwarranted complacency.

Selective EFM produces equally good outcomes as routine EFM.

One study of 35,000 women was not quite a randomized controlled trial, but it is, perhaps, more representative of how EFM versus intermittent listening might work out practically.[15] In this U.S. study, hospital staff alternated between routine EFM and EFM for specific indication on a monthly basis. Indications included oxytocin use, abnormal fetal heart rate, premature labor, and various maternal medical conditions such as hypertension and diabetes. A little over one-third of women had EFM in the selective-EFM months versus three-quarters in the routine EFM months. Newborn outcomes, including seizure rates, were the same in both groups.

Intermittent EFM produces equally good outcomes as continuous EFM.

In one trial, researchers randomly assigned over 4,000 low-risk women to either intermittent external EFM interspersed with intermittent listening during the dilation phase of labor or to continuous external EFM going to internal EFM at membrane rupture.[12] All women had continuous EFM during the pushing phase. When oxytocin was used to stimulate labor or the mother had an epidural in the intermittent group, continuous EFM was done until the oxytocin dose was determined or for one hour after the epidural was administered and thirty minutes after repeat doses. About one-quarter of the women in each group experienced "suspicious" fetal heart rate patterns, which may have been because half of them had oxytocin, which can cause overly long, overly strong contractions. The epidural rate was under 20 percent in both groups. Cesarean rates were low, about 2 percent overall in both groups, with half being for fetal distress. All measures of newborn condition were similar.

Stimulating the baby's scalp can usually replace fetal scalp blood sampling as a follow-up test.

Two studies of scalp stimulation in a combined total of over 200 babies with nonreassuring heart rate patterns during labor found that every baby whose heart rate speeded up in response to scalp stimulation had a scalp blood pH within normal range.[2,8] A third study in a large hospital with 16,300 births annually noted that the use of scalp blood sampling virtually disappeared between 1987 and 1992 without any increases in cesarean rate for fetal distress or babies born in poor condition.[9] They attribute this to substituting fetal scalp stimulation for scalp blood sampling. Another study of 188 babies with nonreassuring patterns got similar results by buzzing the mothers' bellies with an electronic larynx, which startles the baby.[6] Many nonresponders, however, will have normal blood pH, so scalp blood sampling may still be useful in this group.

REFERENCES

1. Blair E and Stanley FJ. Intrapartum asphyxia: a rare cause of cerebral palsy. *J Pediatr* 1988;112(4):515–519.
2. Clark SL, Gimovsky ML, and Miller FC. The scalp stimulation test: a

clinical alternative to fetal scalp blood sampling. *Am J Obstet Gynecol* 1984;148(3):274–277.

3. Curzen P et al. Reliability of cardiotocography in predicting baby's condition at birth. *Br Med J* 1984;289:1345–1347.

4. Dennis J et al. Acid-base status at birth and neurodevelopmental outcome at four and one-half years. *Am J Obstet Gynecol* 1989;161(1): 213–220.

5. Dijxhoorn MJ et al. The relation between umbilical pH values and neonatal neurological morbidity in full term appropriate-for-dates infants. *Early Hum Develop* 1985;11:33–42.

6. Edersheim TG et al. Fetal heart rate response to vibratory acoustic stimulation predicts fetal pH in labor. *Am J Obstet Gynecol* 1987;157(6): 1557–1560.

7. Elimian A, Figueroa R, and Tejani N. Intrapartum assessment of fetal well-being: a comparison of scalp stimulation with scalp blood pH sampling. *Obstet Gynecol* 1997;89(3):373–376.

8. Enkin M. Letter to author, Nov 13, 1993. In: Goer H. *Obstetric Myths versus Research Realities.* Westport, CT: Bergin and Garvey, 1995.

9. Goodwin TM, Milner-Masterson L, and Paul RH. Elimination of fetal scalp blood sampling on a large clinical service. *Obstet Gynecol* 1994; 83(6):971–975.

10. Grant A et al. Cerebral palsy among children born during the Dublin randomised trial of intrapartum monitoring. *Lancet* 1989;2(8674): 1233–1236.

11. Havercamp AD et al. The evaluation of continuous fetal heart rate monitoring in high-risk pregnancy. *Am J Obstet Gynecol* 1976;125(3):310–320.

12. Herbst A and Ingemarsson I. Intermittent versus continuous electronic monitoring in labour: a randomised study. *Br J Obstet Gynaecol* 1994; 101(8):663–668.

13. Keegan KA, Waffarn F, and Quilligan EJ. Obstetric characteristics and fetal heart rate patterns of infants who convulse during the newborn period. *Am J Obstet Gynecol* 1985;153(7):732–737.

14. Kierse MJNC. Electronic monitoring: who needs a Trojan horse? *Birth* 1994;21(2):111–113.

15. Leveno KJ et al. A prospective comparison of selective and universal electronic fetal monitoring in 34,995 pregnancies. *N Engl J Med* 1986; 315(10):615–619.

16. Lissauer TJ and Steer PJ. The relation between the need for intubation at birth, abnormal cardiotocograms in labour and cord artery blood gas and pH values. *Br J Obstet Gynaecol* 1986;93:1060–1066.

17. Low JA et al. The association of intrapartum asphyxia in the mature fetus with newborn behavior. *Am J Obstet Gynecol* 1990;163(4):1131–1135.

18. MacDonald D et al. The Dublin randomized controlled trial of intrapartum fetal heart rate monitoring. *Am J Obstet Gynecol* 1985;152(5): 524–539.

19. Murphy KW et al. Birth asphyxia and the intrapartum cardiotocograph. *Br J Obstet Gynaecol* 1990;97(6):470–479.

20. Nelson KB et al. Uncertain value of electronic fetal monitoring in predicting cerebral palsy. *N Engl J Med* 1996;334(10):613–618.
21. Newton HR, Prihoda TJ, and Gibbs RS. Logistic regression analysis of risk factors for intraamniotic infection. *Obstet Gynecol* 1989;73(4):571–575.
22. Phelan JP and Ock Ahn M. Perinatal observations in forty-eight neurologically impaired term infants. *Am J Obstet Gynecol* 1994;171(2):424–431.
23. Richmond S et al. The obstetric management of fetal distress and its association with cerebral palsy. *Obstet Gynecol* 1994;83(5 Pt 1):643–646.
24. Ruth VJ and Raivio KO. Perinatal brain damage: predictive value of metabolic acidosis and the Apgar score. *Br Med J* 1988;297:24–27.
25. Shy KK et al. Effects of electronic fetal-heart-rate monitoring, as compared with periodic auscultation, on the neurologic development of premature infants. *N Engl J Med* 1990;322(9):588–593.
26. Soper DE, Mayall CG, and Froggatt JW. Characterization and control of intraamniotic infection in an urban teaching hospital. *Am J Obstet Gynecol* 1996;175(2):304–309.
27. Steer PJ et al. Interrelationships among abnormal cardiotocograms in labor, meconium staining of the amniotic fluid, arterial cord blood pH and Apgar scores. *Obstet Gynecol* 1989;74(5):715–721.
28. Sykes GS et al. Fetal distress and the condition of newborn infants. *Br Med J* 1983;287:943–945.
29. Thacker SB, Stroup DF, and Peterson HB. Continuous electronic fetal heart monitoring during labor. In Neilson JP et al., eds. *Pregnancy and Childbirth Module of the Cochrane Database of Systematic Reviews,* updated June 1996.
30. Thacker SB, Stroup DF, and Peterson HB. Efficacy and safety of intrapartum electronic fetal monitoring: an update. *Obstet Gynecol* 1995; 86(4 Pt 1):613–620.
31. van den Berg P et al. Fetal distress and the condition of the newborn using cardiotocography and fetal blood analysis during labour. *Br J Obstet Gynaecol* 1987;94:72–75.
32. Vintzileos AM et al. A randomized trial of intrapartum electronic fetal heart rate monitoring versus intermittent auscultation. *Obstet Gynecol* 1993;81(6):899–907.
33. Yudkin PL et al. Clustering of perinatal markers of birth asphyxia and outcome at age five years. *Br J Obstet Gynaecol* 1994;101:774–781.

Chapter 6
When Doctors Break the Membranes:
If It Ain't Broke, Don't Break It

Amniotomy shortens labor by only a modest amount and is a minor variable in determining the length of labor.

An analysis of data from seven trials in which women were randomly assigned to routine early amniotomy versus late or selective amniotomy found that early amniotomy shortened labor by somewhere between a half an hour and two and a quarter hours.[2] The effect was seen in both first-time mothers and in women with prior births. The difference amounted to a 7 percent to 40 percent reduction of the time remaining in labor. However, other factors have much more effect on the length of labor. A study of over 2,550 women concurred that the fastest labors were those with spontaneous rupture, followed by amniotomy, followed by intact membranes. Nonetheless, this study also reported that the circumstances and timing of membrane rupture and whether the mother had given birth before only accounted for 25 percent of the variance in labor length.[13] Moreover, the real question to ask about shortening labor is "Does it have any value?"

Amniotomy may not prevent or correct poor progress.

Early amniotomy may not prevent poor progress. In a trial where researchers randomly assigned 925 women to early amniotomy or conserve membranes groups, they found that amniotomy had less effect on labor duration in women less than 3 centimeters dilated at time of rupture than on women who had amniotomies later.[5] More importantly, amniotomy before 3 centimeters dilation did not reduce the incidence of women diagnosed as making poor progress.

One study suggests that amniotomy may look like it generally speeds up labor, but in fact it only increases dilation rate in women who don't need it while actually slowing progress in women who do.[15] This study analyzed the relationship between amniotomy and labor rate in 450 first-time mothers who had vaginal births. Half had amniotomies of whom 29 percent had oxytocin to stimulate stronger contractions. Amniotomy nearly doubled the rate of dilation in women not destined to receive oxytocin—in other words, those whose labors progressed at a normal rate—but virtually brought labor progress to a standstill in women who eventually had oxytocin, the problem amniotomy was supposed to prevent. Overall, women dilating slowly before amniotomy continued at the same rate whereas nearly half of women dilating at average or faster than average rates dilated faster after amniotomy.

Even when amniotomy to correct poor progress succeeds in reducing labor duration, it may not reduce cesarean rates, which is the point. A study randomly assigned 120 first-time mothers whose labors had come to a halt to either oxytocin stimulation alone or oxytocin plus amniotomy.[14] Despite the fact that time from random assignment to vaginal birth was shorter in the amniotomy group, cesarean rates were similar.

Amniotomy can cause fetal heart rate patterns indicative of fetal distress.

The effects reported in these studies probably represent minimum adverse effects because with the exception of a study of labor *induction*, all of the studies selected healthy women carrying healthy, full-term babies. These babies would be best able to compensate for the stress of a diminished oxygen supply. And as I mentioned in the chapter, many women in the conserve membranes groups had amniotomies.

An analysis of data pooled from seven trials that randomly assigned women to routine early versus late or selective amniotomy did not find increased incidence of episodes of abnormal fetal heart rate in the early amniotomy group.[4] However, a reanalysis of data from 750 women in one of the larger trials did when it took into account that amniotomy shortened labor.[8] Instead of comparing number of episodes, the authors calculated episodes per hour and found that early amniotomy doubled the average number of episodes per hour of severe variable decelerations, an abnormal heart-rate pattern associated with umbilical cord compression. It also increased the average number of late decelerations per hour, another abnormal fetal heart-rate pattern. Epidural and oxytocin rates, potential confounders because both can cause fetal distress patterns, were similar between groups.

Other trials have also found differences in the incidence of abnormal fetal heart-rate patterns. Researchers in one trial randomly assigned 460 laboring women in the middle of labor to amniotomy or not, although one-fourth of the conserve membranes group eventually had an amniotomy.[7] One-fourth of women in the routine amniotomy group had a totally normal fetal heart-rate tracing during the dilation phase of labor versus one-third of the no amniotomy group. Two-thirds of the amniotomy group versus half of the no amniotomy group experienced mildly to moderately abnormal patterns and twice as many (8 percent versus 4 percent) experienced severely abnormal patterns. In another study, researchers randomly assigned over 200 women to induction of labor with oxytocin and early amniotomy or amniotomy performed at or after 5 centimeters' dilation.[11] Four times as many early amniotomy–group members as late amniotomy–group members (12 percent versus 3 percent) experienced recurrent moderate to severe fetal heart rate patterns emblematic of umbilical cord compression.

Amniotomy increases the risk of cesarean section, especially for fetal distress.

An analysis of data from seven trials that randomly assigned women to routine early versus late or selective amniotomy found that early amniotomy increased the likelihood of cesarean by 20 percent.[2,4] Statistical calculations did not find this overall increase to be *significant*, meaning that the results could have been due to chance. However, in every trial, the early amniotomy group had more cesareans. As mentioned in the main chapter, the authors of one trial explain that the odds of this happening by chance are the same as the odds of flipping seven coins and getting seven "heads."[9] Statistical calculations of the likelihood that results were due to chance depend on the number of cases and the size of the differences between groups. In the seven trials, few women had cesareans and differences in cearean rates between groups were small. This limitation could explain why statistical calculations did not find results to be significant when, in fact, a real difference probably exists. However, even if the association is spurious and amniotomy does not increase cesarean rates, the studies prove that early amniotomy does not *reduce* cesarean rates, which supposedly is its major benefit. And, as I said in the chapter, many of the women in the selective or late amniotomy groups had amniotomies, which minimizes differences between groups.

Two other trials not included in this analysis also report more cesareans in the early amniotomy group. You might say that we have now flipped nine "heads" in a row.

The data reanalysis mentioned in the previous section suggests that the difference in cesarean rates may be due to more women having cesareans for fetal distress. The study reported that 7 percent of women in the early amniotomy group had a cesarean for either fetal distress or fetal distress plus lack of labor progress versus 3 percent of women in the late amniotomy group.[8]

Early amniotomy may increase the risk of maternal infection.

Several studies have found an association between early amniotomy and maternal infection. One randomly assigned over 200 women to induction of labor with oxytocin and early amniotomy or amniotomy performed at or after 5 centimeters' dilation.[11] Doctors diagnosed uterine inflammation (*chorioamnionitis*) in nearly one-quarter of the early amniotomy group versus 7 percent of the late amniotomy group. Another randomly assigned 120 first-time mothers whose labors had come to a halt to either oxytocin stimulation alone or oxytocin plus amniotomy.[14] Four women in the amniotomy group developed postpartum uterine infections versus no women in the intact membranes group. Researchers in a third study randomly assigned 300 first-time mothers to routine early versus selective amniotomy groups and reported maternal infection rates of 5 percent in the routine group versus 3 percent in the selective group.[3] This difference was not statistically *significant*, meaning the difference was attributed to chance. However, nearly 60 percent of the selective group had amniotomies too, which narrows the differences between the groups. Similarly, in two studies that found no association between amniotomy and infection, half the women in the "conserve membranes" group had amniotomies.[1,5]

Yet another group of researchers offer an explanation for why early amniotomy might increase infection rates.[9] They conducted a randomized controlled trial of routine versus selective amniotomy in 1,550 women. Women in the routine group averaged more vaginal exams after membrane rupture. Every exam to check cervical dilation carries up bacteria that normally live harmlessly in the vagina and deposits them on the cervix. Once membranes are ruptured, the uterine barrier is gone. The more vaginal exams a woman has after ruptured membranes, the greater the chances of starting an infection. This is not the only study to find a strong relationship between ruptured membranes, time, number of vaginal exams, and infection (see page 230).

Amniotomy may precipitate umbilical cord prolapse.

Two studies analyzed a series of instances of umbilical cord prolapse. In one, in ten out of seventy-nine cases prolapse occurred with amniotomy and resulted in one case in the death of a full-term, head-down baby (cord prolapse is more likely in preterm babies and breech presentations).[10] The other looked at a series of thirty-seven cases.[12] Amniotomy precipitated cord prolapse in nine of them. In six of these nine, obstetricians performed amniotomy to verify suspected fetal distress by instituting internal electronic fetal monitoring. In some cases they also intended to start amniotic fluid replacement for symptoms of umbilical cord compression. This suggests that the baby was in trouble because the umbilical cord had slipped between its head and the mother's pelvis (*occult prolapse*). The authors seem to think that the motive in these six cases justifies the catastrophe that followed. You can't know what would have happened had doctors not intervened, but there is at least the possibility that the cord would have moved out of the way. At the very least, doctors converted a concerning situation into an emergency. And, of course, what about the other three cases? Finally, five out of eight cases of cord prolapse in a series of 11,800 births occurred in women with head-down babies who had amniotomies.[6]

REFERENCES

1. Barrett JF et al. Randomized trial of amniotomy in labour versus the intention to leave membranes intact until the second stage. *Br J Obstet Gynaecol* 1992;99(1):5–9.
2. Brisson-Carroll G et al. The effect of routine early amniotomy on spontaneous labor: a meta-analysis. *Obstet Gynecol* 1996;87(5 Pt 2):891–896.
3. Cammu H and Van Eeckhout E. A randomised controlled trial of early versus delayed use of amniotomy and oxytocin infusion in nulliparous labour. *Br J Obstet Gynaecol* 1996;103(4):313–318.
4. Fraser WD et al. Amniotomy to shorten spontaneous labour. In: Neilson JP et al., eds. *Pregnancy and Childbirth Module of the Cochrane Database of Systematic Reviews*, updated November 1995.
5. Fraser WD et al. Effect of early amniotomy on the risk of dystocia in nulliparous women. *N Engl J Med* 1993;22;328(16):1145–1149.
6. Fullerton JT and Severino R. In-hospital care for low-risk childbirth: comparison with results from the National Birth Center Study. *J Nurse Midwifery* 1992;37(5):331–340.
7. Garite TJ et al. The influence of elective amniotomy on fetal heart rate patterns and the course of labor in term patients: a randomized study. *Am J Obstet Gynecol* 1993;168(6 Pt 1):1827–1832.
8. Goffinet F et al. Early amniotomy increases the frequency of fetal heart rate abnormalities. *Br J Obstet Gynaecol* 1997;104(5):548–553.
9. Johnson N et al. Randomised trial comparing a policy of early with selective amniotomy in uncomplicated labour at term. *Br J Obstet Gynaecol* 1997;104(3):340–346.
10. Levy H et al. Umbilical cord prolapse. *Obstet Gynecol* 1984;64(4):499–502.
11. Mercer BM et al. Early versus late amniotomy for labor induction: a randomized trial. *Am J Obstet Gynecol* 1995;173(4):1321–1325.
12. Roberts WE et al. Are obstetric interventions such as cervical ripening,

induction of labor, amnioinfusion, or amniotomy associated with umbilical cord prolapse? *Am J Obstet Gynecol* 1997;176(6):1181–1185.

13. Rosen MG and Peisner DB. Effect of amniotic membrane rupture on
    length of labor. *Obstet Gynecol* 1987;70(4):604–607.

14. Rouse DJ et al. Active-phase labor arrest: a randomized trial of cho-
    rioamnion management. *Obstet Gynecol* 1994;83(6):937–940.

15. Seitchik J, Holden AE, and Castillo M. Amniotomy and the use of ox-
    ytocin in labor in nulliparous women. *Am J Obstet Gynecol* 1985;
    153(8):848–854.

16. UK Amniotomy Group. A multicentre randomised trial of amniotomy
    in spontaneous first labour at term. *Br J Obstet Gynaecol* 1994;101(4):
    307–309.

Chapter 7
Slow Labor: Patience Is a Virtue

Nonmedical factors often determine the diagnosis and treatment of slow labor.

A labor support professional describes the glaring discrepancies between
nursing notes and mothers' recall versus physicians' notes for five clients'
previous cesareans.[42] She writes that these cases are typical.

Case 1: the nurse charted complete cervical dilation, a head engaged in
the pelvis, and the mother pushing well. The obstetrician wrote he performed
the cesarean because the mother was 6 centimeters dilated and the head was
high. The father remembered overhearing the obstetrician tell someone on
the telephone to go ahead to the party; he would be there soon.

Case 2: the doctor told the mother she was too short for vaginal birth. In
labor, he said she was not progressing satisfactorily and insisted that she have
an epidural in case a cesarean was necessary. The nurse noted that she started
the mother pushing before complete dilation and that she had been pushing
for thirty-five minutes when the doctor decided on the cesarean. He recorded
that she was fully dilated yet still had a cervical rim and that she had been
pushing for two hours. The author comments that the nurse likely started
the mother pushing early to try to forestall the cesarean.

Case 3: the doctor's notes contained nonsense statements such as "the
patient never even separated." The nurse charted the baby's head as being 2
centimeters below what the doctor's notes indicated. The mother had a cesarean after only an hour of pushing, even though she had had an epidural
(epidurals slow pushing progress).

Case 4: the mother comments that she agreed to the cesarean only because
she was told she had not dilated when, in fact, the nursing notes state she
achieved 3–4 centimeters' dilation.

Case 5: the mother felt no urge to push until they sat her up to do an
epidural preparatory to a forceps delivery. They ignored her when she said
she now had to push and continued with the epidural. The forceps attempt
failed, and the doctor proceeded to a C-section.

Virtually all hospitals plot labor progress on a graph that has centimeters dilation on the vertical axis and time on the horizontal axis. Researchers found that changing how data looked on the graph could alter obstetrician recommendations.[13] They gave sixteen obstetricians six hypothetical equivocal cases sufficiently separated in time that the doctors would not realize they were seeing the same cases twice. In three cases, researchers made it appear that labor was taking longer by increasing the distance between time marks on the horizontal axis in one of the pair. In the other three cases, they either graphed early labor along with active labor or graphed active labor only and described early labor in the case notes. Out of ninety-six decisions, the presentation that visually suggested longer labor resulted in fourteen more recommendations for C-section, five more for instrumental delivery, and eleven more for giving oxytocin.

Intervention rates vary according to the individual practitioner's personal approach. Researchers looked at management according to whether eleven obstetricians had a low, medium, or high cesarean rate.[15] Cesarean rates for poor progress ranged from 3 percent to 16 percent in low-risk first-time mothers despite similar maternal and infant characteristics. While doctors in the low cesarean-rate group induced labor less often and started oxytocin later in labor, they also used oxytocin more often and in higher doses. From this the authors conclude that oxytocin is the key to reducing cesareans, which, as midwifery statistics attest, isn't so. Another study grouped 550 first-time mothers according to whether their doctor's cesarean rate for poor progress was low (6–7 percent) or high (9–15 percent).[27] Women in both groups were equally likely to have epidurals, oxytocin, and to have doctors rupture membranes, all factors influencing progress. However, doctors in the high cesarean-rate group were more than three times as likely (2.5 percent versus 8 percent) to perform a cesarean for poor progress during pushing. Eight babies in the low cesarean-rate group had broken collarbones or facial nerve injuries from forceps deliveries. The authors comment that these might have been avoided by allowing more time to push.

Cesarean rates also vary by practice type (see also page 257, "Active management is at worst . . ."). A study of clinic and private obstetricians at a single hospital found that among 200 healthy, first-time mothers, the cesarean rate for poor progress was 1 percent on the clinic service and 20 percent on the private service, although women were equally likely to have epidurals (42 percent in both groups).[41] Women not having epidurals were *more* likely to have oxytocin on the private service (32 percent versus 20 percent), yet they were fourteen times more likely to have cesareans compared with clinic women not having epidurals. Women having epidurals with private doctors were as likely to have oxytocin as clinic women, yet, they too were fourteen times more likely to have a cesarean. Researchers in another study compared cesarean rates at a hospital that had private doctors, clinic doctors serving low-income women, and HMO doctors working shifts.[37] So that poor progress would be the main reason for cesareans, they looked at low-risk first-time mothers. Rates were 21 percent for private physicians, 17 percent for clinic physicians, and 15 percent for HMO physicians. After taking epidural use into account, women with HMO doctors were less than half as likely to have a cesarean as women with private obstetricians. Interestingly, the study was done a year after the HMO formed. Two years later, there had been a "marked" increase in HMO cesarean rates, which suggests that hospital cultural climate affected practice.

Convenience is a factor. A study of cesarean for poor progress in 4,200 first-time mothers found that more cesareans were performed in the evening than at night during sleep hours or during the day when obstetricians had office hours and scheduled surgeries.[22] A study comparing first-time (*primary*) cesarean rates among three hospitals with private physicians and one with salaried physicians working shifts found that fewer cesareans for poor progress were done at two of the private hospitals at night than during the day or evening.[19] This did not occur at the hospital where doctors worked shifts or at the other private hospital. Cesarean rates were 6 percent at the hospital with shifts versus 9 percent at the private hospital where time of day did not matter and 11 percent at the hospitals where it did.

High-dose oxytocin regimens pose risks.

The major risk of high-dose oxytocin regimens is *uterine hyperstimulation*, that is, overly long, frequent, and strong contractions along with overly high uterine-muscle tension between contractions. Hyperstimulation reduces the baby's oxygen supply, which can cause fetal distress. Researchers at a hospital using a high-dose protocol found that babies were twice as likely to be born with low blood pH, a symptom of oxygen deprivation in labor, when the mother had oxytocin.[32] Several comparisons of high-dose versus low-dose protocols and protocols with short intervals between dose increases versus protocols that have longer intervals between dose increases have found that more women experience hyperstimulation and fetal distress with high-dose and/or short-interval regimens (see also page 229).[20,33,47] In one trial of active management, seven women, more than one-third, experienced hyperstimulation, and one had a cesarean for fetal distress.[5] In another trial, staff ignored a case of hyperstimulation, and the baby died.[53] The National Maternity Hospital obstetricians conducted a large study (13,000 labors) of electronic fetal monitoring in which they found that newborn seizures, the strongest evidence of oxygen deprivation in labor, were associated with oxytocin use and longer labors, the very labors for which active management prescribes oxytocin.[38] In another active managment study, nurses did not turn down the oxytocin as protocol dictated in 4 percent of the women experiencing hyperstimulation. If staff ignore hyperstimulation 4 percent of the time in a hospital with a standardized protocol, what might the percentage be under less controlled circumstances?[1]

Oxytocin-caused hyperstimulation may be a particular problem when the baby has passed large amounts of stool (thick meconium) into the amniotic fluid. The danger with meconium is that the baby will inhale it and develop a life-threatening pneumonia. Researchers studied 250 women with thick meconium whose labors stopped and whose babies were not in distress.[40] Over 40 percent of women given oxytocin who later had a cesarean for fetal distress had babies who inhaled meconium versus 6 percent of babies of mothers given oxytocin who went on to vaginal birth, a percentage comparable to the 5 percent who had cesareans and no oxytocin. The authors speculated that when oxytocin caused uterine hyperstimulation, the baby's oxygen level dropped, causing the baby to reflexively gasp in meconium.

Active management is at worst ineffective, and at best unnecessary.

While several before-and-after studies have shown statistically significant (meaning unlikely to be due to chance) reductions in cesarean rates with high-dose oxytocin regimens, four random-assignment (randomized controlled) trials have not.[10,23,35,44] It is a truism that treatments almost always look better in nonrandomized trials because randomized controlled trials eliminate many sources of bias. For example, with before-and-after trials, the intent to lower the cesarean rate and the belief that the new protocol will work can become a self-fulfilling prophecy.

Two analyses of outcomes from multiple randomized controlled trials (*meta-analysis*) agree that rupturing membranes and aggressive use of oxytocin offer no benefits. In one, researchers evaluated data from trials of the components of active management to determine their efficacy.[52] Rupturing membranes (*amniotomy*) shortened labor somewhat but didn't lower cesarean or instrumental delivery rates. Early use of oxytocin increased pain and uterine hyperstimulation, but conferred no benefits. Combining liberal oxytocin use with rupturing membranes shortened labor, but still didn't decrease cesarean or instrumental deliveries. By contrast, a female labor companion (*doula*) reduced the use of pain medication, instrumental delivery, and C-section and improved the condition of babies at birth. The authors concluded that female labor companions appeared to be the effective component of active management. In the other meta-analysis, researchers collected twelve trials of active management versus usual care totalling 5,100 women.[21] They, too, found a reduction in labor length but no reduction in instrumental or cesarean delivery rates with active management. Some of the trials suggested that active management increased epidural and hemorrhage rates.

A developer of active management analyzed the usefulness of active management and concluded that active management shortened labor overall by shortening early labor, which normally proceeds at a leisurely pace. Active management had no effect on active labor, the phase of labor where a slow-down or halt indicates a possible problem.[9] Undeterred, he and his co-author converted this to a benefit by declaring slow dilation in early labor to be "inefficient" and correctable by application of active management.

Taken together, two small randomized controlled trials, 169 women in all, show that compared with less aggressive management, active management also fails as treatment for longer delays in progress than one hour, the usual delay that triggers oxytocin use.[6,21] Overall, the cesarean rate was 20 percent in the active management group versus 19 percent in the conservatively managed group.

A randomized controlled trial of active management in first-time mothers illustrates how cesarean rate depends largely on physician philosophy.[35] Overall cesarean rates differed only slightly between active management and usual care groups: 11 percent in the active management group and 14 percent in the standard care group. A critique of this study points out that the cesarean rate in first-time mothers the year before the study was 23 percent.[45] This means merely doing the study decreased cesarean rates by 40 percent in women receiving usual care. Furthermore, active management only bene-fited patients of private physicians. The cesarean rate in clinic patients was 9 percent in both active management and standard care groups. The cesarean rate in clinic patients had been 17 percent the year before, so while active management didn't reduce the cesarean rate in low-income women, doing a study halved it. Incredibly, the trial's authors explained the difference be-tween private and clinic patients by saying that active management seemed "especially effective" in private patients, "a group recognized as being at increased risk" for dysfunctional labors. Since all participants, rich or poor, were healthy, first-time mothers who started labor on their own, the authors are claiming that having enough money to afford private care causes dys-functional labor.

Giving women more time works just as well at reducing cesareans. In another randomized controlled trial of first-time mothers, cesarean rates did not differ even though women were more likely to have an epidural in the usual care group.[23] What differed was that women were three times more likely to have labors lasting more than twelve hours in the usual care group (26 percent versus 9 percent).

Active management does not eliminate the adverse effects of epidurals.

Half of the first 1,000 first-time mothers to give birth at the Dublin National Hospital in 1992 had epidurals versus 1 percent of the first 1,000 first-time mothers in 1973. The cesarean rate, which was 5 percent in 1973, had doubled to 10 percent in 1992.[8] Another study of 9,000 first-time moth-ers giving birth at the Dublin National Hospital in 1990–1994 reported that while the overall cesarean rate was 11 percent, it was 24 percent among women having prolonged labor of whom 90 percent had epidurals.[36] An additional 40 percent of women with prolonged labor had an instrumental delivery (the active management protocol limits pushing phase to two hours). Having an epidural increased the likelihood of having a prolonged labor six-fold, forty-two-fold if the epidural was placed early in labor. Another study of active versus standard management in 400 first-time mothers found that even though active management helped women with epidurals somewhat, the cesarean rate was still 11 percent versus 3 percent in women not having an epidural.[43] Over 85 percent of all cesareans were in women who had epi-durals.

Simple, noninvasive strategies may safely and effectively enhance labor progress during the dilation and pushing phases of labor as well as make for a more pleasant labor.

I have five studies that compared walking and staying upright in labor with lying in bed and two studies comparing walking with oxytocin aug-mentation for slow labors. All that can be said for certain is that none found any harm in allowing freedom of activity and position, a statement that can-not be made of oxytocin, and that women who walked liked it—99 percent in a large study that asked women about this.[7] Beyond that it is difficult to draw firm conclusions because the studies all have problems. For example, one major confounding factor is that women could choose whether and how long to walk. The reasons why women would agree or decline to walk and how long they walked would undoubtedly have to do with the kind of labor they were having, which, in turn, could affect whether walking seemed to help or not. It could go either way. Women having more painful, nonprogressive labors with, say, a posterior baby might prefer to lie down as might women in intense, rapidly progressing labors. A recent, large trial randomly assigning women to walk or not found that women who declined walking had *shorter* labors, which suggests that the second possibility was the case.[7]

Three studies concluded that walking had benefits, two of them that first-time mothers had the most to gain. Two trials, one of 370 women and one of only 40 women, that assigned women to walk or to bed-rest groups found that first-time mothers who walked shortened labor by about one and a half hours compared with the group assigned to bed rest.[3,16] A third study analyzed the effect of walking and staying upright in 1,700 women attended by midwives.[2] Women who stayed upright had half the rate of instrumental and cesarean delivery combined (3 percent versus 6 percent). Labor was not shortened, but the midwives recommended walking to women making slow progress.

The two largest studies, both random assignment trials, found no benefit. The first, of 630 women, found no reductions in oxytocin use, instrumental delivery, or cesarean section.[29] However, only about half of women in the walking group walked in early labor and virtually none walked in late labor. The other, involving 1070 women, found no differences in length of labor, use of oxytocin or pain medication, or instrumental or cesarean delivery.[7] This held true for both first-time mothers and women with prior births. However, in the walking group, nearly one-quarter never walked at all, and of women who walked, half walked less than an hour.

Both studies of walking versus oxytocin for slow labor showed benefits. In one, fourteen women were assigned to either walking or oxytocin.[43] In the first hour, all eight walking women made progress in dilation and descent of the fetal head versus three of six women having oxytocin. In the second hour, one woman in the walking group gave birth and the rest made further progress versus four women in the oxytocin group. Oxytocin increased pain whereas walking lessened it or made no difference. The second study, of 57 women, found that 60 percent of women in the walking group gave birth without requiring oxytocin.[31] Women in the oxytocin group reported more pain and experienced more excessively strong contractions.

Researchers in one study randomly assigned 84 women to labor augmentation either by nipple stimulation via breast pump or oxytocin.[49] Nipple stimulation alone succeeded in half the women and achieved similar average labor duration and fewer cesareans compared with oxytocin. This was despite lower contraction pressures in the nipple stimulation group, a potential advantage in that lower pressures could minimize pain and the possibility of fetal distress. (See also page 228.)

Of five studies of women randomly assigned to either upright or lying-down pushing positions, four reported some benefit. In the one that didn't, only six first-time mothers and five mothers with prior births actually squatted, numbers too small to draw any conclusions.[28] The other studies all involved at least 300 participants. All three studies that evaluated pain and preference found that women liked the upright position and experienced less pain.[14,24,54] One study found less genital injury.[24] Two found that upright positioning shortened pushing phase and one that it resulted in fewer instrumental deliveries (9 percent versus 16 percent).[24–25] One in which upright women used a birthing stool reported more blood loss in the upright group, but the authors acknowledged that blood-loss estimates are subjective.[54] On the birth stool, blood collected in a bowl under the stool whereas in bed, some blood soaked into pads and sheets. In a sixth study, in one practice, researchers randomly selected case records of women who squatted to push and compared outcomes with randomly selected records from another practice offering similar labor care except that women gave birth semi-sitting.[26] Researchers found less genital injury, shorter pushing phase, and less use of instrumental delivery in first-time mothers (8 percent versus 17 percent) in the squatting group.

I have six studies evaluating warm tub baths in labor. A randomized trial of 110 first-time mothers found a significant improvement in cervical softening and effacement and a trend toward faster dilation in the bath group.[12] Compared with nonbathers, bathing stabilized pain intensity for about half an hour before it began to rise again. Eighty percent of bathers said the bath soothed pain and relaxed them, and 90 percent would want to bathe in a future labor. Women also tended to have oxytocin less often. Another study compared outcomes between 88 women taking a 1½ to 2 hour bath with 72 similar women who chose not to bathe.[34] Bathers dilated twice as fast in the bath. They hurt more before the bath and experienced greater pain relief from the bath compared with nonbathers. Nonbathers were more likely to have narcotic pain relief and twice as likely to have oxytocin. However, this study did not involve random assignment, so there may well be confounding factors. In the third study, researchers compared 89 bathers with 89 similar nonbathers and found that bathers were less likely to receive oxytocin or to have pain medication, but this may be because bathers were participants in a study of in-hospital homestyle care whereas nonbathers received standard care.[55] Researchers in a fourth study randomly assigned 800 women to be offered a bath or not.[46] Only half the women in the bath group actually bathed and these were more likely to be first-time mothers with less cervical dilation. This may explain why bathing did not shorten labor or lessen oxytocin use. Bath-group women were 25 percent less likely to use pain medication. Bathers reported that the tub relieved pain and helped them relax. The fifth study found no benefit in 45 women who bathed in labor versus 48 who didn't.[48] In the sixth study, researchers randomly assigned two hundred women to bathe either early, before 5 cm dilation, or late, after 5 cm dilation.[18] The early bathers averaged longer labors. However, there were more first-time mothers in the early bath group (72 percent versus 60 percent), and early bathers were more likely to have epidurals (27 percent versus 9 percent), both factors that make for slower labors. And if there were an effect, it could be either that early bathing slowed labor or late bathing speeded it up.

None of these six studies plus a seventh that only evaluated infection rates in 540 bathers versus 850 nonbathers found an increased risk of maternal or infant infection.[17] This was despite the fact that all women had ruptured membranes in three of the studies.[12,17,55]

Women admitted to the hospital in early labor or prelabor may be more likely to have labor interventions.

Researchers found that among 600 healthy, first-time mothers, women laboring slowly who arrived at the hospital earlier in labor were more likely to have a diagnosis of difficult delivery (12 percent versus 3 percent), oxytocin augmentation (45 percent versus 30 percent), instrumental delivery (14 percent versus 9 percent), and C-section (16 percent versus 4 percent) than women laboring slowly who came later in labor.[30] For women making rapid progress, time of arrival made no difference. "Protracted labor" was the reason for cesarean in seven early comers but no late comers regardless of progress rate. Researchers in another study compared outcomes in 3,800 first-time mothers at four hospitals.[50] Cesarean rates ranged from 12 percent to 20 percent, of which three-quarters were done for poor progress. Forty percent of all cesareans were done in early labor. The authors concluded that if doctors would stop doing cesareans before active phase labor and for poor progress in the absence of fetal distress, the average cesarean rate could be halved. A third study found that use of oxytocin to augment labor declined linearly from over 75 percent of women admitted at 1 centimeter's dilation or less to less than 20 percent of women admitted at 5 centimeters' dilation or more.[11] Epidural use was also strongly and inversely associated with both dilation at admission and labor augmentation. The authors of a random assignment trial in first-time mothers noted that the cesarean rate for women admitted at less than 3 centimeters' dilation was 10 percent versus one-tenth that percentage in women admitted at 3 centimeters' dilation or more.[10]

Two other studies have also reported that women who experience "false" labor are more likely to have oxytocin induction, augmentation, and cesarean section.[4,51] Their authors concluded that women experiencing "false" labor were at high risk for dysfunctional labor. An equally plausible explanation is that impatience leads to a diagnosis of prolonged labor and inappropriate intervention, including cesarean section.

Finally, a trial in which over 200 women with prelabor or early labor contractions were randomly assigned to hospital admission or to be sent home found that women who were sent home were less than half as likely to be given oxytocin.[39] While cesarean rates overall were not *significantly* different, meaning the difference was considered due to chance, one-quarter (2 of 8) of the cesareans were done for dysfunctional labor in the group sent home versus three-quarters (8 of 11) of the cesareans in the admitted group. This occurred despite the fact that 16 percent of women in the "admit" group actually got sent home, and most women had epidurals in both groups, factors that would tend to flatten out differences between them.

REFERENCES

1. Akoury HA et al. Oxytocin augmentation of labor and perinatal outcome in nulliparas. *Obstet Gynecol* 1991;78(2):227–230.
2. Albers LL et al. The relationship of ambulation in labor to operative delivery. *J Nurse Midwifery* 1997;42(1):4–8.

3. Andrews CM and Chrzanowski M. Maternal position, labor and comfort. *Applied Nursing Res* 1990;3(1):7–13.
4. Arulkumaran S et al. Obstetric outcome of patients with a previous episode of spurious labor. *Am J Obstet Gynecol* 1987;157(1):17–20.
5. Bidgood KA and Steer PJ. A randomized control study of oxytocin augmentation of labour. 1. Obstetric outcome. *Br J Obstet Gynaecol* 1987; 94:512–517.
6. Blanch G et al. Dysfunctional labour: a randomised trial. *Br J Obstet Gynaecol* 1998;105(1):117–120.
7. Bloom SL et al. Lack of effect of walking on labor and delivery. *N Engl J Med* 1998;339(2):76–79.
8. Boylan P, Robson M, and McParland P. Active management of labor. *Am J Obstet Gynecol* 1993;168(1 Pt 2):295.
9. Boylan PC and Parisi VM. Effect of active management on latent phase labor. *Am J Perinatol* 1990;7(4):363–365.
10. Cammu H and Van Eeckhout E. A randomised trial of early versus delayed use of amniotomy and oxytocin infusion in nulliparous labour. *Br J Obstet Gynaecol* 1996;103(9):939–940.
11. Cammu H et al. Epidural analgesia in active management of labor. *Acta Obstet Gynecol Scand* 1994;73:235–239.
12. Cammu H et al. 'To bathe or not to bathe' during the first stage of labor. *Acta Obstet Gynecol Scand* 1994;73:468–472.
13. Cartmill RSV and Thornton JG. Effect of presentation of partogram information on obstetric decision-making. *Lancet* 1992;339:1520–1522.
14. de Jong PR et al. Randomised trial comparing the upright and supine positions for the second stage of labour. *Br J Obstet Gynaecol* 1997; 104(5):561–571.
15. DeMott RK and Sandmire HF. The Green Bay cesarean section study. II. The physician factor as a determinant of cesarean birth rates for failed labor. *Am J Obstet Gynecol* 1992;166(6 Pt 1):1799–1810.
16. Diaz AG et al. Vertical position during the first stage of the course of labor, and neonatal outcome. *Eur J Obstet Gynecol Reprod Biol* 1980; 11:1–7.
17. Eriksson M et al. Warm tub bath during labor. A study of 1385 women with prelabor rupture of the membranes after 34 weeks of gestation. *Acta Obstet Gynecol Scand* 1996;75:642–644.
18. Eriksson M, Mattsson LA, and Ladfors L. Early or late bath during the first stage of labour: a randomised study of 200 women. *Midwifery* 1997;13:146–148.
19. Evans MI et al. Cesarean section: assessment of the convenience factor. *J Reprod Med* 1984;29(9):670–676.
20. Foster TCS, Jacobson JD, and Valenzuela GJ. Oxytocin augmentation of labor: a comparison of 15- and 30-minute dose increment intervals. *Obstet Gynecol* 1988;71(2):147–149.
21. Fraser W et al. Effects of early augmentation of labor with amniotomy and oxytocin in nulliparous women: a meta-analysis. *Br J Obstet Gynaecol* 1998;105(2):189–194.
22. Fraser W et al. Temporal variation in rates of cesarean section for dys-

tocia: does "convenience" play a role? *Am J Obstet Gynecol* 1987; 156(2):300–304.

23. Frigoletto FD et al. A clinical trial of active management of labor. *New Engl J Med* 1995;333(12):745–750.

24. Gardosi J, Hutson N, and B-Lynch C. Randomized controlled trial of squatting in the second stage of labour. *Lancet* 1989;2(8654):74–77.

25. Gardosi J, Sylvester S, and B-Lynch C. Alternative positions in the second stage of labour: a randomized controlled trial. *Br J Obstet Gynaecol* 1989;96:1290–1296.

26. Golay J, Vedam S, and Sorger L. The squatting position for the second stage of labor: effects on labor and on maternal and fetal well-being. *Birth* 1993;20(2):73–78.

27. Guillemette J and Fraser WD. Differences between obstetricians in caesarean rates and the management of labour. *Br J Obstet Gynaecol* 1992; 99(2):105–108.

28. Gupta JK, Brayshaw EM, and Lilford R. An experiment of squatting birth. *Eur J Obstet Gynecol Reprod Biol* 1989;30:217–220.

29. Hemminki E and Saarikoski S. Ambulation and delayed amniotomy in the first stage of labor. *Eur J Obstet Gynecol Reprod Biol* 1983;15:129–139.

30. Hemminki E and Simukka R. The timing of hospital admission and progress of labour. *Eur J Obstet Gynecol Reprod Biol* 1986;22:85–94.

31. Hemminki E et al. Ambulation versus oxytocin in protracted labour: a pilot study. *Eur J Obstet Gynecol Reprod Biol* 1985;20:199–208.

32. Herbst A, Wolner-Hanssen P, and Ingemarsson I. Risk factors for acidemia at birth. *Obstet Gynecol* 1997;90(1):125–130.

33. Lazor LZ et al. A randomized comparison of 15- and 40-minute dosing protocols for labor augmentation and induction. *Obstet Gynecol* 1993; 82(6):1009–1012.

34. Lenstrup C et al. Warm tub bath during delivery. *Acta Obstet Gynecol Scand* 1987;66(8):709–712.

35. Lopez-Zeno JA et al. A controlled trial of a program for the active management of labor. *N Engl J Med* 1992;326(17):450–454.

36. Malone FD et al. Prolonged labor in nulliparas: lessons from the active management of labor. *Obstet Gynecol* 1996;88(2):211–215.

37. McCloskey L, Petitti DB, and Hobel CJ. Variations in the use of cesarean delivery for dystocia: lessons about the source of care. *Med Care* 1992; 30(2):126–135.

38. McDonald D et al. The Dublin randomized controlled trial of intrapartum fetal heart rate monitoring. *Am J Obstet Gynecol* 1985;152(5):524–539.

39. McNiven PS et al. An early labor assessment program: a randomized, controlled trial. *Birth* 1998;25(1):5–10.

40. Morel MIG et al. Oxytocin augmentation in arrest disorders in the presence of thick meconium: influence on neonatal outcome. *Gynecol Obstet Invest* 1994;37(1):21–24.

41. Neuhoff D, Burke MS, and Porreco RP. Cesarean birth for failed progress in labor. *Obstet Gynecol* 1989;73(6):915–920.

42. Perez P. The patient observer: what really led to these cesarean births? *Birth* 1989;16(3):130–139.
43. Read JA, Miller FC, and Paul RH. Randomized trial of ambulation versus oxytocin for labor enhancement: a preliminary report. *Am J Obstet Gynecol* 1981;139(6):669–672.
44. Rogers R et al. Active management of labor: does it make a difference? *Am J Obstet Gynecol* 1997:177(3):599–605.
45. Rothman BK. The active management of physicians. *Birth* 1993;20(3): 158–159.
46. Rush J et al. The effects of whirlpool baths in labor: a randomized, controlled trial. *Birth* 1996;23(3):136–143.
47. Satin AJ et al. High- versus low-dose oxytocin for labor stimulation. *Obstet Gynecol* 1992;80(1):111–116.
48. Schorn MN, McAllister JL, and Blanco JD. Water immersion and the effect on labor. *J Nurse Midwifery* 1993;38(6):336–342.
49. Stein JL et al. Nipple stimulation for labor augmentation. *J Reprod Med* 1990;35(7): 710–714
50. Stewart PJ et al. Diagnosis of dystocia and management with cesarean section among primiparous women in Ottawa-Carelton. *Can Med Assoc J* 1990,142(5):459–463
51. Summers PR et al. Pregnancy outcome in patients with repeat visits to the labor observation area near term. *South Med J* 1991;84(4):436–438.
52. Thornton JG and Lilford RJ. Active management of labour: current knowledge and research. *BMJ* 1994;309(6951):366–369.
53. Turner MJ, Brassil M, and Gordon H. Active management of labor associated with a decrease in the cesarean section rate in nulliparas. *Obstet Gynecol* 1988;71(2):150–154.
54. Waldenstrom U and Gottvall K. A randomized trial of birthing stool or conventional semirecumbent position for second-stage labor. *Birth* 1991; 18(1):5–10.
55. Waldenstrom U and Nilsson CA. Warm tub bath after spontaneous rupture of the membranes. *Birth* 1992;19(2):57–63.

Chapter 8
Epidurals and Narcotics:
A Shot in the Dark

Epidurals slow labor.

Three trials in which women were randomly assigned to epidurals or narcotics reported longer labors. Random assignment eliminates the possibility that women having slower, more difficult labors would elect epidurals.[44,64]* Another study ruled out the "difficult labor" factor by starting with

---

*One of the three compared labor length in women actually having an epidural or not rather than the groups as a whole. However, as only 5 of 500 women in the narcotic group had an epidural, they are unlikely to alter results.[57]

women who were already receiving oxytocin for insufficient progress before having pain medication.[5] Here, too, an epidural prolonged labor.

Epidurals increase the use of oxytocin.

An analysis of data from four random-assignment trials found that epidurals increased the use of oxytocin by 450 percent.[26] Epidurals also increase how much oxytocin is needed. One study looked at 200 women who were receiving oxytocin for insufficient progress before having pain medication.[5] All gave birth vaginally without forceps or vacuum extraction, but women who chose epidurals progressed more slowly and required significantly more oxytocin.

Epidurals increase the likelihood of vaginal instrumental delivery.

Studies consistently show that epidurals increase the percentage of vaginal instrumental deliveries, including the random-assignment trials.[61] Random-assignment trials eliminate the argument that difficult births lead to epidurals rather than vice versa.

Low-dose and narcotic epidurals have not solved the problem. All three recent random-assignment trials, one of which used a low-dose epidural versus injected narcotic and two of which used narcotic epidurals versus injected narcotic, reported more instrumental deliveries in the epidural group.[46,57,64] Random-assignment trials have also found that narcotic epidurals didn't reduce instrumental delivery rates compared with plain, low-dose epidurals.[13] One trial found that women were somewhat better off with a spinal epidural than a narcotic epidural, but rates were extremely high in both groups (40 percent versus 31 percent).[39]

Epidurals can increase the likelihood of cesarean delivery, especially in first-time mothers.

Studies frequently show that epidurals lead to more cesareans for poor progress even with modern epidural techniques and labor management.[61] Of fifteen studies totalling more than 55,000 women that compared cesarean rates in women having an epidural with women who didn't, twelve found epidurals were associated with more cesareans.[61]

Critics argue that this is because women with difficult labors are more likely to want epidurals. However, studies that attempted to correct for this factor continued to show an excess of cesareans in the epidural group. Researchers reported in one that the cesarean rate for lack of progress in 450 first-time mothers who had an epidural for labor pain was 10 percent, but it was only 4 percent in 270 first-time mothers who did not.[63] The gap remained after excluding women with big babies and women whose labor pattern was abnormal prior to having an epidural. Researchers in another study grouped 1,700 first-time mothers according to their predicted likelihood of having a difficult labor or other factors that might affect the probability of having an epidural. In every subgroup, the women who actually ended up having an epidural were more likely to have a cesarean than the women who didn't.[31]

Three out of the four randomized controlled trials have also shown that epidurals increase cesarean rates. Random assignment to one group or the other eliminates potentially confounding factors such as that women with dysfunctional labors are more likely to want an epidural. Philipsen and Jensen found a three-fold increase in cesarean rate for lack of progress (6 percent to 17 percent) in the women who had epidurals.[41] Thorp and coworkers conducted a randomized controlled trial that was originally planned to have 100 first-time mothers in the epidural and nonepidural groups.[64] They discontinued the trial halfway through when they found that the cesarean rate for lack of progress in the epidural group was 16 percent versus 2 percent in the nonepidural group. They felt it would be unethical to continue assigning women to have epidurals. In this trial, anesthesiologists used low-dose epidurals, cesareans for lack of progress were never performed during early labor, and oxytocin was aggressively used to treat dysfunctional labor, factors that would tend to minimize the number of cesareans attributable to the epidural. Ramin and coworkers studied over 850 women of whom nearly half had given birth before.[46] The combined cesarean and instrumental vaginal delivery rates were 9 percent in the epidural group versus 5 percent in the narcotic group. However, about one-third of the epidural group never had an epidural and one-third of the narcotic group did. The authors then looked at outcomes based on actual treatment. The overall cesarean rate for women having epidurals was 9 percent versus 4 percent in women having narcotic, and the rate for poor progress was 5 percent in the epidural group versus 1.5% in the nonepidural group.* After adjustment for confounding factors, this calculated out to a 250 percent increase in the risk of cesarean section for poor progress in first-time mothers and nearly a 400 percent increase in women who already had children.** This was despite the fact that the average dilation was 5 centimeters when the epidural was placed, and oxytocin was used freely, as with Thorp and colleagues, factors that would tend to blunt the effect of epidurals on cesarean rates. Combined together, these three trials encompass nearly 1,100 women and show that epidurals increase the risk of cesarean by 250 percent.[61]

Epidurals needn't necessarily increase the cesarean rate, though. Sharma et al., a trial in which 700 women were randomly assigned to epidural versus injected narcotic, did not find more cesareans in the epidural group. Even so, having an epidural prolonged labor, again, despite using low-dose narcotic epidurals and liberal oxytocin use.[57] This only proves the point I make on page 267: "Whether an epidural increases the odds of cesarean depends on the caregiver's philosophy."

Having an epidural early in labor, when dilating slowly, or when the head is still high in the pelvis increases the risk of cesarean for poor progress, probably at least partly because epidurals inhibit rotation of the baby from posterior to anterior.

Because it prolongs labor, persistent posterior position (baby's back toward mother's back) is the hidden factor in many cesarean sections for poor

---

*You would expect to see lower cesarean rates because, unlike the other two randomized controlled trials, many women in this trial were not first-time mothers. Women with prior vaginal births rarely have cesareans for lack of progress.

**Women with prior births look worse because women with prior births rarely have cesareans for poor progress. When the base percentage is tiny, it doesn't take much change to quadruple it.

progress (see page 108). Epidurals increase the incidence of persistent posterior babies by 450 percent according to an analysis that pooled data from two trials in which women were randomly assigned to epidural anesthesia or not.[26] Random assignment eliminated the possibility that women laboring with posterior babies are more likely to want epidurals.

The following studies illustrate the consequences of opting for an epidural before the baby rotates. Keep in mind as you read them that slow dilation despite strong contractions, a head that remains high in the pelvis, and excessive pain that might lead a woman to want an epidural, especially an early epidural, are all emblematic of a posterior baby.

One study found that the slower the mother was dilating, the more likely having an epidural would result in a cesarean.[62] In particular, the cesarean rate for poor progress quintupled in women dilating slowly who had an epidural compared with women dilating slowly who didn't have one. The study also found that the earlier in dilation the epidural was started, the more likely a cesarean for poor progress. Two other studies also found an increased risk of cesarean with early epidural placement: five-fold in one and two-fold in the other.[31,39] One of these studies also found the likelihood increased 2½ times if the head was still high in the pelvis at time of placement.[39] Yet another study found that having an epidural while the head was still high strongly predicted a nonanterior baby at delivery.[50]

I must also point out that while it helps, having an epidural when dilating more rapidly or later in labor doesn't eliminate the increased risk of cesarean. The first study mentioned found that even if the epidural was administered at 5 centimeters' cervical dilation or more, the cesarean rate for lack of progress was 11 percent, and it was 6 percent in women dilating at average or faster than average compared with 2 percent in all women—slow and rapid dilators together—who never had an epidural.[62] The study that found a five-fold increase with early epidural placement still found a three-fold increase with later placement compared with the nonepidural group.[31]

Note: Anesthesiologists often dispute the risk of early epidurals by citing a study they believe proves that timing doesn't matter.[11] The study claims to compare first-time mothers receiving an early versus a late epidural. However, even women in the early group had to be at least 3 centimeters dilated before being assigned to a group, and both groups of women actually received their epidurals at 4–5 centimeters' dilation.

Whether an epidural increases the odds of cesarean depends on the caregiver's philosophy.

Researchers compared cesarean rates for 200 healthy first-time mothers managed by the resident staff and 400 similar women at the same hospital who had private physicians.[40] Forty-two percent of each group had an epidural, but the cesarean rate for lack of progress on the clinic service, which had a long-standing commitment to minimize the number of cesareans, was 1 percent versus 20 percent on the private service. Three studies compared cesarean rates before and after introduction of an epidural.[19,22,34] None found an effect on cesarean rates or rates for lack of progress. But the cesarean rates at these hospitals during the "before" periods were around 10 percent in an era when the U. S. cesarean rate was over 20 percent. Clearly, the practitioners at these hospitals had a commitment to keeping cesarean rates low. The random assignment trial mentioned under "Epidurals can increase the likelihood of cesarean delivery . . ." (page 265) that found no increase in cesareans likewise had a low cesarean rate in both groups.

Epidurals cause complications, including life-threatening complications, even with experienced anesthetists using correct procedures and despite taking proper precautions.

A review of 26,500 cases of epidural anesthesia found 1 in 3,000 instances of depositing the anesthetic inward of the epidural space or injection of the anesthetic into a vein.[15] This caused loss of consciousness, convulsions, cardiac arrest, severely low blood pressure, or maternal respiratory difficulty or fetal distress. In one out of three of these cases, there was a "relatively protracted period of real concern." Injecting a test dose prior to instilling the full dose did not prevent these events, and all occurred with experienced anesthesiologists. In another study, researchers sent questionnaires asking about serious complications of epidural anesthesia to all United Kingdom obstetric units.[54] Overall, most of the units responded, providing data on 505,000 epidurals. Respondents reported three cases of cardiac arrest, one causing brain damage, twenty cases of convulsions, eight cases of injection into the wrong space (high or total spinal) causing respiratory paralysis, and one case of allergic shock. In a follow-up project to this second study, researchers sent forms to 79 obstetric units and asked them to keep track of serious complications over a two-year period.[55] This design generally produces more accurate information than after-the-fact questionnaires, although underreporting is still an issue. Respondents reported on 123,000 epidurals and spinals. Potentially life-threatening reactions occurred in 1 per 4,000 cases.

As for serious, but not life-threatening, complications, all three studies also reported instances of these, a few of which caused permanent damage. Complications falling into this category included nerve injury, sensations of numbness or weakness, abcess, severe backache, severe headache, and urinary problems. Another researcher investigated the incidence of abnormal sensations and muscle function in nearly 24,000 women after birth. Incidence rates were 36 per 10,000 in women with epidurals versus 2 per 10,000 in women who had no pain relief medication.[42] All the women recovered fully with therapy.

Other studies show that precautions can fail. One technique is injecting a test dose of *epinephrine* (adrenaline) before injecting the anesthetic. Theoretically, if epinephrine enters the bloodstream it will increase the heart rate, which should detect whether the needle has pierced a blood vessel. A study in which a small amount of epinephrine was deliberately injected into a vein in healthy, unmedicated laboring women showed, however, that the effect was difficult to detect in practice because the stress of contractions also increased maternal heart rate.[30] A review of 4,000 epidurals revealed that pulling back on the plunger to see if blood flows into the syringe and giving the anesthetic in small amounts can fail to detect that the needle is in a vein.[28] By marking the epidural catheter in centimeters, researchers have studied whether looping and taping it to the mother's back keeps it from moving.[45] They found that in more than one-third of cases the catheter migrated inward of the epidural space, which could potentially cause life-threatening complications.

Epidurals cause fevers, increasing the likelihood that the baby will be kept in the nursery, subjected to diagnostic tests (septic workup), and given preventative intravenous antibiotic treatment.

Studies have consistently found that epidurals elevate temperature over time. One study of 33 laboring women found that maternal temperature increased steadily over time at an average rate of 1.8°F per seven hours.[20] Another study inserted a temperature probe vaginally and found that fetal skin temperatures during labor exceeded 100.4°F in nearly one-third of the 33 mothers who had epidurals.[37] The authors estimated this meant that in approximately 5 percent of fetuses, internal temperatures exceeded 104°F. Researchers in a third study found that epidural anesthesia increased the odds by 25 percent that the newborn would have a fever when its temperature was first taken.[66] Lieberman et al. studied 1,650 women and found that 14.5 percent of women with epidurals ran fevers of 100.4°F or more versus 1 percent of women not having an epidural.[32] Seven percent of women with epidurals whose labors lasted six or fewer hours ran fevers, increasing to more than one-third of women whose labors lasted over eighteen hours. Finally, a study of over 3,000 women found that epidural anesthesia increased the odds of developing a fever four-fold.[24] Of the 39 women who ran persistent fevers after birth, 36 had an epidural in labor.

Fever in labor is a possible symptom of uterine infection, which can pose a serious threat to the baby. For this reason, having an epidural during labor markedly increases the odds of doctors keeping the baby in the nursery for observation, ordering diagnostic tests (*septic workup*)—which usually includes multiple blood tests and a spinal tap—and treating the baby with intravenous antibiotics as a preventative measure until cultures come back negative. Compared with newborns whose mothers didn't have epidurals, newborns whose mothers had epidurals in Lieberman et al.'s study were over four times more likely (34 percent versus 10 percent) to have antibiotic treatment.

Some data suggest that epidurals may actually predispose to postpartum infection. In the study of over 3,000 women, less than one woman in five had an epidural, but nearly three-quarters of the 18 infants with potentially serious infections had mothers who had epidurals. Epidurals could increase the risk of newborn infection by prolonging labor. Prolonged labor with ruptured membranes increases the risk of infection because women are more likely to have multiple vaginal exams, internal electronic fetal monitoring, and a cesarean section.

Epidurals may cause long-term, even chronic problems.

Data conflict on whether epidurals lead to long-term backache. A survey of 11,700 women revealed that 18 percent of women who had epidurals for labor versus 10 percent of women who did not have an epidural developed a backache for the first time that lasted at least six weeks.[35] The backache did not appear to be a direct consequence of the epidural because women having epidurals for planned cesareans did not experience increased incidence of backache. The authors speculated that muscle relaxation in combination with the abolition of pain allowed the mother to remain in positions harmful to her back. Another survey of 1,000 women found almost the exact same differences—18 percent versus 12 percent—in the percentage of women reporting new onset of backache after childbirth lasting six months or more.[53] About one-quarter of the women attended a clinic to evaluate their pain. In most cases the pain was not severe and did not interfere with daily activities. Yet another study of 329 women found that 14 percent of women who had an epidural versus 7 percent of women who didn't reported low back pain six weeks after birth.[36] On the other hand, the authors of the smaller survey followed up on women already participating in a study of epidurals and compared the incidence of backache with a nonepidural group.[52] Percentages of women with new, long-term backache were virtually identical, and fewer women had this complaint than other studies have found. Moreover, the authors also found selective recall among respondents. Of seven women reporting new backache but who had complaints of backache in their prenatal records, six had epidurals. This casts doubts on surveys trusting only to memory months or years after the fact.

The larger survey also reported that inadvertent puncture of the dura, the first membrane covering the spinal cord, led to spinal headache, an incapacitatingly painful headache, in 4 per 1,000 women who had epidurals.[35] Although spinal headache is believed to subside within a week even without treatment, nine women reported spinal headache lasting over six weeks, and five women reported a duration longer than one year.

Epidural anesthetics "get" to the baby, as does the narcotic component of narcotic epidurals.

Studies have shown that bupivacaine, the anesthetic most commonly used in epidurals, crosses the placenta and is absorbed into fetal tissues and that the fetal dose rises with epidural duration.[48] Researchers have measured umbilical vein levels of bupivacaine at one-third that of maternal levels.[1,33,48] The narcotic components fentanyl and sufentanil have been measured at one-third and four-fifths of maternal blood levels, respectively.[33]

Far from protecting babies from fetal distress, epidurals can cause profound disturbances of the fetal heart rate.

Epidurals don't protect against fetal distress. Two trials in which women were assigned to epidural or no-epidural groups showed a trend toward higher cesarean rates for fetal distress in the epidural group: 4 percent versus 2 percent in a trial of over 850 women and 8 percent versus 0 percent in a trial of over 90 women.[46,64] Randomized trials eliminate the possibility that results are biased by factors such as women with more difficult labors tending to choose epidurals. Remember, too, that most of the women in the nonepidural group had narcotics, which can also adversely affect fetal status.

In fact, epidurals cause fetal distress. Eleven percent of the babies of healthy mothers in uncomplicated labor in one study developed fetal heart rate patterns alarming enough to prompt fetal scalp blood sampling to measure oxygenation,[12] and 11 percent of the babies of mothers in normal labor in another study experienced a fall in fetal heart rate of 50 beats per minute or more lasting for three or more minutes (the normal fetal heart rate ranges between 120 and 160 beats per minute).[59] Yet another study recorded that nearly three-quarters of the babies of healthy mothers in normal labor had episodes of slowing of the heart rate (*decelerations*), a symptom of fetal distress, after having an epidural.[17] Half of these occurred shortly after either administering a top-up dose or increasing the infusion rate of the anesthetic, which suggests that the anesthetic was, indeed, responsible. Finally, a study reported that 8.5 percent of babies experienced an average decline of 64 beats per minute lasting an average of six to seven minutes after their mothers had an epidural.[60]

A precipitous drop in the mother's blood pressure (*hypotension*) may also compromise fetal well-being. One study reported a hypotension rate of 10 percent,[12] another reported a 22 percent rate, although only 2 percent required drug treatment.[46] It should also be noted that while epidurals are recommended for laboring women with high blood pressure (*hypertension*) specifically because they lower blood pressure, an episode of overly low blood pressure is particularly dangerous when the baby is already compromised.

Epidurals may have adverse effects in the newborn.

Two studies comparing the newborns of women who had epidurals in labor with those whose mothers did not have shown adverse effects on newborn behavioral and motor functions when the mother had an epidural.[38,56] However, one study was published in 1981 and was thus likely to represent the effects of higher doses, and although the other was published in 1992, the women received much higher concentrations of anesthetic than usually given today. Modern types of epidurals may not have the same effects, although some data suggest they might. A recent study found lower neurologic scores at twenty-four hours in babies who had a modern narcotic (fentanyl) epidural compared with a sufentanil epidural and a plain, low-dose epidural.[33] This is all the more concerning because the test researchers gave is only intended to detect drug effects on muscle tone and so it would miss subtle deficits that would be picked up on tests of behavioral competencies. Moreover, the study compared drug to drug, not drug to unmedicated. An experiment in monkeys showed behavioral differences weeks after birth in baby monkeys whose mothers had been given epidurals.[21] Lactation consultants report that newborns whose mothers had epidurals have difficulty breastfeeding, but we have no published studies and "anecdotal data" are the very weakest kind of evidence. Epidurals also have indirect effects that could affect the baby and the early mother-baby interactions as well, namely, increased likelihood of having oxytocin, instrumental delivery, cesarean delivery, and of babies being separated from their mothers after birth.

Lower dosages and newer techniques have not reduced the adverse effects of epidurals.

Comparisons of continuous infusions of anesthetic with intermittent top-up doses report similar vaginal instrumental delivery rates, cesarean rates, bladder catheterization rates for inability to void, and similar percentages of women experiencing low blood pressure and babies experiencing abnormal heart rate.[8,17,58]

Low-dose epidurals—the so-called "light" epidural—have not kept women from having an excess number of vaginal instrumental deliveries or cesarean sections.[64] In fact, in a trial of an "ultra-light" epidural—an epidural where the dose was so low that many women could walk—versus a narcotic epidural, the cesarean rate in both groups was 21 percent and the vaginal instrumental delivery rates were 16 percent and 14 percent respectively.[9]

Adding narcotic and reducing the concentration of anesthetic (*narcotic epidural*) doesn't reduce adverse effects either. A study of narcotic epidurals versus standard low-dose epidurals reported a 15 percent cesarean rate with a standard epidural and an 18 percent rate with a narcotic epidural.[13] Another study of the same thing found similar spontaneous birth rates with both types.[51] Close to one-quarter of babies in both groups were delivered by cesarean, forceps, or vacuum extraction for fetal distress. Narcotic epidurals also do not decrease the incidence of low blood pressure. Sixteen percent of women having a narcotic epidural in one study required medication to treat hypotension.[41] In another, nearly one-third of women having a narcotic epidural experienced low blood pressure versus no women having injected narcotic.[57] Moreover, narcotic epidurals introduce new side effects: itching and nausea.[13,39,51]

The latest wrinkle, the combined spinal epidural, doesn't solve epidural-related problems either. Researchers compared 760 first-time mothers receiving a narcotic epidural with women receiving a spinal epidural.[39] They found no differences in cesarean rates, but women receiving spinal narcotic were much more likely to itch (8 percent in the epidural narcotic group versus nearly half of the spinal narcotic group). Other studies have found that spinal narcotics cause itching and nausea as well.[14,16,25] Spinal epidurals also exacerbate an old problem: spinal headaches. Spinal headaches occur in roughly 4 per 1,000 women who have a standard epidural but in 3 to 5 per 100 women who have the combined technique.[3,10,27] Severe maternal respiratory depression or respiratory arrest can occur when injecting a spinal narcotic as four case reports attest.[2,7,18,43]

Note: Walking with an epidural may be advantageous. In the ultra-light epidural trial described above, few women chose to walk. However, a study of 760 first-time mothers comparing women receiving narcotic epidurals with women receiving ultra-low epidural anesthetic with spinal narcotic found that women with spinal epidurals who walked (women with the narcotic epidural lacked the muscle control) tended to have somewhat fewer cesareans and instrumental deliveries.[39]

Narcotics adversely affect the baby's oxygenation before birth, can cause breathing problems at birth, and interfere with early breastfeeding.

A study looking at factors associated with poor oxygenation at birth as measured by blood pH (*acidemia*) found that meperidine (Demerol) doubled the risk of low blood pH in the newborn.[23] Researchers in another study randomly assigned 100 women to receive butorphanol (Stadol) or fentanyl (Sublimaze) for labor pain.[6] Sixteen percent of the babies of mothers receiving butorphanol required an injection of naloxone (Narcan), a drug that counteracts the action of narcotics, at birth, as did more than one-quarter of the babies whose mothers had fentanyl. Five babies in the fentanyl group required breathing assistance. Another study randomly assigning 100 women to meperidine or fentanyl found that nearly one in five babies in both groups required breathing assistance.[47] Thirteen percent of the meperidine group and 2 percent of the fentanyl group needed naloxone.

As for breastfeeding, researchers compared newborn behavioral abilities at twelve hours and three days of age in women receiving Demerol and women having no drugs in labor.[29] Demerol clearly adversely affected newborn behavioral competency. A study comparing fentanyl to Demerol found they had similar neurobehavioral effects in the newborn.[47] In another study, researchers observed 72 newborns left on their mothers' abdomens at birth.[49] Of the newborns whose mothers had no narcotic (pethidine), 72 percent spontaneously crawled up their mother's trunk, latched on, and suckled correctly versus 20 percent of the newborns whose mothers had had pethidine during labor.

Sterile water injections are a safe, effective means of relieving intense back pain.

In two trials, of 45 and 272 women, respectively, researchers randomly assigned women experiencing severe back pain in labor to either pure water or saline injections at four sites on the lower back.[4,65] (The pure water is irritating, the saline is not.) In both trials, pure water produced profound relief of back pain lasting more than an hour compared with the saline injections. Ader, Hansson, and Wallin's report contains instructions on how to perform the procedure and a drawing showing the locations for the injections.[4]

REFERENCES

1. Abboud TK et al. Continuous infusion epidural analgesia in parturients receiving bupivacaine, chloroprocaine, or lidocaine—maternal, fetal, and neonatal effects. *Anesth Analg* 1984;63:421–428.
2. Abouleish E. Apnoea associated with the intrathecal administration of morphine in obstetrics. *Br J Anaesth* 1988;60:592–594.
3. Abouleish E et al. Intrathecal morphine 0.2 mg versus epidural bupivacaine 0.125% or their combination: effects on parturients. *Anesthesiology* 1991;74(4):711–716.
4. Ader L., Hansson B, and Wallin G. Parturition pain treated by intracutaneous injections of sterile water. *Pain* 1990;41:133–138.
5. Alexander JM et al. The course of labor with and without epidural analgesia. *Am J Obstet Gynecol* 1998;178(3):516–520.
6. Atkinson BD et al. Double-blind comparison of intravenous butorphanol (Stadol) and fentanyl (Sublimaze) for analgesia during labor. *Am J Obstet Gynecol* 1994;171:993–998.
7. Baker MN and Sarna MC. Respiratory arrest after second dose of intrathecal sufentanil in labor. *Anesthesiology* 1995;83(1):231–232.
8. Bogod DG, Rosen M, and Rees GAD. Extradural infusion of 0.125% bupivacaine at 10 M1 H^{-1} to women during labour. *Br J Anaesth* 1987;59(3):325–330.
9. Breen TW et al. Epidural anesthesia for labor in an ambulatory patient. *Anesth Analg* 1993;77:919–924.

10. Caldwell LE, Rosen MA, and Shnider SM. Subarachnoid morphine and fentanyl for labor analgesia. Efficacy and adverse effects. *Reg Anesth* 1994;19(1):2–8.

11. Chestnut DH et al. Does early administration of epidural analgesia affect obstetric outcome in nulliparous women who are in spontaneous labor? *Anesthesiology* 1994;80(6):1201–1208.

12. Chestnut DH et al. The influence of continuous epidural bupivacaine analgesia on the second stage of labor and method of delivery in nulliparous women. *Anesthesiology* 1987;66:774–780.

13. Chestnut DH et al. Continuous infusion epidural analgesia during labor. A randomized, double-blind comparison of 0.0625% bupivacaine/0.0002% fentanyl versus 0.125% bupivacaine. *Anesthesiology* 1988;68:754–759.

14. Cohen SE et al. Intrathecal sufentanil for labor analgesia—sensory changes, side effects, and fetal heart rate changes. *Anesth Analg* 1993;77(6):1155–1160.

15. Crawford JS. Some maternal complications of epidural analgesia for labour. *Anaesthesia* 1985;40(12):1219–1225.

16. D'Angelo R et al. Intrathecal sufentanil compared to epidural bupivacaine for labor analgesia. *Anesthesiology* 1994;90(6):1209–1215.

17. Eddleston JM et al. Comparison of the maternal and fetal effects associated with intermittent or continuous infusion of extradural analgesia. *Br J Anaesth* 1992;69:154–158.

18. Eisenach JC. Respiratory depression following intrathecal opioids. *Anesthesiology* 1991;75(4):712.

19. Fogel ST et al. Epidural labor analgesia and the incidence of cesarean delivery for dystocia. *Anesth Analg* 1998;87:119–123.

20. Fusi L et al. Maternal pyrexia associated with the use of epidural analgesia in labour. *Lancet* Jun 3, 1989;1250–1252.

21. Golub MS. Labor analgesia and infant brain development. *Pharmacol Biochem Behav* 1996;55(4):619–628.

22. Gribble RK and Meier PR. Effect of epidural analgesia on the primary cesarean rate. *Obstet Gynecol* 1991;78(2):231–234.

23. Herbst A, Wolner-Hanssen P, and Ingemarsson I. Risk factors for acidemia at birth. *Obstet Gynecol* 1997;90(1):125–130.

24. Herbst A, Wolner-Hanssen P, and Ingemarsson I. Risk factors for fever in labor. *Obstet Gynecol* 1995;86:790–794.

25. Honet JE et al. Comparison among intrathecal fentanyl, meperidine, and sufentanil for labor analgesia. *Anesth Analg* 1992;75(5):734–739.

26. Howell CJ. Epidural vs non-epidural analgesia in labour. In: Neilson JP et al., eds. *Pregnancy and Childbirth Module of the Cochrane Database of Systematic Reviews,* updated September 1997.

27. Kartawiadi L et al. Spinal analgesia during labor with low-dose bupivacaine, sufentanil, and epinephrine. A comparison with epidural analgesia. *Reg Anesth* 1996;21(3):191–196.

28. Kenepp NB and Gutsche BB. Inadvertent intravascular injections during lumbar epidural anesthesia. *Anesthesiology* 1981;54:172–173.

29. Kuhnert BR et al. Effects of low doses of meperidine on neonatal behavior. *Anesth Analg* 1985;64(3):335–342.

30. Leighton BL et al. Limitations of epinephrine as a marker of intravascular injection in laboring women. *Anesthesiology* 1987;66:688–691.

31. Lieberman E et al. Association of epidural analgesia with cesarean delivery in nulliparas. *Obstet Gynecol* 1996;88(6):993–1000.

32. Lieberman E et al. Epidural analgesia, intrapartum fever, and neonatal sepsis evaluation. *Pediatrics* 1997;99(3):415–419.

33. Loftus JR, Hill H, and Cohen SE. Placental transfer and neonatal effects of epidural sufentanil and fentanyl administered with bupivacaine during labor. *Anesthesiology* 1995;83:300–308.

34. Lyon DS et al. The effect of instituting an elective labor epidural program on the operative delivery rate. *Obstet Gynecol* 1997;90(1):135–141.

35. MacArthur C, Lewis M, and Knox EG. Investigation of long term problems after obstetric epidural anaesthesia. *BMJ* 1992;304:1279–1282.

36. MacArthur A, MacArthur C, and Weeks S. Epidural anaesthesia and low back pain after delivery: a prospective cohort study. *BMJ* 1995; 311(7016):1336–1339.

37. Macaulay JH, Bond K, and Steer PJ. Epidural analgesia in labor and fetal hyperthermia. *Obstet Gynecol* 1992;80(4):665–669.

38. Murray AD et al. Effects of epidural anesthesia on newborns and their mothers. *Child Develop* 1981;52:71–82.

39. Nageotte MP et al. Epidural analgesia compared with combined spinal-epidural analgesia during labor in nulliparous women. *N Engl J Med* 1997;337:1715–1719.

40. Neuhoff D, Burke MS, and Porreco RP. Cesarean birth for failed progress in labor. *Obstet Gynecol* 1989;73(6):915–920.

41. Newton ER et al. Epidural analgesia and uterine function. *Obstet Gynecol* 1995;85(5 Pt 1):749–755.

42. Ong BY et al. Paresthesias and motor dysfunction after labor and delivery. *Anesth Analg* 1987;66:18–22.

43. Palmer CM. Early respiratory depression following intrathecal fentanyl-morphine combination. *Anesthesiology* 1991;74(6):1153–1155.

44. Philipsen T and Jensen NH. Epidural block or parenteral pethidine as analgesic in labour: a randomized study concerning progress in labour and instrumental deliveries. *Eur J Obstet Gynecol Reprod Biol* 1989;30: 27–33.

45. Phillips DC and Macdonald R. Epidural migration during labour. *Anaesthesia* 1987;42:661–663.

46. Ramin SM et al. Randomized trial of epidural versus intravenous analgesia during labor. *Obstet Gynecol* 1995;86(5):783–789.

47. Rayburn WF et al. Randomized comparison of meperidine and fentanyl during labor. *Obstet Gynecol* 1989;74(4):604–606.

48. Reynolds F et al. Effect of time and adrenaline on the feto-maternal distribution of bupivacaine. *Br J Anaesth* 1989;62(5):509–514.

49. Righard L and Alade MO. Effect of delivery room routines on success of first breast-feed. *Lancet* 1990;336:1105–1107.

50. Robinson CA et al. Does station of the fetal head at epidural placement affect the position of the fetal vertex at delivery? *Am J Obstet Gynecol* 1996(4 Pt 1);175:991–994.

51. Russell R and Reynolds F. Epidural infusion of low-dose bupivacaine

and opioid in labour. Does reducing motor block increase the spontaneous delivery rate? *Anaesthesia* 1996;51(3):266–273.

52. Russell R, Dundas R, and Reynolds F. Long term backache after childbirth: prospective search for causative factors. *BMJ* 1996;312(7043): 1384–1388.

53. Russell R et al. Assessing long term backache after childbirth. *BMJ* 1993; 306:1299–1303.

54. Scott DB and Hibbard BM. Serious non-fatal complications associated with extradural block in obstetric practice. *Br J Anaesth* 1990;64:537–541.

55. Scott DB and Tunstall ME. Serious complications associated with epidural/spinal blockade in obstetrics: a two-year prospective study. *Int J Obstet Anesth* 1995;4:133–139.

56. Sepkoski CM et al. The effects of maternal epidural anesthesia on neonatal behavior during the first month. *Develop Med and Child Neurology* 1992;34:1072–1080.

57. Sharma SK et al. Cesarean delivery: a randomized trial of epidural versus patient-controlled meperidine analgesia during labor. *Anesthesiology* 1997;87(3):487–494.

58. Smedstad KG and Morison DH. A comparative study of continuous and intermittent epidural analgesia for labour and delivery. *Can J Anaesth* 1988;35(3):234–241.

59. Stavrou C, Hofmeyr GJ, and Boezaart AP. Prolonged fetal bradycardia during epidural analgesia. *S Afr Med J* 1990;77:66–68.

60. Steiger RM, Nageotte MP. Effect of uterine contractility and maternal hypotension on prolonged decelerations after bupivacaine epidural anesthesia. *Am J Obstet Gynecol* 1990;163:808–812.

61. Thorp JA and Breedlove G. Epidural analgesia in labor: an evaluation of risks and benefits. *Birth* 1996;23(2):63–83.

62. Thorp JA et al. Epidural analgesia and cesarean section for dystocia: risk factors in nulliparas. *Am J Perinatol* 1991;8(6):402–410.

63. Thorp JA et al. The effect of continuous epidural analgesia on cesarean section for dystocia in nulliparous women. *Am J Obstet Gynecol* 1989; 161(3):670–675.

64. Thorp JA et al. The effect of intrapartum epidural analgesia on nulliparous labor: a randomized, controlled, prospective trial. *Am J Obstet Gynecol* 1993;169(4):851–858.

65. Trolle B et al. The effect of sterile water blocks on low back labor pain. *Am J Obstet Gynecol* 1991;164(5):1277–1281.

66. Vinson DC, Thomas R, Kiser T. Association between epidural analgesia during labor and fever. *J Fam Prac* 1993;36(6):617–622.

Chapter 9
Episiotomy: The Unkindest Cut

Episiotomies don't prevent tears into or through the anal sphincter.

Studies consistently show strong associations between midline episiotomy and anal tears. One study, evaluating perineal outcomes in over 1,250 women, found that women were over four times as likely to experience anal tears with an episiotomy.[44] Another, reviewing records for 6,500 first-time mothers, found that after taking factors influencing anal tears into account, episiotomy increased the odds of tears 350 percent.[26] Between 1976 and 1994, the episiotomy rate at one hospital fell from nearly 90 percent to 10 percent.[3] During that time the anal tear rate declined from 9 percent to 4 percent. A study paired 205 women who had episiotomies with 205 similar women who did not.[13] The 2 percent of women who had anal tears all had episiotomies. Two studies looked at the factors associated with anal tears. One, in 2,700 women, found 13 percent of women experienced an anal tear, nearly all of which were episiotomy extensions.[16] After adjusting for factors influencing the anal tear rate, episiotomy increased the risk of such tears nine-fold. The other, in 24,100 women, found an anal tear rate of 8 percent in first-time mothers and 1.5 percent in women with prior births.[36] After adjusting for other factors, episiotomy increased the risk four-fold in first-time mothers and thirteen-fold in mothers with prior births. Finally, in the only randomized controlled trial of midline episiotomy, 700 women were randomly assigned to liberal versus restrictive episiotomy groups. Eight percent of women had anal tears, all but one an episiotomy extension.[23] After adjusting for other factors, episiotomy increased the odds of anal injury twenty-two-fold.[24]

Mediolateral episiotomies don't predispose to anal tears, but they don't prevent them either. Two randomized controlled trials of liberal versus restrictive use of mediolateral episiotomy found little difference in anal tear rates. One studied 1,000 women.[38] Half the women in the liberal group had episiotomies versus 10 percent in the restricted group. Four women, less than half a percent, experienced anal injuries or a tear in the upper vagina of which three were in the restricted group and one in the liberal group. The other trial used the same design and studied 2,600 women.[2] Episiotomy rates were 30 percent and 83 percent, respectively. A little over 1 percent of women experienced severe trauma rates in both groups. The fact that mediolateral episiotomies don't predispose to anal tears should not be taken as reason to substitute them for midline episiotomies. They have other serious drawbacks compared with midline episiotomy (see the comparison on page 154).

Episiotomies don't prevent relaxation of the pelvic floor muscles, urinary incontinence, herniations of the bladder into the vagina, or vaginal or uterine prolapse, or preserve sexual satisfaction during intercourse.

Neither of the randomized trials of restricted versus liberal use of episiotomy that evaluated pelvic floor strength found that liberal use of episiotomy preserved pelvic floor strength.[24,38] In the midline episiotomy trial, the incidence of urinary and pelvic floor symptoms were similar three months after birth regardless of whether the mother had an intact perineum, a spontaneous tear, or an episiotomy.[24] Women with intact perineums had the strongest pelvic floors followed by women who sustained spontaneous tears. Women who had an episiotomy, especially those whose episiotomy extended, had the weakest pelvic floors. The authors point out that women with the strongest pelvic floors at three months after birth would be "highly unlikely" to develop the weakest functioning later. In a mediolateral episiotomy trial, one in five women in both groups reported occasional urinary incontinence three months after birth.[38] A follow-up study three years later found that one-third of the women in both groups experienced urinary stress incontinence.[37] Nine percent and 8 percent, respectively, had to wear a pad. Yet another study of mediolateral episiotomy measured pelvic floor strength eight weeks postpartum by the ability to retain vaginally a weighted cone while standing.[34] Women with intact perineums and spontaneous tears did similarly; women with episiotomies did worse. A follow-up study of the effects of midline episiotomy thirty years later in 150 women found that three-fourths of them had urinary incontinence whether they had vaginal births with episiotomies or cesarean sections.[31]

Since weak pelvic floor muscles lead to herniations and prolapse, these complications would be most likely in women who had episiotomies. And since sexual satisfaction depends on good vaginal muscle tone, the episiotomy group would be the losers here too.

Episiotomies don't prevent brain damage.

Two studies, one of 97 very-low-birth-weight babies and the other of 439 low-birth-weight babies, evaluated whether episiotomy reduced the incidence of brain hemorrhage.[27,42] Neither one concluded that it helped. As for oxygen deprivation, the larger study compared Apgar scores, a measure of the baby's condition at birth, and found episiotomy made no difference there either. The randomized controlled trials of liberal versus restricted use of episiotomy also haven't found any differences in newborn outcomes.[2,23,38]

Episiotomies don't cause less pain than tears.

The only randomized controlled trial of midline episiotomy found that among 700 women, women with intact perineums experienced the least pain on days 1, 2, and 10 after birth; spontaneous perineal tears hurt less than episiotomies; and episiotomies that extended into or through the anal sphincter hurt worst.[24] Three months later, one-tenth of women with intact perineums experienced chronic perineal pain, compared with one-third of women with spontaneous tears, approaching half of women with episiotomies, and over half of women whose episiotomies extended. No woman with an intact perineum reported "horrible" or "excruciating" pain versus 1 in 10 women with spontaneous tears and 1 in 5 women with either episiotomies or episiotomy extensions. Mediolateral episiotomies are well known to cause more pain than midline episiotomies.

Episiotomies, especially when they extend into the anus, increase the risk of pain during intercourse. In the midline episiotomy trial, three-quarters of women with intact perineums had resumed intercourse six weeks after birth versus less than two-thirds of women with spontaneous tears or episiotomies and somewhat more than half of women with anal tears, all but one of which was an episiotomy extension.[24] At three months after birth, 5 percent of women with intact perineums rated their sex lives as unsatisfactory versus three times as many women with spontaneous tears or episiotomies and five times as many women with anal tears. In the trial of mediolateral episiotomy, more than one-third of the "restrict episiotomy" group resumed intercourse by a month after birth versus one-quarter of the "liberal episiotomy" group.[38]

At three months, 1 in 5 women in both groups reported pain during inter-course. (It would be interesting to know whether these were the women who had episiotomies.)

Episiotomies don't appreciably shorten second-stage labor.
In the randomized controlled trial of midline episiotomy, first-time moth-ers in the liberal-episiotomy group had a nine-minute-shorter second stage.[23] Since first-time mothers take twice as long on average to push out a baby as do women with previous vaginal births, this may be considered the maximum savings.

Primarily, but not entirely because they predispose to anal tears, episiotomies increase the risk of infection, delayed healing, wound breakdown, the formation of an opening between the vagina and the rectum (rectovaginal fistula), and gas or stool incontinence.
One study evaluated tissue healing one to two weeks after birth in 370 women, none of whom had instrumental deliveries and half of whom had a midline episiotomy.[29] In the episiotomy group, 8 percent of women experi-enced delayed healing versus 2 percent of the no-episiotomy group. The dif-ference persisted when women with intact perineums (half) were removed from the no-episiotomy group, which means spontaneous tears healed faster than episiotomies. None of the four anal tears that occurred without episi-otomy exhibited delayed healing versus five of the twenty-seven anal injuries that occurred as episiotomy extensions. Both infections occurred in women with episiotomies. By comparison, among women having instrumental deliv-eries, 1 in 3 experienced anal injuries and 1 in 5 had delayed healing.
Fortunately rare—one article reported that incidence ranged from 0.1 per-cent to 2 percent—episiotomy repair breakdown is as nasty and unpleasant an experience as you would imagine it to be.[32] If it goes deep enough, it can create an opening (*fistula*) between the vagina and the rectum. One study reviewed the medical literature to evaluate the relationships among episiot-omy, wound breakdown, and vaginal-rectal openings.[19] The key factor in breakdown is infection. Infection occurs somewhere between 0.5 percent and 3 percent of the time. Tears into or through the anal sphincter are strongly associated with vaginal-rectal openings, and midline episiotomy strongly as-sociates with anal tears. The authors calculated that one vaginal-rectal open-ing will occur in one out of 1,881 midline episiotomies and one out of ninety-six anal tears. Another study evaluated outcomes in thirty-four women who sustained anal injuries.[44] Six women (18 percent) developed infections of which two developed fistulas. In another study of fifty-nine women with anal injury, two had infections and one developed a fistula.[17]
Until recently, obstetricians thought that repaired anal sphincter tears did not cause long-term problems. However, follow-up ultrasound imaging and strength measurement studies show that muscle disruptions and weakness persist,[17,22,39–41] which means even symptom-free women could be headed for trouble down the line when aging and further childbearing take their toll on anal sphincter strength. And a disturbing percentage of women are not symptom-free. Among eighty-one women examined three months after sus-taining an anal sphincter tear during childbirth, six (7 percent) had stool incontinence and a further ten (12 percent) had gas incontinence.[43] Fifty-nine

women responded to a questionnaire two to seven years after anal injury during childbirth.[17] One-third of the women reported incontinence especially of gas, 8 percent reported pain during intercourse, and 7 percent reported perineal pain. Researchers compared outcomes two or more months after birth between thirty-four women who sustained anal injury and eighty-eight similar women who didn't.[41] Nearly half the women with tears experienced incontinence or defecation urgency compared with about 1 in 10 women in the control group.

Episiotomies increase blood loss.

A study investigating factors associated with postpartum hemorrhage found that mediolateral episiotomy increased the risk of hemorrhage more than 450 percent and midline episiotomy by 33 percent.[8]

Forceps deliveries greatly increase the risk of tears into or through the anal sphincter compared with vacuum extractions.

Three trials randomly assigning women requiring instrumental delivery to forceps or vacuum extraction all found more maternal injuries with forceps. In one trial of 640 women, 3 in 10 women in the forceps group versus 1 in 10 women in the vacuum-extraction group sustained anal tears.[5] Women in the vacuum-extraction group were also less than half as likely to have episiotomies: less than one-third, versus two-thirds of the women in the forceps group. The second trial totalled 260 women.[21] Twelve percent of women having forceps deliveries experienced anal tears, versus half that number in women having vacuum extraction, and 8 percent versus one-quarter that number experienced deep vaginal tears. The third trial, in 607 women, found that women having vacuum extractions had 40 percent less risk (11 percent versus 17 percent) of experiencing anal sphincter damage or upper vaginal tears.[20]

Selective episiotomy reduces perineal injury rates during instrumental vaginal deliveries.

All three studies that looked at selective episiotomy with instrumental delivery found that it improved perineal outcome. In a study of 400 women in which only 40 percent of them had episiotomies, half of first-time mothers who had an episiotomy versus 1 in 5 women who didn't had anal tears. Among women with previous births, 1 in 5 had anal tears with an episiotomy versus 1 in 10 without one.[18] After adjusting for other factors influencing anal tears, episiotomy increased the risk of anal injury 240 percent. In a study of over 2,800 women, two-thirds had midline episiotomies, one-quarter had mediolateral episiotomies, and the rest had no episiotomy.[9] Three in 10 overall had anal injuries. Women who had either no episiotomy or mediolateral episiotomy fared the same. After adjusting for other factors, midline episiotomy increased the risk of anal tears eight-fold. A third study of 2,050 women compared episiotomy rates and outcomes between 1984, when virtually all women had episiotomies for instrumental deliveries, and 1994, when one-third of women had them.[11] The decline more than halved the percentage of tears through the anal sphincter (*fourth degree*) (12 percent versus 5 percent). Tear rates into but not through the sphincter (*third degree*) did not change, but the authors note that practitioners also switched from mostly mediolateral to mostly midline episiotomies and that this could account for the lack of change. (Midline episiotomies are much more likely to extend.) At the very least, women were at equal risk with no episiotomy than with one. The authors also note that vaginal tears increased, but that vaginal tears were not graded according to severity, so it isn't known how many were minor injuries. In any case, vaginal tears do not have the prognosis for long-term serious problems that anal tears appear to have.

Breathing and pushing according to the mother's natural inclinations and giving birth in an upright position, or at least not on one's back or with legs spread wide apart, produces the best perineal and infant outcomes.

Five studies have looked at infant outcomes in relation to how the mother pushed. All found that when not directed otherwise, most women expelled air when they pushed by grunting and groaning. When women did hold their breaths, they rarely held it more than six seconds. Most took several breaths between pushing efforts. Twenty years ago, a study reported that when women bore down long and hard, electronic fetal monitors recorded heart rate tracings indicative of distress, and babies had lower umbilical cord blood pH at birth, a symptom of oxygen deprivation.[7] By contrast, pushing spontaneously had no adverse effects. Two later studies observed a total of eighty women allowed to push as they pleased.[33,35] All babies were born in good condition. Two other studies randomly assigned a combined total of twenty first-time mothers to directed or spontaneous pushing.[4,45] The first found no differences in Apgar scores or length of labor. All five women in the directed pushing group had episiotomies and one episiotomy extended. Among the five women pushing spontaneously, one had an episiotomy, and one woman needed a small tear stitched. The second study found that women pushing spontaneously tended toward slightly longer labors but their babies had higher cord blood pHs at birth, which signifies better oxygenation. Two of five babies in the directed pushing group, the ones whose mothers pushed longest and hardest, experienced a profound drop in fetal heart rate shortly before birth. This would usually prompt an episiotomy.

As for pushing position, four studies found an association between both episiotomy and perineal injury and birth in the on-the-back, legs-in-stirrups (*lithotomy*) position.[1,6,28,30] However, the significance of this is hard to judge because doctors would be more likely to use the lithotomy position for forceps deliveries and midwives might use it when an episiotomy is anticipated. Practitioners more prone to perform episiotomies might also be more likely to require the lithotomy position for birth. Three studies ranging in size from 300 to over 500 women, including two randomized controlled trials, looked at squatting versus semi-reclining or side-lying positions.[10,12,14] All found upright positioning conferred benefits, including substantially reduced episiotomy rates (8 percent versus 51 percent, 7 percent versus 20 percent), instrumental delivery rates (7 percent versus 17 percent, 9 percent versus 16 percent), anal tear rates (1 percent verus 14 percent), and increased intact perineum rates (46 percent versus 18 percent, 46 percent versus 32 percent). Upright positioning also shortened second stage an average of twenty-three minutes in first-time mothers and thirteen minutes in women with prior births in one study and eleven minutes in first-time mothers in another. This is a greater effect than performing an episiotomy (see page 279).

Women who exercise regularly have stronger pelvic floors and appear less likely to have anal tears when they have episiotomies.

Researchers grouped seventy women according to whether they exercised regularly, did postpartum exercises only, or never exercised, and measured the strength of their pelvic floor muscles one year after childbirth.[15] Regular exercisers fared best, postpartum exercisers fell in between, and nonexercisers had the weakest pelvic floors. Exercise regimens included fitness classes, walking, jogging, running, dancing, swimming, and yoga. In another study, researchers evaluated perineal and pelvic floor outcomes in 460 first-time mothers according to how much they exercised.[25] Women engaging in weight-bearing exercise more than three times weekly were equally likely to have an episiotomy, but 16 percent experienced anal injury, compared with more than one-quarter of those exercising less often.

REFERENCES

1. Albers LL et al. Factors related to perineal trauma in childbirth. *J Nurse Midwifery* 1996;41(4):269–276.
2. Argentine Episiotomy Trial Collaborative Group. Routine vs. selective episiotomy: a randomised controlled trial. *Lancet* 1993;342:1517–1518.
3. Bansal RK et al. Is there a benefit to episiotomy at spontaneous vaginal delivery? A natural experiment. *Am J Obstet Gynecol* 1996;175 (4 Pt 1):897–901.
4. Barnett MM and Humenick SS. Infant outcome in relation to second stage labor pushing method. *Birth* 1982:9(4):221–230.
5. Bofill JA et al. A randomized prospective trial of the obstetric forceps versus the M-cup vacuum extractor. *Am J Obstet Gynecol* 1996;175(5): 1325–1330.
6. Borgatta L, Piening SL, and Cohen WR. Association of episiotomy and delivery position with deep perineal laceration during spontaneous delivery in nulliparous women. *Am J Obstet Gynecol* 1989;160(2):294–297.
7. Caldeyro-Barcia R. The influence of maternal bearing-down efforts during second stage on fetal well-being. *Birth Fam J* 1979;6(1):17–21.
8. Combs CA, Murphy EL, and Laros RK. Factors associated with postpartum hemorrhage with vaginal birth. *Obstet Gynecol* 1991;77(1):69–76.
9. Combs CA, Robertson PA, and Laros RK. Risk factors for third-degree and fourth-degree perineal lacerations in forceps and vacuum deliveries. *Am J Obstet Gynecol* 1990;163(1 Pt 1):100–104.
10. de Jong PR et al. Randomised trial comparing the upright and supine positions for the second stage of labor. *Br J Obstet Gynaecol* 1997; 104(5):567–571.
11. Ecker JL et al. Is there a benefit to episiotomy at operative vaginal de-

livery? Observations over ten years in a stable population. *Am J Obstet Gynecol* 1997;176(2):411–414.

12. Gardosi J, Hutson N, and B-Lynch C. Randomized trial of squatting in the second stage of labour. *Lancet* 1989;2(8654):74–77.

13. Gass MS, Dunn CD, and Stys SJ. Effect of episiotomy on the frequency of vaginal outlet lacerations. *J Reprod Med* 1986;31(4);240–244.

14. Golay J, Vedam S, and Sorger L. The squatting position for the second stage of labor: effects on labor and on maternal and fetal well-being. *Birth* 1993;20(2):73–78.

15. Gordon H and Logue M. Perineal muscle function after childbirth. *Lancet* 1985;2:123–125.

16. Green JR and Soohoo SL. Factors associated with rectal injury in spontaneous deliveries. *Obstet Gynecol* 1989;73(5 Pt 1):732–738.

17. Haadem K et al. Anal sphincter function after delivery rupture. *Obstet Gynecol* 1987;70(1):53–56.

18. Helwig JT, Thorp JM, and Bowes WA. Does midline episiotomy increase the risk of third- and fourth-degree lacerations in operative vaginal deliveries? *Obstet Gynecol* 1993;82(2):276–279.

19. Homsi R et al. Episiotomy: risks of dehiscence and rectovaginal fistula. *Obstet Gynecol Surv* 1994;49(12):803–808.

20. Johanson RB et al. A randomised prospective study comparing the new vacuum extractor policy with forceps delivery. *Br J Obstet Gynaecol* 1993;100(6):524–530.

21. Johanson R et al. North Staffordshire/Wigan assisted delivery trial. *Br J Obstet Gynaecol* 1989;96:537–544.

22. Kamm MA. Obstetric damage and faecal incontinence. *Lancet* 1994; 344:730–733.

23. Klein MC et al. Does episiotomy prevent perineal trauma and pelvic floor relaxation? *Online J Curr Clin Trials* 1992;1(Document 10).

24. Klein MC et al. Relationship of episiotomy to perineal trauma and morbidity, sexual dysfunction, and pelvic floor relaxation. *Am J Obstet Gynecol* 1994;171(3):591–598.

25. Klein MC et al. Determinants of vaginal-perineal and pelvic floor functioning in childbirth. *Am J Obstet Gynecol* 1997;176(2):403–410.

26. Labrecque M et al. Association between median episiotomy and severe perineal lacerations in primiparous women. *CMAJ* 1997;156(6):797–802.

27. Lobb MO, Duthie SJ, and Cooke RW. The influence of episiotomy on the neonatal survival and incidence of periventricular haemorrhage in very-low-birth-weight infants. *Eur J Obstet Gynecol Reprod Biol* 1986; 22(1–2):17–21.

28. Lydon-Rochelle MT, Albers L, and Teaf D. Perineal outcomes and nurse-midwifery management. *J Nurse Midwifery* 1995;40(1):13–18.

29. McGuiness M, Norr K, and Nacion K. Comparison between different perineal outcomes on tissue healing. *J Nurse Midwifery* 1991;36(3):192–198.

30. Nodine PM and Roberts J. Factors associated with perineal outcome during childbirth. *J Nurse Midwifery* 1987 May–June;32(3):123–130.

31. Nygaard IE, Rao SSC, and Dawson JD. Anal incontinence after anal

sphincter disruption: a 30-year retrospective cohort study. *Obstet Gynecol* 1997;89(6):896–901.

32. Ramin SM and Gilstrap LC. Episiotomy and early repair of dehiscence. *Clin Obstet Gynecol* 1994;37(4):816–823.

33. Roberts JE et al. A descriptive analysis of involuntary bearing-down efforts during the expulsive phase of labor. *J Obstet Gynecol Neonatal Nurs* 1987;48–55.

34. Rockner G, Jonasson A, and Olund A. The effect of mediolateral episiotomy at delivery on pelvic floor muscle strength evaluated with vaginal cones. *Acta Obstet Gynecol Scand* 1991;70(1):51–54.

35. Rossi MA and Lindell SG. Maternal positions and pushing techniques in a nonprescriptive environment. *Obstet Gynecol Neonatal Nurs* 1986; 203–207.

36. Shiono P, Klebanoff MA, and Carey JC. Midline episiotomies: more harm than good? *Obstet Gynecol* 1990;75(5):765–770.

37. Sleep J and Grant A. West Berkshire perineal management trial: Three year follow up. *Br Med J* 1987;32(3):181–183.

38. Sleep J et al. West Berkshire perineal management trial. *Br Med J* 1984; 289:587–590.

39. Snooks SJ et al. Risk factors in childbirth causing damage to the pelvic floor innervation. *Br J Surg* 1985;72(Suppl):S 15–S 17.

40. Sultan AH et al. Anal-sphincter disruption during vaginal delivery. *New Engl J Med* 1993;329(26):1905–1911.

41. Sultan AH et al. Third degree obstetric anal sphincter tears: risk factors and outcome of primary repair. *BMJ* 1994;(308):887–891.

42. The TG. Is routine episiotomy beneficial in the low birth weight delivery? *Int J Gynaecol Obstet* 1990;31(2):135–140.

43. Walsh CJ et al. Incidence of third-degree perineal tears in labour and outcome after primary repair. *Br J Surg* 1996;83(2):218–221.

44. Wilcox LS et al. Episiotomy and its role in the incidence of perineal lacerations in a maternity center and a tertiary hospital obstetric service. *Am J Obstet Gynecol* 1989;160(5 Pt 1):1047–1052.

45. Yeates DA and Roberts JE. A comparison of two bearing-down techniques during the second stage of labor. *J Nurs Midwifery* 1984;29(1): 3–11.

Chapter 10
Elective Repeat Cesarean:
Just Say No

VBAC is safe provided the baby is closely monitored and caregivers can respond promptly to the rare problem with the scar.

Basing my calculations on 37,000 labors after cesarean reported in twenty-nine studies, I calculated that 4 per 1,000 women experienced scar problems during or after labor.[24–53] The scar giving way resulted in neurological injury or the baby's death in 4 per 10,000 labors overall, versus 3 per 10,000 in the 14,700 planned cesareans reported in eleven of those twenty-nine studies. The outcome for the baby depends on how quickly medical staff recognize the problem and perform a cesarean. One analysis of ninety-nine cases of symptomatic scar separation found that all but two of the babies were fine when the cesarean was performed within twenty minutes of the onset of severely abnormal fetal heart rate patterns.[18]* The authors comment that theirs is probably a worst case scenario because their population largely consisted of low-income Hispanic immigrants from countries where *classical vertical uterine incision* (vertical incision of the main body of the uterus as opposed to low-vertical incision) is more common. Classical incisions not only give way more often, but the results are usually immediately catastrophic.

Note: Opponents of VBAC often cite a recent VBAC study that concluded that "major maternal complications" were twice as likely in women laboring compared with women having elective cesareans.[39] However, preeminent VBAC researcher Dr. Bruce Flamm points out that the authors coded wound infections and hemorrhage requiring transfusion as "minor complications," both of which occurred more often in the planned cesarean group.[10] If you make these major complications, the difference between the two groups disappears. Dr. Flamm adds that even without doing this, major complication rates were quite low—a bit less than 1 percent in the planned cesarean group, a bit more than 1 percent in the labor group. I would add that the operative injury rate in the labor group, another "major complication," was more than double that of the planned cesarean (1.3 percent versus 0.6 percent), although I don't know why this should be so, and also, at 60 percent, the VBAC rate was low. As more women have cesareans in the labor group, the balance shifts toward planned cesarean because nearly all complications in the labor group will result from repeat cesareans.

Elective repeat cesarean increases the mother's risk of hysterectomy and death and baby's risk of death in subsequent pregnancies.

Note: I confined myself to hysterectomy and death because they are irreparable. See page 22 for other risks of cesarean section.

The sole maternal death reported in the VBAC trials was avoidable.[42] The doctor felt the scar after vaginal birth but missed a bleeding tear, and staff did not diagnose the hemorrhage before the mother had a cardiac arrest. By contrast, all three deaths in women having planned cesareans were intrinsic to having multiple scars or the surgery itself.[20,31,33]

Overall, the studies report 64 hysterectomies in over 30,000 women with one or more prior cesareans (2 per 1,000). The unplanned hysterectomy rate was 7 per 10,000 VBAC labors versus nearly seven times that many with planned cesareans.

---

*This time frame does not preclude out-of-hospital birth provided the birth center or your home is close enough to a hospital capable of performing emergency cesareans at any time.

One-quarter of those hysterectomies involved *placenta accreta/percreta* (the placenta grows into or through the uterine muscle, sometimes invading other organs) and/or *placenta previa* (the placenta grows over the cervix), both known to be complications that increase markedly with each succeeding cesarean.[6,15,23] According to an analysis of data pooled from many studies, women with one prior cesarean have more than four times the odds, women with two or three prior cesareans have a seven-fold increased risk, and women with four or more prior cesareans have a *forty-five-fold* increased risk of placenta previa compared with women with an unscarred uterus.[1] As for placenta accreta, women with multiple prior cesareans had an eleven-fold increased risk of placenta accreta compared with women with one prior cesarean.[26] Nearly 1 percent of the women with multiple prior cesareans had hysterectomies for placenta accreta versus less than 0.1 percent of the women with one previous cesarean. Placenta accreta and percreta seriously threaten the life and health of mothers and babies. In a study of 109 cases of placenta percreta, 40 percent of women required transfusion of more than ten units of blood, nearly all had hysterectomies, and 9 percent of babies and 7 percent of mothers died.[21] One of the three maternal deaths in my collection of VBAC reports involved placenta accreta in a woman with three prior cesareans.[31]

Elective cesarean increases the baby's risk of breathing difficulties and jaundice.

Researchers matched 700 normal-weight infants born with low 5-minute Apgar scores (a measure of the baby's condition at birth) after healthy pregnancies to similar infants with normal Apgar scores.[4] Infants born after elective cesarean were nearly half again as likely to have low Apgar scores as infants born vaginally. Researchers also compared newborn outcomes between 500 women having planned repeat cesareans and 500 women having labor.[16] Infants born after planned cesarean were more than twice as likely to develop respiratory difficulties, mainly rapid breathing (*tachypnea*), and two versus none in the labor group developed respiratory distress syndrome. They were also three times as likely to develop newborn jaundice. Another study found more need for mechanical ventilation and oxygen in babies born after planned cesarean compared with vaginal birth.[2] Breathing problems and jaundice arise from IV fluid overload caused by giving large amounts of IV fluid preoperatively (see page 241). This means differences may be even greater than they appear because women having vaginal births may well have had epidurals, which also involve giving large amounts of IV fluid in a short time, or they may have been overdosed on fluid in routine IVs (see page 241).

Women should not be disqualified from VBAC because they have an unknown uterine scar type.

A researcher reports that 80 percent to 90 percent of the women having babies at a large Los Angeles institution have unknown scar type.[11] Despite the fact that about 5 percent of these women turn out to have classical vertical incisions because they are mainly immigrants from Latin America, the rate of symptomatic scar separation during or after labor was only 7 per 1,000.[3,42]

Women should not be disqualified from VBAC because they have more than one prior cesarean.

One study, in which over 1,800 women with one or more prior cesareans labored, reported a symptomatic scar separation rate of less than 2 percent.[42] Another study of 435 women reported a rate of less than 1 percent.[26] A third study of 245 women, said only that the rate did not differ from the group with one prior cesarean.[33] The authors of the study of 435 women calculated the vaginal birth rate in a total of nearly 2,700 women with multiple previous cesareans in ten studies (including their own).[26] Overall, two-thirds gave birth vaginally.

Women should not be disqualified from VBAC because they have a low vertical incision.

A recent review reported on outcomes of 372 labors in women with prior low vertical uterine incisions.[19] Four out of five had vaginal births. The scar gave way in four women (1 percent), but only one of these was in a laboring woman with one low-vertical scar. The corrected rate is 3 per 1,000 labors. The authors conclude that women with single low vertical scars should be treated as if they had low transverse scars.

Women should not be disqualified from VBAC because of twins.

Two studies reported outcomes in twin pregnancies after one or more prior cesareans. In a study of over two hundred women, nearly half labored, of whom 70 percent gave birth to both twins vaginally.[20] In another study, fifteen out of twenty-five women labored, and all gave birth vaginally.[13] No woman in either study who labored experienced a serious complication. However, one woman in the first study died of complications of her repeat cesarean, and two required a hysterectomy. In the second study, a woman experienced a bowel obstruction that required further surgery and a subsequent chest infection.

Using intrauterine pressure catheters does not increase the safety of VBAC.

An analysis of seventy-six cases of symptomatic scar separation revealed that in no case did an intrauterine pressure catheter (IUPC) diagnose the problem.[22] Another study simulated scar breakdown in twenty women by recording uterine pressures in laboring women before and after incising the uterus during cesarean section.[7] Researchers tested both fluid-filled and solid IUPCs. Neither type showed a pressure change in any of the women.

Manual exploration of the scar after birth does not increase the safety of VBAC.

In one study of over one thousand women with prior cesareans, fewer scar separations were diagnosed by feeling the scar through the cervix after vaginal birth (*manual palpation*) than were observed during elective repeat cesareans.[12] In two cases, exploratory surgery was performed after doctors thought they felt a scar separation, only to find that one woman had an intact scar. The authors questioned the value of identifying symptomless scar windows because they seem to pose little risk in subsequent pregnancies. In addition, feeling the scar internally could increase the risk of infection and could convert a small, harmless gap into a problem. In the sole reported case of maternal death associated with a scar giving way, the scar had been palpated after the birth, but the rupture was missed.[8] Staff did not pick up the problem until the mother had a cardiac arrest from loss of blood.

Prostaglandin gel to ripen the cervix for induction may be used in VBACs.

A recent review of ten studies reporting the use of prostaglandin gel in a total of 548 women laboring after a cesarean concluded that the procedure was safe.[5] A study published after the review adds another 450 women.[9] It too concluded prostaglandin gel was safe.

Oxytocin to start labor or stimulate stronger contractions may be used in VBACs; however, induction or oxytocin before active labor may increase the risk of symptomatic uterine scar separation.

A review of twenty-six studies comprising about 6,200 women given oxytocin to induce or strengthen labor found no greater incidence of scar problems than in women not given oxytocin.[5] However, one study found a greater incidence of problems in women in dysfunctional labor given oxytocin in excessive amounts or for an excessively long time.[17] These were mostly women given oxytocin before 2 centimeters' dilation because hospital policy forbade sending women with prior cesareans home regardless of whether they were actually in progressive labor. The article describes this as early augmentation, but these were actually inductions, and the difference is more than semantic. Giving a woman oxytocin who was progressively dilating and stopped differs physiologically from giving a woman oxytocin who isn't in labor or who has just begun labor. This is because achieving coordinated contractions that open the cervix depends on several factors besides sufficient oxytocin. In other words, the precipitating factor behind the excessive use of oxytocin and dysfunctional labor that led to scar disruption was inappropriate induction. In confirmation of this, researchers at the same hospital randomly assigned two hundred VBAC candidates who arrived at the hospital with early or prelabor contractions to either admission or to be sent home.[14] Admitted women were given oxytocin after 4 hours with no cervical change. Five women in the admitted group versus none in the expectant management group experienced scar separations (although the only symptomatic scar separation occurred in a woman with a vertical uterine scar). Nearly twice as many women in the admitted group had oxytocin longer than 16 hours (40 percent versus 22 percent).

REFERENCES

1. Ananth CV, Smulian JC, and Vintzileos AM. The association of placenta previa with history of cesarean delivery and abortion: a metaanalysis. *Am J Obstet Gynecol* 1997;177(5):1071–1078.
2. Annibale DJ et al. Comparative neonatal morbidity of abdominal and vaginal deliveries after uncomplicated pregnancies. *Arch Pediatr Adolesc Med* 1995;149(8):862–867.
3. Beall M et al. Vaginal delivery after cesarean in women with unknown types of uterine scar. *J Reprod Med* 1984;29(1):31–35.
4. Burt RD, Vaughan TL, and Daling JR. Evaluating the risks of cesarean

section: low Apgar score in repeat c-section and vaginal deliveries. *Am J Public Health* 1988;78:1312–1314.

5. Chez RA. Cervical ripening and labor induction after previous cesarean delivery. *Clin Obstet Gynecol* 1995;38(2):287–292.

6. Clark SL, Koonings PP, and Phelan JP. Placenta previa/accreta and prior cesarean section. *Obstet Gynecol* 1985;66(1):89–92.

7. Devoe et al. The prediction of "controlled" uterine rupture by the use of intrauterine pressure catheters. *Obstet Gynecol* 1992;80(4):626–629.

8. Farmer RM et al. Uterine rupture during trial of labor after previous cesarean section. *Am J Obstet Gynecol* 1991;165(4):996–1001.

9. Flamm BL et al. Prostaglandin E2 for cervical ripening: a multicenter study of patients with prior cesarean delivery. *Am J Perinatol* 1997; 14(3):157–160.

10. Flamm BL. Once a cesarean, always a controversy. *Obstet Gynecol* 1997;90(2):312–315.

11. Flamm BL. Vaginal birth after cesarean section. In *Cesarean Section: Guidelines for Appropriate Utilization*. Flamm BL and Quilligan EJ, eds. New York: Springer-Verlag, 1995.

12. Gemer O, Segal S, and Sassoon E. Detection of scar dehiscence at delivery in women with prior cesarean section. *Acta Obstet Gynecol Scand* 1992;71(7):540–542.

13. Gilbert L, Saunders N, and Sharp F. The management of multiple pregnancy in women with a lower-segment caesarean scar. Is a repeat caesarean section really the "safe" option? *Br J Obstet Gynaecol* 1988;95: 1312–1316.

14. Grubb DK, Kjos SL, and Paul RH. Latent labor with an unknown uterine scar. *Obstet Gynecol* 1996;88(3):351–355.

15. Hemminki E and Merilainen J. Long-term effects of cesarean sections: ectopic pregnancies and placental problems. *Am J Obstet Gynecol* 1996; 174(5):1569–1574.

16. Hook B et al. Neonatal morbidity after elective repeat cesarean section and trial of labor. *Pediatrics* 1997;100(3):348–353.

17. Leung AS et al. Risk factors associated with uterine rupture during trial of labor after cesarean delivery: a case-control study. *Am J Obstet Gynecol* 1993;168(3):1358–1363.

18. Leung AS, Leung EK, and Paul RH. Uterine rupture after previous cesarean delivery: maternal and fetal consequences. *Am J Obstet Gynecol* 1993;169(4):945–950.

19. Martin N et al. The case for trial of labor in the patient with a prior low-segment vertical cesarean incision. *Am J Obstet Gynecol* 1997; 177(1):144–148.

20. Miller DA et al. Vaginal birth after cesarean section in twin gestation. *Am J Obstet Gynecol* 1996;175(1):194–198.

21. O'Brien JM, Barton JR, and Donaldson ES. The management of placenta percreta: conservative and operative strategies. *Am J Obstet Gynecol* 1996;175(6):1632–1638.

22. Rodriguez MH et al. Uterine rupture: are intrauterine pressure catheters useful in the diagnosis? *Am J Obstet Gynecol* 1989;161(3):666–669.

23. Taylor VM et al. Placenta previa and prior cesarean delivery: how strong is the association? *Obstet Gynecol* 1994;84(1):55–57.

VBAC REPORTS

24. Amir W, Peter J, and Etan Z. Trial of labor without oxytocin in patients with a previous cesarean. *Am J Perinatol* 1987;4(2):140–143.
25. Arulkumaran S, Chua S, and Ratnam SS. Symptoms and signs with scar rupture—value of uterine activity measurements. *Aust NZ Obstet Gynaecol* 1992;32(3):208–212.
26. Asakura H and Myers SA. More than one previous cesarean delivery: a 5-year experience with 435 patients. *Obstet Gynecol* 1995;85(6):924–929.
27. Brody CZ et al. Vaginal birth after cesarean in Hawaii. Experience at Kapiolani Medical Center for Women and Children. *Hawaii Med J* 1993;52(2):38–42.
28. Coltart TM, Davies JA, and Katesmark M. Outcome of a second pregnancy after a previous elective cesarean section. *Br J Obstet Gynaecol* 1990;97(12):1140–1143.
29. Cowan RK et al. Trial of labor following cesarean delivery. *Obstet Gynecol* 1994;83(6):933–936.
30. Duff P, Southmayd K, and Read JA. Outcome of trial of labor in patients with a single previous low transverse cesarean section for dystocia. *Obstet Gynecol* 1988;71(3 Pt 1):380–384.
31. Eglington GS et al. Outcome of a trial of labor after prior cesarean delivery. *J Reprod Med* 1984;29(1):3–8.
32. Flamm BL et al. Elective repeat cesarean delivery versus trial of labor: a prospective multicenter study. *Obstet Gynecol* 1994;83(6):927–932.
33. Flamm BL et al. Vaginal birth after cesarean delivery: results of a 5-year multicenter collaborative study. *Obstet Gynecol* 1990;76(5 Pt 1):750–754.
34. Graham AR. Trial labor following previous cesarean section. *Am J Obstet Gynecol* 1984;149(1):35–45.
35. Hangsleben KL, Taylor MA, Lynn NM. VBAC program in a nurse-midwifery service. Five years of experience. *J Nurse Midwifery* 1989; 34(4):179–184.
36. Holland JG et al. Trial of labor after cesarean delivery: experience in the non-university level II regional hospital setting. *Obstet Gynecol* 1992; 79(6):936–939.
37. Jarrell MA, Ashmead GG, and Mann LI. Vaginal delivery after cesarean section: a five year study. *Obstet Gynecol* 1985;65(5):628–632.
38. Martin JN et al. Vaginal delivery following previous cesarean birth. *Am J Obstet Gynecol* 1983;146(3):255–263.
39. McMahon MJ et al. Comparison of a trial of labor with an elective second cesarean section. *N Engl J Med* 1996;335(10):689–695.
40. Meehan FP and Burke G. Trial of labour following prior section; a 5

year prospective study (1982–1987). *Eur J Obstet Gynecol Reprod Biol* 1989;31:109–117.

41. Meier PR and Porreco RP. Trial of labor following cesarean section: a two year experience. *Am J Obstet Gynecol* 1982;144(6):671–678.

42. Miller DA, Diaz FG, and Paul RH. Vaginal birth after cesarean: a 10-year experience. *Obstet Gynecol* 1994;84(2):255–258.

43. Miller M and Leader LR. Vaginal delivery after caesarean section. *Aust NZ J Obstet Gynaecol* 1992;32(3):213–216.

44. Molloy BG, Sheil O, and Duignan NM. Delivery after caesarean section: review of 2176 cases. *Br Med J* 1987;294:1645–1647.

45. Ngu A and Quinn MA. Vaginal delivery following caesarean section. *Aust NZ J Obstet Gynaecol* 1985;25:41–43.

46. Nguyen TV et al. Vaginal birth after cesarean section at the University of Texas. *J Reprod Med* 1992;37(10):880–882.

47. Phelan JP et al. Vaginal birth after cesarean. *Am J Obstet Gynecol* 1987; 157(6):1510–1515.

48. Schneider J, Gallego D, and Benito R. Trial of labor after an earlier cesarean: a conservative approach. *J Reprod Med* 1988;33(5):453–456.

49. Stovall TG et al. Trial of labor in previous cesarean section patients, excluding classical cesarean sections. *Obstet Gynecol* 1987;70(5):713–717.

50. Veridiano NP, Thorner NS, and Ducey J. Vaginal delivery after cesarean section. *Int J Gynaecol Obstet* 1989;29(4):307–311.

51. Videla FL et al. Trial of labor: a disciplined approach to labor management resulting in a high rate of vaginal delivery. *Am J Perinatol* 1995; 12(3):181–184.

52. Whiteside DC, Mahan CS, and Cook JC. Factors associated with successful vaginal delivery after cesarean section. *J Reprod Med* 1983;28(1): 785–788.

53. Wilf RT and Franklin JB. Six years' experience with vaginal births after cesareans at Booth Maternity Center in Philadelphia. *Birth* 1984;11(1): 5–9.

Chapter 11
Professional Labor Support:
Mothering the Mother

Whether a mother experiences her labor as positive or negative depends on how well supported she feels.

Several studies have found that having a positive experience of childbirth depended on feeling nurtured and supported during labor.[19,21] One of them found that women continued to have vivid and deeply felt memories of satisfaction with the birth or its lack fifteen to twenty years later.[19]

Doulas can decrease the use of medical procedures and treatments for both mother and baby.

An analysis of data from thirteen trials randomly assigning women to doulas or not found that the presence of a doula reduced the use of pain medication in general and epidurals in particular, cesarean section, instrumental vaginal delivery, and the number of babies born in poor condition.[9] Two more random assignment trials have been published since this analysis. One also found a reduction in the use of pain medication (epidurals were not available), cesarean sections, and instrumental vaginal deliveries;[15] the other found a reduction in epidurals.[6] In addition, the analysis did not include another trial that found a marked reduction in cesareans.[11]

Individual studies have found other differences as well. They have found shorter labors,[3,12–14,20] less use of oxytocin to stimulate stronger contractions,[12–13,15,20] fewer instances of rupturing membranes to stimulate stronger contractons,[15] and fewer episiotomies (a cut or snip to enlarge the vaginal opening).[7] And studies have found fewer newborn evaluations for infection and longer than usual newborn hospital stays as well as fewer newborn admissions to intensive care.[12–13] A randomized controlled trial in women in *preterm* labor (before thirty-seven weeks of pregnancy) reported that no baby in the doula group was born in poor condition (5-minute Apgars less than 7) versus one-third (4 of 11) in the control group.[3] This was probably due to doula-group mothers using much less narcotic pain relief but also possibly to doulas reducing maternal distress and anxiety.

For reasons beyond their control, doulas don't always reduce intervention rates.

A Canadian trial randomly assigned 103 healthy, middle-class, first-time mothers to doula support or not.[7–8] Although they came to the hospital later in labor and 40 percent versus 20 percent had no pain medication, women in the doula group were *more* likely to have IV oxytocin to stimulate contractions (43 percent versus 22 percent), equally likely to have cesarean deliveries (20 percent in both groups), and forceps delivery rates were not statistically different (27 percent versus 37 percent). Intervention rates this high in a population of ultra low-risk women reflects their obstetricians' approach. And, in fact, an editorial commentator on this study writes, "One important reason for the lack of effect of a [doula] in this trial is very likely that the practice habits of these private obstetricians utterly swamped any effect of added support during labor and delivery."[18] Similarly, a randomized controlled trial of doula care among over seven hundred low-income, urban, first-time mothers in a Mexican hospital found that one-quarter of the women in both groups had cesareans, even though all women were in active labor and anticipating vaginal birth at the time of study entry.[14]

Epidurals also almost certainly play a role in medical intervention rates. In the Canadian trial, 60 percent of the doula group and 80 percent of the control group had an epidural either as a first resort or after having a narcotic. Epidurals are given as a matter of course in Mexican hospitals, and 85 percent of the Mexican women in both groups had epidurals. In yet a third trial where nurses acting as doulas failed to reduce intervention rates, 84 percent of the doula group and 90 percent of the control group had epidurals.[4] Contrast this with a Houston randomized controlled trial among low-income Hispanic women having a first baby. In this trial, 8 percent of the doula group had a cesarean versus 18 percent of the control group.[12] Only 8 percent of the doula group had an epidural versus over half of the control group. Maternal fever led to most of the infant prolonged hospital stays and workups for infection. Maternal fever was associated with epidural use. Research has since proven that epidurals cause fevers (see page 269).

Doulas improve psychological and social outcomes.

An analysis of data from five trials randomly assigning women to doulas or not and evaulating womens' views of their childbirth experience reported that while the trials measured different aspects, all found benefits for doulas.[9] These included greater satisfaction overall, feeling less tense and anxious, feeling more in control, feeling they coped better with labor, finding mothering easier, and experiencing less postpartum depression in general and less severe depression in particular. One trial published since also found women feeling more satisfied with the labor and that they coped well.[6] In addition, women felt better about their bodies' strength and performance. Another found that first-time mothers scored higher on an evaluation of their mothering skills two months after the birth.[16]

Fathers don't do what doulas do.

A study compared fourteen fathers' labor support activities at labors where doulas were not present with those of three doulas attending twenty-seven women.[1] All women were healthy, first-time mothers. Activities were recorded only when the mother was physically uncomfortable. In both early and late labor, during contractions doulas spent 85 percent of their time within a foot of the mother's body, versus less than one-third of the time for fathers in early labor, dropping to one-quarter of the time in late labor. In early labor, during contractions doulas were actually holding the mother 18 percent of the time versus none of the time for fathers. In late labor, this rose to one-quarter of the time for doulas and remained at less than 1 percent for fathers. Researchers broke down touching into the categories of hand-holding, rubbing/stroking/clutching/holding, other touching, and physical comfort. With the sole exception of hand-holding in early labor, doulas exceeded fathers in all categories. The difference was especially marked for rubbing/stroking/clutching/holding. Doulas spent three-quarters of their time in this activity in both early and late labor versus about 15 percent of the time for fathers.

Doulas complement and enhance the father's care.

Canadian researchers randomly assigned 103 first-time mothers to be accompanied by a doula or not.[7] All women were accompanied by their male partner. Researchers broke down labor support activities into physical comfort measures such as cool cloths or massage, emotional support such as reassurance or encouragement, information/instruction actions such as coaching breathing or suggesting relaxation or comfort techniques, and advocacy actions such as interpreting the woman's needs to staff members or supporting her decisions. Researchers periodically made observations and compared the average number of actions in each category as offered by the doula and husband in the doula group and the nurse and the husband in the control group. Fathers in the doula group averaged more different physical comfort actions than the control group fathers: four versus a little over three. They averaged about the same number of emotional support actions and advocacy activities in both groups. The only major negative change was in giving information/instruction. The average number of activities fell from three in the control group to slightly over one in the doula group.

Labor-and-delivery nurses don't generally offer supportive care.

Two studies of labor-and-delivery nurses' work activities in two different hospitals got the same results.[5,17] Nurses spent less than 10 percent of their time engaged in labor support activities, and half of *that* time was spent giving instructions or advice. Offering verbal and physical comforts and advocating for the mother occupied 3 percent of the average nurse's workday.

In the study cited in the previous section, nurses lagged considerably behind doulas in all labor support categories.[7] Fewer than one-third of the women in the control group reported receiving any physical comfort measures or advocacy actions from a nurse.

REFERENCES

1. Bertsch TD et al. Labor support by first-time fathers: direct observations with a comparison to experienced doulas. *J Psychosom Obstet Gynaecol* 1990;11:251–260.
2. Bryanton J, Fraser-Davey H, and Sullivan P. Women's perceptions of nursing support during labor. *J Perinat Neonat Nurs* 1994;23(8):638–644.
3. Cogan R and Spinnato JA. Social support during premature labor: effects on labor and the newborn. *J Psychosom Obstet Gynaecol* 1988: 209–216.
4. Gagnon AJ et al. A randomized trial of one-to-one nurse support of women in labor. *Birth* 1997;24(2):71–77.
5. Gagnon A and Waghorn K. Supportive care by maternity nurses: a work sampling study in an intrapartum unit. *Birth* 1996;23(1):1–6.
6. Gordon NP et al. Effects of providing hospital-based doulas in health maintenance organization hospitals. *Obstet Gynecol* 1999;93:422–426.
7. Hodnett ED and Osborne RW. A randomized trial of the effects of monitrice support during labor: mothers' views two to four weeks postpartum. *Birth* 1989;16(4):177–183.
8. Hodnett ED and Osborne RW. Effects of continuous intrapartum professional support on childbirth outcomes. *Res Nurs Health* 1989;12: 289–297.
9. Hodnett ED. Caregiver support for women during childbirth (Cochrane Review). In: *The Cochrane Library,* Issue 1, 1999. Oxford: Update Software.
10. Hofmeyr GJ et al. Companionship to modify the clinical birth environment: effects on progress and perceptions of labour, and breastfeeding. *Br J Obstet Gynaecol* 1991;98:756–764.

11. Kennell J and McGrath SK. Labor support by a doula for middle income couples: the effect on cesarean rates. *Pediatr Res* 1993;33:12A.
12. Kennell J et al. Continuous emotional support during labor in a US hospital. *JAMA* 1991;265(17):2197–2201.
13. Klaus MH et al. Effects of social support during parturition on maternal and infant morbidity. *Br Med J* 1986;293:585–587.
14. Langer A et al. Effects of psychosocial support during labor and child-birth on breastfeeding, medical interventions, and mothers' wellbeing in a Mexican public hospital: a randomised clinical trial. *Br J Obstet Gynaecol* 1998;105:1056–1063.
15. Madi BC et al. Effects of female relative support in labor: a randomized controlled trial. *Birth* 1999;26(1):4–8.
16. Martin S et al. The effect of doula support during labor on mother-infant interaction at 2 months. *Infant Behav Develop* 1998;21(Suppl):556.
17. McNiven P, Hodnett E, and O'Brien-Pallas LL. Supporting women in labor: a work sampling study of the activities of labor and delivery nurses. *Birth* 1992; 19(1):3–8.
18. Shearer MH. Commentary: when a monitrice is an outsider. *Birth* 1989: 16(4):183–184.
19. Simkin P. Just another day in a woman's life? Women's long-term perceptions of their first birth experience. Part I. *Birth* 1991;18(4):203–210.
20. Sosa R et al. The effect of a supportive companion on perinatal problems, length of labor, and mother-infant interaction. *N Engl J Med* 1980; 303:597–600.
21. Tarkka MT and Paunonen M. Social support and its impact on mothers' experiences of childbirth. *J Adv Nurs* 1996;23(1):70–75.
22. Wolman WL et al. Postpartum depression and companionship in the clinical birth environment: a randomized, controlled study. *Am J Obstet Gynecol* 1993;168:1388–1393.

Chapter 12
Obstetricians, Midwives, and Family Practitioners: Someone to Watch over You

The midwifery model of care differs from the obstetric model in ways that are beneficial to mothers and babies.

Sakala has written two review papers exploring differences between obstetric management and midwifery care. One review looked at how obstetricians and home birth midwives differed on how to cope with poor progress.[37] Mainstream obstetricians view labor mechanically. It should progress according to a rate determined by a normative curve. Poor progress arises from misfits between the baby's size and the mother's pelvis, weak contractions, or a poorly positioned baby. Inadequate progress requires intravenous oxytocin to stimulate stronger contractions or cesarean section. By contrast, interviews with eleven home birth midwives revealed little concern with rate of progress provided mother and baby were doing well. The midwives believed that labor care and the mother's emotional state could impede or promote progress. For this reason, they encouraged upright positioning, eating and drinking in labor, comfort measures, and relaxation techniques and good labor support to minimize feelings of fear or anxiety. They determined treatment approaches in consultation with the mother and deferred to her preferences. Treatment depended on the mother doing something rather than doing something to her.

The other study looked at coping with labor pain.[36] According to medical textbooks and articles, drugs are the only viable pain relief options and women should be encouraged to use them. By contrast, fifteen home birth midwives offered many strategies, including prenatal preparation (formation of a trust relationship, empowerment through knowledge), physical manipulations (massage, reflexology, acupressure), hydrotherapy (tub baths), oral intake (food and drink, herbal medicines), breathing and relaxation techniques, and psychological techniques (support and attention from those present; positive, supportive language; visualization; creation of a peaceful environment; and vocalization of pain). Midwives believed that pain medication introduced risks and women could cope without it.

Three studies have compared obstetricians' and midwives' views of maternity care. Researchers asked 196 midwives and 114 obstetricians to rate the importance of a long list of components of prenatal care.[17] The two groups differed significantly on half the list. Many more midwives than obstetricians rated aspects of care related to nutrition, education, counseling, women's comfort and convenience (availability of child-care facilities and/or toys, brief waiting times), and joint decision making (discussing birth plans) as "very important."

San Diego researchers surveyed opinions and practices of twenty midwives and fifty-seven obstetricians on twenty-four items known to reduce the frequency of negative outcomes.[12] Many more midwives agreed that social support during labor and birth should be available to all women from friends and family, that social and psychological support should be available to all women from caregivers, and that all women should have unrestricted mother-infant contact after birth. Among other differences, many more midwives agreed that upright positions should be an option during labor and birth, that women should not hold their breath while pushing, that pushing should be delayed when women have epidurals, and that episiotomy should be used restrictively. Many more also believed that external cephalic version to turn the baby head down should be available to all women carrying breech babies. Finally, physicians favored epidurals over narcotics for pain relief.

The same marked differences were found in a Canadian survey of 198 obstetricians, 392 family practitioners, and 70 midwives.[4] Most obstetricians but few midwives felt that women received adequate information about nutrition and exercise and attention to psychological issues, participated fully in decision making about their care, and that women's wishes were respected. Nearly one-third of obstetricians felt that obstetric intervention rates reflected women's requests. Few obstetricians but most midwives felt reducing obstetric intervention rates should be a goal, and nearly half of obstetricians but few midwives felt the nearly 20 percent Canadian cesarean rate was justified. Women obstetricians thought similarly to men.

A survey of over four hundred midwifery practices compared characteristics of hospital care by midwives with physician care at the same hospitals.[38] Over 90 percent of midwifery practices usually offered oral fluids, encouraged walking; offered use of a shower, bath, or hot tub; encouraged alternative positions for the birth; and used intermittent rather than continuous electronic fetal monitoring. By contrast, three-quarters of nonmidwifery patients walked in labor, a little over half were allowed oral fluids or use of a shower, bath, or hot tub; one-third had intermittent electronic fetal monitoring; and one-fourth could choose their position for birth. Similarly, in a trial of midwifery versus physician care at a large, inner-city hospital, the midwives encouraged walking, position of choice for birth, and the companionship of a loved one while the physicians confined women to bed, delivered women on their backs in stirrups (*lithotomy* position) on delivery tables, and rarely allowed labor companions because of "space constraints, lack of assisting personnel, and use of epidural anesthesia."[8]

What medications and procedures you have depends mainly on your caregiver's philosophy, not your medical condition. (See also pages 12 to 21 and page 254.)

From a 1980 national survey, researchers selected a sample of 4,500 women free of risk factors that might lead to the need for medical intervention.[1] They compared electronic fetal monitoring (EFM) rates, labor induction rates, and cesarean rates in this low-risk group with women who had risk factors. Despite the difference in risk status, cesarean rates were virtually identical as were induction rates. The low-risk women were somewhat *more* likely to have EFM. Moreover, the odds of low-risk women having these procedures varied with hospital type. Compared with low-risk women in rural hospitals, low-risk women were half again as likely to have EFM in urban hospitals and 70 percent more likely to have it in large, teaching hospitals. Induction was 70 percent more likely in urban hospitals and nearly 80 percent more likely in teaching hospitals. C-sections were 15 percent more likely in urban hospitals and 25 percent more likely in teaching hospitals. The odds would likely differ were the study to be repeated with more recent data. Nonetheless the fact that risk factors (or their lack) didn't affect intervention rates remains valid today.

A study compared outcomes between a hospital clinic staffed by midwives that served urban low-income women and the mostly white, private patients of the obstetricians who supervised the midwives.[5] The low-income women had more factors predisposing to complications. Despite this, the total cesarean rate in the five hundred clinic women was 13 percent, half the 26 percent rate in the six hundred private patients. The cesarean rate for first (*primary*) cesareans was 11 percent versus 19 percent in private patients. Infant outcomes were similar between the two groups.

Another study compared cesarean rates in two hundred healthy, first-time mothers who were clinic patients cared for by the residency staff and four hundred similar women who were private patients of obstetricians at the same hospital.[29] Epidural rates were identical (42 percent) in both groups, which drops out epidurals as a factor in oxytocin use and in instrumental and cesarean delivery rates for poor progress. Seventy percent of women with epidurals in both groups had oxytocin. Private physicians used oxytocin *more* often in women who did not have epidurals (one-third versus one-fifth). Despite this, the cesarean rate for poor labor progress was 20 percent in the private patients versus 1 percent in the clinic patients.

Two studies looked at factors affecting individual obstetricians' cesarean rates. One found that among eleven obstetricians at a single hospital serving "very-low-risk" private patients, total cesarean rates ranged from one in five to approaching half and rates for first cesareans ranged from one women in ten to one women in three.[14] No differences could be found among patient populations. Similarly, another study of eleven obstetricians revealed that cesarean rates ranged from 6 percent to 20 percent. Again, no differences in patient populations explained this variation.[10]

Researchers who conducted a trial in which they had randomly assigned women to liberal versus restricted use of episiotomy set out to find out why one-third of the doctors agreeing to participate in the trial continued to have 90 percent episiotomy rates in the "restrict episiotomy" group.[26] All women were healthy and at low risk for complications when labor began. Nonetheless, these doctors performed more cesareans, gave more women oxytocin, and performed more episiotomies for impending tear than doctors who viewed episiotomy unfavorably. They also diagnosed fetal distress more often, and the diagnosis became a reason both to keep women from trial participation and to do an episiotomy.

In another study of belief and episiotomy described on page 299 under "Family practitioners tend to be less interventive . . . ," obstetricians defending episiotomy made statements such as, "I think you who don't do episiotomies are lazy, barbaric, and practicing poor obstetrics. [The perineum] doesn't stretch, it tears." And, "Well-timed, properly performed, and carefully repaired episiotomy is one of the most important contributions of modern obstetrics." No research data support these claims.

Researchers compared outcomes between obstetrician and family practitioner management in 800 women with gestational diabetes.[23] The biggest concern with gestational diabetes is an overly large baby. Average birth weights and the percentage of babies weighing over 8 lbs., 13 oz. (4,000 grams) were similar in the two groups. However, the cesarean rate was one in ten women among family practitioners versus one in three among obstetricians. Midwives achieved the same low cesarean rate as the family doctors in a study of 120 gestational diabetics.[32]

The next sections will show that procedure rates vary enormously even in studies of low-risk women.

Midwifery care produces equally good or better maternal and infant outcomes as does obstetric management, with much lower procedure and medication rates.

A study compared infant outcomes of all 153,000 U.S. women in 1991 who had vaginal births of a single baby born between thirty-five and forty-three weeks gestation and who were attended by nurse midwives with a random sample comprising 685,000 similar women attended by doctors that same year.[28] After accounting for differences in social and medical risk factors, infants of mothers cared for by nurse midwives were one-third less likely to die in the first week, 20 percent less likely to die in the first year, and one-third less likely to be of low birth weight.

Several studies compare midwifery care to physician care, including two randomized controlled trials, a practice that eliminates many potential souces of bias. I have graphed their results on pages 300 to 303. The numbers on the horizontal axis refer to the study's number in the reference list. In all cases comparing midwives with doctors, studies included only low-risk women. Infant outcomes were similar, which means intervening more often conferred no benefits. Please note that study #18 is unique in that the doctors' group included both obstetricians and family physicians.

Study #8 has frequently been cited as proving that obstetricians can achieve low cesarean rates in low-risk women. As you can see from the other studies, the issue is not that they can't but that they usually don't. Even so, the other graphs show that obstetricians in study #8 performed more instrumental deliveries, internal electronic fetal monitoring, and episiotomies, and used oxytocin more often than midwives.

Here is a study that differed enough in design from the other comparison studies that I chose not to graph it. Between 1981 and 1992 midwives cared for 36,400 women qualifying for an in-hospital birth center at a large Los Angeles hospital serving low-income women.[16] Two percent of the women had a cesarean and another 2 percent had an instrumental delivery. Only 5 percent had an episiotomy and nearly 60 percent had an intact perineum (no or minimal injury). Newborn outcomes were excellent.

Family practitioners tend to be less interventive than obstetricians, but may intervene more than midwives.

Several studies compare family practice care to obstetric care. I have graphed their results on pages 300 to 303. The numbers on the horizontal axis refer to the study's number in the reference list. Maternal and infant outcomes did not differ between family physicians and obstetricians. In study #20, after statistically adjusting for such factors as the obstetricians having more first-time mothers and more mothers in the obstetrician group having epidurals, women attended by obstetricians were two-thirds more likely to have an episiotomy and half again as likely to have a cesarean. Here are two additional studies that differed enough in design from the other comparison studies that I chose not to graph them.

A study looked at cesarean rates with respect to site and obstetrician versus family physician at each site for 7,350 births at five hospitals.[19] Cesarean rates for family physicians by site ranged from 7 percent to 11 percent, but obstetricians ranged by site from 14 percent to 31 *percent*! Overall, the average cesarean rate for family practitioners was 9 percent versus 16 percent for obstetricians. Because midwives and family physicians might refer high-risk cases to obstetricians, the author recalculated C-section rates limiting the obstetricians' group to women who started care with obstetricians. This *raised* the obstetricians' cesarean rate from an average of 16 percent to 27 percent!

Another study compared outcomes in 850 women attending a practice of midwives and family physicians where birth attendant depended on who was on call.[21] Midwives augmented fewer labors in women with prior children (multiparous women) (9 percent versus 17 percent) but ruptured membranes (*amniotomies*) more often in first-time mothers (59 percent versus 46 percent). Fewer multiparous women (11 percent versus 20 percent) and first-time mothers (31 percent versus 41 percent) had episiotomies, although statistical calculation attributed the latter difference to chance. Fewer first-time mothers had cesareans (8 percent versus 14 percent). The difference lay in cesareans for poor progress (4 percent versus 12 percent). After adjusting for factors that could influence cesarean rates, first-time mothers allotted to family physicians nearly tripled their chances of cesarean section.

Beliefs as well as practices of family practitioners also tend to fall between midwives and obstetricians but closer to obstetricians. Researchers asked sixteen obstetric residents, sixty-seven obstetricians, sixty-seven family practitioners, twenty-four certified nurse-midwives, and twenty-eight direct-entry midwives whether they agreed that episiotomy should be performed for nearly all births, nearly all births in first-time mothers, or for anyone who would tear.[15] One-third of the obstetricians and obstetric residents and 20 percent of the family practitioners agreed with the first statement compared with about 10 percent of the nurse midwives and no direct-entry midwives. All obstetric residents, 80 percent of obstetricians, 70 percent of family practitioners, 30 percent of nurse-midwives, and no direct-entry midwives thought first-time mothers required them. All obstetric residents and nearly all obstetricians, family practioners, and nurse-midwives versus 30 percent of direct-entry midwives thought episiotomies should be done in women who would tear. Similarly, in the Canadian survey described on page 296, family physicians aligned with obstetricians in most responses, although one-third of family practitioners versus half of obstetricians thought all women required an IV in labor and somewhat more family physicians (84 percent versus 74 percent) thought routine episiotomies were unacceptable.[4] Still, only 4 percent of midwives agreed with routine IVs and 90 percent said routine episiotomies were unacceptable.

CESAREAN SECTION RATES

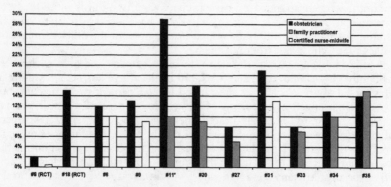

RCT = randomized control trial, meaning women were randomly assiged to one form of treatment or the other, a practice that eliminates many potential sources of bias

*Rates ranged from a disturbing 20 percent to an appalling 46 percent

Instrumental Delivery Rates

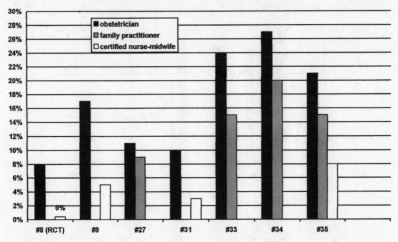

Continuous Electronic Fetal Monitoring Rates

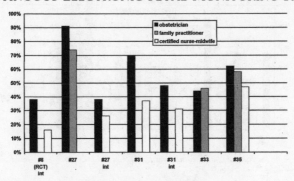

"Int" means internal electronic fetal monitoring

RCT = randomized control trial, meaning women were randomly assigned to one form of treatment or the other.

Percentage Having IVs

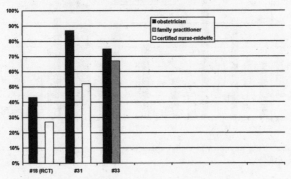

RATES OF RUPTURING MEMBRANES (AMNIOTOMY)

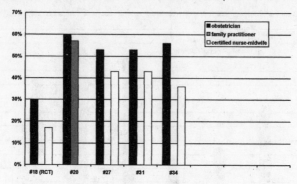

OXYTOCIN USE RATES
(Inductions + Augmentations of Labor)

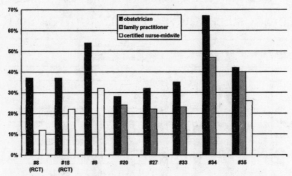

RCT = randomized control trial, meaning women were randomly assigned to one form of treatment or the other.

EPIDURAL RATES

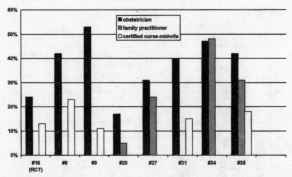

Difference in epidural rates may partially explain the differences in intervention rates seen in the other graphs (see page 132).

EPISIOTOMY RATES

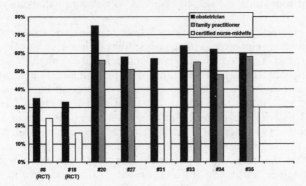

Midwifery-style care may be distorted or limited by a high-tech environment or one where obstetricians dictate policy.

To begin with, look at the procedure and oxytocin rates reported for midwives in the bar graphs and remember that these are *healthy* women carrying *healthy, full-term* babies. In particular, look at study #35, the three-way comparison of obstetricians, family practitioners, and hospital-based midwives. The authors of the three-way comparison speculate that the reason that little differentiates family practitioners from obstetricians is that family-practice residents learn obstetrics from obstetricians and use them for consultation and referral once in practice.[35] Compare, too, the intervention rates in these graphs with those on pages 311 to 313, which include out-of-hospital birth.

Two studies have examined the impact of obstetricians and high-risk care on family physicians. One compared intervention rates in 2,350 low-risk women cared for by family practitioners in one of two high-risk perinatal referral centers or at a third hospital caring mostly for low-risk women.[7] Fewer women in the low-risk hospital had their membranes ruptured (36 percent versus 47 percent), epidurals (42 percent versus 64 percent), labor augmented with oxytocin (9 percent versus 20 percent), continuous electronic fetal monitoring (35 percent versus 53 percent), or episiotomies (45 percent versus 58 percent). They were equally likely to have induced labors (5 percent versus 6 percent), instrumental deliveries (25 percent versus 26 percent), and C-sections (7 percent in both groups). Obstetricians also intervened less often at the low-risk hospital, but the gaps were smaller.

Another study compared intervention rates between 1,750 women admitted to a teaching service supervised by family practitioners and 2,800 women managed on a service supervised by obstetricians.[22] The family practice service only trained family practitioners, but the obstetrician-supervised service trained both obstetric and family practice residents. Women on the family practice teaching service had fewer epidurals (6 percent versus 15 percent), episiotomies (59 percent versus 69 percent), and cesarean sections (8 percent versus 30 *percent*). They had more amniotomies (56 percent versus 49 percent). Use of oxytocin was similar (26 percent versus 29 percent). After adjusting for differences in risk factors, women on the obstetrician-supervised service had four times the risk of cesarean section and half again the risk of episiotomy.

I have no studies of how working where the obstetric model holds sway affects midwives. However, I have two studies of low-risk women cared for by midwives at Yale, a high-risk perinatal referral hospital.[2,30] The studies report electronic fetal monitoring rates of 90 percent and 43 percent, IV rates of 83 percent and 43 percent, and in one, a 69 percent amniotomy rate, a 59 percent episiotomy rate, and a 9 percent anal tear rate. I have a third study of 1,850 low-risk women at a Vermont high-risk center where the cesarean rate was 10 percent.[25] An obstetrician was consulted in nearly half the cases, primarily because women were deemed to have dysfunctional labors. Neither the Yale midwives nor the Vermont midwives saw any problems with their statistics. In one of the Yale studies, the midwives congratulated themselves on their "selective use of technology."[2] The Vermont midwives took the cesarean rate and the frequent need to consult an obstetrician as evidence that birth should always occur in a hospital. I also have a Canadian study whose authors did see a problem.[24] In this pilot study of midwifery care, obstetricians "delegated" nurses, most of whom were midwives, to do births. Midwifery was illegal at the time and the researchers hoped to show its benefits. They compared intervention rates in 79 low-risk women cared for by the nurses with 373 similar women receiving standard care from obstetricians. Somewhat fewer women had amniotomies (33 percent versus 47 percent) and epidurals (34 percent versus 49 percent). Rates were similar for episiotomy (40 percent versus 49 percent), anal tears (13 percent versus 8 percent), and forceps (20 percent versus 16 percent) and cesarean (5 percent versus 7 percent) deliveries. The authors commented that these results underscored the difficulties of practicing under physician supervision.

Female physicians have practice styles and philosophies similar to those of their male counterparts.

Three studies that looked respectively at cesarean rates, vaginal birth after cesarean rates, and beliefs about care found no differences between male and female physicians.[3,4,13]

REFERENCES

1. Albers LL and Savitz DA. Hospital setting for birth and use of medical procedures in low-risk women. *J Nurse Midwifery* 1991;36(6):327–333.
2. Beal MW. Nurse-midwifery intrapartum management. *J Nurse Midwifery* 1984;29(1):13–19.
3. Berkowitz GS et al. Effect of physician characteristics on the cesarean birth rate. *Am J Obstet Gynecol* 1989;161:146–149.
4. Blais R et al. Controversies in maternity care: where do physicians, nurses, and midwives stand? *Birth* 1994;21(2):63–70.
5. Blanchette H. Comparison of obstetric outcome of a primary-care access

clinic staffed by certified nurse-midwives and a private practice group of obstetricians in the same community. *Am J Obstet Gynecol* 1995;172(6): 1864–1871.

6. Butler J et al. Supportive nurse-midwife care is associated with a reduced incidence of cesarean section. *Am J Obstet Gynecol* 1993;168(5):1407–1413.

7. Carroll JC et al. The influence of the high-risk care environment on the practice of low-risk obstetrics. *Fam Med* 1991;23(3):184–188.

8. Chambliss LR et al. The role of selection bias in comparing cesarean birth rates between physician and midwifery management. *Obstet Gynecol* 1992;80(2):161–165.

9. Davis L et al. Cesarean section rates in low-risk private patients managed by certified nurse-midwives and obstetricians. *J Nurse Midwifery* 1994; 39(2):91–97.

10. Demott RK and Sandmire HF. The Green Bay cesarean section study. I. The physician factor as a determinant of cesarean birth rates. *Am J Obstet Gynecol* 1990;162(6):1593–1602.

11. Deutchman ME, Sills D, and Connor PD. Perinatal outcomes: a comparison between family physicians and obstetricians. *J Am Board Fam Pract* 1995;8(6):440–447.

12. Fullerton JT, Hollenbach KA, and Wingard DL. Practice styles. A comparison of obstetricians and nurse-midwives. *J Nurse Midwifery* 1996; 41(3):243–250.

13. Goldman G et al. Factors influencing the practice of vaginal birth after cesarean section. *Am J Pub Health* 1993;83(8):1104–1108.

14. Goyert GL et al. The physician factor in cesarean birth rates. *N Engl J Med* 1989;320(11):706–709.

15. Graham SB et al. A comparison of attitudes and practices of episiotomy among obstetrical practitioners in New Mexico. *Soc Sci Med* 1990;31(2): 191–201.

16. Greulich B et al. Twelve years and more than 30,000 nurse-midwife-attended births: the Los Angeles County + University of Southern California Women's Hospital Birth Center experience. *J Nurse Midwifery* 1994;39(4):185–196.

17. Haertsch M, Campbell E, and Sanson-Fisher R. Important components of antenatal care: midwives' and obstetricians' views. *Aust NZ J Obstet Gynaecol* 1996;36(4):411–416.

18. Harvey S et al. A randomized, controlled trial of nurse-midwifery care. *Birth* 1996;23(3):128–135.

19. Hueston WJ. Site-to-site variation in the factors affecting cesarean section rates. *Arch Fam Med* 1995;4(4):346–351.

20. Hueston WJ et al. Practice variations between family physicians and obstetricians in the management of low-risk pregnancies. *J Fam Pract* 1995;40(4):345–351.

21. Hueston WJ and Rudy M. A comparison of labor and delivery management between nurse midwives and family physicians. *J Fam Pract* 1993; 37(5):449–454.

22. Hueston WJ and Rudy M. Differences in labor and delivery experience in family-physician- and obstetrician-supervised teaching services. *Fam Med* 1995;27(3):182–187.

23. Jackson EA, Francke L, and Vasilenko P. Management of gestational diabetes by family physicians and obstetricians. *J Fam Pract* 1996;43(4): 383–388.
24. Kaufman K and McDonald H. A retrospective evaluation of a model of midwifery care. *Birth* 1988;15(2):95–99.
25. Keleher KC and Mann LI. Nurse-midwifery care in an academic health center. *J Obstet Gynecol Neonatal Nurs* 1986;15(5):369–372.
26. Klein MC et al. Physicians' beliefs and behaviour during a randomized controlled trial of episiotomy: consequences for women in their care. *Can Med Assoc J* 1995;153(6):769–779.
27. MacDonald S, Voaklander K, and Birtwhistle RV. A comparison of family physicians' and obstetricians' intrapartum management of low-risk pregnancies. *J Fam Pract* 1993;37(5):457–462.
28. MacDorman MF and Singh GK. Midwifery care social and medical risk factors, and birth outcomes in the USA. *J Epidemiol Community Health* 1998;52: 310–317.
29. Neuhoff D, Burke MS, and Porreco RP. Cesarean birth for failed progress in labor. *Obstet Gynecol* 1989;73(6):915–920.
30. Nichols CW. The Yale nurse-midwifery practice: addressing the outcomes. *J Nurse Midwifery* 1985;30(3):159–165.
31. Oakley D et al. Processes of care: comparisons of certified nurse-midwives and obstetricians. *J Nurse Midwifery* 1995;40(5):339–409.
32. O'Brien ME and Gilson G. Detection and management of gestational diabetes in an out-of-hospital birth center. *J Nurse Midwifery* 1987; 32(2):79–84.
33. Reid AJ et al. Differences in intrapartum obstetric care provided to women at low risk by family physicians and obstetricians. *Can Med Assoc J* 1989;140:625–633.
34. Rosenberg E and Klein M. Is maternity care different in family practice? *J Fam Pract* 1987;25(3):237–240.
35. Rosenblatt RA et al. Interspecialty differences in the obstetric care of low-risk women. *Am J Public Health* 1997;87(3):344–351.
36. Sakala C. Content of care by independent midwives: assistance with pain in labor and birth. *Soc Sci Med* 1988;26(11):1141–1158.
37. Sakala C. Midwifery care and out-of-hospital birth settings: how do they reduce unnecessary cesarean section births? *Soc Sci Med* 1993;37(10): 1233–1250.
38. Wolfe SM and Gabay M. *Delivering a Better Childbirth Experience.* Washington, D.C.: Public Citizen's Health Research Group, 1995.

Chapter 13
The Place of Birth:
Location, Location, Location

Planned home birth with a trained attendant is safe for low-risk women.

Several strands of evidence support the safety of home birth when the above requirements are met. First, in Holland, a country where home birth never disappeared, researchers compared the *perinatal mortality rate* (deaths of babies around the time of birth) between 1979 and 1982 for various cities and regions with the percentage of home births and found no correlation, although home birth rates ranged from 4 percent to 51 percent.[38] Second, taken together, home birth studies report on over 41,600 women who either planned a home birth or started labor at home.[1–3,6–9,14,18–19,21,24,26–27,33,36–37,39–40,43,45–46] Some are quite large: a U.S. study of 11,788 women,[3] a Dutch study of 6,550 women,[40] a study of 9,800 New Zealand women,[18] which means that if home birth posed risks, they should have shown up even if the excess risk was small. Several of these studies used matching strategies to compare outcomes between women planning hospital births and women planning home births.[1,7,9,18,43–46] Only one study reported what the authors felt was an unduly high perinatal or newborn death rate.[7] The authors calculated that two newborn deaths would occur, and there were eleven. However, only four of those babies were born at home, and in only one of those cases does it appear that a hospital birth might have made a difference. Studies also failed to show excesses of other adverse outcomes such as low Apgar scores (a measure of the baby's condition at birth), the need for resuscitation, or admissions to intensive care units.[1,8–9,36,43,46] Finally, an analysis of data from six home birth studies comprising 24,100 women came to the conclusion that the evidence in no way supports the contention that planned home birth, with a trained attendant backed up by a hospital, poses any excess risk to low-risk women.[29]

Data also support the caveats that birth attendants should have appropriate training and women should be prescreened for risk factors. One Missouri study compared outcomes among planned home births attended by physicians, certified nurse-midwives, midwives belonging to the Missouri Midwives Association, unaffiliated midwives, or family or friends only.[33] There were seventeen newborn deaths versus the statistically expected nine, but the excess came from births attended by nonprofessionals. As for prescreening, a study reported a stillbirth in a baby presenting feet first. Yet another study reported three women who gave birth to surprise twins at home.[7] An ultrasound scan would have detected either situation.

Birth in a freestanding birth center is safe for low-risk women, provided the center has the staff and resources to handle an emergency.

As with home births, we have numerous studies of freestanding birth centers, totalling over 24,000 women in all. None reported abnormally high perinatal or newborn mortality rates.[4–5,10–13,17,30–31,34–35,47] One of them encompassed eighty-four birth centers and 11,800 women so even a slight increase in excess deaths should have shown up.[31] Several studies matched outcomes with low-risk women giving birth in hospitals.[4,13,16,35] Outcomes at birth centers were similar if not superior.

Still, as is true in any setting, quality of care can vary. The overall perinatal mortality rate among the eighty-four birth centers was 1 per 1,000.[31] However, it was 7 per 1,000 at five centers excluded because they did not conform to the study's quality standards.

Although there was no statistical excess of complications, one study of an in-hospital (not a freestanding) birth center concluded that two deaths and three cases of newborn complications could have been avoided by more aggressive care.[42] However, the criticism seems unfounded. In two cases, fetal distress arose hours after transfer to standard care. In a third, the labor and birth proceeded normally and Apgar scores (a measure of the infant's condition at birth) were good. In the fourth case, the authors thought the mother should have been advised to come to the hospital immediately when she reported the baby had not moved for two hours, but two hours of no fetal movement isn't long enough to set off alarm bells in the absence of other symptoms. In the fifth case, the baby suddenly died during labor of unknown causes. The authors thought the outcome "might" have been different with routine electronic fetal monitoring. Maybe it would, but probably not.

Studies show no differences in outcomes between direct-entry midwives and nurse-midwives.

Some of the studies cited in this appendix report on nurse-midwives[2–5,12–13,17,27,30–31,33–35,47] while others report on direct-entry midwives,[1,6,8–9,18,21–22,25–26,33,36–37,39–40,43,46] including nearly all of the non-U.S. studies. None suggest any excess risk based on training. In addition, a study compared outcomes among 6,950 women attended by direct-entry midwives (trained in a state-approved program) who gave birth at home, 14,800 women attended by nurse-midwives in the hospital, 4,050 births attended by nurse-midwives out-of-hospital, and 23,600 women who qualified for midwifery care but were attended in-hospital by physicians.[23] All groups had similar numbers of babies born in poor condition and similar newborn mortality rates.

Out-of-hospital birth attendants achieve equally good outcomes with less use of potentially problem-causing drugs and procedures, especially cesarean section.

To begin with, compare the cesarean rates found in Tables 1 and 2 with those found on pages 300–301 for hospital-based practitioners. Of twenty-three cesarean rates reported in studies of hospital-based practitioners, only one group of obstetricians, one group of family practitioners, and two groups of hospital-based midwives had cesarean rates in the range of those reported for out-of-hospital practitioners. And in the case of all the hospital-based midwives and many of the physician groups, their clients were also low risk. Of course, some of the differences could be because fewer first-time mothers chose out-of-hospital birth. First-time mothers are far more likely to have cesareans. Also, in some studies family physicians and obstetricians cared for higher-risk women. However, I doubt that these factors account for most, let alone all of the gap.

TABLE 1
Cesarean Section Rates: Birth Centers

#10	3%
#47	3%
#11	4%
#31	4%
#42*	4%
# 4	5%
# 5	5%
#30	5%
#34	5%
#35	6%
#13	7%
#17	7%
#22*	7%
#25*	7%

Notes: The study numbers correspond to the reference list at the end of the appendix. The three starred studies are in-hospital, not freestanding birth centers.

TABLE 2
Cesarean Section Rates: Home Births

#40	less than 1%
#21	1%
#36	1%
#43	1%
# 9	2%
#26	2%
#27	2%
#45	2%
# 2	3%
# 3	3%
#24	3%
#39	4%
#46	4%
# 1	6%
# 7	6%

Next, I have graphed other intervention rates, including comparison studies of C-section and other intervention rates, on the succeeding pages. The strongest evidence lies within each comparison study because differences between studies mean you may be comparing apples to oranges. For example, some studies use women beginning labor outside of the hospital and others use women who only *planned* out-of-hospital birth, which would include women who risked out during pregnancy. Still, the bar graphs here and those on pages 300–303 for in-hospital practitioners indicate a clear and consistent trend to intervene more often in the hospital.

The comparison groups are:

#13: women eligible for a birth center at 37 weeks with low-risk women at a nearby hospital

#16: women beginning labor at 84 birth centers with low-risk clients of hospital-based nurse-midwives.

#22: women randomly assigned to an in-hospital birth center with women assigned to standard care

#25: women randomly assigned to an in-hospital birth center with women assigned to standard care

#35: women beginning labor at a birth center with similar women at the back-up hospital

#42: women randomly assigned to an in-hospital birth center with women assigned to standard care

1: women planning home birth with similar women planning hospital birth

7: women planning home birth with all Australian hospital births

#36: women with prior vaginal births planning home birth to similar women planning hospital birth

#43: women planning home births with low-risk women planning hospital birth

Study #16 is worth discussing in detail because both groups were cared for primarily by nurse-midwives. This study compared procedure and medication rates between 11,800 women who began labor at 84 freestanding birth centers and 2,250 women cared for in fifteen practices of hospital-based nurse-midwives serving low-risk clients. Nearly twice as many women (11 percent versus 6 percent) reached or exceeded forty-two weeks of pregnancy in the birth center population, which suggests more hospital clients were induced before forty-two weeks' gestation. The hospital population experienced more pregnancy complications, which could explain at least part of the increased cesarean rate (4 percent versus 8 percent) in the hospital group. (As can be seen in my bar graph, instrumental delivery rates were similar.) However, to compare other procedure rates, the authors looked at the subgroup of 5,150 birth center women and 500 women planning hospital births in whom there were no pregnancy or labor complications. IV, *amniotomy* (rupturing membranes), and *episiotomy* (cutting the vaginal opening) rates in the hospital group considerably exceeded rates at freestanding birth centers.

COMPARATIVE CESAREAN SECTION RATES

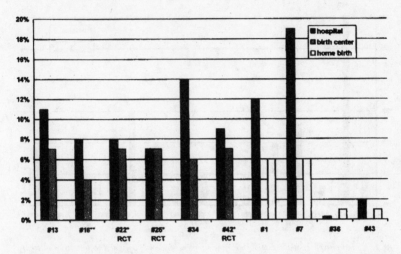

RCT = randomized controlled trial, meaning women randomly assigned to one form of treatment or the other, a practice that eliminates many potential sources of bias.

*In-hospital birth center
**Compares hospital-based nurse midwives to freestanding birth center nurse-midwives.

Notes: The cesarean section rates in #36 are extraordinarily low, probably because the study excluded first-time mothers.

The cesarean section rate for study #42 differs from the one in Table 1. This is because the rate in the bar graph includes women who risked out of the birth center before labor while the table lists rates for women who began care at the birth center.

Instrumental Delivery Rates

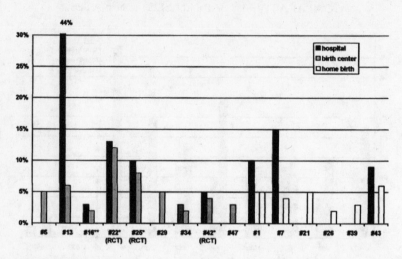

RCT = randomized controlled trial, meaning women randomly assigned to one form of treatment or the other

*In-hospital birth center
**Compares hospital-based nurse-midwives to freestanding birth center nurse-midwives.

Percentage Having IVs

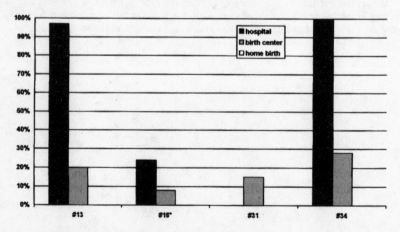

*Compares hospital-based nurse-midwives to freestanding birth center nurse-midwives.

RATES OF RUPTURING MEMBRANES (AMNIOTOMY)

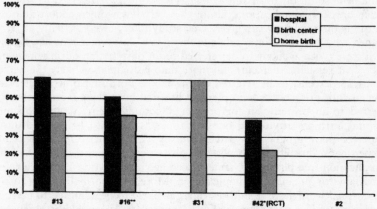

RCT = randomized controlled trial, meaning women randomly assigned to one form of treatment or the other

*In-hospital birth center
**Compares hospital-based nurse-midwives to freestanding birth center nurse-midwives.

EPISIOTOMY RATES

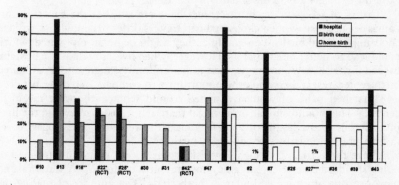

RCT = randomized controlled trial, meaning women randomly assigned to one form of treatment or the other

*In-hospital birth center
**Compares hospital-based nurse-midwives to freestanding birth center nurse-midwives.
***The episiotomy rate in first-time mothers was 2 percent.

In-hospital practitioners tend to see problems that aren't there.

In Holland, midwifery care is the norm and healthy women may elect home or hospital birth. In almost all cases, women are referred to an obstetrician only for complications, although a very few women choose an obstetrician as their primary caregiver. One study interviewed virtually all 1,700 women who gave birth in a single town in 1981.[8] Women choosing hospital birth were twice as likely to be referred to an obstetrician during pregnancy (6 percent versus 12 percent) and more than half again as likely (16 percent versus 26 percent) to be referred during labor. Both first-time mothers and women with prior births who planned hospital birth were more likely to be referred to an obstetrician for pregnancy complications. Women planning hospital birth were two and one-half times as likely to be referred during labor for poor progress (5 percent versus 12 percent). Only twenty-four women chose hospital birth with an obstetrician. Of these, only half had complication-free births, the same percentage as for women referred to obstetricians for pregnancy complications. Moreover, normal babies born in the hospital were more than three times as likely to be admitted to newborn intensive care (3 percent versus about 10 percent). This could be because the babies were sicker (see page 315 "Hospital management may increase . . ."), or perhaps they too were overdiagnosed.

In addition, two studies of freestanding birth centers noted that transfer rates into the hospital fell with increasing out-of-hospital birth experience.[11,17] One of them noted a remarkable 18 percent to 7 percent drop in cesarean rates as well.[17] This suggests that the hospital philosophy and environment powerfully influence the caregiver's perception of problems.

The superior outcomes achieved outside the hospital are not because those women are at lower risk or in any way special or different from women planning hospital births.

Critics of freestanding birth centers have argued that the superior outcomes are because women choosing birth centers differ from low-risk women choosing hospital births. For example, they might be better motivated, which could lead to better health habits. However, when overcrowding at a hospital caused low-risk, low-income women to be randomly assigned to its affiliated birth center, researchers took the opportunity to compare outcomes between 148 matched pairs of women assigned to and women choosing the birth center.[34] They found similar or identical maternal transfer rates into the hospital during labor, cesarean rates, newborn transfer rates, and Apgar scores (a measure of the baby's condition at birth).

I have three trials in which low-risk women were randomly assigned to either standard care or care in an in-hospital birth center.[22,25,42] Maternal and newborn outcomes were similar in both trials. The authors of one of the studies profess to find avoidable factors in the birth center group in the complications experienced by three babies and the deaths of two, but this could be disputed (see page 307 "Birth in a freestanding birth center is safe . . ." for details).[42] An analysis of five such trials totalling nearly 8,000 women failed to find differences in rates of newborn resuscitation, prolonged newborn hospital stay, or newborn admission to intensive care.[20] The author notes a trend toward more stillbirths and neonatal deaths in the birth center group, but a look at the actual studies reveals that they occurred in cases transferred to standard care before labor or transferred in labor for complications.[22,25] Once these deaths are removed, the difference disappears. In fact, birth center babies were 30 percent less likely to experience abnormal fetal heart rate patterns, which may reflect less use of pain medication or merely that electronic fetal monitoring was used less often (fetal monitors over-diagnose fetal distress).

Hospital management may increase fetal and newborn complication rates.

It may be chance, subtle differences between populations, or differing definitions, but several comparison studies have shown higher complication rates in the in-hospital population. One study compared low-risk clients of hospital-based nurse-midwives with similar women attended by nurse-midwives at birth centers.[16] The babies of women laboring in the hospital were more likely to experience "sustained fetal distress" (7 percent versus 2 percent) and "great effort required to establish respiration" (1 per 100 versus 4 per 1,000). Women in the hospital were more likely to have narcotics, which can cause heart rate disturbances and difficulty breathing. Although rare, hospital women were ten times more likely to experience umbilical cord prolapse, a life-threatening emergency in which the umbilical cord slips into the vagina and gets pinched between the baby and the mother's pelvis during contractions (2 per 1,000 versus 3 per 10,000). In five of the eight cases of prolapse, caregivers had ruptured the membranes (*amniotomy*) (see page 252). One-quarter of the babies in another study versus 5 percent were diagnosed as having abnormal fetal heart rate, which may relate to in-hospital women having electronic fetal monitoring and epidurals.[13] The babies were also more likely to have thick *meconium*, the baby's first stool, in the amniotic fluid (18 percent versus 5 percent). (If inhaled, meconium can cause pneumonia.) Newborns were more likely to be admitted to intensive care (6 percent versus 1 percent) as well. Yet another study found slightly more incidence of shoulder dystocia, a potentially life-threatening situation in which the baby's head is born but the shoulders are stuck, in the hospital population even though more big babies were born at the birth center.[35] Delivering women flat on their backs or with forceps predisposes to shoulder dystocia. Finally, an analysis of data from six studies comparing home birth with hospital birth found that about twice as many babies in the hospital group were born in poor condition.[29]

Risk-out and transfer rates vary markedly among studies, but home birth rates generally are lower than freestanding birth center rates.

I have transfer rate data from nine birth centers, three of which were in-hospital birth centers, as well as data from three studies of multiple birth centers, comprising 11, 16, and 84 centers.[5,10–11,15,22,25,30–31,34,42,47] Rates for women who risked out before labor (*antepartum transfer rates*) ranged from 10 percent to 18 percent (except for one small study with a 3 percent antepartum rate and one of the in-hospital birth centers with a 32 percent rate). Rates for women transferred during labor (*intrapartum transfer rates*) ranged from 8 percent to 25 percent, and rates for women or babies transferred after birth (*postpartum maternal and infant transfer rates*) ranged from 2 percent to 7 percent. Total transfer rates for women who began labor at the center and their babies ranged from 10 percent to 31 percent. Some of these differences can be explained by variations in risk factors in the populations using the centers and perhaps in distance of the center from the back-up hospital. Still, much of the difference must be due to practitioner philosophy and birth center guidelines. For example, two birth centers risked out clients whose bag of waters broke and whose labor did not start within as little as twelve hours.[16,47]

I have data from fifteen home-birth studies, almost all of which were multiple practices, including one U.S. study of ninety nurse-midwife practices and 11,100 women and another of twenty-nine nurse-midwifery practices and 1,200 women.[1-3,7-9,14,21,24,26-27,36,39,45-46] Transfer rates before labor ranged from 2 percent to 12 percent, transfer rates in labor ranged from 3 percent to 16 percent, transfer rates after birth for mothers and babies ranged from 1 percent to 4 percent. Total transfer rates for women who began labor at home and their babies ranged from 2 percent to 20 percent.

Notice that while ranges overlap, home-birth transfer rates tend to be lower than birth centers.

- transfer rates before labor: 10–18% at birth centers versus 2–12% for home births
- transfer rates during labor: 8–26% at birth centers versus 3–16% for home births
- transfer rates after birth: 2–7% at birth centers versus 1–4% for home births
- total transfer rates for women beginning labor out-of-hospital: 10–31% at birth centers versus 2–20% for home births

One possible explanation is that more first-time mothers chose birth centers and more women with prior vaginal births choose home birth. If so, this would tend to raise risk-out and hospital transfer rates for freestanding birth centers and lower them for home birthers because first-time mothers are much more likely to experience problems. Nonetheless, the fact that both freestanding birth centers and home-birth practitioners serve low-risk women suggests that differences in home birth practitioner philosophy and policy played a part.

Out-of-hospital birth attendants are more likely to use comfort measures.

Women having home births, of course, have all the comforts and freedoms that one enjoys in one's own home. Some studies of freestanding birth centers have looked at how well birth centers do in this regard or how they fare with respect to hospitals. One survey of thirty-nine freestanding birth centers compared the birth center with non-midwife clients using the birth center's back-up hospital and got these results:[44]

light refreshment during labor:	100% versus 3%
oral fluids during labor:	100% versus 40%
room to walk about during labor:	100% versus 46%

friends allowed to attend:	100% versus 57%
use of shower, bath, or hot tub:	100% versus 37%
freedom of position for the birth:	100% versus 9%
breastfeeding on demand:	100% versus 77%
no separation of mother and infant:	100% versus 17%
unlimited family participation:	100% versus 11%

A study evaluated care given to 11,800 women who labored at 84 free-standing birth centers. Nearly one-third of women with previous children had their children with them.[32] Over one-third of the women were accompanied by other family members or friends in addition to the baby's father or other partner. Over half had clear fluids only and 40 percent either ate solids or had nonclear fluids in addition. Only 5 percent neither ate nor drank. Nearly one-quarter took tub baths and more than one-quarter took showers. Only 20 percent of women giving birth in birth centers gave birth flat on their backs.

Even women planning hospital births with midwives may not have the comfort measures available to women experiencing out-of-hospital births. A study compared the women in the study above with 2,250 women planning birth with hospital-based nurse midwives.[16] They found that 20 percent of women planning births at freestanding birth centers versus 40 percent of women planning hospital births gave birth flat on their backs or on their backs with legs in stirrups. They then narrowed the comparison to 5,150 women who experienced no complications before or during labor at freestanding birth centers and 500 similar clients of the hospital-based nurse midwives and found that 15 percent versus 11 percent had solid food during labor and 40 percent versus 24 percent had a shower or bath during labor. Nearly all women in both groups had oral fluids during labor.

Women prefer midwifery-style, home-like care.

Two trials in which women were randomly assigned to an in-hospital birth center or standard hospital management evaluated their satisfaction. One was in Sweden, the other in England, which means midwives provided care in both settings. This means styles would probably be more alike than if doctors managed labor in the standard hospital setting. Nevertheless, in the Swedish study, nearly 80 percent of women assigned to the birth center gave the highest satisfaction rating to labor care versus about half of the standard hospital group.[41] Birth center women rated both physical (medical supervision and/or treatment) and psychological (how midwives responded to the women's thoughts and emotions) aspects of their care higher than standard care women. Ninety percent of the birth center group preferred the birth center for future births whereas less than half the hospital group wanted standard hospital management for future births. In the British study, three-quarters of those assigned to the birth center were "very satisfied" versus 60 percent of the standard management group.[25] In a U.S. study in which over-crowding led to low-risk women being assigned to the hospital's affiliated freestanding birth center, women assigned to the center liked the care so much that they returned for subsequent babies and referred friends and family.[34] An analysis of five studies randomly assigning women to in-hospital birth center or standard care found that women assigned to birth center care were half as likely to report they were "less than satisfied" with labor care.[20]

REFERENCES

1. Ackermann-Liebrich U et al. Home versus hospital deliveries: follow up study of matched pairs for procedures and outcome. *BMJ* 1996; 313(7068):1276–1277.

2. Anderson R and Greener D. A descriptive analysis of home births attended by CNMs in two nurse-midwifery services. *J Nurse Midwifery* 1991;36(2):95–103.

3. Anderson RE and Murphy PA. Outcomes of 11,788 planned home births attended by certified nurse-midwives. *J Nurse Midwifery* 1995;40(6): 483–492.

4. Baruffi G et al. A study of pregnancy outcomes in a maternity center and a tertiary care hospital. *Am J Public Health* 1984;74(9):973–978.

5. Bennetts AB and Lubic R. The freestanding birth centre. *Lancet* 1982; 1:378–380.

6. Burnett CA et al. Home delivery and neonatal mortality in North Carolina. *JAMA* 1980;244(24):2741–2745.

7. Crotty M et al. Planned homebirths in South Australia 1976–1987. *Med J Aust* 1990;153:664–671.

8. Damstra-Wijmenga SM. Home confinement: the positive results in Holland. *J R Coll Gen Pract* 1984;34(265):425–430.

9. Duran AM. The safety of home birth: the Farm study. *Am J Public Health* 1992;82(3):450–453.

10. Eakins PS et al. Obstetric outcomes at the Birth Place in Menlo Park: the first seven years. *Birth* 1989;16(3):123–129.

11. Eakins PS. Freestanding birth centers in California: program and medical outcome. *J Reprod Med* 1989;34(12):960–970.

12. Faison JB et al. The childbearing center: an alternative birth setting. *Obstet Gynecol* 1979;54(4):527–532.

13. Feldman E and Hurst M. Outcomes and procedures in low risk birth: a comparison of hospital and birth center settings. *Birth* 1987;14(1):18–24.

14. Ford C, Iliffe S, and Franklin O. Outcome of planned home births in an inner city practice. *BMJ* 1991;303(6816):1517–1519.

15. Fullerton JT et al. Transfer rates from freestanding birth centers. A comparison with the National Birth Center Study. *J Nurse Midwifery* 1997; 42(1):9–16.

16. Fullerton JT and Severino R. In-hospital care for low-risk childbirth: comparison with results from the National Birth Center Study. *J Nurse Midwifery* 1992;37(5):331–340.

17. Garite TJ et al. Development and experience of a university-based freestanding birthing center. *Obstet Gynecol* 1995;86(3):411–416.

18. Gulbransen G et al. Home birth in New Zealand 1973–93: incidence and mortality. *NZ Med J* 1997;110(1040):87–89.
19. Hinds MW, Bergeisen GH, and Allen DT. Neonatal outcome in planned v unplanned out-of-hospital births in Kentucky. *JAMA* 1985;253(11):1578–1582.
20. Hodnett ED. Home-like versus conventional birth settings. In: Neilson JP et al., eds. *Pregnancy and Childbirth Module of the Cochrane Database of Systematic Reviews,* updated May 1996.
21. Howe KA. Home births in south-west Australia. *Med J Aust* 1988;149(6):296–302.
22. Hundley VA et al. Midwife managed delivery unit: a randomised controlled comparison with consultant led care. *BMJ* 1994;309:1400–1403.
23. Janssen PA, Holt VL, and Myers SJ. Licensed midwife-attended, out-of-hospital births in Washington State: are they safe? *Birth* 1994;21(3):141–148.
24. Koehler MS, Solomon DA, and Murphy M. Outcomes of a rural Sonoma County home birth practice: 1976–1982. *Birth* 1984;11(3):165–169.
25. MacVicar J et al. Simulated home delivery in hospital: a randomised controlled trial. *Br J Obstet Gynaecol* 1993;100(4):316–323.
26. Mehl LE et al. Outcomes of elective home births: a series of 1,146 cases. *J Reprod Med* 1977;19(5):281–290.
27. Murphy PA and Feinland JB. Perineal outcomes in a home birth setting. *Birth* 1998;25(4):226–234.
28. Murphy PA and Fullerton J. Outcomes of intended home births in nurse-midwifery practice: a prospective descriptive study. *Obstet Gynecol* 1998;92(3):461–470.
29. Olsen O. Meta-analysis of the safety of home birth. *Birth* 1997;24(1):4–13.
30. Reinke C. Outcomes of the first 527 births at the Birthplace in Seattle. *Birth* 1982;9(4):231–238.
31. Rooks JP et al. Outcomes of care in birth centers: the National Birth Center Study. *N Engl J Med* 1989;321(26):1804–1811.
32. Rooks JP, Weatherby NL, and Ernst EK. The National Birth Center Study. Part II—Intrapartum and immediate postpartum and neonatal care. *J Nurse Midwifery* 1992;37(5):301–330.
33. Schramm WF, Barnes DE, and Bakewell JM. Neonatal mortality in Missouri home births. *Am J Public Health* 1987;77(8):930–935.
34. Scupholme A and Kamons AS. Are outcomes compromised when mothers are assigned to birth centers for care? *J Nurse Midwifery* 1987;32(4):211–215.
35. Scupholme A, McLeod AGW, and Robertson EG. A birth center affiliated with the tertiary care center: comparison of outcome. *Obstet Gynecol* 1986;67(4):598–603.
36. Shearer JM. Five year prospective survey of risk of booking for a home birth in Essex. *Br Med J* 1985;291(6507):1478–1480.
37. Sullivan DA and Beeman R. Four years' experience with home birth by licensed midwives in Arizona. *Am J Public Health* 1983;73(6):641–645.
38. Treffers PE and Laan R. Regional perinatal mortality and regional hospitalization at delivery in the Netherlands. *Br J Obstet Gynaecol* 1986;93(7):690–693.

39. Tyson H. Outcomes of 1001 midwife-attended home births in Toronto, 1983–1988. *Birth* 1991;18(1):14–19.

40. van Alten D, Eskes M, and Treffers PE. Midwifery in the Netherlands. The Wormerveer study: selection, mode of delivery, perinatal mortality and infant morbidity. *Br J Obstet Gynaecol* 1989;96(6):656–652.

41. Waldenstrom U and Nilsson CA. Women's satisfaction with birth center care: a randomized, controlled study. *Birth* 1993;20(1):3–13.

42. Waldenstrom U, Nilsson CA, and Winbladh B. The Stockholm birth centre trial: maternal and infant outcome. *Br J Obstet Gynaecol* 1997; 104(4):410–418.

43. Weigers TA et al. Outcome of planned home and planned hospital births in low risk pregnancies: prospective study in midwifery practices in The Netherlands. *BMJ* 1996;313(7068):1309–1313.

44. Wolfe SM and Gabay M. *Delivering a Better Childbirth Experience.* Washington, D.C.: Public Citizen's Health Research Group, 1995.

45. Wood LAC. Obstetric retrospect. *JR Coll Gen Pract* 1981;31:80–90.

46. Woodcock HC et al. A matched cohort study of planned home and hospital births in Western Australia 1981–1987. *Midwifery* 1994;10(3): 125–135.

47. Zabrek E, Simon P, and Benrubi GI. Nurse-midwifery prototypes: clinical practice and education. The alternative birth center in Jacksonville, Florida: the first two years. *J Nurse Midwifery* 1983;28(4):31–36.

BIBLIOGRAPHY

Introduction

CIMS. "The mother-friendly childbirth initiative." Washington, D.C.: CIMS,1996.

Davis-Floyd R E. *Birth As an American Rite of Passage*. Berkeley: University of California Press, 1992.

Enkin M et al. *A Guide to Effective Care in Pregnancy and Childbirth*. Oxford: Oxford University Press, 1995.

Odent M. The fetus ejection reflex. *Birth* 1987;14(2):45–46.

Rooks J P. *Midwifery and Childbirth in America*. Philadelphia: Temple University Press, 1997.

Wagner M. *Pursuing the Birth Machine*. Camperdown, Australia: Ace Graphics, 1994.

Chapter 1

ACOG. Vaginal birth after previous cesarean delivery. *Practice Bulletin* 1998, No 2.

Albers L L and Savitz D A. Hospital setting for birth and use of medical procedures in low-risk women. *J Nurse Midwifery* 1991;36(6):327–33.

Al-Mufti R, McCarthy A, and Fisk N M. Obstetricians' personal choice and mode of delivery. *Lancet* 1996;347:544.

Annibale D J et al. Comparative neonatal morbidity of abdominal and vaginal deliveries after uncomplicated pregnancies. *Arch Pediatr Adolesc Med* 1995;149(8):862–67.

Astbury J et al. Birth events, birth experiences and social differences in postnatal depression. *Aust J Public Health* 1994;18(2):176–84.

Bibliography

Barrett J F R et al. Inconsistencies in clincal decisions in obstetrics. *Lancet* 1990:336:549–51.

Boylan P et al. Effect of active management of labor on the incidence of cesarean section for dystocia in nulliparas. *Am J Perinatol* 1991;8(6):373–79.

Burns L R, Geller S E, and Wholey D R. The effect of physician factors on the cesarean section decision. *Med Care* 1995;33(4):365–82.

Burt R D, Vaughan T L, and Daling J R. Evaluating the risks of cesarean section: low Apgar score in repeat C-section and vaginal deliveries. *Am J Public Health* 1988;78:1312–14.

Curtin S C and Kozak L J. Decline in U.S. cesarean delivery rate appears to stall. *Birth* 1998;25(4):259–61.

Eakins P S. Freestanding birth centers in California: program and medical outcome. *J Reprod Med* 1989;34(12):960–70.

Enkin M et al. *A Guide to Effective Care in Pregnancy and Childbirth.* 2d ed. Oxford: Oxford University Press, 1995.

Enkin M W, Hunter D J, and Snell L. Episiotomy: effects of a research protocol on clinical practice. *Birth* 1984;11(3):145–46.

Evans M I et al. Cesarean section: assessment of the convenience factor. *J Reprod Med* 1984;29(9):670–76.

Feldman G B and Freiman J A. Prophylactic cesarean at term? *N Engl J Med* 1985;312(19):1264–67.

Flamm B L. Cesarean delivery in the United States: a summary of the past 20 years. In *Cesarean Section: Guidelines for Appropriate Utilization.* Flamm B L and Quilligan E J, eds. New York: Springer-Verlag, 1995.

Flamm B L. "Cesarean rates: is the crisis over?" Presented at Innovations in Perinatal Care: Assessing Benefits and Risks, twelfth conference sponsored by the journal *Birth* and the Boston University School of Public Health, Waltham, MA, June 5–7, 1998.

Francome C and Savage W. Caesarean section in Britain and the United States 12% or 24%: is either the right rate? *Soc Sci Med* 1993;37(10):1199–218.

Fraser W et al. Temporal variation in rates of cesarean section for dystocia: does "convenience" play a role? *Am J Obstet Gynecol* 1987;156(2):300–304.

Gabay M and Wolfe S M. *Unnecessary Cesarean Sections: Curing a National Epidemic.* Washington, D.C.: Public Citizen's Health Research Group, 1994.

Goer H. Not just another way to have a baby. *Baby Talk* 1991;56(11):34–35,41.

Gould J B, Davey B, and Stafford R S. Socioeconomic differences in rates of cesarean section. *N Engl J Med* 1989;321(4):233–39.

Haire D B and Elsberry C C. Maternity care and outcomes in a high-risk service: the North Central Bronx Hospital experience. *Birth* 1991;18(1):33–37.

Hall M H. Commentary: confidential enquiry into maternal death. *Br J Obstet Gynaecol* 1990;97:752–53.

Bibliography

Harlow B L et al. Epidemiologic predictors of cesarean section in nulliparous patients at low risk. *Am J Obstet Gynecol* 1995;172(1):156–62.

Haynes de Regt R et al. Relation of private or clinic care to the cesarean birth rate. *N Engl J Med* 1986;315(10):619–24.

Hemminki E and Merilainen J. Long-term effects of cesarean sections: ectopic pregnancies and placental problems. *Am J Obstet Gynecol* 1996;174(5): 1569–74.

Hook B et al. Neonatal morbidity after elective repeat cesarean section and trial of labor. *Pediatrics* 1997;100(3):348–53.

Hueston W J, McClaflin R R, and Claire E. Variations in cesarean delivery for fetal distress. *J Fam Pract* 1996;43(5):461–67.

Hurst M and Summey P S. Childbirth and social class: the case of cesarean delivery. *Soc Sci Med* 1984;18(8):621–31.

Iglesias S, Burn R, and Saunders L D. Reducing the cesarean section rate in a rural community hospital. *Can Med Assoc J* 1991;145(11):1459–64.

Kahn J. Many doctors favor C-sections for themselves. *Medical Tribune*. http://www.medscape.co . . . 2-23-96.caesarean.html, Feb 23, 1996.

Keeler E B and Brodie M. Economic incentives in the choice between vaginal delivery and cesarean section. *Milbank Quarterly* 1993;71(3):365–404.

Klasko S K. The impact of mandated in-hospital coverage on primary cesarean delivery rates in a large nonuniversity teaching hospital. *Am J Obstet Gynecol* 1995;172(2):637–42.

Korte D. *The VBAC Companion*. Boston: Harvard Common Press, 1997.

Koska M T. Reducing cesareans—a $1 million trade-off. *Hospitals* 1989; 63(5):26.

Lagrew D C Jr. and Morgan M A. Decreasing the cesarean section rate in a private hospital: success without mandated clinical changes. *Am J Obstet Gynecol* 1996;174(1):184–91.

Levine A B et al. Sonographic diagnosis of the large for gestational age fetus at term: does it make a difference? *Obstet Gynecol* 1992;79(1):55–58.

Lidegaard O, Jensen L M, and Weber T. Technology use, cesarean section rates, and perinatal mortality at Danish maternity wards. *Acta Obstet Gynecol Scand* 1994;73(3):240–45.

McCloskey L, Petitti D B, and Hobel C J. Variations in the use of cesarean delivery for dystocia: lessons about the source of care. *Med Care* 1992; 30(2):126–35.

McKenzie L and Stephenson P A. Variation in cesarean section rates among hospitals in Washington State. *Am J Public Health* 1993;83(8):1109–12.

Minkoff H and Schwartz R H. The rising cesarean section rate: can it safely be reversed? *Obstet Gynecol* 1980;56(2):135–43.

Miovich S M et al. Major concerns of women after cesarean delivery. *J Obstet Gynecol Neonatal Nurs* 1994;23(1):53–59.

Mutryn C S. Psychosocial impact of cesarean section on the family: a literature review. *Soc Sci Med* 1993;37(10):1271–81.

Myers S A and Gleicher N. A successful program to lower cesarean-section rates. *N Engl J Med* 1988;319(23):1511–16.

Notzon F C. International differences in the use of obstetric interventions. *JAMA* 1990;263(24):3286–91.

O'Driscoll K and Foley M. Correlation of decrease in perinatal mortality and increase in cesarean section rates. *Obstet Gynecol* 1983;61(1):1–5.

Pascoe J M. The cesarean section rate. *JAMA* 1990;26(8):971.

Pearson J W. Cesarean section and perinatal mortality. *Am J Obstet Gynecol* 1984;148(2):155–59.

Phelan J P. Rendering unto Caesar cesarean decisions. *OBG Management* 1996 Nov:6.

Porreco R P. High cesarean section rate: a new perspective. *Obstet Gynecol* 1985;65(3):307–11.

Porreco RP. Personal communication, Feb 1991.

Quilligan E J. Cesarean section: modern perspectives. In *Management of High-Risk Pregnancy*. 2d ed. Queenan, J T, ed. Oradell NJ: Medical Economics Books, 1985.

Radin T G et al. Nurses' care during labor: its effect on the cesarean birth rate of healthy, nulliparous women. *Birth* 1993;20(1):14–21.

Robson M S, Scudamore I W, and Walsh S M. Using the medical audit cycle to reduce cesarean rates. *Am J Obstet Gynecol* 1996;174(1):199–205.

Rochat R W et al. Maternal mortality in the United States: report from the maternal mortality collaborative. *Obstet Gynecol* 1988;72(1):91–97.

Rock S M. Malpractice premiums and primary cesarean section rates in New York and Illinois. *Pub Health Rep* 1988;103(5):459–63.

Rockenschaub A. Technology-free obstetrics at the Semmelweis Clinic. *Lancet* 1990;335:977–98.

Rooks J P. *Midwifery and Childbirth in America*. Philadelphia: Temple University Press, 1997.

Rostow V P, Osterweis M, and Bulger R J. Medical professional liability and the delivery of obstetrical care. *N Engl J Med* 1989;321(15):1057–60.

Rubin G et al. The risk of childbearing re-evaluated. *Am J Public Health*, 1981;71(7):712–16.

Ryding E L, Wijma B, and Wijma K. Posttraumatic stress reactions after emergency cesarean section. *Acta Obstet Gynecol Scand* 1997;76:856–61.

Sachs B P et al. The risks of lowering the cesarean-delivery rate. *N Engl J Med* 1999;340(1):54–7.

Sanchez-Ramos L et al. Reducing cesarean sections at a teaching hospital. *Am J Obstet Gynecol* 1990;163(3):1081–88.

Sandmire H F and DeMott R K. The Green Bay cesarean section study: IV. The physician factor as a determinant of cesarean birth rates for the large fetus. *Am J Obstet Gynecol* 1996;174:1557–64.

Schuitemaker N et al. Maternal mortality after cesarean in The Netherlands. *Acta Obstet Gynecol Scand* 1997;76(4):332–34.

Sepkowitz S. Birth weight–specific fetal deaths and neonatal mortality and the rising cesarean rate. *J Okla State Med Assoc* 1992;85(5):236–41.

Shearer E L. Cesarean section: medical benefits and costs. *Soc Sci Med* 1993;37(10):1223–31.

Smith J F, Hernandez C, and Wax J R. Fetal laceration injury at cesarean delivery. *Obstet Gynecol* 1997;90(3):344–46.

Socol M L et al. Reducing cesarean births at a primarily private university hospital. *Am J Obstet Gynecol* 1993;168(6 Pt 1):1748–58.

Sokol R J et al. Risks preceding increased primary cesarean birth rates. *Obstet Gynecol* 1982;59(3):340–46.

Stafford R S. Cesarean section use and source of payment: an analysis of California hospital discharge abstracts. *Am J Public Health* 1990;80(3): 313–15.

Stewart P J et al. Diagnosis of dystocia and management with cesarean section among primiparous women in Ottawa-Carleton. *Can Med Assoc J* 1990;142(5):459–63.

Turner M J et al. The influence of birth weight on labor in nulliparas. *Obstet Gynecol* 1990;76(2):159–63

Tussing A D and Wojtowycz M A. Malpractice, defensive medicine, and obstetric behavior. *Med Care* 1997;35(2):172–91.

U.S. Department of Health and Human Services. Rates of cesarean delivery— United States, 1991. *MMWR* 1993;42(15):285–300.

van Ham M A, van Dongen P W, Mulder J. Maternal consequences of cesarean section. A retrospective study of intra-operative and postoperative maternal complications of cesarean section during a 10-year period. *Eur J Obstet Gynecol Reprod Biol* 1997;74(1):1–6.

Ventura S J et al. Births and deaths: United States 1996. *Month Vital Stat Rep* 1997;46(1 Suppl 2).

Videla F L et al. Trial of labor: a disciplined approach to labor management resulting in a high rate of vaginal delivery. *Am J Perinatol* 1995;12(3): 181–84.

Vital and Health Statistics. National Health Survey: Annual Summary DHHS Publications No. (PHS) 95-1782, Series 13 No. 121.

Wagner M. *Pursuing the Birth Machine.* Camperdown, Australia: ACE Graphics, 1994.

Weeks J W, Pitman T, and Spinnato J A 2nd. Fetal macrosomia: does antenatal prediction affect delivery route and birth outcome? *Am J Obstet Gynecol* 1995;173(4):1215–19.

World Health Organization. Appropriate technology for birth. *Lancet* 1985; 2(8452):436–37.

Chapter 2

Chauhan S P et al. Sonographic assessment of birth weight among breech presentations. *Ultrasound Obstet Gynecol* 1995;6(1):54–57.

Cibils L A. Breech presentation. In *Cesarean Section: Guidelines for Appropriate Utilization.* Flamm B L and Quilligan E J, eds. New York: Springer-Verlag, 1995.

Cibils L A. Point/Counterpoint: II. Management of a full-term fetus presenting by the breech. *Obstet Gynecol Surv* 1995;50(11):762.

Confino E et al. The breech dilemma. A review. *Obstet Gynecol Surv* 1985; 40(6):330–37.

Consensus Conference Report. Indications for cesarean section: final statement of the panel of the National Consensus Conference on Aspects of Cesarean Birth. *Can Med Assoc J* 1986;134:1348–52.

Cruikshank D P. Breech presentation. *Clin Obstet Gynecol* 1986;29(2):255–63.

Cunningham F et al. *William's Obstetrics*, 20th ed. Stamford: Appleton and Lange, 1997.

Enkin M et al. *A Guide to Effective Care in Pregnancy and Childbirth*, 2d ed. Oxford: Oxford University Press, 1995.

FIGO Committee on Perinatal Health. Recommendations of the FIGO Committee on Perinatal Health on guidelines for the management of breech delivery. *Eur J Obstet Gynecol Reprod Biol* 1995;58(1):89–92.

Flanagan T A, et al. Management of term breech presentation. *Am J Obstet Gynecol* 1987;156(6):1492–1502.

Gaskin I M, Personal communication, Jun 1, 1998.

Gimovsky M and Hennigan C. Abnormal fetal presentations. *Curr Opin Obstet Gynecol* 1995;7(6):482–85.

Gimovsky M L and Schifrin B S. Breech management. *J Perinatol* 1992;12(2):143–51.

Herbst A, Wolner-Hanssen P, and Ingemarsson I. Risk factors for acidemia at birth. *Obstet Gynecol* 1997;90(1):125–30.

Jordan B. External cephalic version as an alternative to breech delivery and cesarean section. *Soc Sci Med* 1984;18(8):637–51.

Kopelman J N et al. Computed tomographic pelvimetry in the evaluation of breech presentation. *Obstet Gynecol* 1986;68(4):455–58.

Lau T K et al. Predictors of successful external cephalic version at term: a prospective study. *Br J Obstet Gynaecol* 1997;104:798–802.

Mahomed K, Seeras R, and Coulson R. External cephalic version at term. A randomized trial using tocolysis. *Br J Obstet Gynaecol* 1991;98:8–13.

Mehl L. Hypnosis and conversion of the breech to the vertex presentation. *Arch Fam Med* 1994;3(10):881–87.

Myers S A and Gleicher N. Breech delivery: why the dilemma? *Am J Obstet Gynecol* 1986;156:6–10.

National Institutes of Health. *Cesarean Childbirth* NIH Publication No. 82-2067. Washington, D.C.: U.S. Department of Health and Human Services, 1981.

Scorza W E. Intrapartum management of breech presentation. *Clin Perinatol* 1996;23(1):31–49.

Simkin P, Whalley J, and Keppler A. *Pregnancy, Childbirth, and the Newborn*. New York: Meadowbrook Press, 1991.

Smith J F, Hernandez C, and Wax J R. Fetal laceration injury at cesarean delivery. *Obstet Gynecol* 1997;90(3):344–46.

Weiner C P. Vaginal breech delivery in the 1990s. *Clin Obstet Gynecol* 1992;35(3):559–69.

Chapter 3

ACOG. Induction of labor. Technical Bulletin No. 217, 1995.

ACOG. Management of postterm pregnancy. Practice Patterns No. 6, 1997.

ACOG. Ultrasonography in pregnancy. Technical Bulletin No. 187, 1993.

Bibliography

Alcalay M et al. Prelabour rupture of membranes at term: early induction of labour versus expectant management. *Eur J Obstet Gynecol Reprod Biol* 1996;70(2):129–33.

Alfirevic Z and Walkinshaw S A. A randomised controlled trial of simple compared with complex antenatal fetal monitoring after 42 weeks of gestation. *Br J Obstet Gynaecol* 1995;102:638–43.

Arias F. Predictability of complications associated with prolongation of pregnancy. *Obstet Gynecol* 1987;70(1):101–6.

Bakos O and Backstrom T. Induction of labor: a prospective, randomized study into amniotomy and oxcytocin as induction methods in a total unselected population. *Acta Obstet Gynecol Scand* 1987;66:537–41.

Blakemore K J et al. A prospective comparison of hourly and quarter-hourly oxytocin dose increase intervals for the induction of labor at term. *Obstet Gynecol* 1990;75(5):757–61.

Boulvain M and Irion O. Stripping/sweeping of the membranes to induce labour or to prevent post-term pregnancy. In: Neilson J P et al., eds. *Pregnancy and Childbirth Module of the Cochrane Database of Systematic Reviews*, updated September 1997.

Centers for Disease Control and Prevention. Prevention of perinatal group B streptococcal disease: a public health perspective. *MMWR* 1996;45(RR-7):1–24.

Centers for Disease Control and Prevention. Prevention of perinatal group B streptococcal disease. *MMWR* 2002;51(No.RR-11):[inclusive page numbers].

Chauhan S P et al. A randomized study to assess the efficacy of the amniotic fluid index as a fetal admission test. *Obstet Gynecol* 1995;86(1):9–13.

Chia Y T et al. Induction of labour: does internal tocography result in better obstetric outcome than external tocography? *Aust NZ J Obstet Gynaecol* 1993;33(2):159–61.

Davidson K M. Detection of premature rupture of the membranes. *Clin Obstet Gynecol* 1991;34(4):715–21.

de Haan H H et al. Value of the fern test to confirm or reject the diagnosis of ruptured membranes is modest in nonlaboring women presenting with nonspecific vaginal fluid loss. *Am J Perinatol* 1994;11(1):46–50.

Egarter C et al. Is induction of labor indicated in prolonged pregnancy? Results of a prospective randomised trial. *Gynecol Obstet Invest* 1989;27(1):6–9.

Egarter C H, Husslein P W, and Rayburn W F. Uterine hyperstimulation after low-dose prostaglandin E2 therapy: tocolytic treatment in 181 cases. *Am J Obstet Gynecol* 1990;163(3):794–96.

Garite T J and Gocke S E. Diagnosis of preterm rupture of membranes: is testing for alpha-fetoprotein better than ferning or nitrazine? *Am J Perinatol* 1990;7(3):276–78.

Gregor C L, Paine L L, and Johnson T R. Antepartum fetal assessment. A nurse-midwifery perspective. *J Nurse Midwifery* 1991;36(3):153–67.

Hannah M E et al. Maternal colonization with group B Streptococcus and prelabor rupture of membranes at term: the role of induction of labor. *Am J Obstet Gynecol* 1997;177(4):780–85.

Bibliography

Hannah M E et al. Postterm pregnancy: putting the merits of a policy of induction of labor into perspective. *Birth* 1996;23(1):13–19.

Hannah M E et al. Induction of labor compared with expectant management for prelabor rupture of the membranes at term. *N Engl J Med* 1996; 334(16):1005–10.

Hannah M E. Prelabor rupture of membranes (PROM) at term: effects of induction of labor. Presented at Innovations in Perinatal Care: Assessing Benefits and Risks, twelfth conference sponsored by the journal *Birth* and the Boston University School of Public Health, Waltham, MA, June 5–7, 1998.

Hauth J C et al. Uterine contraction pressures with oxytocin induction/augmentation. *Obstet Gynecol* 1986;68(3):305–9.

Hjertberg R et al. Premature rupture of the membranes (PROM) at term in nulliparous women with a ripe cervix. *Acta Obstet Gynecol Scand* 1996; 75:48–53.

Hofmeyr G J. Misoprostol administered vaginally for cervical ripening and labour induction with a viable fetus. In: Neilson J P et al., eds. *Pregnancy and Childbirth Module for the Cochrane Database of Systematic Reviews,* updated December 1997.

Kierse M J N C. Amniotomy or oxytocin for induction of labor. *Acta Obstet Gynecol Scand* 1988;66:731–35.

Kilpatrick S J and Safford K L. Maternal hydration increases amniotic fluid index in women with normal amniotic fluid. *Obstet Gynecol* 1993;81:49–52.

Kolderup L B, Laros R K, and Musci T J. Incidence of persistent birth injury in macrosomic infants: association with mode of delivery. *Am J Obstet Gynecol* 1997;177(1):37–41.

Krammer J et al. Pre-induction cervical ripening: a randomized comparison of two methods. *Obstet Gynecol* 1995;85(4):614–18.

Malik N et al. Clinical amnionitis and endometritis in patients with premature rupture of membranes: endocervical prostaglandin E2 gel versus oxytocin for induction of labor. *Obstet Gynecol* 1996;88(4):540–43.

Mercer B M et al. Early versus late amniotomy for labor induction: a randomized trial. *Am J Obstet Gynecol* 1995;173(4):1321–25.

Mittendorf R et al. The length of uncomplicated human gestation. *Obstet Gynecol* 1990;75(6):929–32.

Moldin P G and Sundell G. Induction of labour: a randomised clinical trial of amniotomy versus amniotomy with oxytocin infusion. *Br J Obstet Gynaecol* 1996;103(4):306–12.

Morel M I et al. Oxytocin augmentation in arrest disorders in the presence of thick meconium: influence on neonatal outcome. *Gynecol Obstet Invest* 1994;37(1):21–24.

Nathanielsz P W. A time to be born: implications of animal studies in maternal-fetal medicine. *Birth* 1994;21(3):163–69.

Otto C and Platt L D. Fetal growth and development. *Obstet Gynecol Clin North Amer* 1991;18(4):907–31.

Peralta-Carcelen M et al. Impact of maternal group B Streptococcal screening on pediatric management in full-term newborns. *Arch Pediatr Adolesc Med* 1996;150:802–8.

Rooks J P. *Midwifery and Childbirth in America.* Philadelphia: Temple University Press, 1997.

Russell K P and Anderson G V. The aggressive management of ruptured membranes. *Am J Obstet Gynecol* 1962;83(7):930–37.

Sandmire H F and DeMott R K. The Green Bay cesarean section study. IV. The physician factor as a determinant of cesarean birth rates for the large fetus. *Am J Obstet Gynecol* 1996;174(5):1557–64.

Sandmire H F and Woolley R J. Macrosomia: can we prevent big problems with big babies? *Birth* 1998;25(4):263–7.

Soper D E, Mayhall C G, and Froggatt J W. Characterization and control of intraamniotic infection in an urban teaching hospital. *Am J Obstet Gynecol* 1997;175(2):304–10.

Stoll B J et al. Changes in pathogens causing early-onset sepsis in very-low-birth-weight infants. *N Engl J Med* 2002;347(4):240–7.

Summers L. Methods of cervical ripening and labor induction. *J Nurse Midwifery* 1997;42(2):71–85.

Chapter 4

ASA. "Anesthesia & You . . . Planning Your Childbirth." 1992.

Carvalho J C and Mathias R S. Intravenous hydration in obstetrics. *Int Anesthesiol Clin* 1994;32(2):103–15.

Dumoulin J G and Foulkes J E B. Ketonuria during labour. *Br J Obstet Gynaecol* 1984;91:97–98.

Enkin M et al. *A Guide to Effective Care in Pregnancy and Childbirth,* 2d ed. Oxford: Oxford University Press, 1995.

Foulkes J and Dumoulin J G. The effects of ketonuria in labour. *Br J Clin Pract* 1985;39:59–62.

Gonik B and Cotton D B. Peripartum colloid osmotic pressure changes: influence of intravenous hydration. *Am J Obstet Gynecol* 1984;150(1):99–100.

Greulich B et al. Twelve years and more than 30,000 nurse-midwife-attended births: the Los Angeles County + University of Southern California Women's Hospital Birth Center experience. *J Nurse Midwifery* 1994; 39(4):185–96.

Haire D. Personal communication, Feb 18, 1993.

Haire D B and Elsberry C C. Maternity care and outcomes in a high-risk service: the North Central Bronx Hospital experience. *Birth* 1991;18(1): 33–37.

Hawkins J L et al. Anesthesia-related deaths during obstetric delivery in the United States, 1979–1990. *Anesthesiology* 1997;86(2):277–84.

Hazle N R. Hydration in labor: is routine intravenous hydration necessary? *J Nurse Midwifery* 1986;31(4):171–76.

Lind T. Fluid balance during labour: a review. *J Royal Soc Med* 1983;76: 870–75.

Ludka L M and Roberts C C. Eating and drinking in labor. A literature review. *J Nurse Midwifery* 1993;38(4):199–207.

McKay S and Mahan C. Modifying the stomach contents of laboring women: why and how; success and risks. *Birth* 1988;15(4):213–21.

Michael S, Reilly C S, and Caunt J A. Policies for oral intake during labour.

A survey of maternity units in England and Wales. *Anaesthesia* 1991; 46(12):1071–73.

Morton K E, Jackson M C, and Gillmer M D G. A comparison of the effects of four intravenous solutions for the treatment of ketonuria during labor. *Br J Obstet Gynaecol* 1985;92:473–79.

O'Reilly S A, Hoyer P J, and Walsh E. Low-risk mothers. Oral intake and emesis in labor. *J Nurse Midwifery* 1992;38(4):228–35.

O'Sullivan G. The stomach—fact and fantasy: eating and drinking during labor. *Int Anesthesiol Clin* 32(2):31–44.

Singhi S C and Choo Kang E. Maternal fluid overload during labour; transplacental hyponatraemia and risk of transient neonatal tachypnoea in term infants. *Arch Dis Child* 1984;59:1155–58.

Rooks J P, Weatherby N L, and Ernst E K. The National Birth Center Study. Part II—Intrapartum and immediate postpartum and neonatal care. *J Nurse Midwifery* 1992;37(5):301–30.

Wallace D H and Sidawi J E. Complications of obstetrical anesthesia. Suppl 3, Jun–Jul 1997. *William's Obstetrics*, 20th ed. Cunningham F G et al., eds. Stamford, CT: Appleton and Lange, 1997.

Wasserstrum N. Issues in fluid management during labor: general considerations. *Clin Obstet Gynecol* 1992;35(3):505–13.

Chapter 5

American Academy of Pediatrics and American College of Obstetricians and Gynecologists. Use and abuse of the Apgar score. *Pediatrics* 1996;98(1): 141–42.

ACOG. Fetal heart-rate patterns: monitoring interpretation, and management. Technical Bulletin No. 207, July 1995.

Allman A C and Steer P J. Monitoring uterine activity. *Br J Hosp Med* 1993; 49(9):649–53.

Cusick W, Smulian J C, and Vintzileos A M. Intrapartum use of fetal heart rate monitoring, contraction monitoring, and amnioinfusion. *Clin Perinatol* 1995;22(4):875–906.

Editorial. Cerebral palsy, intrapartum care, and a shot in the foot. *Lancet* 1989;2(8674):1251–52.

Enkin M et al. *A Guide to Effective Care in Pregnancy and Childbirth*, 2d ed. Oxford: Oxford University Press, 1995.

Gilfix M G. Electronic fetal monitoring: physician liability and informed consent. *Am J Law Medicine* 1984;10(1):31–90.

Grimes D. Technology follies: the uncritical acceptance of medical innovation. *JAMA* 1993;269(23):3030–322.

Hall D M B. Birth asphyxia and cerebral palsy. *BMJ* 1989;299:279–82.

Jordan B. "Authoritative Knowledge and Its Construction." In *Childbirth and Authoritative Knowledge*, Davis-Floyd R and Sargent C F, eds. Berkeley: University of California Press, 1997.

MacDonald D. Cerebral palsy and intrapartum fetal monitoring. *N Engl J Med* 1996;334(10):659–60.

Mahomed K et al. Randomised controlled trial of intrapartum fetal heart rate monitoring. *BMJ* 1994;308(6927):497–500.

Miller D A and Paul R H. Cesarean section for fetal distress. In *Cesarean Section: Guidelines for Appropriate Utilization.* Flamm B L and Quilligan E J, eds. New York: Springer-Verlag, 1995.

Murphy K W et al. Birth asphyxia and the intrapartum cardiotocograph. *Br J Obstet Gynaecol* 1990;97:470–79.

Nelson K. "Cerebral palsy: reducing the risks." Presented at Innovations in Perinatal Care: Assessing Benefits and Risks, twelfth conference sponsored by the journal *Birth* and the Boston University School of Public Health, Waltham, MA, June 5–7, 1998.

Paneth N and Stark R I. Cerebral palsy and mental retardation in relation to indicators of perinatal asphyxia. *Am J Obstet Gynecol* 1983;147(8):960–66.

Sandmire H F. Whither electronic fetal monitoring? *Obstet Gynecol* 1990; 76(6):1130–34.

Satin A J et al. High- versus low-dose oxytocin for labor stimulation. *Obstet Gynecol* 1992;80(1):111–16.

Schifrin B S. Medicolegal ramifications of electronic fetal monitoring during labor. *Clin Perinatol* 1995;22(4):837–54.

Shyken J M and Petrie R H. The use of oxytocin. *Clin Perinatol* 1995;22(4): 907–31.

SOGC. Fetal health surveillance in labour. Policy Statement No. 41, October 1995.

Ventura S J et al. Report of final natality statistics, 1995. *Monthly Vital Stat Rep* 1997;45(11 Suppl):1–80.

Vintzileos A M et al. A randomized trial of intrapartum electronic fetal heart rate monitoring versus intermittent auscultation. *Obstet Gynecol* 1993; 81(6):899–907.

Chapter 6

Brisson-Carroll G et al. The effect of routine early amniotomy on spontaneous labor: a meta-analysis. *Obstet Gynecol* 1996;87(5 Pt 2):891–96.

Caldeyro-Barcia R et al. Adverse perinatal effects of early amniotomy during labor. In *Modern Perinatal Medicine.* Gluck L, ed. Chicago: Yearbook Medical Publishers, 1974.

El Halta V. Posterior labor—A pain in the back! *ICAN Clarion* 1996;2(1): 6,7–12,13.

Fraser W D et al. Amniotomy to shorten spontaneous labour. In: Neilson J P et al., eds. *Pregnancy and Childbirth Module of the Cochrane Database of Systematic Reviews,* updated November 1995.

Fraser W D et al. Effect of early amniotomy on the risk of dystocia in nulliparous women. *N Engl J Med* 1993;22;328(16):1145–49.

Roberts W E et al. Are obstetric interventions such as cervical ripening, induction of labor, amnioinfusion, or amniotomy associated with umbilical cord prolapse? *Am J Obstet Gynecol* 1997;176(6):1181–85.

Bibliography

Stewart P, Kennedy J H, and Calder A A. Spontaneous labour: when should the membranes be ruptured? *Br J Obstet Gynaecol* 1982;89:39–43.

UK Amniotomy Group. A multicentre randomised trial of amniotomy in spontaneous first labour at term. *Br J Obstet Gynaecol* 1994;101(4):307–9.

Chapter 7

ACOG. *Dystocia and the augmentation of labor.* Technical Bulletin No. 218, 1995.

Albers L L, Schiff M, and Gorwoda J G. The length of active labor in normal pregnancies. *Obstet Gynecol* 1996;87(3):355–59.

Boyd M E, Usher R H, and McLean F H. Fetal macrosomia: prediction, risks, proposed management. *Obstet Gynecol* 1983;61(6):715–22.

Boylan P C. Active management of labor: results in Dublin, Houston, London, New Brunswick, Singapore, and Valparaiso. *Birth* 1989;16(3):114–18.

Cahill D J, Boylan P C, and O'Herlihy C. Does oxytocin increase perinatal risk in primigravid labor? *Am J Obstet Gynecol* 1992;166(3):847–50.

Consensus Conference Report. Indications for cesarean section: final statement of the panel of the National Consensus Conference on Aspects of Cesarean Birth. *Can Med Assoc J* 1986;134:1348–52.

Cavlovich F E. Subgaleal hemorrhage in the neonate. *J Obstet Gynecol Neonatal Nurs* 1995;24(5):397–404.

Drife J O. Choice and instrumental delivery. *Br J Obstet Gynaecol* 1996; 103(7):608–11.

FDA. FDA public health advisory: need for CAUTION when using vacuum assisted delivery devices. *http://www.fda.gov/edrh/fetal/598.html*, May 21, 1998.

Granstrom L, Ekman G, and Malmstrom A. Insufficient remodelling of the uterine connective tissue in women with protracted labour. *Br J Obstet Gynaecol* 1991;98:1212–16.

Hankins G D V and Rowe T F. Operative vaginal delivery—year 2000. *Am J Obstet Gynecol* 1996;175(2):275–82.

Hemminki E et al. Ambulation versus oxytocin in protracted labour: a pilot study. *Eur J Obstet Gynecol Reprod Biol* 1985;20:199–208.

Keller J D et al. Shoulder dystocia and birth trauma in gestational diabetes: a five-year experience. *Am J Obstet Gynecol* 1991;165(4 Pt 1):928–30.

Klaus M H. Intermittent versus continuous support of women in labor. Presented at Innovations in Perinatal Care: Assessing Benefits and Risks, twelfth conference sponsored by the journal *Birth* and the Boston University School of Public Health, Waltham, MA, June 5–7, 1998.

Kitzinger S. The desexing of birth; some effects of professionalization of care; the god-sibs; what matters to women—their words. Presented at Innovations in Perinatal Care: Assessing Benefits and Risks, ninth conference presented by *Birth*, San Francisco, November 1990.

Lucas M J. The role of vacuum extraction in modern obstetrics. *Clin Obstet Gynecol* 1994;37(4):794–805.

Bibliography

Lumley J. Events and experiences in childbirth: is there an association with postpartum depression? Presented at the tenth *Birth* conference, Boston, Oct. 31–Nov. 1, 1992.

Macara L M and Murphy K W. The contribution of dystocia to the cesarean section rate. *Am J Obstet Gynecol* 1994;171(1):71–77.

McDonald D et al. The Dublin randomized controlled trial of intrapartum fetal heart rate monitoring. *Am J Obstet Gynecol* 1985;152(5):524–39.

Menticoglou S M, Perlman M, and Manning F A. High cervical spinal cord injury in neonatres delivered with forceps: a report of 15 cases. *Obstet Gynecol* 1995;86(4 Pt 1):589–94.

Meyer L et al. Maternal and neonatal morbidity in instrumental deliveries with the Kobayashi vacuum extractor and low forceps. *Acta Obstet Gynecol Scand* 1987;66:643–47.

O'Driscoll K and Meagher D. *Active Management of Labour.* 2d ed. London: Bailliere Tindall, 1986.

Olah K. The active management of labour. *Br J Obstet Gynaecol* 1996; 103: 729–31

Rouse D J, Owen J, and Hauth J C. Active-phase labor arrest: oxytocin augmentation for at least 4 hours. *Obstet Gynecol* 1999;93(3):323–28.

Shyken J M and Petrie R H. The use of oxytocin. *Clin Perinatol* 1995;22(4): 907–31.

Siegel P. Does bath water enter the vagina? *Obstet Gynecol* 1960;15:660–61.

Simkin P. Stress, pain and catecholamines in labor: part 2. Stress associated with childbirth events: a pilot survey of new mothers. *Birth* 1986;13(4): 234–40.

Thornton J G and Lilford R J. Active management of labour: current knowledge and research. *BMJ* 1994;309(6951):366–69.

Ventura S J et al. Report of final natality statistics, 1995. *Month Vital Stat Rep* 1997;45(11, Suppl):1–80.

Wainer-Cohen N. Personal communication, Jun 7, 1998.

Williams M C. Vacuum-assisted delivery. *Clin Perinatol* 1995;22(4):933–52.

Chapter 8

ASA. "Anesthesia & You . . . Planning Your Childbirth." 1992.

ASA. "Mom's Pain Relief During Delivery Helps Dad, Too." Oct. 24, 1995.

Atkinson B D et al. Double-blind comparison of intravenous butorphanol (Stadol) and fentanyl (Sublimaze) for analgesia during labor. *Am J Obstet Gynecol* 1994;171:993–98.

Bates R G et al. Uterine activity in the second stage of labour and the effect of epidural analgesia. *Br J Obstet Gynaecol* 1985;92(12):1246–50.

Boschert S. Anesthesiologists defend epidural safety. *Ob Gyn News* Jul 15, 1998; p. 20.

Chazotte C, Maden R, and Cohen W R. Labor patterns in women with previous cesareans. *Obstet Gynecol* 1990;75(3 Pt 1):350–55.

Cheek T G and Gutsche B B. Epidural analgesia for labor and vaginal delivery. *Clin Obstet Gynecol* 1987;30(3):515–29.

Chestnut D H et al. Does early administration of epidural analgesia affect obstetric outcome in nulliparous women who are in spontaneous labor? *Anesthesiology* 1994;80(6):1201–8.

Cohn V. *News and Numbers*. Ames: Iowa State University Press, 1989.

Corke B C and Spielman F J. Problems associated with epidural anesthesia in obstetrics. *Obstet Gynecol* 1985;65(6):837–39.

Crawford J S. Some maternal complications of epidural analgesia for labour. *Anaesthesia* 1985;40(12):1219–25.

Eddleston J M et al. Comparison of the maternal and fetal effects associated with intermittent or continuous infusion of extradural analgesia. *Br J Anaesth* 1992;69:154–58.

Enkin M et al. *A Guide to Effective Care in Pregnancy and Childbirth*. Oxford: Oxford University Press, 1995.

Fuchs A R and Fuchs F. Endocrinology of human parturition: a review. *Br J Obstet Gynaecol* 1984;91:948–67.

Goodfellow C F et al. Oxytocin deficiency at delivery with epidural analgesia. *Br J Obstet Gynaecol* 1983;90(3):214–19.

Hanson B. Pain in labor doesn't have to be intolerable. *http:// members.aol.com/mthrluvok/labortim.html*, 1996.

Harlass F E and Duff P. The duration of labor in primiparas undergoing vaginal birth after cesarean delivery. *Obstet Gynecol* 1990;75(1):45–47.

Hodnett E D. Support from caregivers during childbirth. In: Neilson J P, et al., eds. *Pregnancy and Childbirth Module of the Cochrane Database of Systematic Reviews*, updated November 1997.

Howell C J and Chalmers I. A review of prospectively controlled comparisons of epidural with non-epidural forms of pain relief during labor. *Int J Obstet Anesth* 1992;1:93–110.

Humenick S S and Bugen L A. Mastery: The key to childbirth satisfaction? A study. *Birth* 1981;8(2):84–89.

Humenick S S. Mastery: The key to childbirth satisfaction? A review. *Birth* 1981;8(2):79–83.

Jimenez S. Supportive pain management strategies. In *Childbirth Education: Practice, Research, and Theory*. F H Nichols and S S Humenick, eds. Philadelphia: Saunders, 1988.

Johnson M and Everitt B. *Essential Reproduction*. 3d ed. Cambridge, MA: Blackwell Scientific Publications, 1988.

Katz Rothman B. The social construction of birth. In *The American Way of Birth*. Eakins P, ed. Philadelphia: Temple University Press, 1986.

Klaus M H. Intermittent versus continuous support of women in labor. Presented at Innovations in Perinatal Care: Assessing Benefits and Risks, twelfth conference sponsored by the journal *Birth* and the Boston University School of Public Health, Waltham, MA, June 5–7, 1998.

Lagercrantz H and Slotkin T. The "stress" of being born. *Sci Amer* 1986; 254(4):100–107.

Leighton B L et al. Limitations of epinephrine as a marker of intravascular injection in laboring women. *Anesthesiology* 1987;66:688–91.

Maresh M, Choong K H, and Beard R W. Delayed pushing with lumbar epidural analgesia in labour. *Br J Obstet Gynaecol* 1983;90:623–27.

Morton S C et al. Effect of epidural analgesia for labor on the cesarean delivery rate. *Obstet Gynecol* 1994;83(6):1045–52.

Prince G and McGregor D. Obstetric test doses. *Anaesthesia* 1986;41:1240–49.

Ramin S M et al. Randomized trial of epidural versus intravenous analgesia during labor. *Obstet Gynecol* 1995;86(5):783–89.

Richards M P. Effects of analgesics and anaesthetics given in childbirth on child development. *Neuropharmacology* 1981;20(12B):1259–65.

Rolbin S H et al. Fluid through the epidural needle does not reduce complications of epidural catheter insertion. *Can J Anaesth* 1990;37(3):337–40.

Rolbin S H and Hew E. A comparison of two types of epidural catheters. *Can J Anaesth* 1987;35(5):459–61.

Saberski L R, Kondamuri S, Osinubi O Y. Identification of the epidural space: is loss of resistance to air a safe technique? A review of the complications related to the use of air. *Reg Anesth* 1997;22(1):3–15.

Simkin P. Just another day in a woman's life? Women's long-term perceptions of their first birth experience. Part I. *Birth* 1991;18(4):203–10.

Vause S, Congdon H M, and Thorton J G. Immediate and delayed pushing in the second stage of labour for nulliparous women with epidural analgesia: a randomised controlled trial. *Br J Obstet Gynaecol* 1998;105:186–8.

Wallace D H and Sidawi J E. Complications of obstetrical anesthesia. Suppl 3, Jun–Jul 1997. *William's Obstetrics*, 20th ed. Cunningham F G et al., eds. Stamford, CT: Appleton and Lange, 1997.

Withington D E and Weeks S K. Repeat epidural analgesia and unilateral block. *Can J Anaesth* 1994;41(7):568–71.

Wuitchik M, Bakal D, and Lipshitz J. Relationships between pain, cognitive activity and epidural analgesia during labor. *Pain* 1990;41:125–32.

Chapter 9

ACOG. *Dystocia and the Augmentation of Labor.* Technical Bulletin No. 218, 1995.

Albers L L et al. Factors related to perineal trauma in childbirth. *J Nurse Midwifery* 1996;41(4):269–76.

Avery M D and Van Arsdale L. Perineal massage: effect on the incidence of episiotomy and laceration in a nulliparous population. *J Nurse Midwifery* 1987;32(3):181–84.

Bromberg M H. Presumptive maternal benefits of routine episiotomy. *J Nurse Midwifery* 1986;31(3):121–27.

Carroli G, Belizan J, and Stamp G. Episiotomy policies in vaginal births. In: Neilson J P et al., eds. *Pregnancy and Childbirth Module of the Cochrane Database of Systematic Reviews.* Updated February 1997.

Combs C A, Robertson P A, and Laros R K. Risk factors for third-degree and fourth-degree perineal lacerations in forceps and vacuum deliveries. *Am J Obstet Gynecol* 1990;163(1 Pt 1):100–104.

Consensus Conference Report. Indications for cesarean section: final statement of the panel of the National Consensus Conference on Aspects of Cesarean Birth. *Can Med Assoc J* 1986;134:1348–52.

Cunningham F G et al., eds. *William's Obstetrics*. 20th ed. Stamford, CT: Appleton and Lange, 1997.

Davis-Floyd R E. *Birth As an American Rite of Passage*. Berkeley: University of California Press, 1992.

Flynn P et al. How can second-stage management prevent perineal trauma? *Can Fam Physician* 1997;43:73–84.

Handa V L, Harris T A, and Ostergard D R. Protecting the pelvic floor: obstetric management to prevent incontinence and pelvic organ prolapse. *Obstet Gynecol* 1996;88(3):470–78.

Helwig J T, Thorp J M, and Bowes W A. Does midline episiotomy increase the risk of third- and fourth-degree lacerations in operative vaginal deliveries? *Obstet Gynecol* 1993;82(2):276–79.

Hofmeyr G J and Sonnedecker E W. Elective episiotomy in perspective. *S Afr Med J* 1987;71(6):357–59.

Klein M C et al. Physicians' beliefs and behaviour during a randomized controlled trial of episiotomy: consequences for women in their care. *Can Med Assoc J* 1995;153(6):769–79.

Klein M C et al. Relationship of episiotomy to perineal trauma and morbidity, sexual dysfunction, and pelvic floor relaxation. *Am J Obstet Gynecol* 1994;171(3):591–98.

Lede R L, Belizan J M, and Carroli G. Is routine use of episiotomy justified? *Am J Obstet Gynecol* 1996;174(5):1399–1402.

Legino L J et al. Third- and fourth-degree perineal tears. 50 years' experience at a university hospital. *J Reprod Med* 1988;33(5):423–26.

Lydon-Rochelle M T, Albers L, and Teaf D. Perineal outcomes and nurse-midwifery management. *J Nurse Midwifery* 1995;40(1):13–18.

McCandlish R et al. A randomised controlled trial of care of the perineum during second stage of normal labour. *Br J Obstet Gynaecol* 1998; 105(12):1262–72.

Nodine P M and Roberts J. Factors associated with perineal outcome during childbirth. *J Nurse Midwifery* 1987 May–June;32(3):123–30.

Piper D M and McDonald P. Management of anticipated and actual shoulder dystocia. Interpreting the literature. *J Nurse Midwifery* 1994;39(2 Suppl): 91S–105S.

Roberts J and Woolley D. A second look at the second stage of labor. *JOGNN* 1996;25(5):415–23.

Shiono P, Klebanoff M A, and Carey J C. Midline episiotomies: more harm than good? *Obstet Gynecol* 1990;75(5):765–70.

Shipman M K et al. Antenatal perineal massage and subsequent perineal outcomes: a randomised controlled trial. *Br J Obstet Gynaecol* 1997;104: 787–91.

Sultan A H et al. Anal-sphincter disruption during vaginal delivery. *New Engl J Med* 1993;329(26):1905–11.

Thacker S B and Banta H D. Benefits and risks of episiotomy: an interpretive review of the English language literature, 1860–1980. *Obstet Gynecol Surv* 1983;38(6):322–38.

Thompson D J. No episiotomy?! *Aust NZ J Obstet Gynaecol* 1987;27(1): 18–20.

Thorp J M and Bowes W A. Episiotomy: Can its routine use be defended? *Am J Obstet Gynecol* 1989;160(5 Pt 1):1027–30.

Vital and Health Statistics. National Health Survey: Annual Summary DHHS Publications No. (PHS) 95-1782, Series 13 No. 121.

Wood E. Personal communication, 1998.

Woolley R J. Benefits and risks of episiotomy: a review of the English-language literature since 1980. Part I. *Obstet Gynecol Surv* 1995;50(11): 806–20.

Woolley R J. Benefits and risks of episiotomy: a review of the English-language literature since 1980. Part II. *Obstet Gynecol Surv* 1995;50(11): 821–35.

Chapter 10

ACOG. Vaginal birth after cesarean section. Report of a 1990 survey of ACOG's membership. 1990.

ACOG. Vaginal delivery after previous cesarean birth. *Practice Patterns* 1995; No. 1.

ACOG. Vaginal birth after previous cesarean delivery. *Practice Bulletin* 1998, No 2.

Chazotte C, Maden R, and Cohen W R. Labor patterns in women with previous cesareans. *Obstet Gynecol* 1990;75(3 Pt 1):350–55.

Chua S and Arulkumaran S. Trial of scar. *Aust NZ J Obstet Gynaecol* 1997; 37(1):6–11.

Enkin M et al. *A Guide to Effective Care in Pregnancy and Childbirth*, 2d ed. Oxford: Oxford University Press, 1995.

Farmer R M et al. Uterine rupture during trial of labor after previous cesarean section. *Am J Obstet Gynecol* 1991;165(4 Pt 1):996–1001.

Flamm B L and Goings J R. Vaginal birth after cesarean section: is suspected fetal macrosomia a contraindication? *Obstet Gynecol* 1989;74(5):694–97.

Flamm B L. Once a cesarean, always a controversy. *Obstet Gynecol* 1997; 90(2):312–15.

Flamm B L. Vaginal birth after cesarean section. In *Cesarean Section: Guidelines for Appropriate Utilization*. Flamm B L and Quilligan E J, eds. New York: Springer-Verlag, 1995.

Flamm B, MacDonald D, Shearer E, and Mahan C S. Roundtable discussion: should the electronic fetal monitor always be used for women in labor who are having a vaginal birth after a previous cesarean section? *Birth* 1992;19(1):31–35.

Harlass F E and Duff P. The duration of labor in primiparas undergoing vaginal birth after cesarean delivery. *Obstet Gynecol* 1990;75(1):45–47.

Jackson R, Reid J A, and Thorburn. Volume preloading is not essential to prevent spinal-induced hypotension at caesarean section. *Br J Anaesth* 1995;75(3):262–65.

Johnson S R et al. Obstetric decision-making: responses to patients who request cesarean delivery. *Obstet Gynecol* 1986;67(6):847–50.

Joseph G F, Stedman C M, and Robichaux A G. Vaginal birth after cesarean section: the impact of patient resistance to a trial of labor. *Am J Obstet Gynecol* 1991;164(6 Pt 1):1441–47.

Kirk E P et al. Vaginal birth after cesarean or repeat cesarean section: medical risks or social realities? *Am J Obstet Gynecol* 1990;162(6):1398–1405.

Kline J and Arias F. Analysis of factors determining the selection of repeated cesarean section or trial of labor in patients with histories of prior cesarean delivery. *J Reprod Med* 1993;38(4):289–392.

Lomas J et al. Opinion leaders vs audit and feedback to implement practice guidelines. *JAMA* 1991;265(17):2202–7.

Martins M. Vaginal birth after cesarean delivery. *Clin Perinatol* 1996;23(1):141–53.

Macara L M and Murphy K W. The contribution of dystocia to the cesarean section rate. *Am J Obstet Gynecol* 1994;171(1):71–77.

McClain C S. Patient decision making: the case of delivery method after a previous cesarean section. *Cult Med Psychiatry* 1987;11(4):495–508.

Norman P, Kostovcik S, and Lanning A. Elective repeat cesarean sections: how many could be vaginal births? *Can Med Assoc J* 1993;149(4):431–35.

Penso C. Vaginal birth after cesarean section: an update on physician trends and patient perceptions. *Curr Opin Obstet Gynecol* 1994;6(5):417–25.

Phelan J P et al. Previous cesarean birth. Trial of labor in women with macrosomic infants. *J Reprod Med* 1984;29(1):36–40.

Phelan J P. Rendering unto Caesar cesarean decisions. *OBG Management* 1996 Nov:6.

Rocke D A and Rout C C. Volume preloading, spinal hypotension and caesarean section. *Br J Anaesth* 1995;75(3):257–59.

Sachs B P et al. The risks of lowering the cesarean delivery rate. *N Engl J Med* 1999;340(1):54–7.

Shapiro M C et al. Information control and the exercise of power in the obstetrical encounter. *Soc Sci Med* 1983;17(3):139–46.

Ventura S J et al. Report of final natality statistics, 1995. *Monthly Vital Stat Rep* 1997;45(11 Suppl):1–80.

Videla F L et al. Trial of labor: a disciplined approach to labor management resulting in a high rate of vaginal delivery. *Am J Perinatol* 1995;12(3):181–84.

Weinstein D et al. Vaginal birth after cesarean section: current opinion. *Int J Gynaecol Obstet* 1996;53(1):1–10.

DATA SOURCES FOR THE ODDS OF VBAC

These studies are in addition to studies listed under "VBAC Reports" on page 290–291.

Chazotte C and Cohen W R. Catastrophic complications of previous cesarean section. *Am J Obstet Gynecol* 1990;163(3):738–42.

Chua S et al. Trial of labour after previous cesarean section: obstetric outcome. *Aust NZ J Obstet Gynaecol* 1989;29(1):12–17.

Finley B E and Gibbs C E. Emergent cesarean delivery in patients undergoing a trial of labor with a transverse lower-segment scar. *Am J Obstet Gynecol* 1986;155(5):936–39.

Peterson C M and Saunders N J. Mode of delivery after one cesarean section: audit of current practice in a health region. *BMJ* 1991;303(6806):818–21.

Pickhardt M G et al. Vaginal birth after cesarean delivery: are there useful and valid predictors of success of failure? *Am J Obstet Gynecol* 1992:166(6 Pt 1):1881–19.

Pruett K M, Kirshon B, and Cotton D B. Unknown uterine scar and trial of labor. *Am J Obstet Gynecol* 1988;159(4):807–10.

Chapter 11

Bertsch T D et al. Labor support by first-time fathers: direct observations with a comparison to experienced doulas. *J Psychosom Obstet Gynaecol*, 1990;11:251–60.

Chapman L. Searching: expectant father's experiences during labor and birth. *J Perinat Neonat Nurs* 1991;4(4):21–29.

Hodnett E D and Osborne R W. A randomized trial of the effects of monitrice support during labor: mother's views two to four weeks postpartum. *Birth* 1989;16(4):177–83.

Hodnett E D and Osborne R W. Effects of continuous intrapartum professional support on childbirth outcomes. *Res Nurs Health* 1989;12:289–97.

Hodnett E D et al. A strategy to promote research-based nursing care: effects on childbirth outcomes. *Res Nurs Health* 1996;19:13–20.

Hodnett E D. Caregiver support for women during childbirth (Cochrane Review). In: *The Cochrane Library*, Issue 1, 1999. Oxford: Update Software.

Klaus M et al. Maternal assistance and support in labor: father, nurse, midwife, or doula? *Clin Consult Obstet Gynecol* 1992;4(4):211–17.

Klaus M H. Intermittent versus continuous support of women in labor. Presented at Innovations in Perinatal Care: Assessing Benefits and Risks, twelfth conference sponsored by the journal *Birth* and the Boston University School of Public Health, Waltham, MA, June 5–7, 1998.

Klaus M, Kennell J, Klaus P. *Mothering the Mother: How a Doula Can Help You Have a Shorter, Easier, and Healthier Birth*. New York: Addison-Wesley, 1993.

Klaus M H and Kennell J H. The doula: an essential ingredient of childbirth rediscovered. *Acta Paediatr* 1997;86:1034–36.

Perez P and Snedeker C. *Special Women*. Seattle: Pennypress, Inc., 1990.

Simkin P. Just another day in a woman's life? Women's long-term perceptions of their first birth experience. Part I. *Birth* 1991;18(4):203–310.

Chapter 12

ACNM. Personal communication, Dec 16, 1998.

ACOG. "Joint Statement of Practice Relationships between Obstetrician/Gynecologists and Certified Nurse-Midwives." Nov 1, 1982. (Unchanged as of September 1997.)

ACOG. Ultrasonography in pregnancy. Technical Bulletin No. 187, 1993.

Administration orders safeguards for Medicare patients. *San Jose Mercury News*. June 23, 1998.

Creevy D. In *Obstetric Myths Versus Research Realities*, Goer H. Westport, CT: Bergin and Garvey, 1995.

Declercq E. Midwifery care and medical complications: the role of risk screening. *Birth* 1995(2):68–73.

Ewigman B G et al. Effect of prenatal ultrasound screening on perinatal outcome. *N Engl J Med* 1993;329(12):821–27.

Humenick S S and Bugen L A. Mastery: the key to childbirth satisfaction? A study. *Birth* 1981;8(2):84–89.

Humenick S S. Mastery: the key to childbirth satisfaction? A review. *Birth* 1981;8(2):79–83.

Leeman L. Letter. *Birth* 1995;22(4):236.

Lumley J. "Events and experiences in childbirth: is there an association with postpartum depression?" Presented at Innovations in Perinatal Care: Assessing Benefits and Risks, tenth conference presented by *Birth*, Boston, Oct. 31–Nov. 1 1992.

Rooks J P. *Midwifery and Childbirth in America*. Philadelphia: Temple University Press, 1997.

Scupholme A and Kamons A S. Are outcomes compromised when mothers are assigned to birth centers for care? *J Nurse Midwifery* 1987;32(4):211–15.

Simkin P. Just another day in a woman's life? Women's long-term perceptions of their first birth experience. Part 1. *Birth* 1991;18(4):203–10.

Tew M and Damstra-Wijmenga S M I. Safest birth attendants: recent Dutch evidence. *Midwifery* 1991;7:55–63.

Turnbull D et al. Randomised controlled trial of efficacy of midwife-managed care. *Lancet* 1996;348(9022):213–18.

Wolfe S M and Gabay M. *Delivering a Better Childbirth Experience*. Washington, D.C.: Public Citizen's Health Research Group, 1995.

Chapter 13

ACOG. *Alternative birth centers*. Dec. 3–4, 1982. (This policy still in force as of December 30, 1997.)

APHA. Guidelines for licensing and regulating birth centers. *Am J Public Health* 1983;73(3):331–34.

Arya R et al. Outcome in low risk pregnancies. *Arch Dis Child Fetal Neonatal Ed* 1996;75(2):F97–102.

Bennetts A B and Lubic R. The freestanding birth centre. *Lancet* 1982;1:378–80.

Declercq E R, Paine L L, Winter M R. Home birth in the United States, 1989–1992. A longitudinal descriptive report of national birth certificate data. *J Nurse Midwifery* 1995;40(6):474–82.

DeVries R G. Image and reality: an evaluation of hospital alternative birth centers. *J Nurse Midwifery* 1983;28(3):3–9.

Dye N S. The medicalization of birth. In *The American Way of Birth*. Eakins P, ed. Philadelphia: Temple University Press, 1986.

Eakins P S. Freestanding birth centers in California: program and medical outcome. *J Reprod Med* 1989;34(12):960–70.

Garite T J et al. Development and experience of a university-based freestanding birthing center. *Obstet Gynecol* 1995;86(3):411–16.

Goer H. More women choosing birth centers. *Childbirth Forum* Summer 1992:1,4–5.

Klein M et al. Care in a birth room versus a conventional setting: a controlled trial. *Can Med Assoc J* 1984;131:1461–66.

Levy B S, Wilkinson F S, and Marine W M. Reducing neonatal mortality rate with nurse-midwives. *Am J Obstet Gynecol* 1971;109(1):50–58.

Lowe N K. Maternal confidence in coping with labor: a self-efficacy concept. *JOGN* 1991;20(6):457–63.

NACC. Personal communication, Dec 15, 1998.

Odent M. The fetus ejection reflex. *Birth* 1987;14(2):45–46.

Pantin C G. A study of maternal mortality and midwifery on the Isle of Man, 1882 to 1961. *Med History* 1996;40:141–72.

Rooks J P. *Midwifery and Childbirth in America*. Philadelphia: Temple University Press, 1997.

Saldana L R et al. Home birth: negative implications derived from a hospital-based birthing suite. *South Med J* 1983;76(2):170–73.

Silver L and Wolfe S M. *Unnecessary Cesarean Sections: How to Cure a National Epidemic*. Washington D.C.: Public Citizen Health Research Group, 1989.

Simkin P. Stress, pain, and catecholamines in labor: Part 1. A review. *Birth* 1986;13(4):227–33.

Spitzer M C. Birth centers. Economy, safety, and empowerment. *J Nurse Midwifery* 1995;40(4):371–75.

Tew M. Do obstetric intranatal interventions make birth safer? *Br J Obstet Gynaecol* 1986;93(7):659–74.

Tew M. Place of birth and perinatal morality. *J R Coll Gen Pract* 1985; 35(277):390–94.

Wertz R W and Wertz D C. *Lying-in: A History of Childbirth in America*. New York: Schocken Books, 1977.

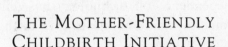

The Mother-Friendly Childbirth Initiative

*The First Consensus Initiative of the Coalition
for Improving Maternity Services*

MISSION

The Coalition for Improving Maternity Services (CIMS) is a coalition of individuals and national organizations with concern for the care and well-being of mothers, babies, and families. Our mission is to promote a wellness model of maternity care that will improve birth outcomes and substantially reduce costs. This evidence-based mother-, baby-, and family-friendly model focuses on prevention and wellness as the alternatives to high-cost screening, diagnosis, and treatment programs.

PREAMBLE

Whereas:

- In spite of spending far more money per capita on maternity and newborn care than any other country, the United States falls behind most industrialized countries in perinatal morbidity and mortality, and maternal mortality is four times greater for African-American women than for Euro-American women;

- Midwives attend the vast majority of births in those industrialized countries with the best perinatal outcomes, yet in the United States, midwives are the principal attendants at only a small percentage of births;

- Current maternity and newborn practices that contribute to high costs and inferior outcomes include the inappropriate application of technology and routine procedures that are not based on scientific evidence;
- Increased dependence on technology has diminished confidence in women's innate ability to give birth without intervention;
- The integrity of the mother-child relationship, which begins in pregnancy, is compromised by the obstetrical treatment of mother and baby as if they were separate units with conflicting needs;
- Although breastfeeding has been scientifically shown to provide optimum health, nutritional, and developmental benefits to newborns and their mothers, only a fraction of U.S. mothers are fully breastfeeding their babies by the age of six weeks;
- The current maternity care system in the United States does not provide equal access to health care resources for women from disadvantaged population groups, women without insurance, and women whose insurance dictates caregivers or place of birth;

Therefore,

We, the undersigned members of CIMS, hereby resolve to define and promote mother-friendly maternity services in accordance with the following principles:

PRINCIPLES
We believe the philosophical cornerstones of mother-friendly care to be as follows:

NORMALCY OF THE BIRTHING PROCESS
- Birth is a normal, natural, and healthy process.

- Women and babies have the inherent wisdom necessary for birth.
- Babies are aware, sensitive human beings at the time of birth, and should be acknowledged and treated as such.
- Breastfeeding provides the optimum nourishment for newborns and infants.
- Birth can safely take place in hospitals, birth centers, and homes.
- The midwifery model of care, which supports and protects the normal birth process, is the most appropriate for the majority of women during pregnancy and birth.

EMPOWERMENT

- A woman's confidence and ability to give birth and to care for her baby are enhanced or diminished by every person who gives her care, and by the environment in which she gives birth.
- A mother and baby are distinct yet interdependent during pregnancy, birth, and infancy. Their interconnectedness is vital and must be respected.
- Pregnancy, birth, and the postpartum period are milestone events in the continuum of life. These experiences profoundly affect women, babies, fathers, and families, and have important and long-lasting effects on society.

AUTONOMY

Every woman should have the opportunity to:
- Have a healthy and joyous birth experience for herself and her family, regardless of her age or circumstances;
- Give birth as she wishes in an environment in which she feels nurtured and secure, and her emotional well-being, privacy, and personal preferences are respected;
- Have access to the full range of options for pregnancy, birth, and nurturing her baby, and to accurate information on all available birthing sites, caregivers, and practices;

- Receive accurate and up-to-date information about the benefits and risks of all procedures, drugs, and tests suggested for use during pregnancy, birth, and the postpartum period, with the rights to informed consent and informed refusal;
- Receive support for making informed choices about what is best for her and her baby based on her individual values and beliefs.

DO NO HARM

- Interventions should not be applied routinely during pregnancy, birth, or the postpartum period. Many standard medical tests, procedures, technologies, and drugs carry risks to both mother and baby, and should be avoided in the absence of specific scientific indications for their use.
- If complications arise during pregnancy, birth, or the postpartum period, medical treatments should be evidence-based.

RESPONSIBILITY

- Each caregiver is responsible for the quality of care she or he provides.
- Maternity care practice should be based not on the needs of the caregiver or provider, but solely on the needs of the mother and child.
- Each hospital and birth center is responsible for the periodic review and evaluation, according to current scientific evidence, of the effectiveness, risks, and rates of use of its medical procedures for mothers and babies.
- Society, through both its government and the public health establishment, is responsible for ensuring access to maternity services for all women, and for monitoring the quality of those services.
- Individuals are ultimately responsible for making informed choices about the health care they and their babies receive.

These principles give rise to the following steps which support, protect, and promote mother-friendly maternity services:

TEN STEPS OF THE MOTHER-FRIENDLY CHILDBIRTH INITIATIVE
For Mother-Friendly Hospitals, Birth Centers, and Home Birth Services

To receive CIMS designation as "mother-friendly," a hospital, birth center, or home birth service must carry out the above philosophical principles by fulfilling the Ten Steps of Mother-Friendly Care:

A mother-friendly hospital, birth center, or home birth service:
1. Offers all birthing mothers:
    * Unrestricted access to the birth companions of her choice, including fathers, partners, children, family members, and friends;
    * Unrestricted access to continuous emotional and physical support from a skilled woman—for example, a doula, or labor-support professional;
    * Access to professional midwifery care.
2. Provides accurate descriptive and statistical information to the public about its practices and procedures for birth care, including measures of interventions and outcomes.
3. Provides culturally competent care—that is, care that is sensitive and responsive to the specific beliefs, values, and customs of the mother's ethnicity and religion.
4. Provides the birthing woman with the freedom to walk, move about, and assume the positions of her choice during labor and birth (unless restriction is specifically required to correct a complication), and discourages the use of the lithotomy (flat on back with legs elevated) position.
5. Has clearly defined policies and procedures for:

- collaborating and consulting throughout the perinatal period with other maternity services, including communicating with the original caregiver when transfer from one birth site to another is necessary;
- linking the mother and baby to appropriate community resources, including prenatal and post-discharge follow-up and breastfeeding support.

6. Does not routinely employ practices and procedures that are unsupported by scientific evidence, including but not limited to the following:
   - shaving;
   - enemas;
   - IVs (intravenous drip);
   - withholding nourishment;
   - early rupture of membranes;
   - electronic fetal monitoring;

other interventions are limited as follows:
   - Has an oxytocin use rate of 10% or less for induction and augmentation;*
   - Has an episiotomy rate of 20% or less, with a goal of 5% or less;
   - Has a total cesarean rate of 10% or less in community hospitals, and 15% or less in tertiary care (high-risk) hospitals;
   - Has a VBAC (vaginal birth after cesarean) rate of 60% or more with a goal of 75% or more.

7. Educates staff in non-drug methods of pain relief, and does not promote the use of analgesic or anesthetic drugs not specifically required to correct a complication.
8. Encourages all mothers and families, including those with sick or premature newborns or infants with congenital problems, to touch, hold, breastfeed, and care for their babies to the extent compatible with their conditions.

*Author's note: This criterion is currently under review.

9. Discourages non-religious circumcision of the newborn.
10. Strives to achieve the WHO-UNICEF "Ten Steps of the Baby-Friendly Hospital Initiative" to promote successful breastfeeding:
    1. Have a written breastfeeding policy communicated to all health care staff;
    2. Train all health care staff in skills necessary to implement this policy;
    3. Inform all pregnant women about the benefits and management of breastfeeding;
    4. Help mothers initiate breastfeeding within an hour of birth;
    5. Show mothers how to breastfeed and how to maintain lactation even if they should be separated from their infants;
    6. Give newborn infants no food or drink other than breast milk unless medically indicated;
    7. Practice rooming in: allow mothers and infants to remain together 24 hours a day;
    8. Encourage breastfeeding on demand;
    9. Give no artificial teat or pacifiers (also called dummies or soothers) to breastfeeding infants;
    10. Foster the establishment of breastfeeding support groups and refer mothers to them on discharge from hospitals or clinics.

RATIFIED BY THESE MEMBERS OF THE COALITION FOR
IMPROVING MATERNITY SERVICES (CIMS), JULY, 1996

ORGANIZATIONS
(names of organizations' officers may have changed since ratification)

Academy of Certified Birth Educators (Olathe, KS), Linda M. Herrick, RNC, BSN, CCE, CD; and Sally Riley, BSEd, CCE, CD, & Judie C. Wika, RNC, MSN, CNM, CCE, Co-Directors

American Academy of Husband-Coached Childbirth (The Bradley Method™), (Sherman Oaks, CA), Jay and Marjie Hathaway, Executive Directors

American College of Nurse-Midwives (Washington, DC), Joyce Roberts, CNM, PhD, FACNM, President

American College of Domiciliary Midwives (Palo Alto, CA), Faith Gibson, CPM, Executive Director

Association of Labor Assistants and Childbirth Educators (Cambridge, MA), Jessica L. Porter, President

Association for Pre- & Perinatal Psychology and Health (Geyserville, CA), David B. Chamberlain, PhD, President

Association of Women's Health, Obstetrics, and Neonatal Nurses (Washington, DC), Joy Grohar, RNC, MS, President

Attachment Parenting International, (Nashville, TN), Lysa Parker, BS, & Barbara Nicholson, MEd, Co-Founders

Birthworks, Inc. (Medford, NJ), Cathy E. W. Daub, RPT, CCE, President

Center for Perinatal Research & Family Support (River Vale, NJ), Debra Pascali-Bonaro, Executive Director

Doulas of North America (Seattle, WA), Barbara A. Hotelling, RN, BSN, CD, FACCE, President

The Farm (Summertown, TN), Ina May Gaskin, President

Global Maternal/Child Health Association (Wilsonville, OR), Barbara Harper, RN, President

Informed Home Birth/Informed Birth & Parenting (Ann Arbor, MI), Rahima Baldwin Dancy, CPM, President

International Association of Infant Massage (Oak View, CA), Ellen Kerr, RN, BSN, MST, CIMI, President

International Childbirth Education Association (Minneapolis, MN), Cheryl Coleman, RN, BSN, ICCE, President

International Lactation Consultant Association (Chicago, IL), Karen Kerkhoff Gromada, MSN, RN, IBCLC, President

La Leche League International (Schaumburg, IL), Carol Kolar, RN, Director of Education & Outreach

Lamaze International (formerly ASPO/Lamaze). (Washington, DC), Deborah Woolley, CNM, PhD, FACCE, President

Midwifery Today (Eugene, OR), Jan Tritten, TM, Editor

Midwives Alliance of North America (Newton, KS), Ina May Gaskin, President

Midwives of Santa Cruz (Santa Cruz, CA), Roxanne Potter, CNM, Kate Bowland, CNM, Co-Directors

National Association of Childbearing Centers (Perkiomenville, PA), Susan Stapleton, MSN, CNM, President

National Association of Postpartum Care Services (Edmunds, WA), Gerri Levrini, RN, MSN, CNAA, President

North American Registry of Midwives (San Francisco, CA), Sharon Wells, Coordinator

Wellness Associates (Afton, VA), John W. Travis, MD, MPH, & Meryn G. Callander, ME, BSW, Co-Directors

INDIVIDUALS

Sondra Abdulla-Zaimah, MN, CNM, CPM, College Park, GA

Shannon Anton, CPM, San Francisco, CA

Susanne Arms, Bayfield, CO, *Immaculate Deception*

Gini Baker, RN, MPH, IBCLC, FACCE, Escondido, CA

Maggie Bennett, LM, CPM, Seaside, CA

Brian Berman, Bainbridge Island, WA

Mary Brucker, CNM, DNSc, Dallas, TX

Raymond Castellino, DC, RPP, Santa Barbara, CA

Robbie Davis-Floyd, PhD, Austin, TX, *Birth As an American Rite of Passage*

Henci Goer, BA, ACCE, Sunnyvale, CA, *The Thinking Woman's Guide to a Better Birth*

Dorothy Harrison, IBCLC, Edmunds, WA

Jack Heinowitz, PhD, San Diego, CA, *Pregnant Fathers*

Tina Kimmel, MSW, MPH, Berkeley, CA

Marshall Klaus, MD, Berkeley, CA, *Bonding—Building the Foundation for Secure Attachment and Independence*

Phyllis Klaus, CSW, MFCC, Berkeley, CA, *The Amazing Newborn*

Judith Lothian, RN, PhD, FACC, Brooklyn, NY

Susan Sobin Pease, MBA, CIMI, CMT, San Francisco, CA

Paulina G. Perez, RN, BSN, FACCE, Houston, TX, *Special Women*

James W. Prescott, PhD, San Diego, CA, *Brain Function and Malnutrition*

Mayri Sagady, RN, CNM, MSN, San Diego, CA

Karen N. Salt, CCE, Coconino Community College, Flagstaff, AZ

Irene Sandvold, DrPH, CNM, Rockville, MD

Roberta M. Scaer, MSS, Boulder, CO, *A Good Birth, A Safe Birth*

Betsy K. Schwartz, MMHS, Coconut Creek, FL

Penny Simkin, PT, Seattle, WA, *Pregnancy, Childbirth, and the Newborn: The Complete Guide*

Suzanne Suarez, JD, RN, Tallahassee, FL

Sandy Szalay, ARNP, CCE, Seattle, WA

Marsden Wagner, MD, MSPH, Copenhagen, Den, *Pursuing the Birth Machine*

Diony Young, Geneseo, NY

A PARTIAL LIST OF ORGANIZATIONS AND INDIVIDUALS ENDORSING THIS INITIATIVE (FOR CURRENT LIST SEE WEB SITE LISTED BELOW)

Academy for Guided Imagery, Mill Valley, CA, Martin Rossman, MD, Co-Director · American Holistic Nurses Association · The Boston Women's Health Book Collective, Boston, MA · C/Sec, Inc., Ocean City, NJ · Canadian Soc. for the Prev. of Cruelty to Children, Midland, Ont, E. T. Barker, MD, DPsych, FRCP(C), Pres. · The Compleat Mother, Minot, ND, Jody McLoughlin, Editor · Doctors Opposing Circumcision, Seattle, WA, George C. Denniston, MD, MPH, President · International Cesarean Awareness Network, Redondo Beach, CA, April Kubachka, President · The Massachusetts Friends of Midwives, Boston, MA · National Association of Parents and Professionals for Safe Alternatives in Childbirth, Marble Hill, MO, Lee F. Stewart, CCE, and David Stewart, PhD, Executive Directors · National Center for Violence Prevention, Francis E. Andrew, JD, and Ellen Craine, Co-Directors · The Nurturing Parent Journal, Prescott, AZ, Jacqueline De Laveaga, Publisher · Touch The Future, Nevada City, CA, Michael Mendizza, Executive Director. *Individuals:* Thomas Armstrong, PhD, *The Radiant Child* · Elizabeth N. Baldwin, JD, North Miami Beach, FL · Elisabeth Bing, RPT, FACCE, *Six Practical Lessons for an Easy Childbirth* · David Bresler, PhD, Associate Clinical Professor of Anesthesiology, UCLA School of Medicine, Elliott E. Dacher, MD, *Whole Healing* · Larry Dossey, MD, *Prayer Is Good Medicine* · Murray W. Enkin, MD, FRCS(C), Prof. Emeritus, Depts of Ob/Gyn, Clin. Epid., & Biostatistics, McMaster Univ., Hamilton, Ont, *A Guide to Effective Care in Pregnancy and Childbirth* · Eunice K. M. Ernst, CNM, MPH, Mary Breckinridge Chair of Midwifery · Sharron S. Humenick, PhD, RN, FAAN, Editor, *Journal of Perinatal Education* · Laura Huxley, *Children Are Our Ultimate Investment* · Dorothy J. Jongeward, PhD, *Born to Win* · Risa Kaparo, PhD, California Inst. of Integral Studies, San Francisco, CA · John H. Kennell, MD, *Mothering the Mother* · George Leonard, *Mastery* · Jean Liedloff, *The Continuum Concept* · Ashley Montagu, PhD, *Touching* · Michel Odent, MD, *Birth Reborn* · Kathy Oriel, MD, Asst. Prof. Dept Family Medicine, U. of Wisc, Madison, WI · Jeffery J. Patterson, DO, Prof, Dept Family Medicine, U. of Wisc, Madison, WI · Joseph Chilton Pearce, *Magical Child* · Kent Peterson, MD, FACPM, FACOEM, *Handbook of Health Risk Appraisal* · Jane Pincus, *Our Bodies, Ourselves* · Judith Rooks, CNM, MPH, MS, FACNM · Martin F. Rubin, MD, Clinical Faculty, UC San Francisco, School of Medicine, Medical Director, Sonoma County (CA) Dept of Mental Health · Regina Sara Ryan, MA, *Wellness Workbook* · Patty Stuart-Macadam, PhD, Dept. Anthropology, U. of Toronto, Toronto

HELP CIRCULATE THIS INITIATIVE

CIMS (pronounced "KIMS") is a coalition of individuals and organizations volunteering their time to make childbirth a safer, more natural experience. We ask your help in disseminating this Initiative. Publish it, give it away, send it to your newspaper editor, give it to government representatives, mention it on talk shows, etc. (please include attribution). We urge you to mail copies (or forward the Web address below) to all appropriate friends/acquaintances along with a personal note requesting that they also forward it to as many people as possible.

GET FREE ELECTRONIC COPIES OF THIS INITIATIVE

Free copies of the document can be downloaded from <http://www.healthy.net/cims>. There are several versions, a word processing file; one that you can print with this same layout (pdf) on four sheets of paper, or a computer file for 11" × 17" paper, that you can download and take to a copy shop to print on a single large sheet of paper like this.

GET INEXPENSIVE PAPER COPIES OF THIS INITIATIVE

For single copies, send $3 ($4 Canada/Mexico, $5 all others) or bulk: 25 copies/$10 ($12 Can/Mex, $15 all others); 100 copies/$20 ($25Can/Mex, $30 all others) to CIMS, 2120 L St, NW, Suite-400, Washington, DC 20037. U.S. dollars only, prepayment required.

MORE INFORMATION AND DISCUSSION

An online discussion forum is planned help support people in many aspects of Mother-Friendly Childbirth. Check our Web site <http://www.healthy.net> for current information.

We also welcome comments and suggestions at the Web site (if about the *contents* of the Initiative, please cite evidence-based material).

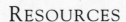

RESOURCES

BOOKS

Active Birth by Janet Balaskas
Birthing from Within by Pam England and Rob Horowitz
The Birth Partner by Penny Simkin
Easing Labor Pain by Adrienne Lieberman
Gentle Birth Choices by Barbara Harper
A Good Birth, A Safe Birth: Choosing and Having the Childbirth Experience You Want by Diana Korte and Roberta Scaer
Mothering the Mother: How a Doula Can Help You Have a Shorter, Easier, and Healthier Birth by Marshall Klaus, John Kennell, and Phyllis Klaus
The Nurturing Touch at Birth by Paulina Perez
Pregnancy, Childbirth and the Newborn by Penny Simkin, Janet Whalley, and Ann Keppler
The VBAC Companion by Diana Korte

ORGANIZATIONS

American College of Nurse Midwives (ACNM)
818 Connecticut Avenue, NW, Suite 900
Washington, DC 20006
(202)728-9860
(888)MIDWIFE
http://www.midwife.org

Association of Labor Assistants and Childbirth Educators (ALACE)
PO Box 382724

Cambridge, MA 02238
(888)222-5223
http://www.alace.org

Birthworks
PO Box 2045
Medford, NJ 08055
(888) TO-BIRTH
http://hometown.aol.com/birthwkscd/bw.html

The Bradley Method of Natural Childbirth
Box 5224
Sherman Oaks, CA 91413-5224
(800)4-A-BIRTH
http://www.bradleybirth.com/

Coalition for Improving Maternity Services (CIMS)
P.O. Box 2346
Ponte Vedra Beach, FL 32004
(888)282-CIMS
http://www.motherfriendly.org

Doulas of North America (DONA)
1100 23rd Avenue East
Seattle, WA 98112
(206)324-5440
http://www.dona.com

International Cesarean Awareness Network (ICAN)
1304 Kingsdale Avenue
Redondo Beach, CA 90278
(310)542-5368
http://www.childbirth.org/section/ICAN.html

International Childbirth Education Association (ICEA)
PO Box 20048
Minneapolis, MN 55420
(612)854-8660
http://www.icea.org/

La Leche League
1400 North Meacham Road
Schaumberg, IL 60173-4048
(847)519-7730
(800)LALECHE
http://www.lalecheleague.org/

Resources

Lamaze International
1200 19th Street, NW, Suite 300
Washington, DC 20036-2422
(202)857-1128
http://www.lamaze.org

Maternity Center Association
281 Park Avenue South, 5th Floor
New York, NY 10010
(212)777-5000
http://www.maternity.org

Midwives Alliance of North America (MANA)
PO Box 175
Newton, KS 67114
http://frank.mtsu.edu/~mhgreene/mana.htm

National Association of Childbearing Centers (NACC)
  (Write and enclose $1.00 for guidelines and brochure.)
3123 Gottschall Road
Perkiomenville, PA 18074-9546
http://www.BirthCenters.org

WEB SITES

ABCs of Parenting
http://www.abcparenting.com

BabyCenter
http://www.babycenter.com

Childbirth.org
http://www.childbirth.org

Cochrane Collaboration
http://www.cochrane.org

Marilyn's Midwifery Page
http://www.midwifery2000.com

Midwifery Today
http://www.midwiferytoday.com

National Library of Medicine: Pubmed and Internet Grateful Med
http://www.nlm.nih.gov/databases/freemedl.html

On Line Birth Center
http://www.efn.org/ndjz/birth/birthindex.html

Parents Place
http://www.parentsplace.com

Pregnancy and Childbirth
http://pregnancy.miningco.com/mbody.htm

Sabrina's Pregnancy Page
http://www.fensende.com/Users/swnymph

Index

Index

Index

North American Registry of Midwives (NARM), 191, 213
Nothing by mouth, 75, 76–78, 83
NPO *(non per os)*. *See* Nothing by mouth
Nurse-midwifes, 189–90
Nurses versus doulas, 177, 186

OBG Management, 164
Obstetricians
　choosing, 5–8, 187–88, 193–97
　complications, not transferred, 192
　cons of, 1–5, 192
　control over midwives or labor and delivery policies, 189
　for high-risk women, 189–90
　literature on, 200
　medical coverage for, 197–98
　pros of, 192
　qualifications, 190
　risks introduced from, 1–5, 188–89
　satisfaction with, 190
　as surgical specialists, 192
　See also Philosophy of caregivers
Obstetric Myths Versus Research Realities: A Guide to the Medical Literature (Goer), 10
Occiput posterior position, 108–9
Odent, Michael, 5, 206
Out-of-hospital births, 217. *See also* Birth centers, freestanding; Home births
Oxytocin
　for breech babies, 46
　challenge test, 57–58
　electronic fetal monitoring (EFM) for, 94
　and epidurals and narcotics, 132, 133, 146
　for induction of labor, 50–51, 60, 65–67, 73
　reducing with doulas, 179, 186
　for slow labor, 111–12, 113, 114, 117, 121
　and vaginal birth after cesarean (VBAC), 172, 176

Perez, Polly, 178
Perinatal mortality, 14–15, 20, 203
Perineum, 13, 149. *See also* Episiotomy
Peterson, G., 27
PGE1 (misoprostol), 59, 64–65
PGE2. *See* Prostaglandin E2

Philosophy of caregivers
　on amniotomy (rupturing membranes), 99–100
　on cesareans, 12–14
　on cesareans, elective repeat, 163–66
　on electronic fetal monitoring (EFM), 89
　on epidurals and narcotics, 126–29
　on episiotomy, 13, 149–50, 152–54
　on labor, slow, 107–14, 122
　medications and procedures, 3–5
Phlebitis, 23
Pitocin ("Pit"). *See* Oxytocin
Placenta
　accreta, 25, 168
　percreta, 25
　previa, 19, 25, 168
Placental abruption, 88
Place of birth, 201–18
　direct-entry midwives versus nurse-midwives, 212–13, 218
　history, 202–5
　interview questions, 213–16
　literature on, 217–18
　out-of-hospital birth advice, 217
　perinatal mortality rates, 203
　transfer rates, 216, 217, 218
　See also Birth centers, freestanding; Home births; Hospital births
Posterior baby, rotation of, 104–5, 120–21, 122
Pregnancy, Childbirth and the Newborn (Simkin, P. et al.), 34
Prelabor rupture of membranes, 52–55, 68–71, 69–70, 74
Prepidil. *See* Prostaglandin E2
Professional labor support. *See* Doulas
Prostaglandin E2 (PGE2)
　for induction of labor, 59, 64–65, 66, 74
　and vaginal birth after cesarean (VBAC), 172, 176
Psychological issues
　of cesareans, 24–25, 26–27
　doulas for support, 179, 180–81, 186
　from epidurals and narcotics, 134
　of slow labor, 109, 119–20
　of vaginal birth after cesarean (VBAC), 174
Public Citizen's Health Research Group, 15, 189–90
Pulmonary embolism, 23

366

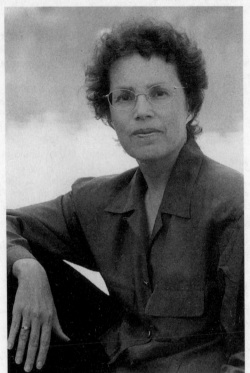

Henci Goer

I'm going to write the best story ever. It's called - okay, I don't know what it's called. But I have a fantastic premise!

It's a world where everyone knows how they're going to die!

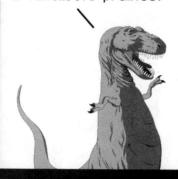

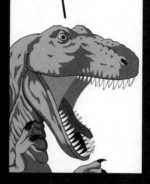

You can go in to a doctor and he takes a blood test, and then his machine spits out a piece of paper that says "exploded" or "drowned" or "poisoned apple" and that's it. No dates, no details! And so people who are to die from drowning spend the rest of their lives avoiding swimming pools, but they end up drowning anyway. Part of the fun would be seeing how!

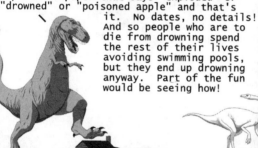

This story sounds pretty morbid, T-Rex!

Morbidly INTERESTING!

True!

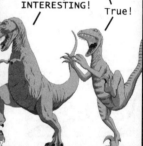

I guess the only safe one would be if the paper said "old age".

Nope, cause then you could be killed by an old guy! This machine delights in ironically vague deaths.

"Natural causes"?

Hit on the head by a falling koala bear!

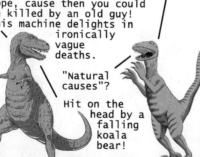

It would also work on animals, but all the ones for cows would say "made into delicious cheeseburger".

Not that the cows could understand!

Friggin' cheeseburgers!

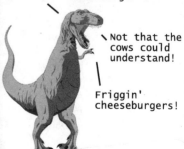

For ebook and audiobook downloads, visit
MACHINEOFDEATH.NET

Cover design by Justin Van Genderen
2046DESIGN.COM

Book design by Ryan Torres
RYANTORRESDESIGN.COM

This book is typeset in ITC New Baskerville and DIN

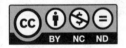
Published by Bearstache Books, Venice, CA
2554 Lincoln Blvd #214 • Venice, CA 90291
BEARSTACHE.COM

First Edition : Third Printing, November 2010.

ISBN-13: 978-0-9821671-2-0

10 9 8 7 6 5 4 3

Printed in the United States of America

FLAMING MARSHMALLOW
FUDGE † TORN APART AND DE-
VOURED BY LIONS † DESPAIR †
SUICIDE † ALMOND † STARVATION
† CANCER † FIRING SQUAD † VEG-
ETABLES † PIANO † HIV INFEC-
TION FROM MACHINE OF DEATH †
NEEDLE † EXPLODED † NOT WAV-
ING BUT DROWNING † IMPROP-
ERLY PREPARED BLOWFISH †
LOVE AD NAUSEUM † MURDER
AND SUICIDE, RESPECTIVELY

MACHINE OF DEATH

CANCER † ANEURYSM † EXHAUS-
TION FROM HAVING SEX WITH
A MINOR † AFTER MANY YEARS,
STOPS BREATHING, WHILE
ASLEEP, WITH SMILE ON FACE
† KILLED BY DANIEL † FRIENDLY
FIRE † NOTHING † COCAINE AND
PAINKILLERS † LOSS OF BLOOD
† PRISON KNIFE FIGHT † WHILE
TRYING TO SAVE ANOTHER † MIS-
CARRIAGE † SHOT BY SNIPER †
HEAT DEATH OF THE UNIVERSE
† DROWNING † ? † CASSANDRA

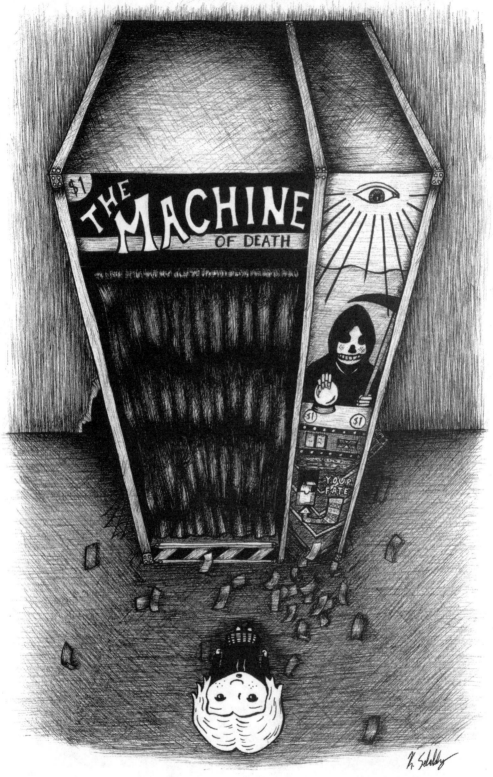

Machine of Death

A collection of stories about people who know
how they will die

Edited by Ryan North, Matthew Bennardo & David Malki !

BEARSTACHE BOOKS VENICE CALIFORNIA

Table of Contents

The illustration on the preceding page is by Katie Sekelsky.

Preface

THIS BOOK, UNLIKE MOST OTHERS, STARTED ITS LIFE AS AN OFFHAND COMMENT MADE BY A BRIGHT GREEN TYRANNOSAURUS REX. This particular dinosaur is the main character in Ryan North's "Dinosaur Comics," and just a few pages ago, you saw how excited he got about his story idea.

And he was far from alone! After Ryan published the comic in which T-Rex laid out his "machine of death" concept, readers immediately began to speculate about this machine and the world it might inhabit. So we posted an open call for submissions, inviting writers to take the idea and run with it however they liked. Now, a few years later, here are thirty of our favorite submitted stories, as well as four by us, that explore that premise. It turns out that T-Rex was right: it's a fantastic premise indeed.

Of course, some of the oldest stories in the world are about the dangers of knowing too much about the future, and a lot of these deal specifically with how people are going to die. (T-Rex would probably point out that he beat Shakespeare and the Greeks to the punch by at least 65 million years, but we're still waiting for the dated documentary evidence to back that up.)

But the funny thing is that these kinds of stories have a way of always being compelling. If we're honest, we'd all have to admit that we'd like to know at least some things about the future—no matter how often we say we don't want to. Yet none of us really have any say in the matter one way or another. We will never get to stand in front of an oracle or a blood-testing machine and have to choose between knowing and not knowing.

Perhaps that's why so many of these stories end badly for the characters who do want to know. We all want perfect knowledge of the future, but we can't have it, so we make up stories to convince ourselves that we shouldn't want it. Sour cosmic grapes. But don't think for a moment that this is a book full of stories about people meeting their ironic dooms. There is some of that, of course. But many more of the stories take the premise as an invitation to explore all kinds of different and surprising worlds. All told we received 675 submissions from writers on five continents, amateurs and professionals alike, ranging across adventure, horror, mystery, fantasy, sci-fi, humor—every existing genre and a few new ones as well.

You'd think that after the first 500 stories or so, we'd have seen it all. But right up until the very end of the reading period, we were still discovering gems—new insights, new characters, new worlds, new twists to the premise. As editors, our biggest challenge soon became picking stories that not only were all excellent (that was the easy part), but that also represented the true diversity of ideas and approaches that we received.

So sit back and take a moment to look over the table of contents. Start at the beginning or just pick the title that sounds most intriguing to you. Either way, there's no telling for sure exactly what you'll get. Prepare to have your tears jerked, your spine tingled, your funny bone tickled, your mind blown, your pulse quickened, or your heart warmed. Or better yet, simply prepare to be surprised. Because even when people do have perfect knowledge of the future, there's no telling exactly how things will turn out.

— Ryan North, Matthew Bennardo & David Malki !

Introduction

THE MACHINE HAD BEEN INVENTED A FEW YEARS AGO: A MACHINE THAT COULD TELL, FROM JUST A SAMPLE OF YOUR BLOOD, HOW YOU WERE GOING TO DIE. It didn't give you the date and it didn't give you specifics. It just spat out a sliver of paper upon which were printed, in careful block letters, the words "DROWNED" or "CANCER" or "OLD AGE" or "CHOKED ON A HANDFUL OF POPCORN." It let people know how they were going to die.

The problem with the machine is that nobody really knew how it worked, which wouldn't actually have been that much of a problem if the machine worked as well as we wished it would. But the machine was frustratingly vague in its predictions: dark, and seemingly delighting in the ambiguities of language. "OLD AGE," it had already turned out, could mean either dying of natural causes, or being shot by a bedridden man in a botched home invasion. The machine captured that old-world sense of irony in death: you can know how it's going to happen, but you'll still be surprised when it does.

The realization that we could now know how we were going to die had changed the world: people became at once less fearful and more afraid. There's no reason not to go skydiving if you know your sliver of paper says "BURIED ALIVE." But the realization that these predictions seemed to revel in turnabout and surprise put a damper on things. It made the predictions more sinister: yes, skydiving should be safe if you were going to be buried alive, but what if you landed in a gravel pit? What if you were buried alive not in dirt but in something else? And would being caught in a collapsing building count as being buried alive? For every possibility the machine closed, it seemed to open several more, with varying degrees of plausibility.

By that time, of course, the machine had been reverse-engineered and duplicated, its internal workings being rather simple to construct. And yes, we found out that its predictions weren't as straightforward as they seemed upon initial discovery at about the same time as everyone else did. We tested it before announcing it to the world, but testing took time—too much, since we had to wait for people to die. After four years had gone by and three people died as the machine predicted, we shipped it out the door. There were now machines in every doctor's office and in booths at the mall. You could pay someone or you could probably get it done for free, but the result was the same no matter what machine you went to. They were, at least, consistent.

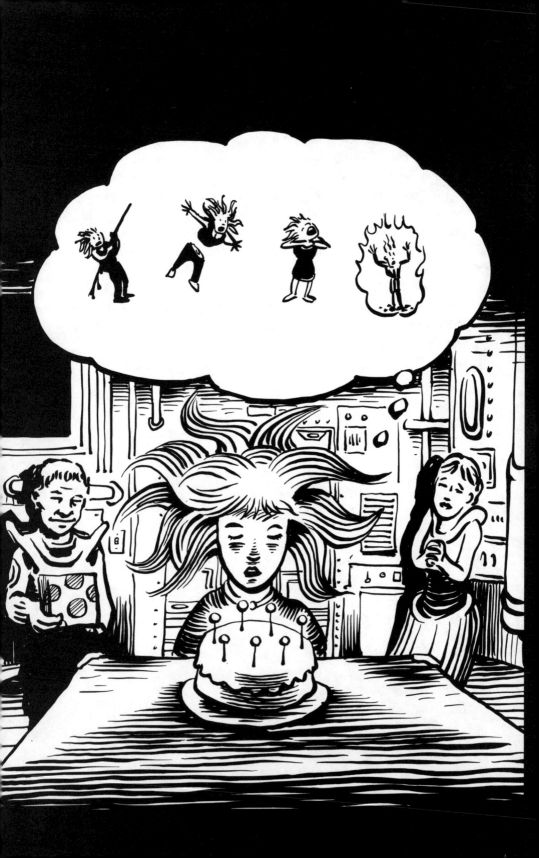

FLAMING MARSHMALLOW

I'M SO FREAKING EXCITED I CAN HARDLY STAND IT.

Tomorrow. Tomorrow is my birthday, *the* birthday. The birthday everybody waits and waits for and until you get there you just hate that all your old friends already got theirs and you're the only one without it yet, and sometimes you think *holy-freaking-eff, I'm never going to turn sixteen,* but then you do.

At first I'm afraid I won't be able to sleep. I turn off the light, but after lying in the dark for half an hour, I turn it back on. I look at the calendar hanging on the wall above my bed. I reach up, lift it off its nail with one hand and snuggle back under the covers, taking the calendar with me and running a finger over all the red Xs marked over all the days leading up to this one. It's a little cold out, and the last thing in the universe I want to do is catch an effing cold the week of my birthday, so I snuggle down into the warmth of my flannel sheets even more. I know there're going to be parties this weekend, and I'm going to want to go.

This is what I've been waiting for all these months. All these years, I guess, though before my friends started getting theirs, it didn't seem like such a big deal. We were all No-Knows then.

Tomorrow, I'm finally going to feel like I belong.

Tomorrow, I'm going to find out how I die.

"Carolyn! Yo, grrl, wait up!"

At the sound of my name I turn around. It's Patrice. I can see her bounding up across the commons toward me. Her super-long hair is braided today, and as she runs it whips around at the sides of her head like two angry red snakes with ribbons tied to their tails.

"Hey, Patrice," I say, and clutch my books closer to my chest. I try to walk a little faster, thinking maybe she'll get the hint. She doesn't.

"Today's the Big Day, huh?" she says.

I nod.

She turns her head away, bites her lip. "Lucky," she says.

I shrug, speed up even more. It's not my problem she's one of the smartest kids in our class and they moved her up a grade, like, four years ago. It's not my fault she's going to be a No-Know for another whole year.

Out of the corner of my eye, I can see Brad Binder. He is so effing cool—a burner, they say. *That's hot*, I think, and then I laugh to myself.

"What's so funny?" asks Patrice. We're at my locker, so I balance my books on my knee with one hand while I fumble my combo-lock with the other. I pretend I don't hear her, but she sees me flicking sly glances in Brad Binder's direction.

"Not *him*," she says, rolling her eyes. "You can't be serious."

"Shhh!" I try to shut her up. I wish I had some kind of freaking super power or something. I wish I could just concentrate really hard and make her go away.

Brad Binder pulls his letter jacket out of his locker, which is so close to mine, three other girls have asked to trade lockers with me. He shrugs his perfect—so effing perfect!—shoulders into his jacket and takes out just a notebook with a pencil shoved in its rings. No computer, no books, no nothing. God, that's so effing cool. Just like a burner.

As Brad walks away, Patrice fixes me with one of those stares of hers. "He's not that great, you know. I heard he kisses like a dead lizard."

I guess you'd know, I almost say, but I stop myself. I don't want to stoop to her level, be so childish. I'm sixteen today and after school my dad's taking me to the mall to get that slip of paper, and then I'll know where I really belong. So I shrug again instead, let it slide off me, like egg off Teflon. "He's a burner," I say. "They're pretty cool."

Patrice snorts. "You know what his slip said? 'Flaming Marshmallow'. That doesn't sound like a real burner cause-of-death to me, no matter what he says. He should probably be hanging out with the chokers, instead. You wouldn't think he was so tough then."

I've had enough of Patrice. "You wouldn't understand," I tell her, and walk away toward Geometry class. Maybe Cindy Marshall will be nice to me today, it being so close to me getting my c-of-d slip. Maybe I'll end up being a crasher, like her.

If only!

I'm almost late getting to class. Mrs. Tharple looks at me extra-sour, but I don't give a flying eff. I slide into my seat right as the bell rings, and catch Cindy Marshall's eye. I smile.

"Don't even look at me, you No-Know," she says to me, low under her breath as Mrs. Tharple starts handing out our pop-quiz. The other two girls behind her snicker. I can feel their eyes darting against my skin, sharp like the teeth of weasels.

"It's my birthday," I say.

She turns in her seat and looks at me full-on. I try to understand the look in her eyes, but I can't. I feel like it's something really obvious, like she's trying to tell me something so, so, so obvious, I should already know it.

I feel really stupid.

Mrs. Tharple walks between us, places our blank quizzes face-up on the desks in front of us, glides on by to the next row and toward the front of the room again.

I look down at my Geometry quiz, try to concentrate, try to ignore the heat in my cheeks and the tips of my ears and on the back of my neck.

"Hey, you," hisses Cindy Marshall.

I look up.

"So did you get your slip yet?"

I shake my head. "After school," I tell her.

She narrows her eyes. I can sense the other girls, crashers both, also watching me, but I play it cool. I hope.

She nods. "If you get your c-of-d, and it's crashing—anything: plane, car, bike, hot-freakin'-air balloon, whatever—you come talk to me again. Tomorrow."

I have to bite the insides of my cheeks to keep from smiling. I try to look like this isn't the best offer I've gotten all morning. I try to look tough. I want to be crasher material, I really do.

"Tomorrow," I say, and she nods again, once.

Not one of those girls acknowledges my existence the entire rest of the class, but I don't care. Everything will be different tomorrow.

Tomorrow, my life can begin.

Lunch isn't what I'd hoped for.

I've spent all this time counting down to my birthday, thinking, *this is the day everything changes*, but it isn't. I don't feel like a No-Know anymore, even though technically, I still don't actually know. I'm under eighteen, so I have to have my parent or legal guardian with me to get my slip. If I could've, I would have ditched lunch today, gone to the mall, gotten the whole thing over with. Instead, I have to wait for my dad to get off work. It's so unfair.

So, even if I get my slip tonight, nobody but me is going to know my cause-of-death until tomorrow. Well, my parents will know, and my little brother, I guess. And I'm sure I could call Patrice and tell her, but why? After tomorrow, I'll have new friends to hang out with.

But for today, I'm still stuck in No-Know-ville.

I grab my tray and slide onto the bench at the end of the table. Patrice waves me down further toward her end, but I pretend I don't see her. I line up my eight extra packets of mustard and start tearing the corners off one by one, slowly squeezing out the sharp yellow and gooping it all over the top of my synthesized proteins and pressed vegetable shapes.

Covertly, I scan the room, wondering, fantasizing about where I might be allowed to sit tomorrow. Who's going to welcome me with open arms? It all depends on my c-of-d.

A ruckus is going on over in the corner. Of course it's the burner kids, cracking each other up, starting a food fight. The burners, the drowners, the crashers, the live-wires, and the fallers—all the violent accidentals—they sit in mingled clumps along the two tables in the corner. That's the coolest corner, and I'm pretty sure I'll get to sit there tomorrow, or at least close. The next couple tables out wouldn't be so bad; you've got the med-heads and the sharpies and the bullets—mostly malpractice and murder, right?—though some kids sneak in there who should probably be over with the suicides. I can see those from here, all dressed in black and with pale faces. They look like a bunch of crows, pecking at their food.

Just please don't let me be at one of the last two tables: sickness and old age. Ugh. They look boring even eating lunch. That would be my c-of-d if I was forced to sit at that table: Bored to Death.

"Happy birthday, Carolyn."

I'm so startled I squeeze a mustard packet too hard and it squirts all down the front of my dress. I start to dab it with a napkin, but I'm just turning bitter yellow clumps into bitter yellow smears.

"I'm, I'm so sorry, Carolyn...*eff.* I—I—"

I look up into Jamie's face. We used to be friends, a long, long time ago. He lives just down the street, and we used to ride bikes together every single day. I can still taste the sun and summer dust on my tongue, just looking at him. We stopped hanging out when his parents joined the Anti-MoD League. Sometimes, on the way home from school, I see his mom standing out in front of the mall with her placard and her sandwich board. "Lives are for Living" say her signs some days. Others, "People Against Machines of Death" or even, "Don't Ask, Don't Know—You Have a Choice!"

Jamie's almost eighteen, and he's still a No-Know. I'd just die if that were me. I'd just die.

"It's okay, Jamie," I tell him. "Don't worry about it."

He has a couple of napkins in his hands, and he's dipping them in his water and holding them out to me. He started to dab one on my breast, but figured out in time it probably wouldn't be such a good idea.

I try to stifle a sudden memory of me and him kissing behind the convenience store dumpster. I was probably about twelve or thirteen, and he was fourteen or so; right before his parents joined the League. I remember he tasted like strawberries.

I hope Jamie doesn't see my ears and neck turn red. He's one of the few people who knows me too well for me to hide it.

"Your mom picking you up after school?" he asks.

I keep dabbing, shake my head. "My dad."

He nods. He's watching the motions of my hands as I rub the damp napkins on my lap, on the fabric stretched across my ribs, but he's not really seeing me.

"I'm sorry," he says again, and I don't think he's talking about mustard.

By the time Dad picks me up, I'm mentally exhausted.

He kisses the top of my head when I get into the car. "Hey kid! Happy special day."

"Thanks."

I throw my stuff in the back seat and fasten my lapbelt.

Dad's just sitting there with a loppy-sided smile on his face. "You want to go get an ice cream first, or something?" he says. "You want pizza? A movie?"

How can he be so freaking clueless? I want to tell him what a moron he's being, but when I look at him something feels like it slips sideways in my stomach. For the first time, I'm looking at the forty-something man with the glasses and the stubbled cheeks and the ugly sweater, and I don't see my dad.

I mean yes, of course, I see my dad; the middle-aged med-head c-of-d (accidental overdose) with the over-expensive house and the boring job and the two kids and last-year's-last-year's car, bought cheap with high mileage from a rental fleet...

But I also see a guy. I see a guy who loves me so much, he can't even put it into words. It never occurred to me to think this might be a big deal for him, the day I get my slip. He looks tired, I think. More tired than usual.

I reach out and put my hand on his where it's resting on the steering wheel.

"Sure, Dad," I say. "Whatever you want."

He covers my hand with his other one, so it's kind of like a hand-sandwich, my fingers and knuckles pressed between two layers of his. His eyes look a little bright for a second, but I decide it's only my imagination as he places my hand back in my own lap and starts the car and pulls out from the curb.

I watch the school get smaller and smaller in the side mirror as we drive away.

I finish off the last of my ice-cream cone, and so does Dad. We wipe our sticky fingers on the wet-wipes and throw those away, and I get up from our food-court table and gather all my bags as I stand. Dad's bought me a new pair of shoes, two new books, and a hat he says I look great in, but which I know I'll never, ever wear again in a million billion. All I'm missing is the partridge in a pear tree.

"So...what next, Birthday Girl? Need some new gloves? Music? You used to love the music store."

He's walking over to the mall directory, studying the list of stores. I walk up to him, set down my bags of books and shoes, and touch his arm. "Dad," I say. "It's time."

He doesn't look at me right away. He takes off his glasses and starts to clean them on the edge of his sweater. I can see he's just making them all linty and smeary, so I take them from him and clean them on the inside hem of my dress, instead. When I hand them back they're considerably cleaner, and I pick up my bags and start walking in the direction of the slip kiosk. I don't have to look up the location on the mall directory; I know exactly where it is. There's not a fifteen-year-old in the country who doesn't know the location of the nearest machine. I know its hours of operation (regular mall open-hours: ten a.m. to nine p.m.), I know how much it costs (nineteen-ninety-five-plus-tax), I even know the brand (Death-o-Mat, by DigCo.; "We Give the Same Results—For Less!").

The only thing I don't know is what's going to be on that strip of paper when it scrolls out of that slot.

It's getting kind of late, and the mall's going to close soon. Most of the stores are empty. It's a school night, so nobody my age is around. It's mostly tired-looking shop clerks with achy feet, and straggly-haired moms pushing heavy strollers.

The machine kiosk is in a darkish corner over by the restrooms. The janitor has the door propped open to the ladies', and even though I kind of have to go, I'm not about to brave the janitor and his stinky mop. Besides, I don't want to put this off anymore. I need to know.

Dad pauses when we get to the machine. He fumbles with his wallet, pulls out his identity and credit cards. He clears his throat, but doesn't say anything, doesn't look at me.

I thought Dad's hand shook a little when he slid his cards into their proper slots and keyed in his and my social security numbers and other information, but I'm sure I was imagining things. It was probably just my brain buzzing. That's what it feels like inside my head right now; like all the curves and loops and folds of my brain are buzzing with tiny bees, or maybe electric currents. I guess brains *are*, after all, though. Filled with electric currents, that is, not tiny bees.

The machine's green light comes on and an arrow points to the small, shiny, self-cleaning divot in the otherwise dull metal. I set my bags down at my feet, slowly reach one finger toward the indention—

"Carolyn!"

I jump, look up into Dad's face.

He pushes his glasses back on the bridge of his nose, fumbles it a little, blinks.

"Uhm...for an extra five dollars, it will tell you your blood type, your glucose levels, and whether or not you're pregnant." He points to the list printed on the machine's face. Then he frowns, distracted. "Hey, there's no way you might be pregnant, is there?"

I close the tiny distance between us and wrap my arms around his waist. He hugs me back, and for a second, as I breathe in the warm fuggy-sweatered dadness of him, I feel like the most precious and important thing in the universe.

Without letting go of Dad or giving him any warning, I reach behind him and jab my finger into the shiny divot. Dad flinches, and presses my face closer to his chest.

A tiny slicing pain flits across my finger, then numbness as the machine sprays its analgesic and disinfectant.

I pull back from Dad, and he clears his throat and lets me go. The machine spits out Dad's two cards from their slots, and my slip scrolls out from the single slot below. Dad and I both reach for it, but when I freeze he pulls back. I've got to do this, and he knows it. He plucks his plastic from the machine and slides the cards into his wallet while I uncurl my slip and read.

I read it three times. Four times. I'm on my fifth when Dad, unable to contain himself, gently tugs the paper from my stiff fingers and reads aloud.

"Death by Millennium Space Entropy," he says.

"But..."

Dad wraps both arms around me and swings me up into the air like he hasn't done since I was a very, very little girl. I keep my arms stiff, but let my legs and body go limp, and Dad twirls me in a circle, laughing, joyous.

He finally sets me down, and I have to reach out a hand to steady myself against the edge of the machine. I'm a little dizzy. Dizzy, and confused.

"Millennium space entropy," says Dad, shaking his head, unrolling the slip and reading it again. "That's amazing, Carolyn. It's fantastic! You'll be nearly a thousand years old by the next millennium. Maybe you live to be a thousand! Just think, medical breakthroughs all the time, vastly extended lifespans... It could happen, sweetheart. It could really happen."

Dad, grinning, crushes me to his chest again, and I can hear the rumble of his happiness somewhere deep inside. "I just want you to have a long and happy life, Carolyn. A very long, long, long and happy life."

"But Dad," I say into the nubby wool of his sweater, "where will I sit tomorrow at lunch?"

Story by Camille Alexa
Illustration by Shannon Wheeler

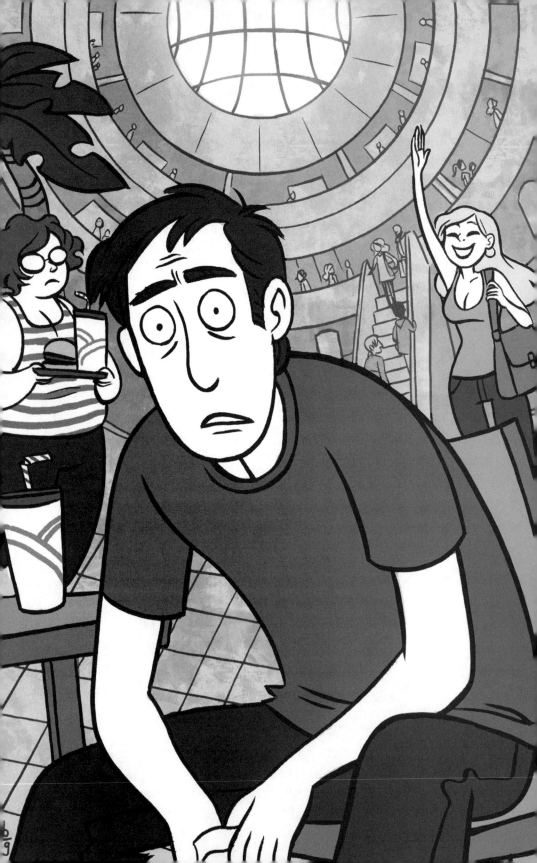

FUDGE

TO ANY OF THE COUNTLESS SHOPPERS PASSING BY, THE KISS WOULDN'T HAVE SEEMED LIKE MUCH. Longer than a peck, sure, but nothing overlong or excessive. It didn't appear to be anything special. But for Rick it was something else entirely. Any time he touched Shannon he managed to get lost in the moment, swept up like the hapless lead in some cheeseball Hallmark special.

"Bye, baby," she said, giving him a little wave. "Don't spend too much!"

"Not too little either," he fired back, and her grin widened before she flipped her hair and walked away. As Rick watched her go he noticed more than one set of eyes doing the same, but he was used to that. When you're engaged to a beautiful woman, it comes with the territory. Best to take it as a compliment, because at the end of the day she was coming home with him, not anybody else.

Busy schedules had left them with no choice but to be here at the mall so close to Christmas. Over the next hour he managed to find a few things for under their tree: a bottle of her favorite perfume, the scent of which stirred him in all the right regions; an earring set with sapphires that would match her eyes; fuzzy green footie pajamas, which on her would be sexier than the flimsiest of négligées; an outstanding chef's knife, razor sharp, which was a bit of a boomerang gift—he loved to cook too. A quick glance at his watch informed him that their time apart was due to end soon, and he began heading toward the fountain where they'd agreed to meet.

A sign in the window of a bulk candy store caught his eye. In bold white letters against a black background, it proclaimed 'WE HAVE THE MACHINE HERE!'

Rick stopped in his tracks, then edged up to the glass and peered in. They had a Machine? A Death Machine?

He was fuzzy on the details—he'd skimmed an article on it in the Sunday *Times Magazine* on his way to losing another bout with the crossword puzzle—but the nuts and bolts of it, he remembered, were that you stuck your finger in a hole in the Machine where it took a blood sample. Imagine the first guy who volunteered for that! Then it would spit out a piece of paper marked with a couple of words, or maybe only one. If the stories were true, that little slip would tell you how you'd die. Not when, not where, but the manner in which you'd meet your demise, although the writer of the article had cryptically added that there always seemed to be a bit of a gray area.

There were also websites devoted to following predictions with a level of obsession that bordered on the ghoulish, and Rick wasn't so proud that he could claim he hadn't visited a few from time to time. If one were willing to accept that an inanimate object could be capable of such a thing, it seemed undeniable that the Death Machines had a healthy sense of irony. One girl drew 'BOAT,' so she immediately gave up sea travel—which did her no good two years later when a truck towing a cabin cruiser jackknifed in front of her on the freeway. Some dude got 'BAT' and started avoiding baseball and caves, but he found out what it meant when the husband of the woman he was having an affair with used one—of the wooden variety, not the kind with wings and sonar—against the side of his head. Of course the story that came up most often was the junkie who got 'CRACK.' The guy managed to break his addiction, clean himself up, find a job, and start a new life. One day on his way to work, he tripped over a break in the sidewalk—a crack, if you will—and dashed his head out against the concrete. Or so the story went.

They made for good lunchtime reading, but Rick wasn't quite sure how much faith he put into tales told on the Internet. Still, he'd always been intrigued by the whole concept of the Death Machine, but too lazy and embarrassed to make an appointment at his doctor's office. Moving over to the store's entrance, Rick spotted a short queue in the far corner. A sign proclaimed: 'THE MACHINE! $20'

As he watched, two girls in their early teens wheeled away from the front of the line. The shorter of the two was consumed by high-pitched giggles, but her wispy friend was ghost-white. As they moved past, the giggler took a deep breath and said, "Oh, Robin! Don't take it so seriously! It's probably not true!"

Rick watched and saw the other knuckle at her eyes. "But what if it is?" she said. "I can't believe he'd..." Then they drifted out of his earshot.

When he looked back at the corner, someone else was walking his way, a tall guy about his age. When he saw Rick staring he broke into a sheepish grin and shrugged, waving a slip of paper in a matter-of-fact way. "Fifth time I've taken the test, fifth time I've gotten this answer." His smile vanished, and his face clouded over. "Still not quite sure what it means, you know?"

Before Rick could say anything—or get a look at the prediction, which, to be honest, was what he wanted to do—Mr. Five-Times had moved past and was swallowed by the mall traffic. Now the store was empty but for two kids filling a bag with jelly beans, and two figures under the Machine sign. One, presumably an employee, had a hand-ful of bills in his hand; the other was a middle-aged woman with her index finger in her mouth. A few moments later her head jerked down, and she stepped a little to her right—giving Rick his first live look at a Death Machine.

It was...*cute*, that was the only word for it. Squat and stout, with stubby little legs. The hole for your finger was larger than he'd expected, and its location made the unit look like a little gunmetal-gray piggy.

He couldn't help looking back up at the woman's face as she read her slip, her eyes widening for a second before she stuck the paper in her pocket and wandered off toward the chocolate section. Rick sur-mised that the slip hadn't said "FUDGE." As he watched, she paused to draw her prediction out again, staring as if it might have changed in the last few seconds. Her brow furrowed, one finger idly tapping her chin, eyes a million miles away.

"Twenty bucks."

The employee's voice, bored and impatient, snapped Rick from his observation. "Huh?"

An exasperated sigh. "Twenty bucks, for the Machine. Or are you just going to stand there and block the line?"

Embarrassed, Rick set his bag down and reached for his wallet, turning to apologize to the people behind him. Nobody there. He was the line in its entirety.

Pulling out a trio of fives and a bunch of singles—he had a twenty, but the kid had annoyed him—he thrust them out, saying, "Pretty funny. What comedy clubs are you working at?"

Snatching the money away, the guy scowled as a flush spread under his bad skin. "Whatever, dude. I get tired of people standing in front of the Machine all day while they decide whether or not to go through with it."

"Yeah, must be really draining. I bet you didn't hesitate at all, right?"

"Me? I'm not doing that thing, not ever." He shook his head and gave the Machine a look of complete and utter disdain. "I mean, it's cool if people pay me to get themselves all freaked out, but that's not something I wanna know, 'kay?" After a pause he added, "No refunds."

"None wanted," Rick replied with a snarl, thoroughly nettled by the attitude. "I'm not afraid."

"Go right ahead, then," was the answer as his bills were added to a sizable wad. No credit cards for the Death Machine, it appeared. After the money was tucked away the guy looked at him with a questioning glance. "You going to go today, or maybe you want a rain check?"

That was it. "Okay, I want to talk to to your manager."

"Ha! Don't have one."

Rick looked over at the girl behind the counter, ringing up candy purchases. "What about her? She your boss?"

This prompted another laugh, along with a sneer. "I'm the boss. This is my Machine, I just rent a spot from the store. So, did you want to register a complaint? Because I promise I'll get my best people on it right away."

"You own this? And it's real?"

"Yeah, it's real, and yeah, it's mine. I bought it from the company that makes them, you know? Anyone can. I was tired of cutting lawns and flipping burgers." He leaned back against the wall and smiled. "Smartest thing I ever did." After a few seconds his haughty expression eased a bit. "Listen, you gotta do it or move on. There really are people behind you now."

From the murmuring behind him Rick knew it was true, so without another word he shoved his finger into the piggy's mouth, down into the bowels of the Machine.

At once it began to hum. It wasn't as cold as he'd expected, but rather disturbingly warm and soft, almost as if his digit was being suckled. That sensation was interrupted by a sharp prick, to draw blood. The vibrations began to increase, and Rick realized with no small measure of alarm that he couldn't pull free. But before he quite panicked, the Machine stopped dead and ejected his finger.

A piece of paper spat out of a slot on the side, and without any real conscious thought Rick grabbed it and stepped aside, shoving his bag over with his leg. He could sense the Machine owner's glare at his sudden clumsiness, but Rick wouldn't give him the satisfaction of eye contact. He gathered up his previous purchases and walked out, slip still clutched, unread, in his other hand.

Outside the shop he fought his way through a suddenly heavy current of shoppers, making his way to a group of tables in the middle of the corridor. One table was occupied by a young woman trying to get a squalling infant to take a bottle. Rick moved to the other table furthest away, dropping into a chair that gave him a view of where he'd just come from, as if he had to keep watch for a sneak attack by the Death Machine, clomping after him on those ridiculous little stems, those leg-ettes, coming to take another blood sample, a much larger one.

A piercing wail from the nearby child snapped Rick from his fugue, and with a start he realized he'd crushed the piece of paper in a fist. Putting down his bag, he stared at his closed hand. It would be easy—simple, even—to walk away from it right now. Just toss the crumpled paper into the nearest garbage can. Hell, even dropping it on the floor would do just as well. He'd wasted twenty bucks on much sillier things before, so what would this matter?

He tapped his knuckles together, kneaded the empty hand over the other. If the stories were true, even if he threw this one away, he'd still get the same answer some other time. So there was no reason to obsess about it now. He should go find Shannon, kiss those full, inviting lips, make a lewd suggestion as to what they could do when they got home and instead of being offended she'd top his offer with something even better. Rick felt himself smile. With her in his life, why would he even *want* to know how he was going to die? A real no-brainer. Easy decision.

But instead, he opened his fist, then the paper.

There was no special font, no borders, no color. In simple black lettering was written a single word: 'LOVE.'

Rick turned the paper over to see if he'd missed something. Nothing but LOVE. His brow furrowed and he shook his head, confused. "What the hell is that supposed to mean?"

He looked around but saw no answers, only the mother cooing to her now-pacified child. How could he die from love? Too much love? Too little? Someone else's, like that psycho ex-boyfriend of Shannon's? He'd threatened to kick Rick's ass the one time they'd met—how much, or how little, would it take for that nut to go for a knife? Or what about that loony chick Shannon had been living with when she and Rick first started dating—what was her name? Kerry? Kara?

She'd bawled her eyes out when Shannon handed her back her keys; what was that all about? Stared absolute daggers at Rick the whole time. He'd made a point to politely refuse her offer of coffee. Was *she* still lurking around somewhere?

Or maybe it had nothing to do with anyone else. Did the Machine mean love in an emotional sense, or was something going to happen during sex? Were he and Shannon going to have a break-up so crushing that he'd only find solace at the end of a knotted rope? Or would the jilted one seek a sense of closure with some dramatic, foolhardy, violent act?

LOVE. Rick looked at his future, his demise, one more time before crumpling the paper in his hand and dropping it. He was a man, not a child, and his life wasn't going to be ruled by some ludicrous prediction from a machine he knew nothing about, owned by a smart-ass punk who probably got his rocks off screwing with people's heads. What Rick had with Shannon was a good thing, a powerful thing, the best thing ever. No would-be oracle was going to change that. She didn't need to know about it, and he'd never tell her—so the matter was settled as far as he was concerned. Their life together could go on like before, a slice of heaven on earth, two people made for one another.

As if on cue, a pair of arms wrapped around him from behind, enveloping him in a familiar scent as her hair spilled over his shoulder. "Hey handsome," Shannon purred in his ear, "you want some company?" She punctuated her question with a kiss on the side of his neck.

Rick shuddered.

Story by Kit Yona
Illustration by Vera Brosgol

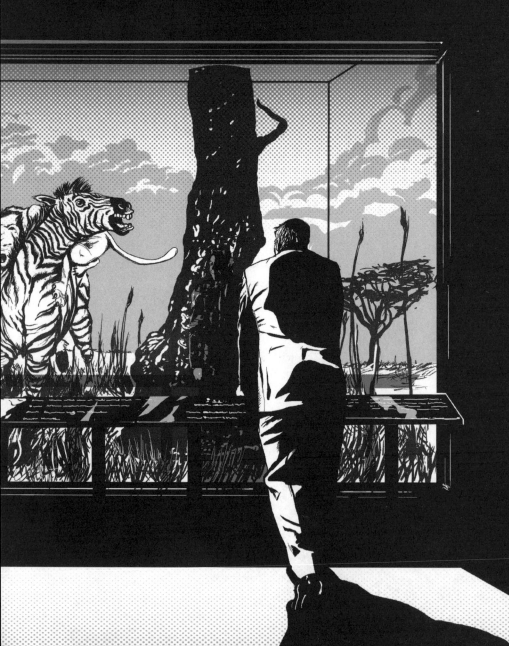

TORN APART AND DEVOURED BY LIONS

"Missus Murphy, I will have you know that I am to be torn apart and devoured by lions."

Simon Pfennig was fully aware of how strange he must sound.

He had no choice. It was too exciting not to share.

There came a startled pause on the other end of the line. As might well be expected, thought Simon. He imagined her there, sitting in her parlor (did people even have "parlors" anymore?) listening to the salesman on the other end of the line droning on and on about Company X's jolly new life insurance policy for citizens over 50, about the security it would bring to your family were you to suddenly keel over stone dead and how content you'd be, as the final darkness was falling, that you'd at least managed to avoid becoming a big fat financial burden and suddenly, *bam*, out of the blue, he drops a line like that. Damn straight she should be startled.

Eventually, the silence on the other end of the line was broken. "...Excuse me?" Mrs. Murphy eventually managed.

"I," said Simon, "am to be torn apart and devoured by lions."

"I'm sorry," said Mrs. Murphy. "Weren't you just talking to me about insurance a moment ago?"

"I was," said Simon. "Now I'm talking about lions."

"Oh," said Mrs. Murphy, apparently unsure of what to make of all this.

"Did you know that an adult male lion can consume up to seventy-five pounds of meat in a single meal? And that said meal will often have to last him an entire week?"

"I, er, did not."

"That'd be two whole meals, out of me alone!" said Simon. "I'm guesstimating a bit, because I am not made *entirely* of meat."

"Well. Who is?" replied Mrs. Murphy, gamely.

"Exactly. For one thing, there's the matter of bones. I'm not quite certain how much my bones weigh. Lions don't eat bones; they leave them behind for the hyenas to consume. But, you see, that doesn't matter as much to me, Missus Murphy. Because I am to be torn apart and devoured by lions, not by hyenas."

"So you said."

"I will be long dead," said Simon, "before the hyenas ever get ahold of me."

"Ah...hah."

"Naturally, though, I don't expect myself to last the whole two weeks. Far from it! After all, as you know, I am to be torn apart and devoured by *lions*, plural, not 'a lion.' And it is uncommon for male lions to travel together, unless they're roaming the savannah in unwed bachelor groups." Simon leaned back in his chair and studied the single fluorescent fixture mounted above his tiny cubicle, imagining it for a moment to be the red-hot sun of the Serengeti. "No," he continued, "far more likely, I am to be torn apart and devoured by lionesses, a group of huntresses intent on bringing food back for their leonine patriarch."

"I...see."

"As you might expect," Simon went on, "I've given this some thought, and I have eventually come to the conclusion that the word 'lions' doesn't necessarily refer to the male of the species exclusively. Good news for me, you understand, because I must confess to harboring this romantic notion of how it will all play out."

Mrs. Murphy smiled into the phone; you could hear it in her voice. "Just got your prediction today, did you?"

"Actually," said Simon, "it's been seven weeks now."

"Oh," said Mrs. Murphy.

"But, I'm sorry, you're quite right. We should probably go back to talking about life insurance now." Simon cleared his throat, straightened his tie and put his salesman voice back on. It was a good salesman voice, keen and enthusiastic, and it bore shockingly little resemblance to the one he'd been using his entire workaday life up until that day about two months ago, the day Simon now liked to call "Torn Apart And Devoured By Lions Day." "Missus Murphy," the new, exciting Simon began, "did you know that in the event of your sudden, accidental death, your family might incur miscellaneous costs of upwards of—"

"Ah, see, there," said Mrs. Murphy. "I'm sorry, I was waiting for something just like that. I'm to kick off from colon cancer, lad, not a stroke or a heart attack or anything quick like that. Plenty of time to get my affairs in order."

A common response, these days. Simon knew the company rote. "Many of our potential customers come to us with this same story, Missus Murphy," said Simon. "Truth to tell, though you may believe that you know the circumstances surrounding your eventual demise based on your prediction alone, the fact of the matter is that the specifics can often be surprising. To both you and your loved ones."

Mrs. Murphy chuckled. "Come now," she said. "Have you ever heard of anyone crossing the street one day and getting hit by a runaway colon cancer?"

Simon had to admit that he had not.

"I'm fairly certain that I'm destined to pass away peacefully in a hospital bed, lad," said Mrs. Murphy. "All shrouded in white and surrounded by my family. Probably in some pain, too, mind, but there's little helping that."

"Missus Murphy, if I might—"

"Lad," said Mrs. Murphy, "I have my fantasy, just as you have yours. And I am unwilling to cheapen it by banking on the possibility that the chips might not fall that way." Her voice smiled again. "You clearly have one of your own. And I think that if you think about it," she said, "you'll understand."

Simon thought about it. And he did.

"Well," he said, after a moment. "Good day to you, then."

"To you as well," said Mrs. Murphy. "May God bless. And say hello to the lions for me."

"Will do, Missus Murphy," said Simon. There was a click as Mrs. Murphy disconnected the line, and then a low, steady drone. Dutifully, Simon's auto-dialer started in on another number.

"Dude," said Scott, the guy in the cubicle next door. "You gotta cut that out. Armbruster is going to be mighty horked if he ever catches you in the middle of that."

Simon pulled his chair closer to his desk, fully intending to ignore his wall-mate, as per usual. After all, he had insurance to sell.

"You can't let this Death Machine crap run your life, man," continued Scott, heedless, as Simon waited for his line to pick up. "I mean, geez, look at you. Ever since you did that stupid prediction thing, you've gone, like, totally mental on us. With the suit, and the tie, and—"

Simon's line picked up; it was an answering machine. Simon dropped his headset to his neck for a moment and rolled his chair back. "Customers can hear the tie, Scott," said Simon. "Just like they can hear a smile."

"Uh huh," said Scott. "So d'ya suppose they can hear this little stain here on my shirt, too?"

"I believe they can," said Simon.

"Wow," said Scott, with feigned amazement. "Those are some really keen ears right there, Simon." He snickered and spun his chair around a couple of times. "Dude, you have lost it, man," he said.

Simon pulled himself back to his desk, replacing his headphones just in time to hear the answering machine disconnect. "To each," he said, with measured patience, "his own."

"I'm sorry, what?" said Scott. "I couldn't hear you there, dude. Between my stain and your tie there's just too damn much noise goin' on around here."

Simon just shook his head as the auto-dialer worked its magic again, preparing to serve him up another golden opportunity. It was hard to get too angry with Scott about his little jibes. After all, thought Simon, Scott was likely bored and a bit depressed and was probably compensating for it by taking his frustrations out on the people around him. But he was fundamentally a good guy. He just needed a life goal or two; it would fix him right up.

It had certainly fixed Simon right up. He himself had two life goals: (1) being torn apart by, and (2) being devoured by, lions.

And that had made all the difference, really.

The morning rolled on in a series of polite refusals, and soon it came time for lunch. Standing by the break room microwave, Simon marveled at how quickly the day was going. It was to be a short lunch; Simon had been thinking of ways to improve the company's sales script, and since the auto-dialer gave him only limited opportunities to hash them out on work-time, he was thinking of devoting some of his break to the task.

"Hey, Simon," said one of his co-workers, coming up from behind. Brad. Blue-eyed, fair-haired and a bit on the pudgy side. Simon and he had joined up with the company about the same time, and Brad had quickly latched on to him as a conversational partner. Simon didn't mind; Brad was, also, a fundamentally good guy. "I'm'a head to Mickey's in a minute. You want I should pick you up some fries or something?"

"Not today, Brad!" said Simon, twirling an empty little coated cardboard box in his hands, the erstwhile contents of which were now warming pleasantly in the microwave nearby. "Today I'm having Rosemary Chicken with Vegetables."

"Rosemary," said Brad, frowning. "Is that an herb or something?"

"Indeed it is," replied Simon.

Brad thought about this for a moment. "So you're eating herbs now?" he said, eventually.

"Yep," said Simon. "It's only polite, I figure. After all, you are what you eat. Right, Brad?"

"Well, I guess I pretty much gotta be a triple-stacker roast beef melt by now," said Brad.

"Quite possibly," said Simon, diplomatically. "But for me? No." Simon smiled to himself, his eyes going distant. "No, Brad, from here on in, I intend to make myself exceptionally, even exquisitely, healthy. And, if possible," he added, "herb-flavored."

Brad narrowed his eyes. "Wait a sec," he said. "This isn't the thing about being eaten by the lions again, is it?"

"It will always be the thing about being eaten by the lions, Brad. From here on in, until it occurs."

"You're obsessed, guy."

Simon grinned. "Perhaps," he said.

"Totally!" called out Scott from his corner table. He sneered at them around and through a mouthful of sandwich.

"Hey, shut up," said Brad.

"Make me, fatboy," Scott replied. Then he chucked a piece of onion at him.

"Little snot," muttered Brad, picking the onion out of his hair. "Look, Simon," he said, putting his hand on Simon's shoulder. "Little friendly advice. You don't have to be a Machine of Death slave like this. Don't be trapped by it. Use it to free yourself." Brad spread his arms wide, exposing his substantial midsection. "I mean, look at me."

"Can't not," said Scott, swallowing his latest bite. "You take up our entire visual field."

"Hmph," said Brad, raising both his chins in a dignified fashion and turning his back to Scott's table. "Look at me, Simon. Here I am, going to die in a car crash or something. So, I don't worry about the roast beef melts anymore. I don't worry about the soda refills. And I don't worry about getting the chili and the cheese on the fries instead of going healthy and eating them without." He smiled amiably. "You see?" he said. "Little changes. I know it won't matter what I eat, so I eat what I want. And I'm happier for it."

Brad shook his head, then. "But you, Simon. You're thinking about this thing all the time now. It can't be good for you."

"I *want* to think about this thing all the time, Brad," said Simon, earnestly. "I am looking forward to it. Like you wouldn't believe."

"For Pete's sake, Simon," said Brad. "Why?"

"Because," Simon replied, his pale brown eyes as wide as the veldt itself, "it will be the most exciting thing that's ever happened to me."

Brad shrugged. "Suit yourself," he said. "But I read in this self-help book my mom gave me that you shouldn't sacrifice your now just because you're looking forward to being eaten by a bunch of lions at some point in the future."

"Don't worry," said Simon. "I'm not sacrificing my now. I'm happier, healthier, and more vital than I've ever been." He smiled. "The thing is, Brad," he said, "everything I do for my lions? It makes my life better too."

There came the sound of a throat clearing from the door of the break room. Simon looked up.

"Pfennig," said Paul Armbruster (Vice President In Charge Of Targeted Media Solicitation), leaning into the room. "When you have a moment. My office, please."

Silence. Simon gathered his smile. "Certainly, sir," he said, tossing the box from his frozen dinner into a nearby waste container and stepping toward the door.

"After lunch is fine," said Mr. Armbruster. The tips of his moustache lifted in a tiny grimace, as though someone had invisibly popped by with an eyedropper full of lemon juice and given him a bit. "But soon. We need to talk about your...performance."

Simon's smile did not falter. "'Performance' in the sense of 'how I'm doing relative to the quota'?"

"No," said Mr. Armbruster, sucking on his tongue thoughtfully. "'Performance' in the sense of 'Ooh, ooh, look at the dancing bear; now look, he's riding a little unicycle.' That type of performance. Specifically," he added, "your performance earlier this morning, Pfennig."

"Right," said Simon, his smile still adamant. "After lunch, then?"

"Yes," said Mr. Armbruster. "If you please." He then vanished from sight.

The subsequent quiet was broken only by the noise of Scott sniggering quietly to himself in the corner.

Brad smiled at Simon, sheepishly.

The microwave went 'ding.'

"Pfennig," said Mr. Armbruster, motioning to the chair opposite his desk with one hand and taking a moment to fine-tune his rather heroic combover with the other. "Sit down, please."

"You wanted to speak with me, sir?" said Simon, taking a seat.

"That is, in fact, why you are sitting in my office right now," said Mr. Armbruster.

A moment passed as Armbruster sucked on his tongue again for a bit. Then he leaned forward and nudged a small brass dish out from behind a fancy little wooden desk clock and over toward Simon.

"Malted milk ball?" he asked.

"Don't mind if I do," said Simon, cheerfully helping himself to one.

Armbruster regarded Simon as he sat, there, crunching. "You understand," he began, "why I brought you in here today."

"I think so," said Simon, swallowing his candy. "You're about to tell me a piece of bad news."

Armbruster sighed. "Simon," he said. "I want to start by telling you that I've been really quite pleased with your new-found gumption and enthusiasm for selling insurance policies over the telephone. You show a level of dedication that is...well, let's say, uncommon in these halls. You remind me a bit of myself when I was your age."

"Thank you, sir," said Simon.

"That having been said," said Armbruster, leaning forward even further, "I need you to stop describing to our potential customers, in gruesome detail, how you're planning on going to Africa and getting eaten by a lion."

"Lions," corrected Simon, politely.

"My point," said Armbruster, "remains a salient one."

"I see," said Simon, biting his lip. "'Gruesome' detail, though, sir?" he asked, then. "I mean, I realize that I've been a bit chatty on the fact to some of them, but—"

Armbruster reached beneath his desk and produced a portable cassette player. He clicked at a button. "—organ meats!" came Simon's voice. "Not as desirable as the muscle meats, mind you, which are frequently claimed by the dominant male of the pride, but certainly full of good, nutritious—"

Armbruster clicked the 'stop' button.

The clock on the desk ticked a handful of times.

"Well...yes," said Simon. "I can see where you might—"

"I don't know if I'm imparting the proper gravity to this situation, Simon," Mr. Armbruster interrupted. "So I will make it perfectly clear to you that I have no desire to see Consolidated Amalgamated Mutual become known as 'That Place With The Guy Who's Always Going On About Lions.' To this end, I am warning you that I absolutely, positively will not tolerate any further behavior of this sort. Do we understand one another, Mister Pfennig?"

"Mm hm!" said Simon, cheerily.

Armbruster narrowed his eyes at Simon. "Let me try this again," he said, picking up a pencil in an attempt to add emphasis to his words. "We are talking about you *losing your job with us,* Simon. You don't want to be unemployed in this city. Not in this economic climate. Trust me."

Simon nodded brightly. "I understand, sir," he said.

"You don't seem like you understand," said Mr. Armbruster. "I'm looking for a little solemnity or something."

Simon pondered for a moment. "Permission to speak freely, sir?"

"This isn't the military, Simon," said Mr. Armbruster.

"Well," said Simon. He gathered himself. "The thing is, sir, it's really hard for me to get worked up at the prospect of losing my job, sir." He raised a hand against Armbruster's objection. "Now, I don't mean that," he continued. "I will try to restrain myself from talking about my lions to the customers from here on in. But if I can't...?" Simon shrugged. "Well, another job will be on the way. After all, I have to fund my African safari *somehow.*" He smiled. "These are more than just idle hopes and dreams now, Mister Armbruster," he said. "They're part of my destiny."

Armbruster regarded Simon for a moment, then shook his head. "You are a strange little guy," said Armbruster. "If you were any less of a salesman, I'd be handing you your pink slip now and personally ushering your behind out of this building while I instructed Stacy to prepare an invoice charging you for the milk ball. But for every lion mutilation story I've got on tape, there're two or more instances of you winning over a stubborn customer on attitude alone. And that's the kind of attitude we need around here. Desperately."

"'Desperately,' sir?" inquired Simon.

Armbruster tapped his pencil on the desk a couple of times. "I don't know if I should even be talking with you about this," he said. "According to the last Board of Directors meeting, Consolidated Amalgamated Mutual isn't doing so well. It's not bad," he added, quickly. "But comparing our first-quarter sales to how we were doing two years ago, well, it's sobering. To say the least. And that's company-wide, Simon. It's not just Targeted Media Solicitation. It's across the board."

He sighed, deeply, and tossed his pencil back into the little cup on his desk. "It's this damn Machine of Death thing, Simon," he said. "We're in the uncertainty business, here. All we've got to offer the world is protection against the frightening, unpredictable future. You give the people something, anything, to latch on to, something that gives them a sense of control—even a false one—and suddenly, well, they don't need us anymore."

"I'm sure we'll come through this all right," Simon volunteered.

"Oh, I know," said Armbruster, pushing his chair back and rising to a stand. "I know. We weathered that damn 'no-call list' thing all right, and I suppose we'll pull through this, too." Armbruster rounded the desk and patted Simon on the back; Simon stood, sensing his cue. "But to do it," said Armbruster, "we're going to need all our salesmen giving us one hundred and ten, or perhaps fifteen, percent. Can you do that for me, Simon?"

"Yes, sir!" said Simon.

"Good," said Armbruster, ushering him to the door. "Now get back out there and sell us some policies, all right?"

"Will do, sir!" said Simon, disappearing out the door.

"And NO LIONS!" added Mr. Armbruster, calling after him. But if Simon Pfennig had a response to this, Mr. Armbruster did not hear it.

He sat back against the corner of his desk for a while after Simon had gone, listening to the whirr of the air-handler and the steady ticking of the clock.

"Wish I were looking forward to my heart attack like that," said Mr. Armbruster.

Night. Home. Simon stood at the sink, washing the last few remnants of tonight's dinner of lamb and parmesan orzo out of his good dishes. In fact, Simon only *had* good dishes, nowadays. He had long since donated the bad ones, and even the slightly dodgy ones, to the local thrift shop. The window over his sink was open to the cool night air, and the crickets outside yammered excitedly among themselves, unable to contain their enthusiasm that evening had arrived again, right on schedule. The dishes had been a bit crusty, as they had been left sitting for several hours, and it felt good to Simon to get them all cleaned up. Easier, perhaps, to have tackled them right after dinner, but Simon had run out of time to wash them before his show had come on the television, and the show took clear precedence because it happened to be all about lions tonight. Simon had, naturally, enjoyed every minute of it.

And Simon knew how ridiculous this all must seem, this arrangement of his entire life around the concept of being Torn Apart And Devoured By Lions. Particularly ridiculous, he felt, was the poster (lionesses, of course) he had tacked to the ceiling—preteen-girl style— right above his bed, so it'd be the last thing he saw at night every night of his life. The lion-themed comforter, too, he knew, went a bit beyond the pale. But really, honestly? The whole thing. Ridiculous.

And, as always, Simon had to conclude that there really was no choice.

It was just too exciting.

The dishes done and dripping in their wire rack, Simon moved on to an invigorating workout on the shiny new exercise bicycle he'd purchased at the mall, and from there on to a relaxing shower. Thusly cleaned up for bed, Simon dressed himself in his lion-print pajamas, snuggled down beneath his leonine blankets, and waited for sleep to come. And, as ever, the last sight that greeted him before he finally shut off his bedside lamp was of his lionesses, all in a row, waiting patiently for him and him alone.

At night he dreamed of them, low and tawny, their eyes luminous in the charcoal African dusk. He welcomed them to him like he might a lover, inviting them in to the limits of his light, inviting them to feed.

"Come, beautiful ones," he whispered to them as they circled close. "Come."

Story by Jeffrey Wells
Illustration by Christopher Hastings

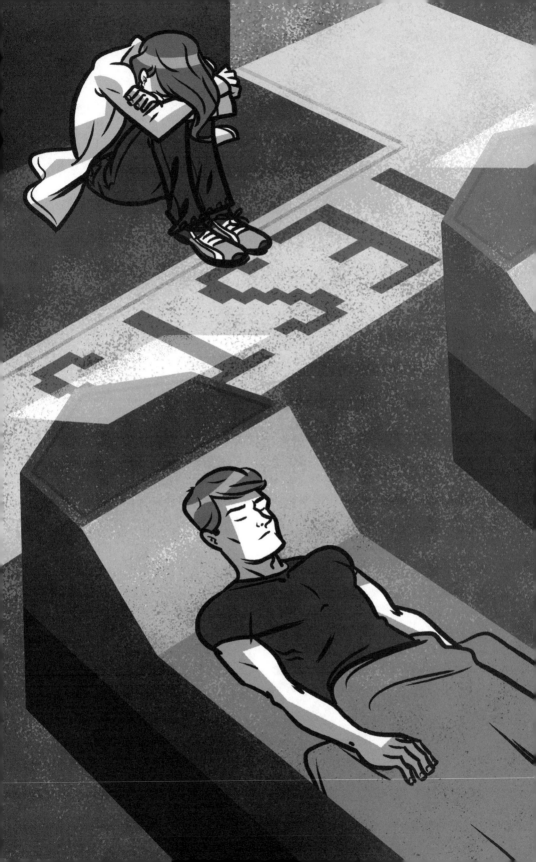

DESPAIR

THEY DIED ANYWAY. Of course they did, that's what those little cards are good for.

The security guards here have a league table of the most impressive death predictions reported in the UK press: "The Cool List," they call it. They got me to phone the doctor whose machine predicted that an eighty-three-year-old bedridden Cardiff woman would die of STUNT PLANE CRASH. I used to feel sick looking at the list, because for a moment a bit inside me would laugh in wonder at the improbabilities written there, and then the moment would pass and I would begin to imagine the Cessna tumbling from the sky, falling down, down, down onto a slate roof under which an old lady was sleeping. The top of the list at the moment is SOLAR FLARE. I have no idea how that one will turn out.

The first one came in twenty-one hours ago, just as I'd started my shift. In the early morning the emergency waiting room was intolerably bright, and I squinted out of the windows—clean enough at midday, but blindingly dirty against the low sun. The call that the ambulance was coming in had been taken by the guy who'd just gone off shift, and I didn't really know what to expect. In theory there is supposed to be some kind of chain of responsibility to keep us all prepared, but in practice, doctors have long shifts and want to go home more than they want to tell you that a middle-aged man is coming in suffering from severe pain and passing blood in his urine.

This is the procedure now: A vehicle comes into the bay, paramedics pull a body out on an unfolding trolley, and a nurse meets them and asks them for the card. Sometimes she smiles, and you know that this one might well walk out of the hospital. Sometimes she gets a stony look on her face and you know that her eyes have flicked across to the patient to see who's going to die. Sometimes—rarely, but sometimes—she frowns. As Nurse Kealing did with that first one.

We doctors don't like to look at the cards. Once upon a time all doctors sounded like Hawkeye Pierce. Death was our enemy, and if you can't point to your enemy, your crusade is noble. You are fighting against the odds, snatching a few more years, months, weeks of life for your patients, defeating your endless foe. But of course, we don't fight that fight anymore. We fight a stiff piece of card, and we know that ultimately we are going to lose. What could be more ignominious than to be defeated by a few grams of wood pulp?

I examined the patient. Late forties, according to the driving license that the paramedics had found, but looking like he might be in his thirties. I had seen people like him at the speed-dating evening the previous Friday, divorcees taking their shot while they still had the time, boring and desperate. He could so easily have been there, and as I directed him to be moved into a nearby observation room I suddenly felt sorry for them. They were alive, and they deserved their chance at a little happiness.

"Marianne," Nurse Kealing said, by my elbow. The other doctors don't like to be called by their first name, but I let the nurses do it because it endears me to them, and they don't complain as much when I land them with paperwork that I should really be doing myself (which I do shamelessly).

"What's the verdict?" I asked her.

"I...uh..." She held out the card to me, and I know that I recoiled, because I haven't touched a card other than my own in five years. "You'd better look for yourself."

I stared at the card without reaching for it, and Nurse Kealing flipped it up so that I could see.

TESTS.

"Shit." I ran back to the doors that lead to the ambulance parking area. The two paramedics that had brought in my patient were trying to manoeuvre out past another ambulance, and as I cleared the doors the driver spotted me and leant on his horn in an effort to scare the other vehicle out of the way. I was too fast for them, though, ducking around the accidental roadblock and intercepting one ambulance as it swerved around the back of the other. They screeched to a halt a few feet in front of me, and I strode over and pulled open the door.

"Before you ask, we didn't do any tests!" The paramedic in the passenger seat cried. The driver, who looked afraid for his life (and in truth I myself felt like pulling him out of his seat and beating him), cringed away from me and nodded.

"You'd better not have," I snarled, and slammed the door shut.

We could barely do anything without the tests, of course. For two hours after he was brought in we watched my patient get weaker and weaker. He passed blood in his urine, but we were too scared to take even that for analysis. That is what the machines have done to us:

they've left us second-guessing reality. We gave him an analgesic to keep him as comfortable as possible, but we all knew that we were not dealing with something that would pass if we treated the obvious symptoms. Something was wrong with him—injury, possibly, more likely a viral or bacterial infection—something that would kill him. But if we tried to discover what was wrong and he died, we would be outside the NHS rules. Clause 14 of the revised patients' charter: Medical staff or hospital trust employees will take no action likely to hasten or lead to a predicted death.

"Realistically," Nurse Kealing argued, "there's no way that testing the blood in his urine can kill him, surely?"

"You know what those fucking machines are like," Doctor Jamison said, shaking his head. "You could trip while carrying the test results back in and stab the poor bastard with a needle." He leaned down and reached for the sheet covering our patient.

"What are you doing?" I asked sharply.

"Nothing."

"It doesn't look like nothing," I told him.

"I'm taking a look, all right? A look, not a fucking test, a look!" I stepped back, and he peered under the sheet at the patient's back. After a few seconds, he stood up again. "Kidneys rather than bladder, definitely."

"So it's going to kill him," I said.

"Yes," he said, in a quiet flat voice.

The second and third ones came in almost together, although I didn't know about the second one until much later. I found out about the third one from Doctor France, who saw me standing at the vending machine in the lobby. I was deciding whether to have a Crunchy or a packet of Nik Naks, and had been trapped in that deci-sion-making process for three minutes. Perhaps I wanted to make a difference to something, however trivial.

"Hello Marianne," he said. "Are you doing anything tomorrow night?"

"Going out with my boyfriend," I lied. I don't have a boyfriend. I occasionally fuck one of our security guards in the supply closet –an ex-policeman who was fired because his card read SHOT. The Northampshire police force have one of the lowest reported incidents of gun crime in the UK, and it would have been a terrible public relations blow to have a policeman shot on duty. I like him because he keeps himself in shape, and because he has an ex-wife and a child who take up all the emotional energy that he would otherwise spend developing feelings for me.

Doctor France flinched. Perhaps he knows, I thought.

"Anyway," he said, plastering on a smile. "I've got something a bit interesting, thought you might enjoy wrestling with a little problem. We've got a young woman in with blood in her urine, probably simple urinary tract infection." An ice sheet spread out from my spine. "Thing is, her card says..."

"TESTS," I interrupted him.

He looked at me quizzically.

"How did you know?"

Patient Two was in a room at the other end of the ward, being treated by one of the junior doctors. Patients Four and Five we found by calling the emergency admissions at Kettering, and Patient Six, a thin middle-aged woman in old clothes, came in a few hours later. I could see instantly that she could understand the way things were headed, because she was arguing strenuously in Italian with her husband and in somewhat less eloquent English with the two grown-up daughters that accompanied them. She wanted to go home, and she must have understood what we did, that her devoted family's wish to help might be the death of her.

We gave her painkillers and I talked to them, individually and as a group. But for bad timing I think she would have persuaded them to let her go home, but about a quarter of an hour after they arrived, I noticed that she was beginning to fade somewhat, and five minutes later she fell unconscious. At that point we had to give her the same care we were giving the others, and we moved all four of the local patients into the same ward. Doctors France and Jamison argued endlessly with me over the treatments we could give, but all of our arguments came to nothing.

Without knowing the cause of the distress, any actions we took were more likely to be harmful than helpful (and more likely still to have no effect at all other than to waste time).

I got desperate and handed the details of the patients over to Joe (my occasional tryst)—strictly against hospital policy, because security staff do not generally need access to confidential medical records, or indeed any kind of patient information. I thought he might be able to shed some light on a possible connection between the unfortunate four patients at our hospital—and if he had found one I might have been able to persuade our equivalent numbers at Kettering to hand over the equivalent information about their unfortunates. Despite a bit of help from some old friends of his at the local police station it was all dead ends. The six people lived near each other, but not near enough to form a cluster for the purposes of determining some environmental cause.

There were no common work links, and no social connection. There was a moment of excited hope when he discovered that the serial numbers on the back of two of the cards showed identical mistakes in the printing, but neither of the other two cards showed any similar signs. So two of the patients had been diagnosed by the same machine—probably at roughly the same time—but that was the only connection we could find.

"Almost certainly a coincidence," he told me sadly. "I mean, I'll keep looking if you like, but don't rely on me to turn up anything useful anytime soon."

"Fine," I said, and left him to it. I was grateful to him for trying, for giving me that moment of hope that we might find some way to cheat the machines (if only for today), but I couldn't show it. That wasn't the way it worked between us.

We got the two patients from Kettering transferred over by ambulance—it was easy, no one wanted responsibility for them. Even with all six of the sufferers together we could find out no extra information.

It was Doctor France who finally said it.

"What if we just start," he said quietly.

"We can't."

"We have to do something, what we can't do is just let them die." He shot me a sullen look. "I can't, anyway."

"What's that supposed to mean?"

"Nothing." He shook his head. "Look, I'm tired. I know it's not good, but we have to start some kind of tests. They're not going to last much longer."

"Just one then," Jamison interjected.

"What?"

"You know what those damn machines are like. TESTS could mean a completely different thing for everyone here. Maybe only some of them are at risk from the tests we might do. God, we do tests all the time."

"And people die from them. Even people without cards. If we start," I spoke slowly and calmly, "we know what will happen."

The three of us stood silent, watching the six patients and listening to the muted sounds of bustle and activity coming from the corridor outside the ward. A strange sensation came over me, as though the world were receding—as though I were looking at it through a long tunnel. My hands were hard to move, as though I had slept in the cold, my muscles stiff and unresponsive. With an effort, I walked to the foot of Patient One and read out the details at the top of his chart.

"Brian Felton, 47." I turned it sideways. In the margins of the chart, Nurse Kealing had written in pencil. "Wife and two children," I read aloud.

Replacing the chart, I moved to the next bed.

"Simon Lines, 23. Girlfriend brought him in."

"Janice Greg," said France without looking at the chart. "She's 31, unmarried, a schoolteacher." He turned to the fourth bed, the old woman transferred from Kettering. "Maud Carver, 63. You'd guess from the name, wouldn't you—who calls anyone Maud anymore?" He looked down at the chart again. "Widowed."

Doctor Jamison picked up the fifth and sixth charts, one in each hand. From the left: "Louise Burdon, 28. One kid." From the right: "Emilia Strabbioli, 51. Married, two daughters, one son, one grandson." He put the charts back on their hooks, and we stood back and looked at the six bodies laid out before us.

"Are we really considering this?" Jamison asked.

"No, we can't consider it," I said. The others looked at me. "We have to just do it."

"It can't be Brian or..." France pointed to the fifth one.

"Louise," Jamison supplied. "Or Emilia. No one with children."

"Janice is young," France said. "Simon, too."

They looked at me.

"So we're going to kill Maud because she's the oldest?" I asked.

"She hasn't got any..." France began, but Jamison interrupted him.

"We're not going to kill her at all. We're going to test her."

"And the tests are going to kill her," I nodded. "Have the balls to admit it."

He sighed, shrugged, and walked over to pick up the chart. "Says here she had a stroke two years ago."

"So? Look, she made it two years, who's to say she won't make it another thirty?"

"Plus," said France carefully, "that's exactly the kind of thing that makes me nervous. Given her stroke, I'd be a bit careful what tests I did on her anyway." He walked over and took the chart away from Jamison, scanned it, then put it back on the hook. Then he turned back to the third patient. I could tell he was thinking something that he didn't like, and I realised what it was going to be. She was his patient, of course, he had been charged with making her well again. "Perhaps we should consider Janice."

Jamison picked up the schoolteacher's chart.

"She's healthy," France continued. "Least likely to have any trouble with the tests, I'd say." He smiled. "Hey, I've just thought of something. She's a teacher, right? Perhaps the stress of grading is what's going to get her! It could be nothing to do with this at all. Of all of them, she's the most likely to survive, right?" He nodded at Jamison and me, trying to convince himself by convincing us.

I ignored his pleading and pointed to my own patient. "Why save Felton?" I asked.

"He has kids."

"He's a shit," I spat. "He beats them. He screws around, and he's given his wife the clap."

"Jesus, Marianne!" France slapped my hand down. "He might be able to hear you! That's not funny!"

I saw Jamison's eyes flick down to my balled fists.

"No, wait." He pulled France back by the shoulder.

"She's..." France protested.

"I see what she means," Jamison said, staring past France directly at me. France had believed he was talking to him, of course. "We can't make this decision. We can't just do this based on our prejudices. That's how the cards beat us. They use us against ourselves."

He was wrong, of course, but we had to tell France something to make him listen to sense.

"There's only one thing to do," I told them.

I found the box in the waiting room—there's a little pile of books and toys to keep kids occupied while we talk with the parents. Most of it was for the smaller children, but there was a wooden box of classic games that had a backgammon board. I don't suppose it had ever been used. Half of the white counters were missing, but I found most of the red ones and one of the dice, which I scooped up into my pocket and carried back to our ward.

"We make up something to tell the families, of course," I told France and Jamison, then rolled the die on top of the defibrillator cart. I saw two come face up for a moment, two black sockets in a white face, then it was past and the cube came to a rest.

"Five," said France.

"Louise," Jamison corrected him.

They died anyway. Of course they did, that's what those little cards are good for. The first round of tests showed nothing, so we took more blood from Louise. That's when she began to bleed under the skin around where we'd put the needle in. Pretty soon she was convulsing, and then her vitals began to deteriorate and her heart stopped.

While the tests were coming back, Maud stopped breathing. We revived her, but her brain had been without oxygen for too long. When she stopped breathing again, we couldn't bring her back. Nurse Kealing brought the test results back: some viral activity, but sadly not characteristic enough for us to work out what we were dealing with.

The die rolled five again, then two. So we took blood from Simon. He survived, but we got the same inconclusive results, during which time Brian and Emilia had both gone. We gave the young man antivirals, but his condition deteriorated faster, and he died two hours after Emilia. Finally we watched Janice Greg's heart rate get slower and slower until finally she, too, left us.

We had been watching the six of them for close to a day on and off. France and Jamison looked like corpses themselves, grey-faced and without a hint of emotion. It had drained everything from them—not just the deaths, but what those cards had forced us to do. I left them to it, slipping off quietly to find Joe.

The causes of death were hemorrhagic fever with renal failure, or so the pathologists determined. I didn't feel like anyone was to blame—who could have suspected a hantavirus outbreak in the midlands? No other cases were reported, and the investigators were unable to trace any more connections than we had.

I have Brian's card in my wallet. I keep it next to mine, because that night its prediction came a little bit closer. I take Brian's out when I am alone, and stare at the word. I am still unable to under-stand what it meant. Was it the tests, I wonder, or the lack of tests? Did the word mean the same thing for all of those six? Did it mean hospital tests, exams, what?

The thoughts run through me like water, ever changing. But there is one I come back to: Who was being tested?

Story by K. M. Lawrence
Illustration by Dean Trippe

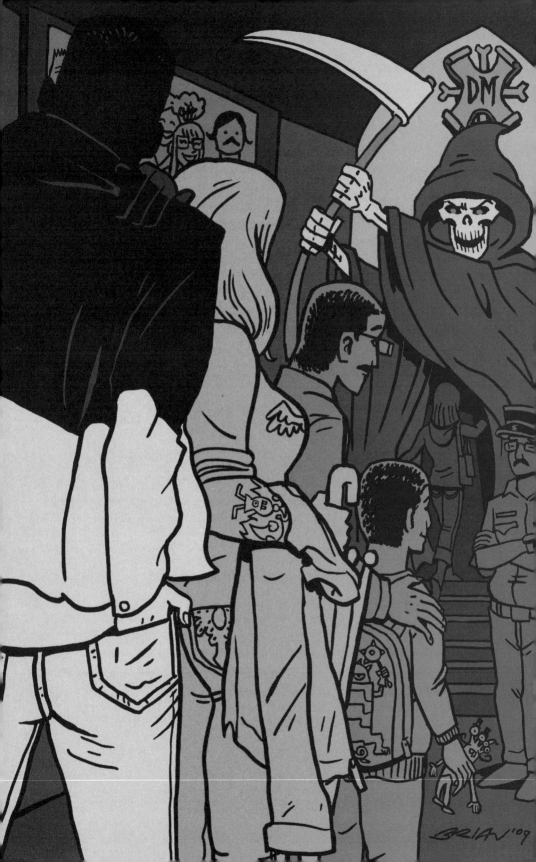

SUICIDE

THE CLERK SET THE GUN ON THE COUNTER.

"There's a seven-day waiting period."

Tommy peeled off an extra couple hundreds and slid them across the counter. The clerk hesitated, then pocketed the bills and loaded the weapon into a brown paper bag.

"Some weeks are shorter than others."

He added a box of bullets to the bag, then rang up the total. "You need any extra ammo?"

"No," replied Tommy. "One box will be plenty."

It was pissing rain on the walk back to his apartment, the first time it had rained in the city for months. The water cut greasy rivers down his cheeks, tasting faintly of gasoline and ash. *At least the city's consistent,* he thought, *even the rain's corrupt.* He ducked into a familiar coffee shop to douse the chill. He ordered what he always ordered and dug in his pockets for exact change.

"Can you believe those freaks?"

Tommy followed the kid's gaze out the front window, across the street. A pack of No-Faters gathered on the corner, their placards bleeding ink as they fought to keep a fire alive in a trash bin. One of them, a chubby white kid with unconvincing dreadlocks, pulled out a white card, the size of the index cards Tommy's students used to cram notes onto before exams, and tossed it into the fire. He stepped back, arms out, relishing the cheers of approval the protesters poured out at him.

"Yeah, you're home free now, asshole," said the kid behind the counter. He finished with Tommy's order and passed the steaming cardboard cup to him. "What's that shit supposed to accomplish?"

Tommy shrugged. "It's a symbol. Rage against the dying of the light, that sort of thing. Just human nature."

"More like rage against getting a job, the stupid hippies." The kid flipped a rag off his apron string and wiped down the counter where Tommy's cup had spilled a few drops. "You wanna know what my card says? Burned to death. Bad news, right? Not exactly the finest hand in the deck, right? But I still smoke. 'Cause what's the point? Way I see it, the way we're gonna die is the way we're gonna die. That's the way it's always been, motherfucking death machine or no motherfucking death machine."

Tommy didn't say anything, just slugged back half the cup of coffee, letting it burn his throat, not caring. Outside, the rain had stopped as the No-Faters tossed another card onto the altar of inevitability.

He dropped the envelope into the mailbox. He'd written it all out, the whole thing, the night before in his motel room. As he watched Mel's address—her new address—swallowed by the box's maw, he marveled at how much life could change with the rearranging of a few letters and numbers. She should get it by the end of the week, but she'd already know by then. She would have heard about it on the news, or someone would have told her. He'd be the name on a thousand pundits' lips before rush hour. Lots of people asking why, but she'd be the only one with the answer. It felt right that way.

As he waited for the crosswalk light to change, he noticed the bar across the street. There was always a bar within walking distance of these places, without fail, or a liquor store. They were like remoras, feeding from the belly of the Death Machine wherever it sprang up. He could see a few of them in there now, heads down, that uniquely blank look on their faces. Some of them had their death cards laid out on the bar, staring as if waiting for the ink to shift, for the universe to hiccup, for destiny to laugh and admit, "Just kidding." Others laughed and caroused, to all appearances celebrating a promotion at work rather than a glimpse at their own end.

Tommy waited in line, smiled at the girl behind the glass partition, and forked over $11.50 for his ticket. The Death Machines were everywhere now—doctor's offices, mall kiosks. They were both wholly remarkable and thoroughly mundane. Not this one, though. This one was the first. The first Death Machine ever, entombed in a glass-and-chrome building that was half museum and half theme park. If you turned Auschwitz into a theme park.

Tommy ignored the huge plasma screens somberly reciting the history of this holy temple, the narrator's voice smooth and comforting as the screens displayed the most famous photograph in the world. The first Death Machine, its creators lined up behind it, grinning with the pride of those who know they've changed the world. He'd heard the rumors, of course, that the whole thing had been an accident, that they'd been trying to create something else and only stumbled ass-over-teacups backward into their discovery. Either way, they were all rich as sin now, at least the ones that were still alive.

Not so the older man with a smile like Norman Rockwell's grandpa, who had eaten a shotgun barrel six months after that photo was taken. Tommy wondered if he'd bothered to look at his death card first. Was it the knowing that drove him to that end, or the not knowing? Did it even really matter?

Tommy joined the queue that snaked its way up to the Machine. It was a weekday, so the crowds were light. It only took a minute or so until he reached the front of the line. The Machine's words greeted him, the same as they always greeted everyone. "Please insert your finger." It was a sentence that had become the punchline to a thousand jokes and monologues and headlines over the past few years, but Tommy didn't think any of them were funny. The least they could have done was polish up the death sentence a little. Maybe hire some *New York Times* bestseller to do a pass, come up with something really snappy, something to bring a smile to your face on the bus ride home.

He winced as the needle pierced his fingertip, sucked at the tiny pearl of blood that peered out. The Machine buzzed, flashed "Thank you," and spit out the card. He took it and moved aside to let the redheaded woman behind him have her turn. She was young, maybe nineteen, and from the way she was shaking, she'd never done this before. He wasn't sure whether to envy her that.

He read the card, just one word. Seven letters, no substitutions. So final, and yet, in a way, so freeing. Tommy had never worried about car accidents or plane crashes or cancer. The same word that doomed him had also rendered him, in a way, untouchable. Was he only here because of the word? Would he have had the courage to do what needed to be done if the word were different? He smeared blood across the card, tossed it into a nearby trash can along with his doubts. He reached in his pocket, felt the shape of the gun, solid and comforting.

The red-haired woman stepped over, her eyes glued to the card, welling up. She was pale as her legs gave out and she lowered herself to the floor. He crouched next to her.

"First time?"

She looked at him, but didn't seem to see him at first. Then her eyes focused, and she brushed at the tears with the back of her hand. "Yeah. I guess I wasn't really ready for it."

Her other hand white-knuckled the card. Tommy could read part of her word, "Explo—", the rest eclipsed by her fingers.

"I haven't met anybody yet who is." He pulled a tissue out of the pocket without the gun and offered it to her.

"It could be wrong."

Tommy smiled. "It could be. They say it's infallible, but it only has to be wrong once, right?"

She smiled back at him, weakly, then looked sick to her stomach. She shook her head. "My mom told me not to get checked. She said it was better not to know. Now there's no taking it back, you know? It's like...now nothing else I do matters."

He stood up, one hand sliding back to his pocket, wrapping around the gun. He offered her his other hand, and she took it, her knees barely finding the strength to stand. For a moment, the curve of her face reminded him of Mel, and he felt his commitment wavering. Did he have the right? But then his eyes turned to the screen above, to the photograph, to the smiling faces. Did he have the right? Did they? They'd killed the whole world. She would die to—just maybe—restore it to life.

"What's your name?" he asked.

"Alice."

His thumb caressed the back of her hand. "Alice, I want you to close your eyes."

On any other day, she might have been suspicious, but today he was human contact, he was comfort, and that was enough. She closed her eyes.

Tommy pulled the gun from his pocket, locked the hammer back. He thought of his word, and her word, and billions of tiny little soulless goddamn cards around the world, each with their own word.

It only had to be wrong once, he told himself. Just once.

He lifted the gun, aiming at the center of her forehead.

Except...

His stomach wrenched as a terrible realization hit him. He envisioned the hammer falling, the spark, the bullet driven forward by the explosion. By the *explosion*. The Machine, the damned Machine, would still win by technicality.

He staggered back away from her, and she opened her eyes, confused. She gasped as she saw the gun in his hand. He spun, back toward the front of the line, toward the sound of the Machine vomiting up a new proclamation of doom. It wasn't too late. He could still beat it. He leveled the gun at the man at the front of the line, trenchcoat and wild hair.

"You!"

He heard screams from the crowd, the squawk of walkie-talkies and the clatter of security guards' booted feet. He only had seconds. He closed the distance, jammed the gun barrel against the man's head.

"What does your card say?"

The man's card lay in the machine's tray, face down, future unwritten. The man was calm—why was he so calm?

Tommy screamed: "Pick it up and tell me what it says!"

The man smiled at him.

Furious, frantic, Tommy grabbed the card, flipped it over, reeled from déjà vu. The card read: "Suicide."

The man shrugged. His trenchcoat hit the floor. Tommy saw the wires circling the man's chest, through the gray claylike bricks, leading up to what looked like a TV remote in the man's hand. Tommy thought it was odd; it looked just like it always did in the movies.

"No fate," said the man, an edge of madness in his eyes.

Tommy wanted to laugh as the man pressed the button. The Machine never said it was *his* suicide.

It only had to be wrong once.

But not today.

Story by David Michael Wharton
Illustration by Brian McLachlan

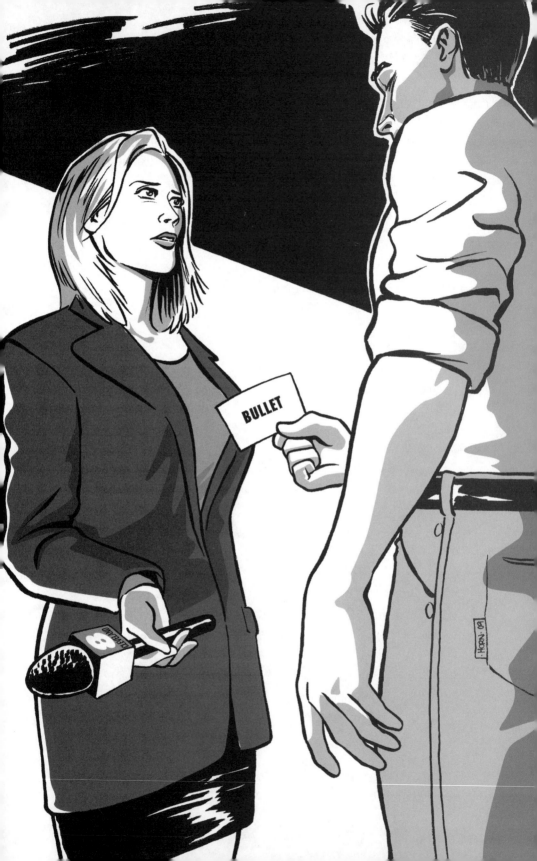

ALMOND

Administration and Maintenance Log, Cleveland Office

Feb 25 - No user requests. Tested samples 1-4. No problems.

Mar 4 - No user requests. Tested samples 1-4. No problems.

Mar 11 - No user requests. Tested samples 1-4. No problems.

Mar 18 - No user requests. Tested samples 1-4. No problems.

Mar 25 - No user requests. Tested samples 1-4. No problems.

Apr 1 - No user requests. Tested samples 1-4. Lab destroyed.

Apr 8 - No user requests. Tested samples 1-4. No problems.

Apr 15 - No user requests. Tested samples 1-97. No problems.

Apr 22 - No user requests. Tested samples 1-4. All predicted death by Mr. Potato Head.

Apr 29 - No user requests. No samples tested. No one is reading this log anyway.

May 6 - No user requests. I am beginning to suspect there's a fundamental problem with a machine that tells people how they're going to die, i.e. no one wants to know. However, we can all sleep soundly tonight knowing that, once again, Sample A dies by CRASH, Sample B dies by HEART, Sample C dies by SUICIDE, and Sample D dies by ALMOND, whatever the hell that means.

May 13 - No requests. How much, exactly, did we pay for this, and why was that money not put toward raises for the lab techs?

May 20 - No requests. Almonds continue to be deadly.

May 27 - Machine continues to predict the deaths of the four test samples. I continue to write entries in a book no one else will ever read. In fact, I asked Paul why he thought we weren't getting any requests, and he said he didn't even realize we had a machine yet. Way to spend the grant money, guys. Does anyone other than me even know we've had this thing since February? The samples were all printed on these neat, white business cards, like the kind you write your phone number on in a bar. "Why don't we get together, baby? Just call me SUICIDE. Please don't say no." You couldn't make me try this thing on myself for a million dollars. I'm certain the result would be MACHINE MALFUNCTION.

Jun 3 - I'm starting to wish I would have taken the job in Tulsa. The sample results on this machine are A) kind of creepy, B) a waste of time, and C) annoyingly vague. These samples are all from people who died already, right? If the guy choked on an almond, shouldn't it say CHOKING? Or was he allergic? The other three are pretty straightforward, although now I think about it, CRASH could be a plane crash or a car crash. Or even a bike crash, I guess. They should send something that says how they died.

Jun 10 - I'm tired of looking at the machine, but there's nothing else to look at. Maybe it's supposed to wear down my defenses and get me to take the test, but I've made my decision. So I sit and stare at it. My planner is black with the blood of my tormented doodles. There is a brick wall outside my window. What's on the other side? My guess is that it's a locker room, and there are dozens of hot naked chicks inside, all with a thing for underpaid lab technicians who could, at the drop of a hat, tell them how they're going to die.

Jul 1 - One request. (!) Results were kept confidential. Tested samples 1-4. No problems.

Jul 8 - No requests. I'm a little intrigued by the idea that someone in town knows how he is going to die. The rest of us are going on with our lives, worrying about paying bills or finding a good school system for the kids, but this one guy is nervously eyeing the mixed nuts aisle in the grocery store, or whatever. He's got that little insight that no one in town (except me) knows about. I'm Alfred to his Batman, except I don't know what's on his card. Just that he knows what's on his card. Unfortunately, I can't think of anyone in comics who knows that someone *has* a secret identity, but doesn't know what it is.

Jul 15 - Four requests. Apparently word is getting around. Three of them, all men, came and left, and I can only wonder what the machine says fate has in store for them. But the woman wanted to show the result to me. It was printed out on the same business card as the test samples, only hers said CANCER. She was really shaken up about it. I felt really bad for her, but then after she left, I thought what the hell, lady, what do you expect? It's going to tell you how you die, right? You should probably be expecting cancer. In fact, it wouldn't be a bad idea for the machine to have a label on it that says "Warning: Expect Cancer." It's not like it says you'll get cancer tomorrow or anything. Seriously, we've had this thing for half a year now, and I see the first real result, and I think the whole machine is a bad idea. Plus, I haven't seen any evidence that it's even right! I'm the resident expert on this destiny-meter by dint of being the only person who's read through the manual, but I don't like it, and I don't know if it works. And I refuse to use it on myself. Tell me that's not screwed up. I wonder if the lab in Tulsa has one of these stupid things.

Jul 21 - From this spot on my chair you can see exactly 64 bricks. Sixty-four is divisible by two, four, eight, sixteen, and thirty-two. That's four to the third power, or two to the sixth power. There are 64 squares on a chess board, of which 32, or one half, are taken up by pieces in the beginning of the game. Every time there's a pawn exchange, one-sixteenth (or 6.25%) of the pieces are removed from the board, thus freeing up one thirty-secondth (or 3.125%) of the board. Just thought I'd share. 64. 64. 64. Oh yeah, and, apparently I wasn't the only one that lady talked to last week. Paul told me today that she *currently* has cancer. She was told by her doctor that it went into remission. I guess I can see why she was so upset. Well, all the more reason not to use the machine. There were another five requests this week, and I got to see a couple. The first was another CANCER (plus, the guy was totally a smoker), but I don't think I was supposed to see it. I just happened to see the card when he looked at it. And then, get this, the other guy got JOY. If you're gonna go, that's the way to do it, I guess. I totally want to hear about this guy getting smothered in an orgy somewhere. Well, I mean, not immediately.

Jul 21 - All right. Being honest here, I guess I was thinking sooner rather than later. Pretty bad, huh? Does spending a long boring day with a death machine make you cavalier about death? Well, the guy will be happy at least.

Jul 22 - I just thought of "Almond Joy". Seriously, this machine is probably sponsored by Hershey's. On the other hand, between ALMOND and JOY, it's predicted cancer and heart attacks. Maybe it's sponsored by a competitor. Nestlé or something. Their new slogan is probably "sometimes you feel like death by a nut, sometimes you feel like some other kind of death." If someone tells me that his cause of death is MOUNDS, I'm swearing off candy bars for good.

Jul 28 - Two people came in for predictions this week, and apparently they didn't want to share their information. Wusses. In the meantime, things here are ridiculously boring. I've spent the last three hours staring at a machine that wants to tell me how I die. Alternatively, I could look out the window, and stare at 64 bricks in a big brick wall. Why put in a window at all? Are there people on the other side of the wall, wondering what's in here? No, because that wall doesn't have any windows. So with the lack of things to do, my mind has gone to dangerous places. I have been sitting here thinking that Dr. Womack had a bloody nose this morning. It would be easy (if a little gross) to fish a tissue out of his garbage can and find out how he dies. I would know, and he wouldn't. And what if it were CHLAMYDIA or something? That's the kind of information I could use to get a corner office. Then I'd have something to look at, and I wouldn't have to sit and think about ways to blackmail my damn coworkers.

Aug 4 - The woman with cancer came back in today. Her name's Beth. Her doctor said that her cancer poses no threat and now she wanted a second opinion from the machine. I told her that part of the machine's maintenance is rechecking the same four test samples and they've never changed. (I did not mention that I've been neglecting my samples testing for a while.) Beth wanted to try again anyway. CANCER, again. So many people are so fiercely private about their cards. It's really awkward that Beth shows hers off to anyone she meets, and then talks about it. It seems so personal. It's like finding your neighbors' secret sex tapes. You're curious as hell to see them, but as soon as you hit play, you know you shouldn't have. And then you give them back to your neighbor, but they see you leave it in their mailbox and they're like, "what did you think about the part with the trampoline," and you wish you'd never heard of videotapes or neighbors or sex in the first place. Probably. Anyway, the conversation with Beth was uncomfortable. She said if she could start over again, she wouldn't have taken the test. She'd prefer not to know. I told her that I'd never seen any indication that this particular machine is accurate. If it were spewing out lies all this time, I'd have no way of knowing. They're just consistent lies, that's all. All I was going on to vouch for its accuracy was the pamphlet that came with the machine. I don't think my argument was as persuasive as her getting the same results twice, though. She wasn't very happy when she left. It's too bad. She seems really nice.

Aug 11 - Things are picking up again. Eight people. And now that Beth is gone, I find that my qualms about knowing other people's deaths have completely disappeared again. I'm just a peeping Tom. Bring on the trampoline!

Aug 18 - Our office has death fever. It's actually less morbid than it sounds. I just mean that a bunch of the folks here suddenly got really interested in finding out how they're going to kick the bucket. All right, maybe it's exactly as morbid as it sounds. I wonder if they all went out for lunch last week and talked about it over drinks or something. I never got invited. I spend my lunches with my good friends Bricky and the Fatal Fortune-Teller. A bunch of people came in as a group to get their death cards, so I got to watch them share. I've got some interesting coworkers: Paul is going to die by FALL, Tammy from HR got LIGHTNING, and Mitch got OVERDOSE. He seemed to think it was pretty funny, but Tammy got a strange look on her face. Mitch had never struck me as the kind of guy who would take drugs irresponsibly, but, you know, there are an awful lot of drugs around here in the office that he has access to. And he took a trip with his girlfriend to Amsterdam last Christmas. Hmmmm... Mike from accounting got the weirdest one: GOVERNMENT. How do you die by government? Will he commit treason? Get drafted? Maybe he'll happen upon who really killed JFK. Paul tried to get me to do it, but I refused. First of all, I still don't want to know. Second, I don't want other people to know. Third, I don't have any proof that this thing works. I don't know if they think this machine is like a party game, or if they all just really want to know how they die, but I stare at this thing every day, and I'm maybe a little scared of it.

Aug 25 - Apparently, getting your death foretold by a machine isn't covered by insurance. Paul was fuming yesterday, but I think he's crazy. Do you really want your insurance company to know how you are going to die? I'd think your auto premiums would skyrocket if your insurance company knew your death card said CRASH. They probably wouldn't cover you at all. In related news, inventory showed that one lab was missing over a thousand dollars' worth of stimulants. That's serious business. Everyone thinks it's Mitch. He looks miserable, but the question is: Is he miserable because he's been caught, or because he's stopped taking stimulants? Or is it possible that he's innocent, and he's miserable because everyone thinks he's stealing from the company?

Sep 1 - Mitch is gone. Whether he stole anything is still uncertain, but he apparently missed a conference when he was in Amsterdam with his girlfriend, and that's the official reason he's canned. Sounds a little trumped-up to me. No one made a big deal out of the conference then. I tried to talk to Paul about it, but he didn't seem concerned. Did he not make the connection between Mitch getting laid off and drawing the card that says OVERDOSE? Or is he just preoccupied by when and where he's going to fall to death? There's been a steady stream of people coming in asking for the test. I guess there was a bit on the news about it last night. Someone in New York took the test, and when she found out it said SUICIDE, she killed herself. Does that justify that the Morbid Medium Machine works? I think it means that people with suicidal tendencies shouldn't use the stupid machine. I was thinking it would be nice if the machine would print the number for a suicide helpline every time someone got SUICIDE, but I guess it would be pretty futile. I mean it doesn't say they'll attempt suicide. It says they'll die by suicide. Someone else got GOVERNMENT yesterday. I wanted to refer him to Mike, but there are confidentiality rules that I would be breaking. I'm like a priest. I store all these confessions, and I'm forbidden to say anything. A priest tells the confessions to God, and I tell the predictions to the maintenance log. Plus, I'm not getting laid, so that's another thing I have in common with priests. I wonder if Batman has a priest. Anyway, maybe Mike already knows this guy from their top secret anti-government cabal.

Sep 8 - Wow. A family came in today, with two kids, and only the father spoke English. He made them all take the blood test. They looked terrified. And every single one of them came up with the same result: FIRE. I told the dad, and he got this weird faraway look in his eyes, and then he got really mad at me. He threw the cards back at me and called me a crook, told me to stay the hell away from him. Then he gathered up the whole family, all of them staring at me, and stormed off. I've been shaking for the last hour. I don't think he's going to tell his family. Well fine, I guess I'd rather not know, so maybe they're better off not knowing. But...how will not knowing help them prevent a fire? Or, if the machine really is accurate, is it too late to prevent it now?

Sep 15 - Well, the machine works, I guess. It's just got a sick sense of humor. The guy whose card said JOY died over the weekend. No orgy, no heart attack from winning the lottery. He was run over walking home from the library. By a woman named Joy. That's really messed up. I'm sort of freaking out over this. How does a machine know the name of the person who runs you over? And why wouldn't it say RUN OVER? The sample card said CRASH, not the driver's name. It's like it was toying with him. Is that what it was? A joke? A machine joking about death? It sounds stupid but why not? I mean, a machine isn't going to die, right? That's the big advantage to being a machine. Finally, after doing every little thing we've told them to do, a machine is lording something over us. Seriously, no wonder it says ALMOND. It delights in being ironically vague. I hate this thing. I'm sleeping with the lights on tonight.

Sep 23 - I had someone come in for a second visit today because—get this—he lost his card and forgot what it said. He forgot. Did I just meet the stupidest person in America? Is this person the reason that my instruction manuals are 60% warnings and all the good TV shows are canceled in favor of pap? I told him he should write it down next time. Speaking of how death makes people stupid, there was a new announcement from Tammy in Human Resources. All new employees will be subject to getting a readout from the death machine. I am required to pass on the results to her. Current employees are strongly encouraged to share their results with Human Resources, but it's not required. I don't like the sound of that. Also, I've gotten a ton of people coming in, with a lot of vague results. The JOY thing has me second-guessing all of them. One man got RAM. He was thinking goat. I'm thinking Dodge. So he'll probably get smashed in a battering ram, just to prove us both wrong. Another one was BLOCKAGE. Will his arteries be blocked? Will his way to the hospital be blocked? Poor Beth is probably going to be killed by someone born in July. And what about Fallin' Paul? I keep wondering if there's a way autumn could kill him. Tammy already knows his card, and Mike's, and a bunch of others. I've been trying to keep an ear to the wall to hear if anyone else who has taken the test will lose their jobs. I've heard that Dr. Caine drew SHIV. If that doesn't spell bad news for your future, I don't know what does.

Sep 30 - Someone managed to stump the machine, from the looks of things. His card said $C◼KLE. What does that mean? Death by aliens? I asked if he had any ideas. He said he was in a really bad car accident, and keeps having dreams about car accidents every night, and wanted to know if that's what would kill him. No, lucky you, you'll be killed by a $C◼KLE, which for all I know could be a new kind of car invented ten years from now. I called our distributor at EndVisions, and they're going to send someone out to see if there's a problem with the machine. I have taken the liberty of hiding this log in my desk, and getting a new one that makes it look like I've been running the same four tests every week and that we've had all kinds of users who always keep their results confidential (except for Mr. $CINKLE). I'm a little worried that I screwed it up somehow. I guess if he gets mad, I'll blame it on the fact that I'm stuck in a room with no view and a death machine, and understandably, it made me temporarily insane.

Oct 7 - Well, I can take comfort in knowing that the EndVisions tech isn't any more knowledgeable than I am. Actually, I take no comfort in this at all. Neil, the rep who came in, had no idea why the machine would say JOY when it meant RUN OVER. Or what it means when the sample says ALMOND. I'm disappointed. I kind of trusted the distributor to know these things. Neil's pretty sure that Mr. $CINKLE won't die from a car accident. He guessed the cause of death was a dollar, a penny, and a nickel, like he'd make a deal with a loan shark but end up being a day late and $1.06 short. So, like I said, Neil's no expert. Maybe this will be a mystery for the ages. He was impressed with my (fake) record-keeping, but even more impressed with the way the office has embraced the machine. He said that most offices don't usually use it on their own employees, much less factor the results into their hiring practices. He was even talking about using our lab as an example of EndVisionary Thinking in the next newsletter. Apparently Neil helps edit it. He asked what my card said, and I lied and told him ELECTROCUTION. His card said STROKE. He seemed proud of that fact. He plans to go skydiving next summer, since he knows it won't kill him. I immediately thought that he'd land in a lake, try to do a breaststroke, get a cramp, and die. I did not mention this to him.

Oct 14 - I was interviewed for a news story. Candace Harrelson, the reporter, wanted me to tell her what some of the stranger results have been, but I didn't tell her much. I said that some of the more typical results are CANCER, CRASH, and HEART. I also mentioned the ALMOND one, and they asked me to verify that one guy whose card said JOY. Candace came in knowing a lot already. I don't think

I was much help to Channel 5 Prime Time News. Apparently the story is going to be about how the machine is sometimes cryptic, but never wrong. They've compiled results from machines throughout the country, and have two dozen predictions that have all come true. Candace even volunteered to find out her own results. They filmed me drawing the blood and everything. She was talking about how easy the process is, and how the results are printed up on a single business card, with the same results every time. I had to just sit there and wait for her to stop talking before I informed her that she's going to die by BULLET. For a second, just for a second, she got this funny look on her face. Then she wrapped up by saying, "A harrowing prediction. Will it come true?" It was completely professional-news-reporter sounding. Totally didn't match the shocked look on her face just a second earlier. My guess is the station will cut that part. She spent the whole report basically convincing the viewers that the predictions always come true, but she gets hers, and suddenly there's a question? I'm sure that part will never air. That's too bad really. So many people come in here, and they're all easygoing until they see the card. Then, suddenly, they're serious. Almost panicked. I'm sure I'll see a rush of people come in here after the story airs. I just wish they'd show that one second, where Candace Harrelson stops reporting the story and starts thinking about her mortality. That's what the real report should be about.

Oct 21 - I was right. I've been swamped. I watched the report, and sure enough, they cut the part where Candace hears how she's going to die. Instead, after the report, Mark the anchorman asked if she took the test herself, and she said, "Maybe. But I'm not telling." I guess she figures I won't squeal, since I wouldn't tell *her* anything. Since the report, I've heard from the media almost as much as I've heard from new customers. The death machine is the talk of the town. It's bigger than Tickle-Me-Elmo. I can only guess how well Tell-Me-How-I-Croak-Elmo would sell. Some people are coming back for a second run. One guy came in with a little silver frame pinned over his breast pocket. When he got the result (HEART), he slipped it into the frame. I asked if he knew that his card would say HEART, and he said he'd taken the test before, but he thoughtlessly threw away the card. Now it's a fashion statement. He's planning to sell the frames with a fake HEART card inside. That way, if people are proud of their deaths, they can stick it in the frame, and if they get, say, BOTCHED PLASTIC SURGERY, no one has to know. If the frames sell well, he's going to try making custom T-shirts.

Oct 28 - There has been a line going outside the door. I've seen so many death cards in the last two days that I can't even remember most of the weird ones. So here's a list of the ones I do remember, FEAR, TRAPEZE, GERALD, RELIGION, MINK, MARSHMALLOW, CAMCORDER, PIE, and RONALD MCDONALD. I want a custom made T-shirt that says RONALD MCDONALD. Seriously, after reading that one I was slightly tempted to try the machine myself. But then I got another visit from Beth. She wanted to try the machine again. We both knew she'd get the same result. It was like watching a car crash, and not being able to do anything about it. She said something to remind me just exactly why I didn't want to take the test. She said, "I'm the same person as I was in July, only now I've emptied my bank account talking to doctors and I have panic attacks in the middle of the night." That warning should be put on the front of the box. I told her so. It was nice to see her again. She told me about a dream she's been having, where the machine is just this spigot that attaches to your arm and slowly drains all of the blood out of you. I had a similar dream, where instead of getting a business card, your death was written on a big cinder block, and I had to swim across the river with it around my neck. Oh, I almost forgot the best card: DISK ERROR. I had to run that one three times before I was convinced that the guy would die from DISK ERROR and there really was nothing wrong with the machine.

October 30 - Another busy week. I actually ran out of blank business cards. I kept fifty people waiting while I sent Paul to pick up a new box from the store. I was waiting here for him to come back when I had my epiphany. Let me set the scene. I'm waiting in the office, alone, with all kinds of people waiting to get in. I'm trying to think of how many words I can make out of "Brick Wall." I cross out the letters as I go, and suddenly, it hits me. **SCNKLE** is one word written on top of another. It's SINK written on top of ICICLE! The guy has two deaths, unless he manages to sink into a pile of icicle. So I thought about that for awhile, and here's my best guess. He said he was in a car accident, right? What if it was a recent car accident? Maybe he had a blood transfusion recently, and the machine tested the blood of two people at one time! How long does it take for blood to acclimate to a person? My guess is that one or the other will disappear in time, but for now, he should probably avoid sinks, sinkholes, and cold climates. I've got him coming in for a second test next month. I am now officially more knowledgeable than the product rep at EndVisions. Hope that knowledge won't give poor Neil a stroke.

Nov 4 - Why on earth is the government killing so many people? Candace over at Channel 5 did a story about it. There were a bunch of people who came forward and said they were disturbed that their card said GOVERNMENT and more than a little distrustful of our elected leaders.

Nov 11 - Neil showed up unexpectedly yesterday. I was excited to tell him about the double printing on **SCNKLE** but he kicked me out of the office, said he needed to make some adjustments to the machine. It was a nice change of pace, to be away from the brick wall and the icy specter of death for a little while. I actually called up Beth, to see how she was doing, and we had lunch together. A good lunch. I like her. But get this: part of me doesn't want to get involved with her because I couldn't deal with it if she died. She'd have her midnight panic attacks, and then I'd get worried that she was dying. It's too stressful. I checked back in to the lab after lunch, and Neil was already gone. Great customer service there, Neil. It didn't take too much investigation to find out what he had changed. Now the machine, the Bucket-Kick-O-Meter, is hooked up to a phone line. His note said that it would make maintenance easier, and I should not unplug it for any reason. I can't believe that the machine of death gets its own phone and I have to share the one in the hallway with Paul. If the machine gets a window with a view better than a brick wall, I'm going to personally start telling people how they're going to die.

Nov 18 - I was talking to Paul about Thanksgiving. Get this: He canceled his ski trip this year. Fear of heights? I told him he's the same person he was back in July, except now he doesn't want to go skiing. I guess it didn't sound as profound as when Beth said it.

Dec 1 - Sad news. Mitch, my former coworker who got laid off, died yesterday. It was really sad. He couldn't get a recommendation from work and couldn't find a job. His wife left him, and he killed himself with aspirin and alcohol. Once again, the machine was correct. If he wouldn't have taken the test, he'd be alive today, I'm sure of it. Tammy and the rest of the HR people aren't beating themselves up about it though. She told me I don't need to report results to her anymore, because now the machine does it automatically. That's why Neil was in before Thanksgiving. If there isn't a database of results already, you can bet your ass that Human Resources is starting one. Then she sent out a memo to the whole office that says everyone needs to retake the test. Dr. Caine is resigning. Seriously. I still don't know if he drew SHIV, but it sure sounds like it. Who is this going to affect? People who drew health problems, like HEART? People who drew deaths that imply they'll happen sooner than later, like FALL? Now I'm thinking about resigning, too.

Dec 8 - Not resigning. I bit the bullet and ran a sample, telling them it was my result. It said ALMOND. They wouldn't lay me off for ALMOND, plus I didn't have to, you know, actually take the test. Of course, this means that from this day forward, I can't test the ALMOND sample anymore, but I've long since given up testing the samples anyway. We closed the office to outside clients for a day so I could test everyone else. I guess I underestimated the contingent that didn't want to be tested. In fact, there were a couple of people who took the test and then threw the card away without looking at it. Mike was really resistant to getting tested again, now that it's a mandatory thing. I feel bad for him, since GOVERNMENT sounds like one of those deaths that HR would get really worked up about. I also retested $ICICLE, but the results are the same. I told him that if he knew who donated blood to him, I could test that person and we'd know which applied to which person. Unless the donor has already died in a tragic icicle accident or something. I found that funnier than he did.

Dec 10 - I just now realized that I told Neil I would die by ELECTROCUTION and I told Tammy I would die by ALMOND. I hope they don't compare notes.

Dec 15 - The powers that be running the lab have been good enough to put off layoffs until after Christmas. Nothing like a little yuletide panic. Last year, our Christmas luncheon had fried chicken, potatoes, a bunch of pies; it was really good. This year, we're getting salads and low-fat, unfrosted angel food cake for dessert. For a healthy new year, they say. Beth called me and asked if I wanted to catch a movie with her. I said no. I just have too much stress in my life right now.

Dec 30 - A local news story made the national news this week. The mayor's cousin (or maybe second cousin) found out that his roommate was sleeping with his girlfriend. He also found out that his roommate's death card said PIE. So this cousin has been slipping

pie crusts and pie filling into the roommate's food, hoping that will be
the pie that kills him. He hasn't done anything to the pie, it's perfectly
normal. The day after Christmas, roommate is eating supper when
he finally notices a hunk of pie under his turkey. He gasps, chokes
on his food, and he really does die. Now the mayor's cousin has been
arrested for murder. All kinds of big-name politicians are in town, all
with their own take on pie murder. The mayor is humiliated. Reporters
from every channel have come in to talk to me this week, and I've
seen myself on three different news programs. It's unreal. I feel like I
shouldn't be interviewed by this many reporters without my own
book coming out, or winning the Super Bowl, or something. After
they turn the cameras off, I've asked each one if they've taken the test.
(I've tested so many people in the last three months, I've honestly lost
track.) Every single one of them said yes.

Jan 6 - Wow, Cleveland is *the* place for controversy, and it's all
because of Murder Pie. Suddenly, Congress wants to talk about the
Buying-the-Farm-Reporter. The Op-Ed pages are filled with pleading
to get the government to pass some death machine laws. The flames
have been fanned by a person who took a bunch of hostages and
died in a shootout in Texas. They tested him posthumously, and
sure enough, the result said "SHOOTOUT." There's been a push to
register people's death cards with local law enforcement, or even the
federal government. I'm trying to get ahold of Tammy to approve
some vacation time quickly, because I do *not* want to be here when the
shit goes down. I've heard people are planning a protest for right outside my building. Why am I in the middle of all this? All I did was read
an instruction manual, for crying out loud.

Jan 8 - Things are crazy. They're protesting right outside and
throwing things at cops. I am not going to sit here and protect the
damn machine. They can have it. I'm getting out of here...

Jan 27 - OK, so it's been a while, but now here I am. Tammy talked

me into coming back, but I really don't know why I came in at all.
Everything has pretty much gone to hell. Here's what's happened:
On January 8 about 2,000 protesters marched through Cleveland,
opposing the death machine. Police showed up in riot gear to try
to keep things civil, but the crowd turned violent. People started
throwing things at cops, a bunch of people got arrested, protesters were burning effigies, cops were getting fire hoses. There was
some kind of blast that took out a bunch of windows, and started
a fire right here. The lab sustained some water damage when the
firefighters showed up, but made it through in pretty good condition. On the other hand, the building next door—the brick building
that was outside my window—was completely destroyed. It was a fire-
trap. The shell of bricks that remained has been torn to the ground.
Apparently, it was thought to be abandoned but was actually hous-
ing a sweatshop, employing illegal immigrants, even kids. I'm
almost certain they included the family that was in here earlier, the
kids who didn't speak any English. The ones whose cards said FIRE.
The remains of 27 people were found inside the building, and six
more, including my coworker Mike, were killed in the protest. I got
out of here just as things were turning really bad. I've been at home,
left alone by the media and this is my first day back in the office. It
is unworldly. I never thought something like that could really happen here. I always thought that chaos and disaster were reserved for
other countries, or at least big cities like New York or Chicago. Even
after all this time, it's like I'm walking in a dream. There is a body-
guard stationed outside my door at all times, but I am still alone
in this room with the damn machine. Now, instead of staring at a
brick wall, I stare at scorched rubble. It's a huge, dirty, gaping pit,
and every time I look up at it, I feel a wave of despair. I think about
those poor kids. There was a sweatshop—a sweatshop in Middle
America—mere inches from this room, and I had no idea. And
now, because whoever was running it didn't give a damn about their

employees, 27 of them are dead. If a machine that can predict death can also bring about so much death, is it really worth it? I don't think anyone can convince me that it is.

Feb 3 - When a single machine is the cause of so much heartbreak and so much risk to human lives, what's the logical next step? Order more machines, of course. I'm aghast. Apparently, I am no longer the sole operator of the Posthumous Predictor in Cleveland. Now, I'm just the senior operator. Meaning I've been taking calls from the Cuyahoga County hospital about installation all day, in addition to handing out SUICIDE and DROWN cards to my morose clients. Someone at Cuyahoga County wanted to know if people traded their actual deaths if they traded their cards. I rolled my eyes and was about to tell her that was the stupidest thing I'd ever heard, but you know, I have no idea. I gave her Neil's number. Let him roll his eyes awhile. The tension here has eased quite a bit. I think the politicians are still talking about the machine, some even talking about making testing mandatory, but the news media have lost interest. Some people apparently saw a nipple on TV over the weekend, so all of their attention has gone elsewhere.

Feb 4 - They were clearing out the debris from the building next door today. It's just a blank lot now, and yes, I can see the next brick building down, but I can also see the sky and the street below. All it took for this window to serve its function was the deaths of a bunch of kids. Over lunch, I grabbed one of the bricks before they cleared them all away, and now it's here on my windowsill. I really don't know why I kept it.

Feb 10 - Guess what I found out today? Paul and Beth are dating. How did that happen? I saw her come in yesterday, thinking she wanted another go-through with the machine. But then she and Paul left holding hands. I've got to admit, I feel weird about that. She didn't even stop in and say hello to me. They looked kind of sweet together, I guess, but I have to admit, when I saw them walking out to her car, I couldn't help but think of two doomed prisoners on their way to the gallows. Or something. She with her cancer, he with his falling, it's like they're on borrowed time. Is Paul more willing to deal with suffering than I am? Or is he just more desperate for sex? Or does he not understand that one day, the cancer will overwhelm her, and he'll be left to face his fall all alone?

Feb 17 - I've seen a couple of those custom shirts in the last couple of weeks. One said EXPLOSION. One said OLD AGE. The public has embraced wearing their death on their sleeve. What's more disturbing, is there's some role-playing game based on the death cards. Apparently a starter pack comes with 60 fake death cards, and you're encouraged to shuffle your own into the deck. Then the characters in the game start dying left and right and the winner is the last person standing. Also, on my way to work, I always pass this building that says "Palm Readings" in the window. Well, they took down the sign a few weeks ago, and now they just put up a new sign that says "Death Cards Explained." At least three private businesses in town have gotten their hands on their own machines. Apparently they're a lot cheaper than they were last year. Now, with the added competition, demand at the lab has dropped considerably. I find that more often than staring out the window, I'm staring at the brick, waiting for someone else to come in. Everyone's getting rich off of death but me.

Feb 24 - Happy first birthday, you freaky pile of circuits and premonitions. I sincerely regret that you're still around.

Mar 3 - I'm in trouble. All of a sudden, Tammy has questions about the card I submitted for myself. Was she talking to Neil? What's so implausible about ALMOND? I finally came to accept it. She wants to bring in the examiner from the hospital to administer the test on me "again." Now what? Plus, Paul's mad at me because I confided in him that I lied about my card. I think I could get into serious trouble here.

I could lose my job for this.

Mar 4 - I got no sleep last night worrying. Dr. Henry from Cuyahoga County is coming in this afternoon. I've been worked up about it all day. I think I'm just going to have to go through with it. I'll tell Tammy I sent her the test card by mistake. Paul probably won't tell her anything. I won't lose my job. But I'm still stressed out because I don't want to know. Let it be a mystery! No one needs to know! I don't need to know. Whatever that card says will just consume me, and those feelings of doom I get when I see Paul or Beth will paralyze me every time I look in a mirror. I wish there was some way to avoid this. I shouldn't have to know if I don't want to!

Mar 4 - Dr. Henry finally left. I took the test six times. I feel like a pincushion. I don't know if there's something wrong with the machine or what. I tried calling Neil, but he's doing installations all over Ohio now. But clearly something is wrong, because every time I took the test, I got the same result: a blank card.

Mar 5 - Didn't sleep well last night either. Big surprise there. So did the machine read my mind? Did it know that I didn't want to see the answer? It knows how people die, maybe it can read my mind. I think I read a study once where a polygraph machine reacted to a tree when someone talked about cutting it down. Maybe this machine knew I was panicked about reading the results and spared me. Or maybe it's screwing with me.

Mar 5 - If I don't get a reading, does that mean I won't die? How is that possible? I've sat next to this machine for a year, and watched it dispense little cards that made people depressed, or angry, or terrified. I've counseled people who didn't like their cards, I humored people who wanted to be retested. I've been the machine's caretaker, and little else. Is there something special about me? Why is it doing this to me?

Mar 5 - No one has come in to use the machine today, so I've used it on myself. Over and over again. I'm covered in dried blood. The cards are all blank.

Mar 6 - I am so tired. Can people die from lack of sleep? Can I die from lack of sleep? Can I die? *Can the machine?*

Mar 6 -

MAR 10 - ENDVISIONS' NOTE: *found maintenance log, missing maintenance entries after april 29 of last year. previous user had been using log as a journal, with the last entry dated march 6. he was found march 7, apparently electrocuted while trying to damage machine with a heavy object, most likely a brick. machine no longer operational. i will be returning it to endvisions to try to salvage. journal entries indicate that user became enraged, possibly delusional when the machine stopped working. apparently, he was unfamiliar with the process of changing the ink cartridge.*

a square of paper was removed from this log and placed on top of the remains of the machine. Written in handwriting that matches this journal was the single word, "me."

Story by John Chernega
Illustration by Paul Horn

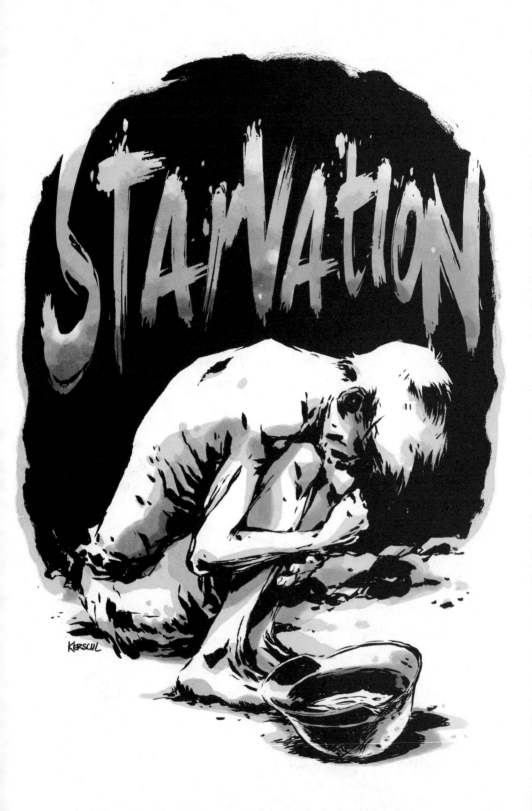

STARVATION

DALTON WAS LOOKING DOWN AT HIS HANDS. They were dirty, and maybe a little bloody, too. One of his thumbnails was split wide open. "I guess I always just figured what the hell, you know?" They were in the jungle now and things were quiet, relatively speaking. They were just sitting there, like nothing happened. Just two guys sitting in the jungle, waiting for the shock to wear off. "I mean, it was gonna happen either way, right?"

Johnny sat still, hugging his legs in his arms. He was younger and smaller than Dalton, just out of basic. The sunburnt skin was still peeling off his bare shoulders. In a few more weeks, he'd be tanned just as deep as everybody else. "Still, man," he said. "The Army?"

Dalton laughed, his lips curling up around his big teeth. "Yeah, I know," he said. "Goddamned stupid kid, huh? Signed up the day after I found out. It's like that where I come from, though. I figured it was there on the streets or here in the jungle. And I sure as hell didn't want to catch it back there. Not without seeing something first, not without doing something." His lips stopped smiling now.

The smile had never reached his eyes anyway. "Never seemed fair."

Johnny rubbed his arms with his hands. There was no reason why he should have been cold, but suddenly he wanted his jacket. But it was back there, back with the others in the clearing. Johnny just hugged himself tighter and shook his head to clear some gnats out of his face. "You ever think anytime that—"

"Only every day, kid." Dalton stood up, stretching his arms over the assault rifle slung across his back. He'd held on to his jacket, his gun, his pack, his helmet. Johnny hadn't thought to take anything with him. He'd just run. But Dalton had somehow managed to keep all his kit. "Every stinking day. Every time those guns started going off, I thought I was done for. But I never knew which way it would come from, so I just kept running. Just kept going the way they told me to."

Johnny watched Dalton pace under the trees. He was a big man, well muscled. Johnny felt like a little kid next to him. Even in fighting form, Johnny still looked scrawny. He had tried everything to bulk up, but he never could.

"Even back there on the chopper," said Dalton. "I thought that was it for sure." He turned suddenly, looming over Johnny like a scarecrow. "Homicide don't mean anything except you get killed by somebody else. It don't have to be on purpose. It can be like that crash back there just as long as it's the pilot's fault."

"You didn't die," said Johnny.

Dalton grinned. "I know it," he said. He squinted down at Johnny a minute. "You ready now?"

Johnny straggled behind Dalton as they came out of the jungle into the clearing. Streaks of fuel burned in the grass, the flames pale and languid in the bright midday sun. But they were still hot and smoky as hell. The smashed chopper was only about twenty yards away, a crumpled aluminum can surrounded by four smoldering lumps of black. The rest of the men.

Dalton brought the nose of his rifle up and put his finger on the trigger. They hadn't seen any enemy fire when they had gone down, but it was hard to be sure. And even if the bad guys hadn't been around before, there was nothing like a crippled chopper to bring them out of cover. "Keep your eyes open," said Dalton. Johnny just grunted, and drew his knife. It was the only weapon he had anymore.

The two men picked their way carefully through the tall grass. A few yards away from the helicopter, an injured snake lay writhing in the grass. Dalton kicked it out of the way with his boot. Then he motioned up to the chopper. "Check if the radio's still working," he said. "I can cover you."

Johnny moved past Dalton, and pushed a clump of reeds out of the way. Suddenly, he drew back, his mouth working involuntarily open and shut. There, on the grass in front of him, lay a severed head still encased in its dented helmet. The eyes and mouth were open. It was Sanchez, or maybe Dallas. Johnny couldn't tell for sure. He couldn't look away either. He just felt terror welling up inside him, his lungs tight and his stomach balled up like somebody had sucker-punched him. He thought he heard somebody screaming and he didn't know if it was coming out of his mouth or if it was just in his brain.

Suddenly a strong hand gripped Johnny's shoulder. He could hear Dalton's voice in his ear. "Don't look at it, kid," said the voice. "Don't look at it, don't think about it. Just keep going. Just keep doing what you gotta do." Somehow, Johnny felt his feet moving. He inched his way closer to the cockpit, but it was still on fire. It was too hot, he couldn't get any closer. The radio was toast for sure. Dalton, standing a couple yards behind him, could see it too. "Forget it, kid," he called. "Come on back. There's nothing left here. It's all gone."

—‡—

That night, Dalton went back to the clearing to get some embers to build a fire. They only had reeds and rotting wood to burn, but they had plenty of time to try to get them burning. There wasn't anything else to do anyway. Johnny watched Dalton blowing gently on the thin licks of flame. He tossed a handful of grass into it and the fire flared up, scattering ashy sparks into the air. Otherwise it wouldn't do better than sputter.

"That'll have to do for now," said Dalton. He leaned back on a big fallen log next to Johnny and clapped his knee with his big hand. "You're one hell of a hiker for such a scrawny guy."

Johnny just nodded, staring at the fire. One of the logs was starting to smolder a little, the bark curling up as it glowed red. Dalton had forced a march after they'd discovered the radio and the rest of the supplies were gone. That's how they found out that they'd crashed on an island. It had a little bit of jungle and the clearing where the helicopter had crashed, and a few miles of beach. On three sides they could see land close by, but as far as they knew they were just more islands. Even if one of those blue outlines were the mainland, they wouldn't have known which one or where they were liable to come ashore. It could be right in the middle of an enemy camp.

"Well," said Dalton. "Here's what we got." He had emptied out his pack. There were rations enough to feed one of them six days, or both of them three days. It didn't take a genius to do that math. Either way, it wasn't long.

"I ain't hungry," said Johnny.

"Don't matter," said Dalton, pushing one of the MREs at Johnny. "You gotta eat something. I'm not gonna carry you around tomorrow if you're too weak."

Johnny laughed. "Yeah, and where are we supposed to go?"

"Gotta find water," said Dalton. "Unless you saw a spring somewhere today."

Johnny leaned back on the log and shook his head. "No," he said. "I didn't." Dalton held out the MRE again and Johnny took it this time. He opened it, looking for stars through the canopy the whole time.

"What are you doing out here anyway?" asked Dalton. He took a swig from his canteen and wiped his mouth with his sleeve. "You don't seem the type. You seem like a smarter guy than this."

"Yeah," said Johnny, "well, I'm not." He picked at his food for a minute in silence. "I couldn't get into school."

"What? High school?"

Johnny looked over at Dalton for the first time. He thought he was maybe making fun of him, bullying him, but it didn't look like it. "College," he said.

"Oh," said Dalton.

"Yeah, well," said Johnny. "I didn't want to flip burgers, so I thought I'd join up and maybe get into school that way. Or at least learn how to do something." He wiped his forehead with the back of his hand and rubbed his wrist into his eye socket. The mosquitos were biting now. Or whatever they were. "I didn't think I'd actually end up here."

"Nobody does," said Dalton. They were quiet for a few minutes. Johnny nibbled a little on the food, and Dalton rearranged the fire as best he could. "I can't get Sanchez out of my head back there," he finally said. "Still in his helmet like that. I mean, how the hell does that even happen?" He lifted one of the logs and tried to get a bit of bark burning. A puff of smoke hit him in the eyes and he sat back, blinking. "That's not even the worst part," he said. "Imagine going through your whole life with *that* on your ticket. I mean, Goddamn." Dalton rubbed the last of the smoke out of his eyes, smearing a line of ash down his cheek in the process. He was still looking at the fire. "I've been meaning to ask you," he said slowly, "what's on your ticket, kid?"

Johnny didn't answer right away. He couldn't answer. As soon as Dalton had mentioned Sanchez, his bowels had all gone weak and his stomach had flopped and risen, forcing all the air out of his lungs. By the time Dalton turned around again, Johnny was already vomiting his dinner back out into his hand. Dalton jumped up to his side and Johnny felt his big hands pressing against his head.

"Oh hey, kid," said Dalton. "I'm sorry about that. I should have never said that stuff about Sanchez. I keep forgetting this is your first time out here."

Johnny didn't feel any better in the morning light. Heavy beads of sweat clung to his forehead, and his skin felt like it was stretched tight across the bones of his face. Dalton had given him the canteen in the night, but he had drunk it dry. He still hadn't eaten anything.

"You okay, kid?" asked Dalton, feeling Johnny's arms and legs for fractures. "You sure you didn't get hurt in the crash? Does anything hurt? You could have been in shock most of yesterday and never even known it."

Johnny shook his head. "No," he croaked. "Just shook up, that's all. I'll be fine in the afternoon." Even as he spoke, he knew it wasn't true. He felt terrible, like he was floating on the surface of a fast-moving stream. He was only wearing his undershirt and his pants, but even so he felt like he was being slowly smothered to death. Like snakes were coiling themselves around his body and biting his bowels. "I think I drank all the water," he said. "Sorry."

Dalton shook his head and picked up the empty canteen. "Don't worry about it, kid. I'll find some more." Dalton stood over Johnny a second longer. He seemed to be thinking hard about something. Then he put the rifle on the ground next to Johnny. "Here, be careful with this," he said. "But I'll probably be gone all morning. If something happens and you need me, let off a round." He stood up again. "And for God's sake, kid, don't shoot me when I come back."

By afternoon, Johnny was a little better. He heard Dalton crunching through the undergrowth and he reached out to push the rifle away. He hadn't even been touching it before, but it was better to be safe than sorry. A minute later, Dalton knelt down next to him, holding the canteen to his lips. The water tasted gritty, but it was cool and wet enough.

"Did you find a spring?" asked Johnny.

Dalton shook his head, squatting on his heels nearby. He picked up his rifle and slung it over his shoulder again. "I ended up collecting the water from leaves." He motioned to the canopy as he took a drink himself. "Dew and stuff, I guess."

"Sounds like that would take a while."

Dalton laughed. "It does." He wiped his forehead. "I just hope I didn't sweat away more than I got." He flashed his big toothed smile again. He had a rough face, swarthy and twisted, but he looked boyish and almost handsome when he grinned that way. "You eat anything?"

"Still not hungry."

Dalton nodded, rocking back on his heels. "Look, Johnny," he said. "We have to have a serious talk." Johnny looked over at him, waiting. "How do you die?"

Johnny shook his head. "What does it matter to you?"

"You know mine," said Dalton. "Homicide, murder, whatever you want to call it. I got a gun, and we each got a knife. I just want to know how this ends, you and me alone here. What chance do we got?"

Johnny's eyes widened. "What are you talking about?"

"Look, kid, we don't know where we are. Maybe we're close by home, and maybe they're looking for us right now, and maybe a chopper'll fly overhead in the next five minutes. Maybe." Dalton scratched the side of his face, stretching his mouth. "But maybe nobody else knows what happened to us. Maybe we're stuck somewhere they can't get to us. Maybe they got other problems."

Johnny just looked at Dalton. He still felt a little feverish. He understood everything Dalton was saying, but it sounded like it was coming from far away.

"We might be here a while," said Dalton. "That's all I'm saying. We got to prepare for that. And if we're going to prepare, then we have to know what we're up against. What do we have to watch out for, you know?" Dalton tapped himself on the chest. "Me, that's murder. Other people. That's what I got to watch out for."

Johnny shook his head and made like he was going to get up. Dalton stopped him.

"I'm not talking about you, kid. You're sick, and I can take you in a fair fight anyway." He patted the stock of the rifle. "And I got the gun right now, so I'm not scared of you. We got no reason to kill each other. But if you're gonna go down homicide too, then maybe we'll get rid of the knives and the gun. Throw them in the ocean or something." Dalton raised his eyebrows and looked down at Johnny. "It's just the two of us here, and if we can keep from killing each other then we'll be okay. As long as we're alone and as long as we both stick together, nothing can happen to us." Suddenly his voice softened and dropped. "We got water and food now, but that's not gonna last. Not the food anyway. If nobody comes for us, we're gonna start getting desperate and I'd just as soon not have any weapons around when it happens." Dalton looked down at his hands. "You see what I'm getting at here? We got to know these things so we can do what we have to do before we get to the point when we start thinking crazy things about each other." Dalton paused for a minute. "So, how do you die?"

Johnny breathed in deep. "You didn't find any food?" Dalton shook his head. "What about those snakes? Or birds?"

"Gotta catch them," said Dalton. "And even then..." He shrugged. "Not much meat on a snake. I didn't even see any fish out there.

Maybe there'll be some that come by later, but who knows."

"And you don't think they're coming for us?"

Dalton pressed his lips together. "I hope they are," he said. "But there're a lot of islands out here, and we're not exactly in friendly territory." His voice trailed off.

Johnny just nodded and sighed. "All right then." He raised his eyes to Dalton's. He could feel the sweat breaking out on his forehead and his upper lip. "I'm supposed to starve to death."

Dalton didn't look surprised. He just looked angry. "Goddamn it!" he shouted. He stood up and walked a few paces around the camp, and then he seemed to calm down a little. He went over to the pack and tossed Johnny an MRE. "Eat something anyway."

Johnny shook his head. "What's the point? Can't you see what's happening? We're done for, here. They're not gonna come and we're not gonna find any food. I don't know. Maybe you make it out okay, but I'm gonna die here for sure."

Dalton sat down, tipping his head back. He looked at Johnny through his knees, his hands dangling clasped above his feet. "Eat it," he said. "If you're right, at least you'll live another day. But you might be wrong. Either way, you might as well eat while you can."

Johnny opened the MRE and took a bite. He hadn't realized how hungry he was. Now that he had food in his hands, it was hard to convince himself to eat slowly. In between bites, he glanced at Dalton. "You're not having one?"

Dalton shook his head. "I ate earlier."

On the morning of the third day, Johnny felt almost better. When he awoke, he was still sore and hungry, but the fever was gone. The back of his neck was cold and slick. His arms and legs ached with tension. The muddy places where his buttocks rested against the earth were wet. Looking down at his body, he saw a spider with long spindly legs climbing up his trousers. Johnny brushed it away and sat up.

"Thirsty?" asked a voice. Johnny jumped. Dalton, of course. He was holding out the canteen. Johnny took it.

"You back already?"

"It's almost noon," said Dalton. He was sitting on his haunches again, watching Johnny like a mother hawk over her chicks. He must have been waiting there awhile. "You want anything to eat?"

Johnny squeezed his eyes shut and stretched his arms and legs. "Better not," he said. "There's only two left, right?"

"Three."

Johnny did the math in his head again. They'd both eaten two so far, so there should be only two left. "You didn't eat yesterday?" asked Johnny. Dalton smiled and shook his head. "You have one then," said Johnny. "I can have one tomorrow."

"What's the point of that?" asked Dalton. "I'm not planning on starving to death, no matter how little I eat. But you need some food if you're gonna get better."

"We'll split one."

In a few minutes, they were eating. After a while, Johnny sat up higher and looked around the little camp that Dalton had built over the past two days. There was a place cleared for the fire with a bit of wood drying nearby. Dalton's blanket was hung across a couple of wires stretched between the trees—a tent or a water collector, maybe. And that was it. That was the whole camp.

"Where's the rifle?" asked Johnny.

Dalton licked his fingers, trying to suck the last bit of grease off them. "Ditched it," he said. "Threw it into the ocean like I said." He leveled a finger at Johnny. "I want to ditch the knives too, both of ours."

Johnny shook his head. "We're gonna need them. You should have kept the gun too. What if there's an animal we could have shot? Or what if somebody shows up?"

"We're running out of food already," said Dalton. "It's like I told you before, things are going to get desperate and who knows what we'll do then. We just gotta keep from killing each other and maybe we'll be okay. Just get rid of the weapons, and we'll be fine."

"You'll be fine," said Johnny darkly. "I'm still gonna starve to death."

"We don't know that. We don't know what's gonna happen."

"Forget it," said Johnny. "I'm keeping my knife. You said yourself that you could take me in a fair fight. I'm sick and I'm not as strong as you. If we get rid of the knives, then I got nothing. This is all I got."

Dalton suddenly stood up, gripping his scalp in his hands. "Don't you get it?" he said. He was kicking the dirt like a mad bull. "I can't kill you! I can't do anything to you at all! I'm bigger and I'm stronger and I'm healthier, but none of that means anything. Even if I still had the gun, it wouldn't make a difference! If I come at you, I'm the only one who's got a chance of getting killed. I'd have to be an idiot to risk it!"

"You thought about it?"

"What?"

"You thought about coming at me?" asked Johnny.

"Dammit, kid. I thought about *everything.*" Dalton looked down at Johnny. His face was harsh. "I thought about every possible way to get us both out of here alive, or one of us, or neither of us. I'm trying to figure this thing out. I'm trying to think up a plan where neither one of us gets hurt. So yeah, I thought about jumping you while you were lying there passed out. But what good would it do? What would be the point? I'd just be risking my neck for nothing. We gotta do this together. It's the only way, and I know I can get us through it. But we gotta get rid of those knives to do it."

"Forget it!" Johnny's voice was loud. He had taken his knife out and was holding it now, squeezing the handle tightly. "If we ditch the knives, then there's even less hope we'll ever eat again. And dammit, Dalton, even if you can't kill me, there're other things you can do."

Seeing the knife out, Dalton drew his, too. "There's no point dragging this out then, is there? Why not just do it now if you're so sure how it all ends?"

"That's what I thought," said Johnny. "You keep pretending that you don't think I'm gonna kill you. You keep pretending you're not afraid of me. But now what? You trust me so much that you want to fight me when I'm sick?" Johnny lurched forward, half rising. The blood rushed to his head and he almost fell over, but he regained his balance. "You want to come at me?" He waved his knife at Dalton. "You want to come at me, then come!"

Dalton looked from his knife to Johnny's. He clenched his fists and let out a howl. Then he turned and stalked into the jungle, slashing at vines and branches as he went. He didn't come back at all that day.

Johnny hardly slept at all that night, but he dozed a little towards dawn. Still sick and weak, he couldn't force himself to keep watch any longer. When he woke, Dalton was sitting calmly on a log at the edge of the camp. He held up his hands to show they were empty.

"You were asleep a long time," said Dalton. "If I'd wanted to do anything, I could have done it easily enough."

Johnny nodded, rolling over. "Where's your knife?"

Dalton jerked his head over his shoulder. "See it?" It was sticking out of a nearby tree. "Can I bring you some water now?"

A few minutes later, the two men were facing one another a couple of yards apart. Johnny still kept his knife, but he had sheathed it. They were talking almost easily again.

"I found a spring yesterday," said Dalton. "It was down in a cave, practically underground. I wasn't going to tell you about it..." He paused a minute, then cleared his throat. His jaw was tight when he spoke again. "It's like I said, though. We do this together or not at all."

Johnny sneered. "Yeah."

"Look, the way I see it, this can still turn out a few different ways. I could have left you here and taken the food and the canteen and not told you about the spring. Then I could have let you chase me all over the island. As long as you never caught up to me, I'd be safe. And eventually you'd starve."

Johnny snorted and looked away. "Is that supposed to scare me?" he asked. "I'd get you sleeping or something."

"You're missing the point, kid. I don't want to do it that way. I don't want to be sitting here trying to think up ways to get rid of you. I want to get us both out. And if I didn't have homicide on my ticket, we wouldn't be at each others' throats like this. It's just because we think we already know how it's going to work out. But maybe we're wrong. That's the point I'm trying to get at. Maybe we're wrong. There's more than one way to look at this yet. It doesn't have to be us fighting until you kill me, and then you starving to death by yourself. So forget about that machine and those damned predictions, and we'll just work this out our own way."

Johnny shuddered and closed his eyes. When he opened them, Dalton was holding out his hand.

"Come on, kid. What do you say? Let's be friends still. We got a chance to get out of this alive, both of us. Let's not give up yet."

Johnny sighed and then nodded. He reached up to take Dalton's hand. They shook. "You found a spring then?"

"Yeah," said Dalton. "If you're strong enough to walk, you can wash off some of that muck."

It had been days since Johnny had been on his feet, and after five minutes of walking he could feel it. The jungle was still sticky and hot, and roots kept tripping him up. Dalton led the way, breaking off branches and clearing a path, but Johnny still recoiled from every leaf and every spider web that brushed against him. His nerves all felt like they were twice as sensitive as usual.

"You okay back there?" asked Dalton. He didn't turn around. Johnny only grunted.

Johnny lost track of time. It could have been an hour or two hours. It could have been twenty minutes. All he knew was that he was taking step after step, his hands moving from tree trunks to vines, trying to steady himself. He hated those palm trees. He'd only ever seen them on TV and movies before he shipped out. They had them in Hollywood and Miami, in glamorous places like that. But looking at them up close, they didn't even look like real trees. They just reminded him that he was going to die thousands of miles from home where everything was different. There were moments when he would have given his right arm for an oak or a maple and an ugly little squirrel. Everybody had to die someday, he knew. But why did it have to happen in a place you hated?

Dalton paused and pointed into the jungle. "Fruit tree," he said. "I don't think they're ripe yet, but it's something." Dalton grinned. It was the first time he had looked at Johnny since they started walking. "So don't give up hope yet, kid."

They pushed on a little while longer, and then Dalton stopped at the lip of small cliff. It led down into a dark chasm about fifteen feet deep. Johnny could only see that the walls were steep, and that it was dark under the canopy and rock below. "How you feeling?" asked Dalton. He didn't even wait for an answer. "It's down there, down at the bottom. That's how I missed it the first time."

Johnny leaned forward, his hands on his knees. He didn't hear any water, but it had to be there. He was exhausted. If he was ever going to make it back to camp, he needed a rest and a drink—and food. "Give me a minute," he said. He didn't even want to think about how he was supposed to get down to the spring. Dalton should never have brought him. He should never have come.

"I'll give you a hand," said Dalton, pressing his palm against Johnny's back.

"Wait," said Johnny. Dalton's hand pushed against him. He took a stumbling step forwards. "Wait." The pressure grew more insistent and Johnny felt himself tipping. He took another stumbling step. The edge of the chasm opened wide before him, stony and dark. Johnny's feet sank into thick carpets of moss.

"Sorry, kid," said Dalton. And suddenly Johnny was moving faster than he thought possible. The ground and the trunks of palms rushed by him, spinning into each other as his feet dragged and scuffed and then lifted entirely into the air and for one breathless moment Johnny was touching nothing. He had no connection to anything except Dalton's hand clutching his shirt, and then that too was gone and Johnny tumbled lightheaded through a cushion of air. His arm brushed something rough and the skin split wide open. He tried to push away but it kept coming at him, pinning his shoulder tight until a stabbing pain sliced through his body. Just when he thought his shoulder must snap, his left leg struck hard against something and he sprung free, spinning through the air again before coming down hard once more on his leg. Something happened in Johnny's ankle and a rush of black swallowed up his eyeballs in a single gulp and left him tingling for a moment.

When Johnny opened his eyes again, there were hands on his body. He thought it must have been three or four pairs, but only Dalton was there. He was stepping back, away from Johnny's body, a knife in his hand. Dalton was sweating hard. Johnny tried to move, but his ankle flared into a throbbing ball of pain. There were brands burning all over his body, sharp points of fire on every muscle and bone.

"Come on, kid," said Dalton. "Listen to me, kid. Did you hit your head?" He was looking down over Johnny, his hands searching his face and head. "Come on, you'll be okay."

Johnny didn't say anything. His mouth was full of blood and rocks. Sharp, hollow pebbles biting into gums. Johnny spit out the blood and the pebbles. Teeth, he knew. Even then he knew. He breathed through his nose. That smelled like blood too.

"I'm sorry," said Dalton. "I'm sorry I had to do it. But I couldn't let you have that knife. I was gonna take it when you were sleeping, but it was too risky. You could have just woken up and stabbed me. You could have just been pretending to sleep. So I had to—I had to. You understand that. I had to do it like this. I knew it wouldn't kill you, so I had to."

Dalton looked down at the knife in his hand. He shook his head and suddenly flung it away, up over the rim of the chasm. "It's gone now," he said. "It's just you and me now. Just us. And we're gonna make it, just like I told you." Dalton crouched down, lowering his face next to Johnny's. "Just trust me, that's all. I'm gonna look out for you. I'm gonna look out for both of us. I'll be back with food and water every day. I promise. I promise I'll be back. I know I can do this."

Dalton stood again. "You were shutting down," he said. "You gave up. You can't do that. I learned that here. Even though you think you're gonna die every minute, you just keep going. You keep doing whatever you can to beat that. And this is what I had to do. And now we'll be okay. You'll see—just trust me, kid. I know I'm not gonna die here. I'm gonna die an old man, murdered warm in my bed. And you too, kid. Both of us, we'll be so old we won't even know what happened."

And then Dalton was gone again, climbing up to the rim of the chasm. Johnny lay there at the bottom alone.

Time passed. A lot of time passed. Dalton came now and then. Or at least Johnny was aware of him now and then. He brought helmets full of water and left them for Johnny. Warm, gritty water. There was no spring in the chasm, of course. That had been a lie, like all of it. Holding the helmet in his good hand, Johnny lapped at it. When the fever was on, the water seemed to be full of crawling and swimming things, tiny snakes and tiny fish. But Johnny drank it anyway and the snakes and fish wriggled around inside his belly. They wriggled through his intestines and down his leg, down into his swollen ankle. It was broken, maybe infected. But it always hurt and Johnny couldn't put any weight on it. His wrist was better, at least. It was just stiff and sore. Johnny could squirm his way from place to place at the foot of the cliff. He could squirm up to the wall and lean against it. He could squirm over to where Dalton left the water. He could squirm to the corner if needed to relieve himself. But he was stuck down there. There was no way he could make his way back up.

Sometimes Johnny was able to fall asleep just before dawn. He would wake a few hours later, the fever gone for a little while. It was then that he felt hungry. The hunger built inside of him, day by day, brick by brick. First it was an emptiness, and then it was a nauseated feeling. Johnny heaved now whenever he awoke to the hunger. It was the hunger that was going to kill him and he didn't want to die. So he woke and he heaved, and nothing came up save some sour juice and a panic that threatened to swallow him.

Every now and then, Dalton brought something to eat. A piece of fruit, a little bit of fish, some grubs. They were in a jungle, for God's sake. There should be food hanging from every tree, washing up on every shore. But day after day Dalton brought only leaves to chew. He was eating plenty, there was no doubt of that. Johnny never could have kept up such activity on the scant food he was getting. No, Dalton was eating everything and only bringing him the scraps he couldn't finish. It should have been the other way around. It should have been Dalton lying in that hole with leaves to chew, and Johnny out filling his belly from the jungle. Dalton wasn't going to starve. Johnny tried telling Dalton this once.

"You were right," said Johnny. He could barely mumble the words. "You were right. You're not going to starve and I'm not going to get stabbed." Johnny's fingers clutched Dalton's sleeve weakly. "I'll give you my knife for the food. You take my knife and give me the food. You won't starve and I won't get stabbed."

Dalton unhooked Johnny's fingers from his arm. "There is no knife," he said calmly. "Now listen to me. No one's coming for us.

They would have been here by now. I need to swim to one of the other islands and see if I can find anybody." Dalton set down the helmet, full to the brim with water. "I'll be gone a couple of days at least, so be careful of the water. Until I get back, that's all there is." Dalton stood and reached up to climb the cliff wall. "And I will be back," he said. "Don't think I won't be."

More time passed. Johnny lapped at the water in the helmet. The hollowness in his stomach grew and sharpened, and then dulled again. He didn't heave anymore when he awoke. The hunger was too familiar. How long had it been since he had eaten? Johnny didn't know. He didn't even know how many days he had been in that hole. He moved his good hand over his body, feeling his arms and legs and ribs and face. He wanted to feel how much flesh had wasted away, how thin he was. He didn't feel like a skeleton yet. There were still some meaty parts on his body. He had seen pictures of people with nothing but skin and bones, so he still had time. Of course he did. Hadn't he read that it takes a month to starve to death as long as you have water? But he didn't have much water. Not anymore.

More time passed. Nobody came. Had Dalton left him there? Had Dalton been killed or captured? Or was he just sitting up above at the rim of the chasm, waiting for Johnny to finally starve to death? Johnny licked a wet rock experimentally. Was that how he was going to live? Was he going to spend a month licking rocks while he slowly deteriorated into a bag of sticks? Johnny's ankle and wrist hardly hurt anymore. He couldn't feel anything beyond the ravening tumult in his stomach. Dalton had done this. Dalton had killed him, had tortured him to death. How long had he been gone? Two days? Three days? If he were coming back, he should be back soon.

Johnny lifted his good leg slowly. Inch by inch, he raised his knee to his chin and curled his body so he could reach the boot. How long had he worn this boot? No doubt his toes were shriveled and black inside. Covered in mold maybe. Infected, gangrenous.

Dalton had done that to him too. Slowly, Johnny picked at his bootlace. It took him ages to untie the knot and pull the lace out of one eyelet. He stopped and rested. His fingers were numb and they felt raw. Johnny pulled at the lace again. For hours, he worked at it, pulling it from eyelet to eyelet, until finally it was free of the boot. He clenched his fingers. The lace was still strong at least—it hadn't rotted. It would hold fast. He would pull it tight, like a noose, and it would hold fast.

More time passed. It passed darkly, mostly in unconsciousness and in fever. Johnny tried to get used to being dead. As he felt himself falling asleep he breathed deep and let death smother him. He fell into darknesses long and still, where no dream troubled him. These were deaths, he told himself. He had died over and over again, thousands of times all through his life. He was always dying, and it was nothing to be frightened of. The only difference was that he had always woken up before. Soon he wouldn't wake up. That was fine. Death was fine. It just meant not waking up. Johnny clutched the bootlace tighter.

He woke with a start. One more death over. One more life begun. But something had woken him. There was a scrabbling and crumbling noise. Something landed near his head. "Johnny, Johnny!" yelled a voice. "Come on, kid, wake up!"

There was a hand under Johnny's head. Water splashed his face and he opened his eyes. The voice called his name again. Johnny couldn't see who it was, but the person had Dalton's voice. That was good enough for him. Water was flowing over his lips now and Johnny swallowed reflexively. He coughed weakly. A head bent down near, and Johnny moved his good arm. He aimed the loop in the bootlace for the head. He tried to catch that throat in his lace, he tried to pull it tight. But he was too weak. He couldn't do anything.

"Hey, careful, kid." Dalton lifted Johnny's torso in his arms. Now Johnny could hear other voices up at the rim of the chasm. Johnny tried again with the lace, but he couldn't see anything. He had wanted to kill Dalton so much, and he couldn't even do that. He couldn't even kill a man who was fated to be murdered. "Don't worry, kid," said Dalton. He wasn't even paying attention to the bootlace, probably didn't even realize what it was for. "There's a little camp on the next island over. I got their medic here. I got food here. You're gonna be okay. They're gonna get us out of here." Dalton hugged Johnny's head in his arms. "I'm sorry, kid. I'm sorry I did that to you, but I told you to trust me. I told you I could do it. I told you, just keep doing everything you can. Oh, Christ." Dalton was almost crying now. "I swear to God I thought they were gonna shoot me when I found them. Friendly fire, after everything we've been through. But we made it, kid. We made it."

A couple of months later, Sarge came to see Johnny in the hospital. His ankle was still mending, but he had finally moved back on to solid food. And his wrist was good enough to write a couple of letters back home. Dalton was right, after all. He was going to make it. He was going to survive. Johnny could hardly believe it.

"So what did they do to him?" asked Johnny.

"Court-martialed," said Sarge. "He'll be in jail awhile, then he'll get a dishonorable discharge." Sarge smiled a little. "They're not gonna shoot him or anything. Too many extenuating circumstances. Nobody wants to be that harsh on a man who came back for his buddy in the end."

Johnny was quiet. Then he looked up at Sarge. "I tried to kill him, too, you know."

"When?"

"When he came back for me with the medic. I was crazy, I guess. I tried to strangle him with my bootlace."

Sarge laughed. "Son, when he brought you back to me, you weren't fit to make a fist, let alone kill anybody."

Johnny nodded. "I tried anyway." He shut his eyes. "It was the worst experience of my life. That hunger was the worst pain I have ever felt." Johnny shook his head. "I never knew what it would be like. I never knew it would hurt so bad."

Sarge patted Johnny's leg under the covers. "It's over now, son. You'll be on your way home before you know it."

Johnny laughed a bitter laugh. "Yeah," he said. What did Sarge care? As soon as Johnny was gone, he wouldn't be responsible for him anymore. He would feel fine. He'd gotten him out of the jungle alive and sent him home to his folks. That was fine for Sarge. But Johnny hadn't been lying. Starving was worse than he had ever imagined it could be. And now—since he had lived—he would have to do it all over again some day.

"Thanks, Sarge," said Johnny, holding out his hand. What the hell? They might as well shake on it.

Story by M. Bennardo
Illustration by Karl Kerschl

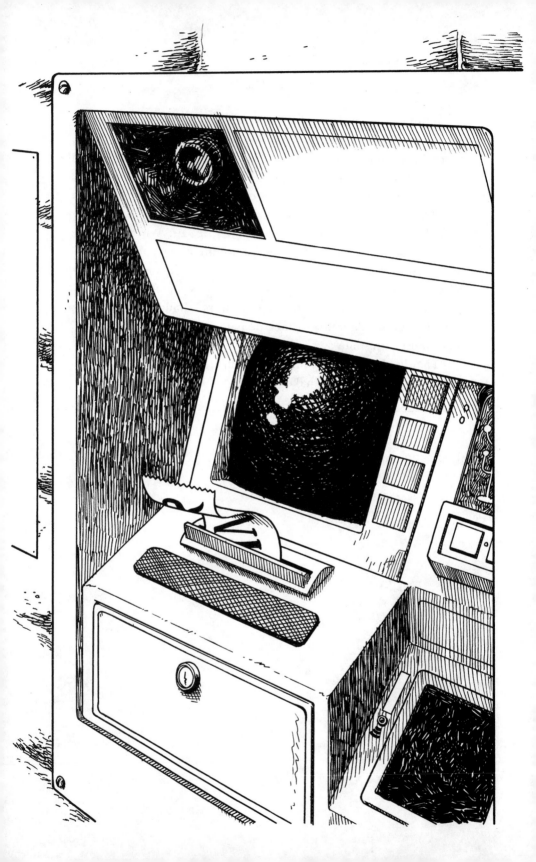

CANCER

IN THE MONTHS AFTERWARD, IN SUBURBAN DINING ROOMS, THE BOHEMIAN BOURGEOISIE DEBATED THE ETHICS OF THE MACHINE. The first had been installed unobtrusively in leading doctors' surgeries, and as they spread across the country, schoolteachers and bank managers and creative consultants and publishers met for cocktail parties, suppers, restaurant lunches, and the conversation turned to the machine, the machine, again and again, the machine. Like the weather, or, in time of war, the latest battle, it provided a constant conversational reference point, came to be something akin to a worldwide obsession, in the West, at any rate.

"I saw one," said Kate Boothroyd, sucking on a cigarette, "on Kensington High Street. There was a line a bloody mile long—madness."

A temporary silence settled over the Broads' dining table, broken by the hostess.

"And would you?"

"What?"

"Use it."

Kate pondered the question a moment.

"No—I don't think so. I mean, human beings, ultimately, don't want to know—do they? Or do they? I mean, didn't somebody write about that?—in trying to avoid the inevitable, you actually bring it about. Who was it, Rory?"

"I don't bloody know, do I?"

Kierkegaard. Nietzsche. Dostoevsky.

The argument continued around the dining table long into the cheese and coffee.

This was the debate, amongst the upper middle classes. Did one really want to know what life held in store? When there was nothing one could do about it at all, when there *was* no happy ending. A blank slip was an impossibility. At best, "old age." At worst, something unspeakably awful, the self-fulfilling prophecy one couldn't do anything about.

But people *were* doing it. Sure enough, in the days after department stores and pharmacies installed "the machine," lines of hundreds formed, eager to know that which could not be avoided. The evening news carried scattered reports of suicides, occasionally *en masse.* Support groups sprang up, devoted to those whose slips had read "suicide," those for whom the specter of whatever horror could drive them to such desperate measures proved too much. Support groups that turned to cults. One weekend, two hundred teenagers, neatly arranged in two rows along an underground railway station platform on the Victoria Line, stepped neatly to their deaths, drugged smiles on their pimply faces. The whole event engineered by means of the Internet—"Facebook Event Invitations" with a difference.

Marion Broad was out shopping in the West End the day of the Victoria Line suicides, the day public transport was crippled and she had to take a cab to Kate's for lunch.

Stringy hair, no makeup, Kate answered her door with a drawn look to her face, lit cigarette between her fingers.

"Jesus," breathed Marion. "You've done it, haven't you?"

She followed her into the house, through a bluish haze of tobacco smoke.

"Emphysema!" barked Kate. "Bloody emphysema!"

The words hung between them, over the John Lewis coffee table.

"Not exactly a surprise, but still... At least I won't be needing to quit anytime soon."

A dry laugh crinkled her darkened eyes, and Marion's heart grew cold.

And so it went on, for months and months. Parliament rejected bids to outlaw the machine, and rejected them again, despite the frenzied speeches of religious groups, political organisations, mothers, fathers, societies for the old, societies for the young, all futile in the face of humanity's child-like curiosity.

Supermarkets quietly erected them, in the entranceways, by the photo booths.

Leaving Selfridge's, Marion saw a well-dressed mother leading her infant daughter out of the curtained booth, tears trickling down, melting away the makeup.

James Broad, good-natured and stoical, steadfastly refused to do it. Late at night, taunted by the faces of her friends, Marion envied her husband's easy sleep, as she tossed and turned. Dinner parties were a grim fandango of fraught nerves, now. Those who had "done it"—euphemisms all round, like it was something dirty— seemed half-dead and half-alive, eyes dull, filling in time until what was predetermined by the fates rolled around. Emphysema. Cancer. Cancer. Suicide. Cancer. Cancer. Cancer.

For the rest, eggshells everywhere. Mentioning the mode of death marked out for anyone at your dinner table was taboo, and the Broads desperately strained to keep the conversation away from illness, disease, and demise. Almost buckling under the strain, like tired horses, never a pleasure, only a chore, they gave up entertaining.

Bars emptied in the suburbs, where stoical stockbrokers bunkered down in semi-detached splendor to await their various tumors and cancers and sleep apneas. In the cities, they filled by night, as cosmopolitan sophisticates drowned their morbid sorrows. On Saturday and Sunday mornings, the lithe young bodies that washed up on the banks of the Thames posed a serious danger to public health.

And then, one afternoon, coming out of the Food Hall at M&S, she stopped, bags over both wrists, and stared solemnly at the new machine in the vestibule. Rebuking herself, she passed by.

That night, in the darkness of the witching hour, across the bedsheets: "Are you ever tempted?"

From the husband, only gentle breathing.

The next morning, unspeakably early, pale and baggy-eyed after a sleepless night, nursing bitterness in the kitchen: Enough! Enough!

On with the jeans and cardigan, and out into the car, down the deserted, cold, early morning city streets, to the nicest place she could find.

She slipped inconspicuously into the booth, inserted the credit card, tapped in the passkey. Pale and wincing, placed her finger under the needle, poised like the sword of Damocles.

Down and up, in and out, she barely felt a thing. The machine churned out its slip, and she turned it over, in fearful, trembling hands.

"Cancer," there, and nothing more.

Marion Broad walked slowly through the empty foyer, towards the car in the empty lot, maneuvered herself into the driver's seat, and drove carefully home.

Letting herself into the grey and silent house, she tiptoed upstairs and into the bedroom, where the light of dawn seeped around the edges of the curtains. Slipping off her trousers and sweater, she drew back the covers and let herself into the bed, and into the small of her husband's back, smiled a secret smile.

Story by Camron Miller
Illustration by Les McClaine

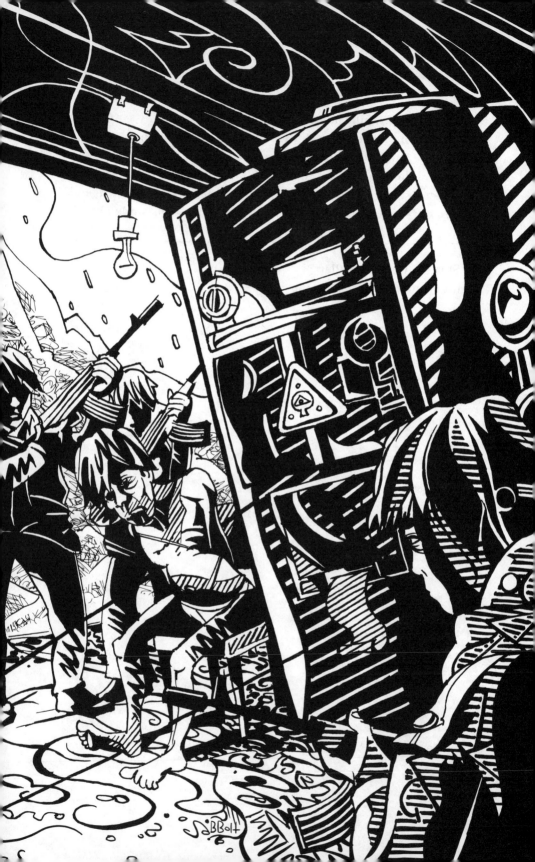

FIRING SQUAD

I HAD DINNER WITH AN OLD HIGH SCHOOL ACQUAINTANCE THE
OTHER DAY. We'd bumped into each other on the street after years
with no contact at all. Even though we hadn't been very close when
we were teenagers, it was a pleasant surprise to see him. After
standing at an intersection chatting through a few cycles of the
traffic light he asked if I was too busy to have a meal and really
catch up. One thing I'm rarely accused of being is busy, so we were
soon at a stylish little restaurant he knew.

Conversation quickly moved from the banal to his travels. It
turned out that after graduating from university he'd spent a long
time out gallivanting through all sorts of parts of the world. He'd
saved up a bit of money and went to countries where it would last
him a long time. That's what this guy was like. He'd always been the
one to do the things everyone wanted to do. As teens it had made
him the dare taker, the gutsy one, and understandably led to him
being much more popular than a nobody like me.

Even as kids when he talked about his adventures he never
sounded like a braggart. That hadn't changed. He'd always been
matter-of-fact in talking about the sorts of scrapes he'd been in and
he came off as brave, instead of filled with bravado. Even though
he lacked a beard, it only took a few minutes for me to settle on a
descriptor: grizzled. He seemed like a veteran of something.

Thinking about this, I asked him if he'd had any experiences out
in his travels that he'd thought he wouldn't make it through, that he
felt lucky to be alive after.

He sat back in his chair a bit, the slice of bread in his hand forgotten while he thought. "Lucky to be alive? It's hard to say. Because of
my emphysema, it's never really bothered me." I was about to offer an
apology when he stopped me. "I mean, I don't have emphysema now,

but that's what my death is going to be. Eventually. I breathe just fine these days so it's hard to feel like that's ever going to affect me."

Fair enough, I thought and prepared for the subject to change, but he surprised me by continuing.

"There was one time out in Asia, though, when I thought that all the emphysema in the world wasn't going to save me. You want to hear it?"

"That's why I asked," I replied. We ordered another round of beers and he began his tale.

—‡—

I was in a country that was undergoing a bit of a revolution at the time, but figured it wouldn't affect me much. I was just a tourist, tramping around the mountains with my backpack, supporting the local economies by staying in little three-house villages and purifying the bottled water I was buying. No problem to anyone. But the revolutionaries had a lot of support in these villages, or at least it seemed like they did from the way their graffiti was scrawled on rocks and buildings.

I didn't pretend to understand the politics of it all, and for most of my travels that didn't give me any trouble. I had no idea what a revolutionary even looked like until I found myself face to face with three of them one evening.

I was in the common room at a little guesthouse, eating lentils and drinking a beer some poor sherpa must have dragged up the mountain on the same slippery little paths I was travelling for adventure. It was spring, so the snow at the lower altitudes was gone, but the weather could still wreak havoc with your schedule if you cared about those kinds of things. And it was still pretty chilly, so these smoky old common rooms at the guesthouses were the perfect places to rest after a day on your feet.

When I looked up from my plate, three young men were sitting on the other side of the rough table, staring at me intensely. None of them were very tall, but they had the tough look of mountain people. Their faces were purple from burst blood vessels—or maybe it was makeup, I'm not going to pass myself off as some expert here. They wore heavy canvas clothes and long, filthy woolen scarves.

So these three guys were sitting there, silently staring while I ate. Kind of unnerving, as you might expect, but I'd gotten used to people staring with abandon and didn't let any annoyance show.

When I finished my meal the one on the left spoke to me. "Do you know where we can get a Machine of Death?"

This surprised me on a few levels. First, his English was good. I'd only learned a couple of words of the local language, and usually struggled to understand the broken English employed by those in the hospitality industry out there. This guy's was accented, sure, but very clear.

Second, a Machine of Death? A bit of a non sequitur there. I would have expected something about how they wanted to be my guides for a great new route to the summit of Angku Norge IV that no Westerner had ever set eyes on (apart from the Swedish couple they took yesterday). He noted my surprise and continued.

"I'm sorry to interrupt but we are from the local, umm...non-governmental organization." He smiled shyly at his joke. "Our operations in this region would be greatly helped if we had access to such a device. It's understood that in the West these machines are to be had in great abundance, but here in the mountains we are sadly deficient in your luxuries. We were hoping you knew where we might be able to find one."

"I'm not sure I do know where to get one," I told them. "It's not really my line. I mean, I'm just a guy, no special connections or any-thing. I don't think I'd be able to help you."

"That's all right," he replied as he and his two friends got up and wrapped their scarves around them, preparing to leave. "But if you could keep your eyes open and remember us, we would greatly appreciate it. My English name is MJ. Like Michael Jackson."

They would have walked out of the guest house right then, but I was curious about one thing. "You do know that a Machine of Death doesn't kill anyone, right?"

They stopped at the blanket-covered doorway and MJ explained with a slightly patronizing air, "We aren't simpletons. Of course we know what the Machine does. We need one for internal use."

"How so?" I was really curious at this point.

"We have some traitors in our group. They are selling informa-tion about us to the government but we don't know who they are. Yet. This is a big problem for our cause. When we find them, we will execute them in the name of revolution." I nodded, and he seemed encouraged by the way I didn't shrink away at this plain talk of death and traitors and such.

"If we had a death machine we would be able to find out who is due to be executed. It would say Firing Squad, because that's how we deal with traitors. With the Machine's verdict we will know who the traitors are. Then we will execute them as such."

It was a very straightforward explanation, and for some reason it impressed me. I thanked MJ for his answer, and promised him that I'd keep an eye open.

"It's kind of weird to think of now," my friend said between mouth-fuls of salad, "but I found their logic oddly appealing. I mean, I really wanted to help them. These poor guys just wanted to get their revolution going without outside interference and needed a common enough device to get on with it."

"Outside interference is kind of par for the course when it comes to revolutions though, isn't it?" I asked. "And besides, I'm pretty sure the Machines don't work like that."

"Well sure, sitting here it seems a little off to see them as foolproof traitor-finding machines. But these guys just seemed so confident their plan was solid and that all that was holding them back was this lack of technology. It's hard to get down on that kind of idealism. I was young at the time." He shrugged, half-smiling, and speared a segment of mandarin orange.

"But this isn't where you felt in danger?"

"Oh no. That only came after I found them a Machine."

It was a couple of weeks later. I'd made my way up through those revolutionary mountain paths and then down to the road where I was about to catch a bus back to the lowlands. There was a bit of a chill in the air but the sun was busy melting away the snowdrifts, all that remained of a blizzard that had delayed me here a few days. I was sitting at a teahouse where I could keep an eye on the road without getting run over, and enjoying the opportunity to let my socks dry out on the cheap plastic table.

I heard sounds of a party coming from a part of the village I couldn't see. It seemed to be a wedding or something, lots of music and cheering and things. It made for a festive background while I sipped my tea. Out of nowhere the music stopped. A few minutes later a bunch of well-dressed young men came out of an alley and dumped what looked like a small refrigerator into the creek that ran next to the road. After a moment of study, I realized it wasn't a fridge at all, but a Machine of Death.

There's no way, I thought to myself. I mean, what are the chances that such a thing would show up unattended so soon? I'd been thinking about the revolutionaries as sort of a quixotic rabble, good for a bit of local colour in my stories, but nothing more. Now here I was, in a position to get them exactly what they desired. It was kind of an odd feeling. I don't think I can remember ever being in such a powerful position before.

Anyway, I paid my bill and went down to the creek to check out the Machine. It was intact, except for the electrical cord, which didn't have a plug anymore. Looked like it had been torn out quite forcibly. No one was coming down to berate me for messing with their property, so after about half an hour I figured it was free for the taking.

I found a young guy and asked him if he'd like to make a bit of money. He was from the town, not the mountains, wearing knockoff plastic sneakers. He understood a bit of English and seemed eager for the cash.

"I need you and maybe a couple of your friends to help me carry this thing to a village," I told him, down by the creek. "It'll take a day or two, but I'll take care of your expenses." The kid hemmed and hawed about it but eventually we negotiated a price for him and three of his friends to help me.

Of course I was going with them. I couldn't remember the name of the village I'd met my revolutionaries in, but knew how to get there. And besides, I wanted to make sure the Machine arrived without being dumped in another mountain stream.

The hike back to the village went quickly. I didn't do any of the carrying but the guys I got did fine. On the walk they ended up telling me how the Machine had arrived in the first place: The richest guy in the village had a daughter who was getting married, and he imported it at fantastic expense for the wedding party. It was sort of a novelty thing, flaunting how rich they were. The groom was the first to find out how he was going to die, and the paper read 'Stabbed in Heart by Jealous Wife.' Not the greatest way to get a marriage started off right. The Machine, disgraced by such an inauspicious announcement, was discarded, as I'd witnessed.

At this my friend stopped his story and contemplated his still half-full bowl of soup.

"So what happened?" I asked. My soup was done—the benefit of listening to a tale over dinner instead of telling, I guess.

"Now, in my mind the plan had been to drop off the Machine somewhere in town and get word to the revolutionaries somehow." He put down his fork and knife and his fingers ran along the rim of his water glass as he explained. "I wasn't demanding any payment for my service, so I didn't really need to see them again. It was barely an inconvenience, or at least, that's what I hoped. I mean, I wasn't doing this to be praised or anything, right?"

I knew what he meant. "You wanted to be able to say, 'Oh this? It was nothing. Don't worry about it.'"

"Exactly! It had cost me the equivalent of, I don't know, four dollars in sherpa fees. Not a big deal at all. But they didn't see it that way."

—‡—

One of my guys tried to explain to the woman at the guesthouse that she should tell the revolutionaries that the plug needed replacing before the Machine could be used. It was taking a while. She was confused about what the Machine did and even though I'd told my translator the details weren't important, it seemed he couldn't stop himself. She was loading wood into the stove while he talked, forcing him to repeat himself over the clatter and roar of the fire.

I was ready to let my inner North American take over and leave for the sake of my schedule. I was done, ready to go catch the bus back down to the lowlands the next day. My bag was on my back when the blanket-door behind me lifted up. I hadn't realized how smoky the stove had made it inside until a shaft of light fell through the room only to be blocked again by three figures walking in.

"It is so nice to see you again," said the one in the centre. It was Michael Jackson and the revolutionaries. "How time flies."

They looked the same as when I'd last seen them. Same old uniforms with the same long, woolen scarves, same earnest expressions.

I guess the only difference in me was a bit more beard, so who was I to talk?

"Hey guys, nice to see you, too. I guess this'll be easier than all these explanations here." I indicated my sherpa and the proprietor woman, and noticed they'd both shut right up when the others entered. The woman had a smile on her face, and the sherpa had a defiantly set jaw. The other three sherpas weren't making any sudden moves, but they kept their hands in their pockets ominously.

I didn't want to get in the middle of a fight, so I told my guy everything was fine and gave him his money. He took it without taking his eyes off the revolutionaries, and then he and his friends left, quickly, like they were trying not to show how badly they wanted to run.

That's when I started to get an inkling that I might not exactly understand everything that was going on.

Once the townies were gone, MJ warmed right up. He beckoned me to sit at the hacked and dented wooden table. "What brings you back to this village?"

"I found you a Machine of Death. It's sitting outside."

The woman brought us tea. The other two revolutionaries stood back by the blanket-door. Something about them seemed a lot more menacing than I'd remembered, as if they'd seen a lot of action in the past few weeks. They weren't old, but they weren't the fresh-faced youths I thought I'd met.

Michael Jackson spoke thoughtfully, "Yes, we saw it when we arrived. I hoped that's what it was." He took a few more sips of tea. "So what do you want for it?" He asked this in the same quiet tone, but I noticed that the two others at the door were watching me closely.

At this point my emphysema sentence popped into my head. These guys weren't going to kill me. I knew that. But I also knew there's a lot of wiggle room in these things. If I said the wrong thing they could possibly make me a prisoner for the rest of my days. Or at least enough of those days to make me severely uncomfortable.

Happily, I didn't have any intention of doing anything to get anyone angry.

"Me?" I asked, smiling as broadly and non-threateningly as I could. "I don't want anything. It's my gift to you. It's a little broken though. The Machine doesn't plug in because the cord is torn. I'm sure you can fix that."

Maybe I was just projecting my own emotions into him, but MJ seemed relieved. Instead of the terse businesslike smile he'd been wearing, a much more peasant-like grin split his face.

"That is excellent! Thank you so much for your help. We cannot possibly repay the magnanimity of your gesture."

"Oh this? It was nothing," I said. "Don't worry about it. In fact I should be on my way back. I have a flight to catch in a week and the buses around here take…"

MJ grabbed my arm in what seemed a friendly gesture. Not a violent restraint, though his grip was strong. "No, you cannot! We may be poor and unable to honour your gift as you deserve, but the one thing we can do is to have a meal. You will come back to our camp and we will have a feast to the now-inevitable success of our cause!"

I tried to demur, to explain about bus schedules, to say I didn't need any sort of feast or honour, to spout clichés about a good deed being its own reward, but he wouldn't have any of it. He promised it would be done that very evening and that I'd lose practically no time at all. His grip on my arm didn't slacken through the whole exchange I desperately didn't want to escalate into an argument. In the end, I gave in, and went back to the revolutionary camp.

—⁑—

The tale was interrupted here by the arrival of our main courses. One bite of his entrée—some sort of duck in a sweet-smelling sauce—and my friend was delighted. "There really is nothing better than a good meal with fine company."

"Very true. Let's have a toast." We raised our glasses of beer. "To chance meetings!" I said.

He nodded and responded, "To civilization!" And we drank.

The restaurant was filling up. The new patrons looked dressed for the theatre. A large group behind me were calling for wine. We ate silently for a few minutes before I brought us back to his story. "I get the feeling the revolutionary camp wasn't quite like this."

"No it wasn't," my friend replied, staring down at his plate.

—‡—

MJ sent one of his companions ahead to get preparations started for the feast, and the other got a series of straps together to help him carry the Machine on his back.

We set off in the direction I'd need to go to get back to the bus, which did alleviate a few of my apprehensions. Soon, though, we left the main path for a narrow muddy trail through the trees. I hadn't realized how I'd been hiking on the equivalent of a freeway the previous weeks. Those main paths had room for you to press up against a cliff face when you met a train of donkeys. But this trail seemed like we were the first to travel it. The density of the trees gave loads of shade, so the snow I'd hiked through and seen melt a few days before here made our way even more treacherous. We were descending, and often I found myself falling on my ass for safety's sake. And I wasn't the one with a Machine of Death on my back.

The walk had been quiet, mostly me cursing at the slopes I was sliding over, but when we arrived at the camp, MJ took charge. Before talking with a crowd of eager kids who'd congregated, he told the guy with the Machine to bring it to a large tarp-covered lean-to. Soon I could hear the sputter of a generator inside.

The camp wasn't large. A dozen canvas tents and a few shanties made out of the local trees held out the snowdrifts. The ground was a mess of wet mud with a few planks thrown down at random. You couldn't see the sun through the needly canopy.

And there were revolutionaries. I hadn't expected them to be so young. Almost all of them were skinny teenagers. They seemed to look up to MJ, and were getting in a lot of questions that seemed to be about me. I've been in enough strange places that being the centre of attention wasn't a novelty anymore, so I let my mind wander.

A young girl brought me a bottle of beer. Like always, the bottle was huge. I took it from her with a smile and my best "thank you" in her language. Instead of the giggle that usually produced, her eyes went wide and she bolted to a group of older girls standing near what looked like a kitchen tent. They all looked nervously across the camp at me. It took a few moments of fumbling with my bottle opener to get that drink into me. This wasn't going how it was supposed to.

MJ finished with his mob and came over, smiling apologetically. "I am so sorry to have to tell you that our leader is out on an operation and will not be able to get back in time to meet you this evening. Unless you would consider staying until tomorrow?"

I explained that I couldn't possibly, but thanked him for the consideration. We wrangled politely for a few minutes but eventually I won. Arrangements would be made to guide me to the nearest guesthouse on the main path after the celebration was over.

Once all those niceties were out of the way we could get down to the tour of the camp. MJ told me how long they'd been encamped and how dedicated they were to the cause of freedom from the tyranny of the capital. He talked about corruption in the towns, how farmers couldn't afford to grow anything and instead had to turn to letting foreigners into their homes, while they bought their food from the outside.

"And now they want us to stop using firewood!" he exclaimed outside the tent where he'd shown me their collection of rifles and ammunition. "'It's bad for the environment to cut down so many trees,' they say. They've never lived through one of our winters. Do you know how much it would cost to use their gas stoves?" I didn't, but was soon informed.

The whole tour had just been a way of killing time while the feast was being prepared. He could have pointed out each tent and told me its contents from almost any point in the little camp. As we moved off from the armoury tent I spotted something off behind it a little ways. It looked like an animal pen of some sort, but the fences seemed a bit high for pigs.

MJ noticed me looking and thought for a second before speaking. "Would you like to see?"

"Yeah, what is it, your chickens?"

"Not exactly."

The pen was the most sturdily built thing I'd seen in the camp. When we got closer I realized that it was in a bit of a gully and the fences were much higher than I'd assumed—maybe ten feet tall— and covered with chicken wire. We stopped on a small ridge where we had a good view over and inside.

Eight people were in the cage.

"Like I said," MJ said in a conversational tone, "we've had some problems with traitors recently. These are our current suspects."

Once one noticed us looking in, all of the prisoners began staring. MJ talked about the reasons why each of them might have betrayed the revolution, but they mostly looked at me. The oldest might have been fifteen. Two of them were girls. I'd imagine none of them had seen a foreigner before. There were a few muddy blankets inside and everything was sodden. I couldn't see even a pit for a toilet.

"And now that you've brought us the Machine, we will be able to tell which of these are guilty," MJ finished up, clearly pleased with the situation. "The innocent ones will, of course, receive the revolution's deepest sympathies and positions of honour."

When he finished with his oration, which because it was in English they had no way of understanding, most of the prisoners started talking at once. They were pleading with MJ, but he replied dismissively, then patronizingly. At least that's how it sounded, but it's so hard to tell when you don't know the language. He turned back to me. "They all say they are innocent, of course, and don't want to be in this cage, but it won't be much longer. I told them how you'd brought the Machine that would exonerate they who truly are innocent."

They were all staring at me with horrible looks. A few deep scowls, some wide-eyed terror, and one calm gaze you could tell was a mask for calculating how to get over that fence and cut my throat.

MJ wasn't the kind of guy who liked silence from his guest of honour. "It's too bad the plug is damaged, or we could get all this justice out of the way tonight." When I kept on staring into the cage, he went on. "We have a few boys who are good with these kinds of things though. They should be able to get it up and running very soon."

And with that we headed back to see if the feast was ready.

—‡—

"How did we get on this story again?" My friend hadn't stopped fidgeting with his water glass for five minutes.

"A time you felt scared, like you might not make it back."

"Right." He stared at his glass for a few more seconds. Somewhere in the restaurant a woman was laughing at what she wanted everyone to know was the funniest thing she'd ever heard.

"They had this feast for me, I sat at the head of the table, got the choice pieces of goat, the whole deal. And through the whole thing everyone's faces looked like those eight prisoners' did. Like they couldn't believe the monster they'd let in to their home. Just scared of me and what I'd brought. They didn't say anything weird, didn't spit at me or anything, but I've never felt so hated in my life. The girl who'd brought me the beer when I arrived wouldn't look anywhere near our direction. I wondered if she had a brother in the cage. That wasn't the worst of it, though.

"The worst thing was fearing that one of those bright kids would come running from the generator tent saying he'd fixed the plug: that the Machine could pass sentences that very night! I ate bits off my goat haunch and smiled at MJ's jokes, just waiting for the horribleness to play out.

"Everyone would have to gather by the generator to witness each judgment in turn. They'd lead each prisoner over, get her drop of blood and wait. Each one of their deaths would say 'Firing Squad.' There's no way around it. I could feel it in the air. It wouldn't matter if they were traitors or the most fervently loyal revolutionaries history had ever known. All of those prisoners were going to die. Because of my good deed they'd be shot by a squad of teenagers.

"And then when the prisoners were all dead, MJ would start to think, 'That was a lot of traitors. More than I'd thought even.' And he'd get inspired to test everyone he'd had any suspicions of. And each of their deaths would say 'Firing Squad'. And then they'd start to run out of suspicious people and have to test everyone. The little girl that brought me my beer, all of his little sycophants, even those two I'd met him with, they'd all be revealed as traitors. By the Machine I'd brought.

"Clearly it would come to just the two of us and he would need to take my blood and I would submit and it would come up 'Emphysema'. He'd give an impassioned speech about how I was the only one who truly understood struggle while the bodies slowly froze around us. Then he'd want to go find his leader and the rest of the revolutionaries to test them and it wouldn't stop until everyone in those mountains was dead. And I'd have to run for home and safety, knowing what I'd set loose.

"So yeah, none of that happened." Both of our plates were gone and dessert menus lay in front of each of us, unread. "In reality we ate a fake-jovial meal and gave toasts all around. Everyone was scared, like they could hear barbarian hordes just over the hill, but there was nothing they could do except eat their bits of goat.

"MJ kept on treating me like an honoured friend right until the end. I wanted to hit him. Hell, I wanted to shoot him and send all those kids home. But I didn't. A kid was my guide to the path after the feast was over. I didn't warn him to get the hell away from that machine. Couldn't have really. I stayed in a guest house, barely sleeping. I took off before dawn and didn't stop until I was on a bus and far away. If I were any sort of human being I would have wrecked the Machine before I left. I didn't do that either."

My friend had let all this out in a quiet rush, much quicker than the measured pace of the rest of his storytelling. He had another gulp of water, and caught his breath. "I guess I've never told this story before." He tried one of his usual self-deprecating smiles. It didn't quite work. "Harder than I thought."

I couldn't let it go there. "But then what happened? Did they get the Machine working? Did they all kill each other?"

He looked hard at me. "I don't know. After I left, I refused to pay any attention to the news from that area. Plenty of other things in the world to care about, right? Besides, maybe I didn't affect anything. The Machine might have done exactly what they thought it would do. Maybe they never got it working. Who knows?

"But I'll tell you this: I'll never go back. If that means I miss a few mountainscapes, so be it. I knocked about in the third world for a few more months but my heart just wasn't in it anymore. I tried keeping clear of revolutions but there are just too many kids out there with guns. Too hard to forget.

"Eventually, of course, I came back to civilization. And here we are."

Here we were indeed.

I stared at my dessert menu and decided on an inconsequential tiramisu.

Story by J Jack Unrau
Illustration by Brandon Bolt

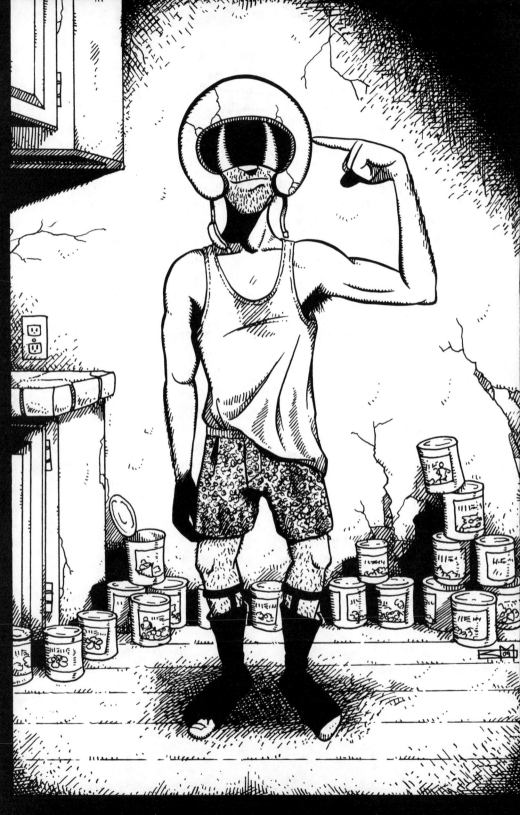

VEGETABLES

"THE BLOKE'S A FUCKIN' WHACK JOB."

Billy, the Director of Marketing, tells me this while he's picking his nose with a paperclip. "He wasn't right to start with; he's the last bastard who should've got that blood test. He's been treading water all his life, but he's sinkin' now."

He straightens the paperclip, then slides it between his thumb and finger to squeegee the snot off. Unimpeded by my *Ugh* face, he wipes his fingers on the fabric of my cubicle wall. In the background a phone has been ringing for five minutes without kicking into voice-mail, and in the next cube, somebody's screaming at a subordinate employee on another line. I want to kill them all and dance to the sounds of their suffering through the junkyard of smashed computers and office plants and overturned desks.

I ask Billy, "What did it say?"

Tilting his head back, throat tight, Billy inserts the straightened paperclip once again into his nostril. He's wearing a tailored Armani suit that probably cost more than I make in two months. This time he keeps pushing, until the wire disappears into his skull.

"It doesn't talk," he informs me. He makes quotation marks with his fingers. "It didn't *say* anythin'."

If I whacked the stub of the wire with the heel of my hand, Billy would be dead in a second. If he took the test, it might say *Paperclip* or *Bastard* or *Whim*. Instead of killing him, I say, "I know it doesn't talk, you facetious prick. I meant what did his ticket say? How's Frank gonna die?"

Billy tilts his neck to a normal angle and looks at me, a half-centimeter of wire emerging from his nose. Frank—the subject of our abject diagnostics—is our mutual friend and colleague, and he's going through a rough patch right now. If I flicked the wire into Billy's face, hard like a fly on a chair arm, I wonder if that would be enough. Then his test might say *Flick* or *Slither*. If he fell backward, he might crack his head on the photocopier or a desk, and then it'd say *Wham!* and he'd become obsessed with George Michael drunk driving or going postal or somebody attacking him with an LP broken into lethal splinters.

This is how it works: The blood test machine just tells you *How*; never *When*.

Billy says, "Vegetables."

"He's gonna die by vegetables?"

He nods. "He took it four times, taking blood from four different parts of his body, and that's all it said every time. *Vegetables*."

My eyes narrow as I visualize random ways to die at the hands of veg, and Billy connects his cheek to his forehead with Scotch tape, pulling it tight so his lip curls into a snarl.

—✠—

Frank lives in a small terrace of red brick houses, in an area begging to be demolished and overhauled. Dogs carry knives, and as it's getting dark, I walk past a gang of ten-year-olds wielding a discarded car bumper, openly discussing whether they could break my shins in one whack.

I knock on Frank's door, then look down the street at somebody burning a fire in a drum. A section of roof is missing off Jack James' house three doors down, and inside the exposed cavity is a shack made of corrugated sheets. Jack used to live in the house, but now lives inside the shack in the roof. He took the blood test, and it told him *Pavement* would be his demise. He never considered that falling off the roof is more probable than the ground swallowing him, but this is none of my business, and something I would be interested in witnessing.

The door opens. Frank is wearing an old, scratched white crash helmet with the visor down. I cringe at his level of mental degradation as the words *Fish* and *Barrel* spring to mind.

Crouching, I wave into the visor and he lets me in.

Frank's kitchen looks like the courtyard in a scaled down model of a castle, with cans of vegetables lined up along the skirting boards like a perimeter fence. For some inexplicable reason, he's stacked the Green Giant brand two high.

"Why?" I ask.

"He's a giant, stupid. Gotta stand taller'n the rest."

"I mean why aren't they in your cupboard with the rest of your food, Mr. Stability?"

I open Frank's cupboards to find other provisions—ravioli, powdered sauces, cornflakes; it seems that only the vegetables have been evicted.

"They can't fall on me from down there," Frank says, tapping his crash helmet to acknowledge his ingenuity.

I briefly visualize a firework getting stuck inside the helmet, resting on the bridge of his nose and blowing the lenses of his small round glasses inward. I want to be in the middle of a city as the world falls off its axis and people melt all round me in the street.

Pulling two chairs out, I make Frank sit and persuade him to take off his cranial protector. His curly brown hair springs out six inches in every direction, except for a strand pasted to his forehead with sweat. Within seconds it bounces to life defiantly, and his eccentric professor appearance returns, with the addition of two new forehead zits since I last saw him.

"Phew," he says.

"Better, huh?"

Frank agrees, and I make us a cup of tea. Every night, I dream of Armageddon.

"Mind if I get logical for a second?" I ask him. He shakes his head and curls his bottom lip, like it's a puzzling question.

"One," I say. "Even the heftiest can of potatoes, falling six inches onto your head, wouldn't kill you. Especially with all that padding. Think straight, Frank. Two: you're more likely to trip over these things and break your neck. When was the last time a can of *anything* fell out of your cupboard?"

Frank looks sufficiently ashamed, and I assist him in returning his food to its rightful location.

"World's gone mad," he says, glaring vengefully at a can of Niblets. "Ever since the Newton Twins, they've been settin' fire to churches all over the country."

I nod understanding and pat his arm, even though inside I scorn our species completely, and wish ill upon almost everybody. The Newton Twins were the first to try to force the machine to be wrong. Both their tickets said *Old Age*, so they committed suicide. Ten times they tried, and ten times they failed.

Gun jammed. Car engine died. Gas ran out. Tree branch snapped—and by now, the media was all over it. They injected HIV, and it just went away. Concrete slippers in the lake, underwater for half an hour—but the medics brought them back to life, pictures of health.

One of the twins, Julie, jumped off the railway bridge, but her sister was scared of heights, so abstained. Nonetheless, she was caught by the tarp on a slow-moving train, and trudged home three days later.

I try to inject some perspective, but it's hard when religion died overnight.

"Look Frank—it doesn't change a thing. It just means science shed new light on it, and our deaths are proven to be pre-destined. We're still gonna die, same way we always have done. Are ya gonna wear a crash helmet and eat nothin' but meat for the next forty years, right up to gettin' run over by a Peapod delivery truck?"

He slumps, dejected, then looks at me with those puppy-dog eyes that broadcast a big and unpleasant request on the way.

"Mick?" he says, his voice quivering for dramatic effect.

I could slap his face, but refrain.

"What?"

"I'm scared. I could live with *Old Age*; that gives you a reasonable chance of having a decent amount of time left. But...how are ya supposed to live with *Vegetables*?"

"Forget about it. It's gonna take ya by surprise, whatever your ticket says. But it's up to you whether ya greet it with a *Fuck You*, or spend the rest of yer life crying over milk that hasn't even spilled yet. We all die; it's hardly a revelation, is it?"

Frank starts crying, so I cave and slap him hard across the face. The sniveling stops, and a white handprint lingers on a bright red cheek.

"Get a *grip!*" I yell. "Are we dying younger cuz of it? No. It's mass hysteria; they've got therapy groups and protestors and are trying to get 'em banned. But they're makin' too much money to ban 'em, and all you repulsive fashion followers takin' the tests and then blubbering about it like you're an unwilling victim seem to have forgotten one thing: Prior to receiving your delivery note, you were *still* slated to croak one day! You weren't immortal just because you didn't think about it or know how. So stop thinkin' about it and it therefore ceases to exist. Okay?"

Frank nods, his eyes still wet but now wide and grateful, and then he asks me, "Will you stay a few days, 'til I get my shit together?"

With every passing hour, I see the potential for many tragic accidents.

"I couldn't say no," I tell the bottom of Billy's shoe as he fishes behind my desk for the box of staples he just knocked off. A euphoric cloud of omnipotence lingers comfortably in the back of my mind, everywhere I go.

TV commercials warn us against the tests. Flip the channel and they tell us, Take the Test Today and Get a 20% Discount! I wonder how many people get *Iraq* or *Antichrist* or *Insanity*. Nobody cares about Tomkat or Brangelina anymore, and even Britney's parenting abilities have gone back to being her own business. Everybody's test-obsessed these days, and since the advent of the machines, life has been draining out of people's eyes piece by piece.

Upside down, Billy grunts something inaudible in a tone that suggests disdain for my weakness, and then humps my mouse as he adjusts his position in the staple hunt. I picture him drooling into a power-outlet, his legs shooting into the air. His ticket would say *Drool* or *Power* or *Idiot*. His shoe is a slip-on, brand new, with a walnut inlay crafted into the shiny black sole. I could snatch it off and club him to death with it in a second. Then he'd get *Shoe* or *Walnut Inlay* or *Contemptuous Colleague*. Instead of killing Billy, I wonder what Jim Morrison's or Mama Cass's tickets would have read.

I also wonder if the machine ever prints names, and if this would stand up as evidence in court.

—⸸—

"Look," I tell Frank, making my best I'm Not Joking face. "Just so you know—this is takin' our friendship too far. You're abusing my good nature, and this is wrecking my important plans for the week. So let me make myself clear, right off the bat. I'm in charge here, or I walk. We're gonna face this stupid fear head-on, or I walk. I'm not wasting my precious time having an arrested-development pajama party with my derailed friend for recreation. This is inconvenient, so if you're not ready to deal with it, I'll get my stuff and come back when you are. Comprendez?"

Frank nods, his lip trembling, and I fling his jacket at him, aiming to snap the sleeve into his eye but missing.

The outdoor market is busy and loud, allowing for nothing faster than a shuffle through the damp, cardboard-smelling cluster-fuck trapped in a repulsive conga line of aged welfare recipients in unwashed brown clothing. We're surrounded by carts piled eight feet high with vegetables, and Frank's face is the color of fresh cauliflower. I can tell the spineless little rodent wants to skitter off and cry—but per *Rule 18* I enforced, pertaining to my conditional residence in his stinking asylum—*When shopping for vegetables, we are handcuffed together at all times.*

The key is in my right sock. Some people are so weak they'll go along with anything you say. Slap them in the face a few times and you could tell them the moon is made of edam cheese. Prior to leaving the house, per *Rule 11*, I made him smoke a joint, and have been whispering paranoia-inducing suggestions into his ear all morning. The poor sap's eyes are pink and perpetually brimming with fear-tears.

"I could reassure you, Frankie," I tell him as we pass between two wheelchairs loaded up with bulging bags full of carrots and cabbages and sprouts. "But it'd completely defeat the purpose of my stay."

In addition to his regular blend of ugly, pathetic, sniveling, disgusting, and completely-at-my-mercy, Frank looks confused.

I get my wallet out, and already he's shaking his head, so I grab his cheeks with my free hand, squeezing hard enough to give him a toothache.

"You need to face this alone," I tell him. "I can't be there forever. You have to build some self-reliance, Frank. Now go buy thirty pounds of whatever veg scares you the most. And before the seller bags them up, I want you to sniff 'em, and inhale the essence of your terror. Look the devil in the eye, Frank. *Now*."

We take the motorway home, *Rule 31* requiring that Frank watch as I tailgate and cut off and drive with reckless abandon around a sixteen-wheeler *Smith's Garden Produce* truck at ninety miles an hour. The sadistic delights are never ending in this vegetable-laden culture. It's raining and the road is slick, and Frank is curled up in the back seat, whimpering and surrounded by sacks of every vegetable we could find. As the truck driver blasts his horn, I flip my middle finger at him, then take a slug from a quart of vodka and start typing a text message on my phone.

Frank starts crying and I grin.

It's late now and Frank's asleep on the sofa.

Earlier on, before he crashed out drunk, he asked me, "Haven't you ever been curious? Hasn't it ever tempted ya?"

I said no, but I was lying. I took the test three weeks ago.

Everybody's curious—it's impossible not to be, but my curiosity was aroused in a different way than most. The testing brought death close and made it seem normal. People realized once again that death is everywhere, all around us all the time. And out of the panic and the closeness came opportunities to assist destiny. I always suspected I was capable of such foul deeds.

Billy's funeral was on Saturday. His ticket in the end would have read *Icy River* or *Cut Brake Lines* or *Betrayal*. I hated that smarmy prick from the moment we met, and my only regret is not seeing his face as he died.

The demented old bastard next door in his piss-stench—I have no idea what his ticket would say, but I beat him to death with his noisy dog and stuffed them both in the oven.

My ticket's worn now, thumbed and crumpled. But as I scoop a handful of cold mashed potatoes from the pan, and get the roll of tape so Frank can't spit it out, I read for the hundredth time: *Electric Chair.*

I screw the ticket up and flick it in the trash, smiling, then walk towards him wielding what he's learned no longer to fear.

Story by Chris Cox
Illustration by Kevin McShane

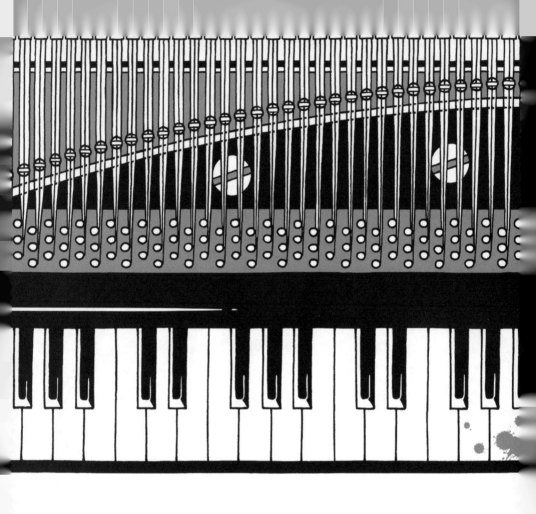

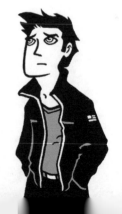

PIANO

PIANO, MAN. CAN YOU BELIEVE IT? FRIGGIN' PIANO. You know what the problem was? I did it when I was sixteen. Friggin' sixteen years old. You don't do that kind of thing when you're sixteen. You're not supposed to know the exact way you're gonna die when you're sixteen! You're supposed to be...friggin' skinning your knee playing street hockey! Reading comics! Getting laid! Not having a blood test to find out you're gonna die by PIANO!

Why why why why did I do it at sixteen? Two reasons:

One, my girlfriend put me up to it. She was that kind of girl, you know. Had that little speck of morbid curiosity. Hell, that's why I was dating her in the first place. She was blonde and morbid. Of course, it wasn't her getting the news. It was the kid in the steel-toed boots and bad haircut.

Two, well...yeah, I was a friggin' kid! People are still waiting in line for a working brain at that age. And I was still holding my number when the Death Machine came out. Whoo! You couldn't miss it. It was the big friggin' summer thing. Stick your arm in, press the button and find out how you're going to die! Everybody was doing it. Stockbrokers, soccer moms, Madonna. It was the latest of the latest. It was in. And when you have sixteen years, steel-toed boots, a bad haircut, and no brain, you want to be in so bad.

I remember everything about that day. It was right there at the mall, between the ice cream stand and Hot Topic, a big hunk of metal with a hole and a slit. There we were, my girlfriend, the voyeur, and I. We went for ice cream, she wiped a spot of vanilla from my forehead with one of those little napkins they give you, and then I did it.

It's incredible, I don't even remember the girl's name, but I still remember what kind of ice cream I got. Vanilla and rocky road. And PIANO. Friggin' PIANO, man.

I didn't know what to make of it, at first. What did it mean? Would a music store collapse on me? Would a kid stab me with a Casio keyboard? Would a piano crush me on the street, and would I stick my head out of the wreckage with black and white keys for teeth? Would I die like Sylvester the Cat?

You try not to think about it, try to live your life like before, when you didn't have to try to not think about it. It wouldn't have been so bad if I didn't live in Manhattan, the skyscraper capital of the world. I was constantly looking up, searching for a crane, a scaffold, a couple of guys holding a rope with a big ol' concert grand swinging back and forth, all the while fingering and twirling that little cardboard rectangle inside my pocket.

"Pay attention to where you're going," my mom used to say. "Get your head out of the clouds." I didn't care. I wasn't going to die from falling into a sewer hole or getting hit by a car. Unless it was a piano-moving truck, of course.

Eventually it got the best of me. The girlfriend dumped me after I had a nervous breakdown watching *Mr. Jones*. You know, Richard Gere. The scene where he takes the girl to the store chock full of... I can't bring myself to say it anymore. And he sits down and plays on one...and then two...I couldn't take it. I snapped.

Hey, she got off easy. She should have seen the drama a couple days later, when *Big* was on and I watched in sheer horror as Tom Hanks danced Chopsticks with his boss.

It was bad. I spent my days cooped up in my room, staring at the Internet and listening to "Bright Eyes" for hours on end. My mom suggested therapy, but I was too embarrassed to discuss it with anyone. It would have been so different if the machine had sentenced me to LANDMINE, or SEPPUKU, or even LOW CABIN PRESSURE.

Those were good ways to go, dude! Manly. But no, the utter ridicu-
lousness of PIANO haunted me night and day.

And the looking up. All the time, everywhere, looking for the
Piano of Damocles swinging over my head.

After three years of thinking about death, facing death, and ultimately waiting for death—just hoping that it would show itself and
rid me of the friggin' question—a thought assaulted me during one
of many sleepless nights. It was a new thought, but at the same time
it was the same old one that whirled around in my mind all the time,
just turned backward. I whacked my forehead at four a.m.

I knew how I was going to die, right? So what did I also know?

How I was not going to die.

I slept like a baby.

I woke up a brand new man. Everything around me was colored
different. Cereal smelled sweeter, the wind felt crisper, and traffic
sounded like chirping birds. Everything changes when you start to
live without fear. I left high school in the dust. I called up friends I
had neglected for too long. And I made a decision about the rest of
my life.

See, it was all the looking up. My head had literally been in the
clouds for three years. And in the sky, I found the love of my life.

I wanted to fly.

Everything fit. I could never be scared of flying at twelve thousand feet, because I knew perfectly well that no plane under my
command would ever crash. I'd find my niche among the aircraft's
buttons, levers, and instruments. As long as none of them were musical instruments, I would be fine.

So I went to flight school. None of my instructors had ever seen
such a confident student. They were used to seeing regular people
shaken or even a little daunted by the complexity of a flying machine.
Not me: I grabbed the controls and took her up like I was riding a

bike. Not a moment of hesitation. If only they knew I had the certainty that nothing would ever go wrong with me at the stick.

The skies became as familiar to me as home. And I was good! It was amazing: knowing I couldn't crash realized and solidified the fact that I would never crash.

Passed every test with flying colors, so to speak. Finally made my mother proud. And how could I fail? I was unafraid. That little card, the one I carried in my pocket everywhere I went, had told me the only thing that could ever kill me. PIANO. Ha! I laughed at the word now. It was just a harmless little word. All I'd had to do was wrap myself in a piano-less world. And planes and pianos do not mix.

I wish I'd known earlier how knowing the exact way I'd die would grant me such happiness and self-confidence. I wanted to kick life in the shin. I became such a daredevil that I joined the military. Yeah, why not? I would go to war. That white card was my carte blanche. It didn't say BULLET, did it? It didn't say BOMB or MISSILE, either. I was unstoppable.

I climbed the ranks like crazy; I made captain like you'd make a hardboiled egg. No one was able to match my piloting skills and daring stunts in the air. I was the envy of the entire service. They trained me to fly helicopters, and I aced that as well. I couldn't wait to get into combat! That's how psyched I was. I even heard they thought I had a deathwish. But death was the least of my concerns. If it wasn't playing the *Cheers* theme song, I said bring it on.

I was the first in line to tour the Middle East. There's always something over here that needs bombing, and I was counting on being the first one off the ground. They even put me in charge of a Black Hawk. A Black Hawk, man! The predator of the sky.

I don't remember the details of this particular mission; I know it went something like this: the Humvees and the .50-cals were supposed to roll into some town somewhere, neutralize the insurgency, and go home. Our four birds were the air support, and I said no worries, dudes. There'll be no Black Hawk Down with me on board, baby. Right?

Wrong.

OK. I hope all this is readable, by the way. I'm writing in the dark on some scrap of cloth I found lying around on the floor of the cell, and you do not want to find out what I'm writing with.

At this point, if anyone ever does read this, you must have figured out there's no happy ending for this one. Obviously I've been taken captive—a hostage to barter with, or perhaps payback for all the Gitmo/Abu Ghraib crap they must have seen on Al Jazeera. That would explain all the cruel-and-unusual we've been subject to for the past...week? Month? I don't even wanna know anymore. This is as far as I want to remember. I'd like to get to the point of all this before I lose the rest of my mind.

I have to think hard about what the point of all this was...I've been having problems gathering my thoughts, lately. It's been hell with the lightbulb, and the mask, and the hi-fi sound system constantly blaring in the background...actually, the foreground when you think of it, since there's nothing over or under it, aft or fore... it smears my days and it haunts my dreams and I know, I know now what it's all come to—I know that music, I know precisely what musical instrument is playing that music, and I have time to think about it too, as I weave and heave and lie here in the darkness, silently contemplating my death...

It's a symphony, it's a concerto, it's "Great Balls of Fire," and yes... whatever it is...it's a *solo*.

Story by Rafa Franco
Illustration by Kean Soo

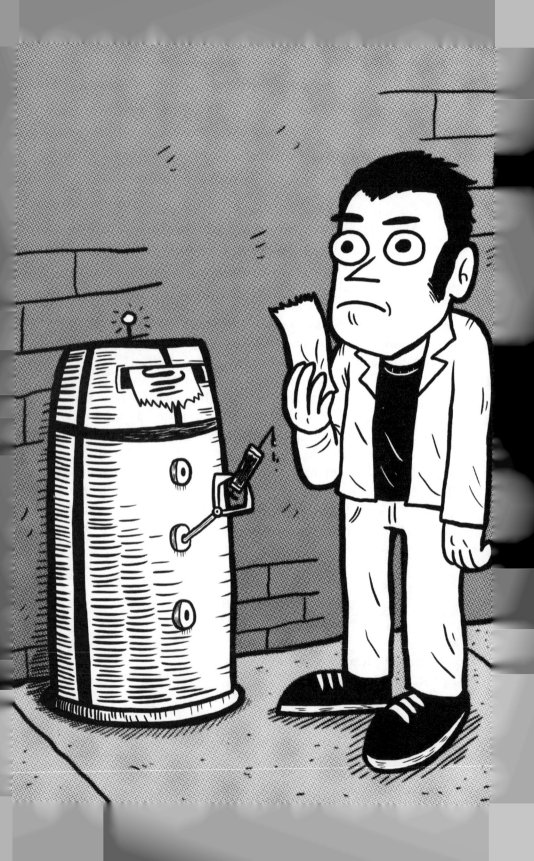

HIV INFECTION FROM MACHINE OF DEATH NEEDLE

"WELL," I thought, "that sucks."

Story by Brian Quinlan
Illustration by KC Green

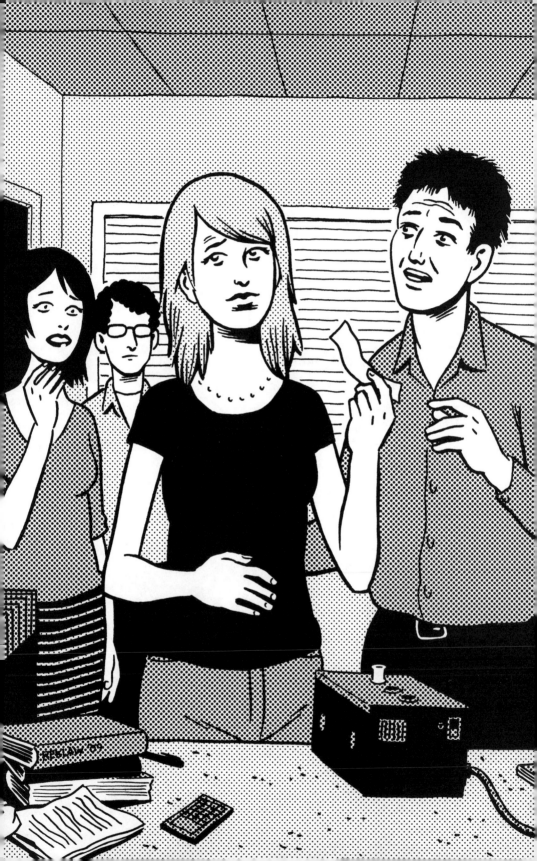

EXPLODED

"Fuck!"

It came from the den. Later I'd learn that it had followed a much quieter, "Oh fuck. Oh—"

My first thought was that it had broken. I was going to spend a lot of time over the next five years wishing that I'd been right about that.

He burst into the room, crunching the door hinges and smacking the handle deep into the plaster. He nearly fell over trying to stop. I didn't say anything, just stared.

"*391!* He was on the train this morning! He was one of the victims!" He stared too. We just stared. *"Look it up!"*

I didn't have to. An electric buzz, as much like actual pain as excitement, jumped from my stomach to my head. I didn't have all our test cases memorised yet, but Mr. 391 I did know: EXPLODED. He was one of the reasons I was sure it wasn't working—his prediction was a joke. He saw I wasn't looking it up, saw me looking at him, and knew I knew, but said it all the same:

"*It fucking works.*"

We were eating.

"Okay, well, it's *on* now." I munched a chip.

"Yeah."

"I mean, it's *on.*" I pointed a chip at him for emphasis.

"Yeah."

"I'm just—"

"*I get that it is on.*"

"Okay." I put my chips down.

I fixed myself a drink.

—⸙—

He came into my office again, calmly this time, through the broken door. My office, his house. We left all the doors open that afternoon, and just walked around doing small, unimportant things, occasionally meeting in the corridors of his big, dusty old house and swapping new thoughts.

"What's the latest count? How many others died?"

"Wikipedia has a hundred now." I told him, underplaying it a little. "Some places have two." They all had two.

"Christ. From one bomb?"

"They think it was a few, and it was on the subway, so…"

"Yeah. Christ." He slouched against the wall and looked up at the cracked ceiling. "This isn't quite how I imagined it working."

"You know we still have to publish our results, right? I mean, that was the point of no return, right there."

"Yeah, yeah, I know. It's just—" He looked at me. "It's going to look like we're profiting off this."

I laughed, then met his eyes. "It's going to look like we're *profiting* from it? Pete, it's going to look like we *did* it. You don't seem to realise how sceptical people are going to be about something like this. You're the only person in the world who has any idea how this box works, and to the rest of us it looks a hell of a lot like a hoax. And when some small-minded prick with a bag of pipe bombs decided commuters were responsible for all the world's problems this morning, it became the most vicious hoax in history. We're going to have protesters on your lawn around the clock, we're going to get ripped to shreds in the press, we're going to be hounded by cameras. We're going to get *mail bombs,* Pete." I sat down, and lowered my voice. "They're gonna try and kill us. Nobody knows yet, but I promise you that at some point in the next eighteen hours, someone Googling the victim names is going to find our prediction list and our lives as they stand will be over." I was realising most of this as I said it. I felt sick. We were fucked.

"We're fucked, aren't we?"

"We're not fucked." I thought about it. We were definitely fucked. "No, we're not fucked."

He shook his head. "We're so fucked."

I sighed. We were so, so fucked.

"I don't, you know," he said suddenly, as we boxed up the prototype.

I frowned. "What?"

"Have any idea how it works. I'm the same as anyone else, except I know it does."

"You *made* it, Pete. I just did your accounts."

"I didn't really. I discovered it. If it had done what I built it to do, if it had been the thing we were trying to make, if it had been the Death Clock—"

"I told you we couldn't call it that."

"—Then I would have made it. But you can't make something like this, it's out there waiting to be found."

"Well, I certainly hope you *can* make it. Because we're going to need a job fucking lot of them."

"You know, this is the best possible way it could have happened."

"What the hell?" I was actually shocked.

"No, I mean, to prove it. You couldn't ask for a more conclusive test." He put up a hand to silence me, "I know, I know loads of people are going to think we blew up a train to sell a box, but this is still going to convince more people than we ever dreamed we would. Your investor friends aren't going to think we blew up San Francisco, they're going to think it works."

"They're not going to like the publicity."

"They don't have to, yet. No one has to know they're investing, and they all know that by the time they come to sell them, the whole world will realise they work." I was the business brain of the operation, but Pete wasn't an idiot. I knew it from the moment he said "391": this would *make* us.

"Did you tell Jen yet?"

"What? Yeah, of course! You didn't tell Cath?"

"Not yet." Honestly, it had only just occured to me.

"Well why the hell not? You've got to tell her, dude." I hate it when he calls me *dude*.

"I just—how do you say it? How did *you* say it?"

"I said 'Jen, it works,' same as I said to you."

"Actually you said *'It fucking works!'*" I mocked, in my best nasal geek voice. "But you told her how we know?"

"Yeah."

"Was she freaked out?"

"Of course. Aren't you?"

"I'm—I've been—" I came clean. "I feel sick. I've been feeling sick for three hours now."

He looked straight at me; I don't talk like that often. "You've got to tell her. Jen'll tell her, and she'll tell her when I told her. You know what they're like, women just find a way to get times into conversations."

"I can't say I'd noticed."

"Well, they do."

I walked into the den. Pete was tinkering again, already. I set his coffee down and took a sip of mine.

"Thanks."

I ignored him. "Here's what we do. You spend the rest of the night packing all this away, everything you need. I hire a van. You hire a hangar. I hire an agent. You draw me up a list of the components that went into the latest prototype—not the ones you *think* you'll need for the new improved version, I know you. The components for *this* one. I'll give the investors the heads-up before the news breaks, and tell them we need the first payment by noon tomorrow. You call every engineer friend you trust and get them on board. Write out a step-by-step assembly guide an idiot could follow in the van on the way, then make sure we don't hire any idiots to follow it. I order us a new pair of phones, we throw these away, and we give the new numbers to *no one* but Cath and Jen unless I say. We disappear. I can sort out accommodation once we're out of here, and a few months down the line we can buy a new place, but right now we have to get as many of these things built and making predictions as possible. The more predictions they make, the more get proved right, the fewer mail bombs we get." I sipped. "What's that?" He was writing something.

"It's a step-by-step assembly guide an idiot could follow." He put it on a thin pile.

"What are those?"

"Well," he leafed through them, "this one's a component list for the prototype, this one's a map to the hangar we've hired, these are the resumés of the three most expensive agents I could find, this one's a printout of a receipt for two iPhones, this one's a fax from the Hyatt confirming our reservation, and these are the keys to our new van." He tossed them to me. I looked around the room, I guess for the first time. It was full of neatly packed boxes.

"What do I do at this company again?"

"It's never really been clear to me." He took a sip of his coffee and went back to writing. "Call the investors!" he shouted after me as I left, forgetting my mug.

"We're not going to get killed by a mail bomb, you know," he said in the van on the way up. It was dark, I was driving, which meant the radio stayed off. "We know that much. Whatever happens with this, it won't kill us. I'm an aneurysm and you're a heart attack, those were the first two tests we ever ran."

"Yeah." I'd been thinking about that a lot since we discovered the box really worked. I wondered what it would feel like. "Christ, what about Cath and Jen?" I'd refused to let either of them be tested.

"We'll have them take it, we have to now." They were coming up tomorrow. The thought of it made me queasy.

"*No,*" I said suddenly. "No. I don't want it hanging over them." Then, feeling the familiar emotional crunch of stepping on Pete's toes when it came to Jen, "Not Cath, anyway."

"We have to."

"You think about it, don't you? What it's going to feel like? Come on, we don't want that for them." He stared at the wing-mirror. "If I looked through your browser cache, I'd find a bunch of sites about aneurysms, right?"

"No." He looked back at the road. We sat in silence for a few minutes, the blank road purring beneath us as a half-tunnel of arched black trees flashed by either side. "I cleared it."

I looked away from the road for the briefest moment. He was smiling.

So that was that day. I persuaded Cath not to take the test, and Jen didn't need persuading: she said over her dead body, and I said we probably wouldn't bother if she was already dead, and she said good, and updated her position to "Not *even* over my dead body." In all of our discussions that night, I don't think Pete or I considered that they'd have a say in it themselves.

But Cath did take it, years later, and it was the beginning of the end. For us, for everything.

We had a few good years before that. I'd thought the heat would die down once everyone realised the machine truly worked, but

I couldn't have been more wrong. Once it became clear just how reliable the predictions were, a huge number of people decided the machine itself was *causing* the deaths. And after we went into hiding that night, we never came out.

We knew fairly early on, I think, that we wanted nothing more to do with the device. We'd only started this company to get rich, and there seemed little doubt we'd achieved that. We thrashed out a deal that would net us a huge lump sum then continue to pay out in royalties no matter what people did with our technology, and sold the rights that first week. We became the elusive guys who just made this inexplicable thing and disappeared, which of course only added to the romance and public fascination with our little box. It wasn't until much later that Pete's scientific curiosity took hold again, and for those intervening years he was as happy as we were to let the world scratch its head at what we'd done, even as it wrote out our cheques.

We each changed hair colour at least once, we went by fake names (I was Chris, Pete was Jason, Cath was Carol and Jen insisted on being Cath, confusing and irritating us all), we only did interviews by email and IM, and we took turns picking the next country to spend a month in. The genius of it was that we'd essentially made our millions by creating something utterly useless. It didn't *help* to know how you would die, precisely because the machine was so accurate—you couldn't avoid it even when you knew it was coming.

Well, not entirely useless. You couldn't avoid the death it predicted, but it was very possible that you'd avoided other deaths simply by consulting the machine. The way Pete explained it to interviewers was this:

Say you're a clumsy skydiver. One day you're going to screw your parachute up and fall to your death. But the machine won't tell you that, because then you'd stop skydiving and it wouldn't come true. Instead, the machine tells you you'll die of a heart attack. You decide to take it easy on the high-stress sports, preferring that your inevitable demise be later rather than sooner, and you live twenty years longer than you would have if you'd never taken the test.

For an electrical engineer, Pete was suspiciously good at marketing. I maintain that it would have been cheaper to produce an empty box with "Don't skydive" written on the side—and usually say so at that point in the interview—but the world seems to prefer his device.

It gets a little more complicated if you're not a clumsy skydiver, of course, but on the whole the machine extends peoples' lives by giving them the chance to stave off their fate for as long as possible—and in the process, miraculously avoiding the many others that ought to have claimed them along the way. None of the deaths it predicts are avoidable, but almost all of them are postponable. *Almost.*

That's why we never felt particularly bad about what we'd done, no matter how much pain and misery it seemed to cause, no matter how many times the police intercepted anthrax and explosives addressed to the old manor. I found those more *offensive* than anything. It's a matter of public record that Pete and I are not scheduled to die from an explosion or a disease, so the authors of these assassination attempts must have known their efforts would only ever hurt innocent people. Not that *we* were even guilty of anything in particular.

In between the people whose lives we saved and the people whose lives we ruined, we got a pretty bizarre set of responses to our mysterious black box—co-licensed and manufactured by over three hundred companies worldwide, to date. A lot of people found the suggestion of inevitability incredibly offensive, and tried to do everything they could to defy it.

In some cases, avoiding death became secondary to disproving the machine: one man gashed his wrists to disprove a slip that told him he'd die of AIDS. He survived, of course—he'd just received his prediction from a machine in a GP's office, so there was help on hand. But he'd used an unsterilised scalpel from a nearby dolly, and with a grim inevitability familiar to anyone who follows special prediction cases, he contracted HIV from that.

Others took the fatality of it all as an excuse for hedonism, either because the manner of their death wasn't related to their passions, or precisely because it was. If it's going to kill you anyway you'd be mad to abstain, went the logic. Both types tended to die quickly. That caused some public concern, but I hardly thought the machine could be blamed for the live fast/die young correlation. Obviously those that overindulged in the vices that were to kill them died from them quickly—even *they* must have seen that coming.

It was the former group that suffered a stranger fate: their heart attacks, tumors and cancer struck quickly, as if eager to get their kill in before the toll of that lifestyle snatched it from them and proved the machine wrong. It looked, in other words, like the machine was killing to prove itself right. Mind you, all statistical anomalies look suspicious if you take them in isolation. That was a tiny group—reckless men with bad habits didn't get slips saying NATURAL CAUSES often.

For the most part, it was just like each of us had a new medical condition, and all of us were hypochondriac about it. Even me. I, like the millions of HEART-ATTACKs out there, never touched red meat again, drank only in moderation, took light, regular exercise and simply left the room if anyone started arguing or stressful decisions needed to be made.

I'd even heard that some particularly ghoulish socialites held parties at which guests were obliged to wear their slips like name-tags, using the nature of their demise as a conversation starter. I never went to one, but a part of me felt like they had the right idea: you can't take this cruel cosmic joke seriously, this blackest of humour, this mockery of fate. The only reasonable response to it is to go up to a stranger and say "Oh, hey, megaloblastic anemia? I hear that one's a bitch."

We could laugh about it, and we could forget it, and we did—lots of both. But it encroached on all our quiet moments: we felt infected. The prediction made it as if our death had already taken root in our bodies, and it was impossible not to visualise it. Memories of health-infomercial graphics haunted me, phong-shaded fat congealing in my arteries and constricting my bloodflow. I could put it to the back of my mind, always, but never entirely out.

The traveling was my idea. I never really knew what to do with the money, after working so long in the pursuit of it. Buying anything extravagant—helicopters, hotels, heroin—seemed to involve an awful lot of effort, and I can't honestly say that the only thing stopping me from buying these things before had been a lack of funds. I didn't want them. I didn't *want* anything, much, just a little safety.

I thought about giving it all to charity—there was even a dedicated one to helping people escape their machine-determined fate, the futility of which made me gape—but I knew I'd regret it. I hadn't done many generous things in my life, and they'd all made me feel terrible. In the end I did give a chunk of it to BrainHelp, a charity devoted to helping the survivors of aneurysms, because it was close enough to home to mean something to me, and useless enough to Pete not to be personally motivated.

But travel was my way of escaping that contentment, fleeing the realisation that we had nowhere else to go in life. We would, instead, go to the places we hadn't yet been. It was one of my better ideas, except for the part where it nearly kills my girlfriend.

I begged her not to do it. Well, pleaded. Well, openly disapproved. A Thai taxi had smashed into our flimsy tuk-tuk on the reeking streets of Bangkok. I, she argued, had been smugly safe in the knowledge that it wasn't going to kill me as we tumbled out onto the sidewalk, while she had been freaking out. I tried to tell her that it wasn't like that, that when something actually *happens* all rational thought about predictions flies from your head, but either she didn't believe me or she didn't care. She was wild, she just had to know.

I should have been a real man about it and stopped her. Or a good man, and supported her. But instead I was an *actual* man about it, which meant that I whined, chided, and made her feel bad about herself without actually helping in any way. She'd come to expect nothing more.

We used the original prototype for it, still under a tarp in that first hangar, and everything we did echoed. Pete and Jen came along for moral support. She replaced the needle with its fresh tube of claret attached, and we waited for the smooth hum of the printout.

She stood up, took it, looked at it, and looked away, almost in one motion. I didn't notice her hand tremble as she passed it to me, but the tip of the slip of paper quavered delicately, giving her away. I looked up at her.

I took it. I read it. It was one word.

I started to sob.

The machine doesn't tell you *when* you're going to die, I'd corrected a hundred interviewers about that. But in this case it had. In this one case, it had done exactly what we originally designed it to do: give an ETD.

We both knew, at the moment each of us saw it, even over the simple horror of that awful word, that it meant nine months at the most. We both knew that it would rend us apart, that we'd never be that close again. Closer in other ways, sure, but not like this, not now that we knew I was going to kill her. We'd already set the wheels in motion. We had nine months, maybe less.

LABOUR. It stared back at us innocently until Cath made me throw the slip away, like it had just wandered out of a perfectly harmless sentence about union disputes. I wanted so badly to be involved in a union dispute right then, for that to be my biggest problem, for that to be what LABOUR meant to me.

I wanted to recall all the machines and tell Pete to redesign them to print in lower case, or Latin, or pictograms, or anything but that giant glaring word burning its way through the bin and my eyelids. And more than anything I wanted to hold her, and I just, *just* couldn't. I couldn't.

I did it anyway. Standing up was like controlling a crane, and she felt cold, tiny, bony against my chest. I'm a weak, mean, small man, and so is Pete—he told me so. But the one thing he and I can do, and I think it's the reason we became friends, the reason we started this company, is the impossible. If there's a good enough reason to do it, we just do it. In my case that was standing up and putting out my arms, and it was the hardest thing I've ever had to do, but goddamn it I had her now and I wasn't letting her go—for minutes, at any rate.

I looked at the machine over her shoulder as my wet face pressed against her warm cheek, and wondered what Pete's reason had been.

It killed him, in the end. I could never understand it, but those seven months—we didn't get the full nine, and I was almost glad of it by the end—hit Pete every bit as hard as they hit us. It was the first time that what we'd done really got to him. He *loathed* the machines, smashed that original prototype—valued at six and a half million dollars on our insurance paperwork—with a crowbar while drunk one night. Have you ever tried hitting anything with a crowbar? They're fucking heavy. Pete's a geek, but that machine was dust when I found it. I was angry then, actually, but I hadn't realised how bad he'd gotten.

That was when he went back to work. He was obsessed with the idea of "fixing it", as he put it. We'd set out to tell people how long they had to live, and by virtue of the now-famous TILT chip—intended to take into account probabilistic factors relating to your lifestyle that might increase the chances of accidental death—we'd ended up spitting out a horrible piece of information that haunted the user for the rest of his and his family's life. At the time we'd thought its popularity meant it was a success, but Pete was right: we'd failed utterly, we'd created a horrible, horrible thing. *He'd* created it. I only got into the habit of taking some of the credit after he made it clear how ashamed he was.

The TILT chip was the problem. It didn't stand for anything, by the way—Pete just named it in all caps because he was really pleased with it at the time. He was like a little kid once you got him hard-coding. It was all I could do to persuade him to leave off the exclamation mark he insisted it deserved. We both loved telling interviewers that story.

He'd spent years, literally years, working on the algorithm that would use actuarial data and hugely sophisticated conditional probabilities to get a rough idea of how likely people's stupid habits were to kill them, and when he'd finally done it, he discovered something odd. Actually, *I* discovered something odd. If he's going to call it a discovery rather than an invention, then I really can take some of the credit. It was me who, through incompetence rather than the spirit of experimentation, first tried using the machine without entering any data. And instead of a ballpark life-expectancy figure, I got "48 45 41 52 54 2d 41 54 54 41 43 4b". Which, Pete reliably informed me, an extraordinary expression on his face I'd never seen before or since, translated to "HEART ATTACK".

The truth was, it didn't even really need the blood sample—we just kept that part in so that people would take it seriously, and to drive up the manufacturing costs to something investors would believe. For the same reason we insisted that all connectors be made of solid 24-carat gold when any old crap from Radio Shack would have worked, and there was a whole circuit full of wildly expensive and important-looking components in there that wasn't even hooked up to the live elements of the machine.

A few technical journals had picked up on that, but no one dared try remove them. You could see where the fanatics were coming from, really: that hard nugget of inescapable truth just came down a wire, almost in our language, and not even its creator knew why. You could also see why Pete was so pleased with himself, and you could even see, years later, after millions of morbid projections proved true, why he was so wretched.

The problem, he suddenly announced once he stopped drinking, was the accuracy. He'd made it far, far too good. You didn't actually *want* a machine that was always right, the machine you really wanted was one that was always wrong. Wrong because you were able to *avoid* the death it predicted, the one you would otherwise have succumbed to, and live happily ever after.

A bad news machine that can't be defied is an inherently unmarketable idea, he told me, trying to speak my language. I decided not to get out my black AmEx card to demonstrate just *how* marketable it had been. So he started work on a spec for the machine's nemesis, the cure, the Final Solution to death itself, what he called Project Idiot.

I would have stopped him, should have, and God damn me for not doing it, but I was just grateful for the distraction. Something to think about other than the ways in which Cath's ever-growing bulge might rip her apart, and how it would make me feel about our daughter, if she survived.

He couldn't do it. He had a dozen brilliant ideas, but it just couldn't be done. The TILT chip defied him with the same silent, sinister smugness it defied those who tried to prove it wrong. He couldn't recreate it, he couldn't modify it, and he couldn't trick it. He discovered that it wasn't even using his actuarial data to make the predictions, it had just incorrectly surmised our purpose in entering them, and pulled the result it imagined we were after from nowhere.

My explanation was that it was quantum, the perfect catch-all for the apparently impossible. But Pete said something over and over that to this day I don't quite get: "It's a function of the future," he said, "not the past." He said it didn't matter what he did to it before it was built, because its predictions were somehow independent of anything that had already happened. I don't know, but he kept saying it.

So it was the future he tinkered with, and he was sure one of his tricks would work. He became fixated on the moment when the patient actually reads his slip: if he takes the test but never reads it, it will say something different than if he'd taken it and read it as normal. The ink doesn't change, it will *always* have said something different—it was the machine's most uncanny and unsettling ability: knowing with total certainty what you will do in response to its prediction.

He talked to a loose society of machine fanatics who kept their unread predictions curled up in tiny silver pendants around their necks, to be opened and read in emergencies to find out if they're about to die. No help. Eventually he built a full prototype of a machine that would email the result to a server in Wyoming that was hooked up to a Geiger counter, and would send the result on to the patient's email address if it registered a radioactive decay within a second of receiving it, or scrub the data from its hard drives if not.

He needed a way of getting the information to the patient without the machine knowing whether it would or not, but every time he tested it it produced the same result as the existing machines. Schrodinger's Idiot, he called that one. He'd decided the physics students who owned the machine in Wyoming were going to get drunk one night and mail out everyone's results, which he was sure they were recording despite his instructions, and he'd been planning to drive out there and do I don't know what the next morning. The morning after I found him.

He was slumped over his desk. I always knew it would be me doing this. I set our coffees down and looked at the clock. Time of death, 22:25—or earlier. I'd pictured him with a soldering iron in hand when I'd played this out in my mind before, hundreds of times, but as I gently lifted his cold, curly-haired head off the bench I saw that it was papers he'd been working on. Printouts from his CAD software, scribbled on in green biro. I couldn't make them out then, but I looked later, and I liked them so much I had them framed.

I never picked up much engineering savvy from Pete, but his margin notes made it plain enough. He'd designed The Idiot, and it would have worked. It had a lookup table of the most common causes of death and it simply discarded the blood sample and picked one at random, weighted toward the most common. It would be wrong, again and again, and even when it was right, it would be avoidable. The Idiot, had he made it, would have exceeded its spec as dramatically as the original machine. I could only think of one way to make it stupider, and I knew Pete always got a kick out of my terrible ideas, so before framing it I wrote "Don't skydive" on the side.

Lisa, we called her. Oh, yeah, she was fine—we knew she would be. We took a blood sample in the second trimester and had it tested: She's going to die of emphysema, so unless she'd been bumming smokes off the placenta in there, we were in the clear. She and I.

She's going to be an interesting case, actually—it's not something that happens quickly, emphysema, so I'll be intrigued to see how I fail *this* woman so utterly that I end up repeatedly exposing her to a toxic gas over the course of enough years that it ultimately destroys her lungs and kills her. Am I just going to forget to tell her, for her entire life, "Oh, and don't smoke"? You have to wonder.

I was already overcompensating—I actually hit a guy last week for pulling out a cigarette at a housewarming party I was hosting at Pete's old place, my old office, the place where it started. He'd left it to Jen, but she'd given it to me when she left the country. She didn't ask for any money and I didn't offer any; Jen and I had a double-share each now, so it made no difference to either of us. We hardly talked, anyway. Tragedy doesn't bring people together, who started that bullshit? It's like nitro-fucking-glycerin.

"Does anyone have a light?" he said.

"No, but I have a...lights out...sandwich?" I almost said, before realising how amazingly lame it was. I'd already hit him by then, too, so I think the point had been made. It was almost a reflex.

I've been steadily losing it for a year now. I should come up with a more peaceful solution, like "Actually I'd rather you smoked outside. *In Kazahkstan.*" But I don't think it's going to come up again, not now.

I was working in my old office when it happened, the crib within arm's reach. He burst into the room, crunching the door hinges and smacking the handle deep into the plaster, and nearly fell over trying to stop. For that split second, when it was just a blur, on my *life* I thought it would be Pete.

It wasn't Pete. He was huge. A big, broken, sad face. I didn't say anything, just stared. He must have been six foot six. He stared too, wild. We stared. He said two low, fragile words, "My son," then trailed off and just pointed it at me.

The words sounded dumb even as I spluttered them: "Please, I have a—"

He dropped the gun, apparently surprised by what he'd done, though from my perspective it was hard to see how it might have been an accident. I couldn't see what was in his other hand, but I had a good guess. He presented it to me timidly, like a receipt for our transaction, and I could see then that this had not been his plan. He must have imagined shoving it in my face, or making me eat it as I died. The whole thing seemed to be surprising him a lot more than it was me. I always figured I had something like this coming.

I was paralysed, I could feel that immediately. My body felt like soft lead, heavy and heatless, as I slumped against the oak-panelled wall, heart pounding, my head bent awkwardly down into my chest as the last twinges of control and sensation faded from my clammy hands. I gurgled like a baby. Blood, I saw, sticky brilliant blood dribbling down my chin. Messy business.

I couldn't take the slip from his hand, but I could read it even through the rivers of sweat trickling into my eyes. And I could see his issue with me—with *us*, but Pete lucked out and died first. I could see how horrible the last three years must have been for this hulking man and his tiny kid, and how much worse that final moment must have been. POISON. One of the machine's bitterest pills. He probably thought it was the worst you could get. I knew better, but I wasn't in a position to argue.

Ah, who knew? Maybe it was. I tried to imagine watching Lisa suckle one of those cold rubber teats I filled Cath's role with, knowing that any given gulp might be infected with a fatal toxin. He must have known that checking his food beforehand wouldn't help, but I knew, now, having Lisa, that it wouldn't have stopped him. Nothing could have stopped him. He probably starved him for a while. Okay, big guy, maybe you're right. You've certainly got me beat. All I had to endure was seven months of knowing that I'd kill the woman I loved. I got off easy. I *deserve* this.

It wasn't until after a few sizable seconds of self-pity that something I'd said over a year ago suddenly drifted through my head again. *"When something actually happens, you forget,"* or words to that effect. I almost laughed. Ha! I just remembered, *I don't die like this!* Screw you and your dead son, asshole! I'm going to get up and kick your ass now, and after that I'm going to raise my goddamn daughter to lead a long, happy life dying of emphysema! If you'll just give me the use of my limbs for a moment.

I managed to cough a bubble of blood, close enough to stain him with a few flecks. Take *that!* My breath stank of, what, money? Dirty loose change, that acid stink. The only thing I could feel was the sweat trickling down my face, nothing below the neck—so much goddamn sweat. Who knew getting shot was such hard work? I was excited now, though, this was my thing. My heart raced. The impossible, you big-boned prick, is my goddamn speciality. You are so fucked. I was just about to stand up, I felt sure, when he slammed an enormous knee into my chest and kept it there, kneeling on me with what must have been all of his gigantic weight.

When I came to I saw, even as the pressure mounted, nothing on my chest. Both the man's knees were walking away from me to investigate a tiny cry from Lisa in the crib. I couldn't see his reaction, I couldn't get up, I couldn't get this invisible fucking thing off my chest, I couldn't *breathe.*

I had just enough time to think, "Oh come on, this hardly counts," before I let out a sad little rasp and it all closed in.

Fuck.

Story by Tom Francis
Illustration by Jesse Reklaw

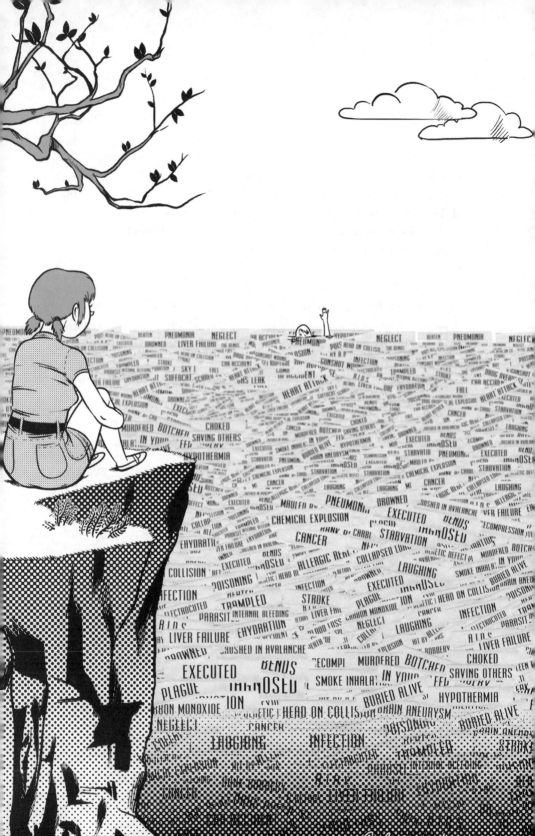

NOT WAVING BUT DROWNING

EVERYONE KNOWS THAT THE FOURTH DAY OF NINTH GRADE IS WHEN YOU GET YOUR RESULTS. I mean, that's the way it happens in our town; other towns do it differently. Amy, who moved here from Atlanta, said that in the big cities they do it when you're born, since they have to take blood from babies, anyhow, to test for HIV and that disease that means you can't drink Diet Coke. (She says she's going to be shot in a botched robbery, but I think she's lying. She also said her aunt is on *Days of Our Lives,* and I don't believe that either.) But here, in our town, all the parents got together and decided that they just couldn't take knowing before we were at least in high school. Tim K. says it's because when you're in ninth grade, your parents find you so annoying that they can actually bear to think about you dying. Allycia thinks it's because when you're our age you think you're immortal and they want to scare it out of us. That might have been true for our parents, or our grandparents, but I don't know anyone our age who hasn't always known that they're really going to die.

The way it works is pretty easy. The first day of ninth grade, in homeroom, the school nurse comes in and takes blood samples. She gives a ten-minute speech about the machine and how it works. (Short answer: nobody knows, but it's never been wrong.) She tells us that she's going to die in a fire. She doesn't even shiver when she tells us that—I guess when you've known for years and get up and talk about it every year, it becomes routine. And I guess as a nurse she knows that more people die from smoke inhalation in a fire than from actually being all burnt up.

It's weird to see other people's blood. Darryn and Mike, the two biggest boys in homeroom, can't even watch. I watch the needle go in, careful not to look away. I might want to be a doctor someday. It's hard to decide what you want to do with your life until you know how it's going to end.

All the blood, each sample in a little barcoded tube, goes into one of those freaky BIOHAZARD mailers, and the nurse seals it in front of us. She has a whole cart of packages. Our homeroom was last.

Then we wait. Of course it's all anyone can talk about. Helen wants to die glamorously, like in a terrorist attack. "Do you know how much money your family gets if you die in a terrorist attack?" Naturally, we all hoot at this—there haven't been hardly any terrorist attacks at all, since the machine. There are still some every once in a while, in really poor places like India and Russia, where people can't afford the test, but it's hard to scare people about terrorism if they know they're going to die because they stuck a fork in a toaster. Kells wants to die of old age, but that sounds awful and boring to me. And everyone knows that it's impossible to get a job in a rock band if you have a test that says "old age." All the record labels are looking for the next Kurt Cobain—death, even when you know it's coming, still bumps up downloads and sales. You know that singer Bryson? She got "drug overdose" and you can't even click on a tabloid page without a picture of her looking wasted. Her music sucks but everyone can't wait to see how she flames out. My brother thinks it's all a big put-on. He thinks she's totally straightedge and "drug overdose" means that some overworked nurse is going to give her the wrong dose eighty years from now when she's in a nursing home. Mylena wants mad cow disease. She says if she gets that it means she'll never die, 'cause she's a vegetarian, and always has been. Her parents are vegetarians and everything.

It's hard to know what to wish for. Old age could be dying in bed, with all of your family around you, just like in a movie, with your daughter holding your hand and a room full of flowers, or it could be horrible Alzheimer's and being tied to a bed so you don't wander off, with no one there at all but you don't care because you can't remember anyone anyway. Car accident could be instant or it could be paralysis or amputation and infected bedsores that give you that staph they don't have antibiotics for anymore. Heart failure could be a dramatic heart attack, the fall-down-clutching-your-chest kind, or it could just be you get old, your heart stops. As I said, it's hard to know.

My mom and dad have the same one. Cancer. They met at a death party in college, where you got paired up with someone who was going to die the same way. They were the only two cancers at the party; by the time the machine came around most cancer was curable. Which sucks for them because they know they're going to have one of the bad kinds of cancer, like ovarian or pancreatic or brain, the really painful kinds. At least now when you get those kinds of cancer the doctors know you're going die from it, and they give you lots of painkillers. It used to be that it was hard to get painkillers, my mom told me. When her grandma died of breast cancer she was in lots of pain but the doctors wouldn't give her drugs in case she got addicted. That's because nobody knew she was going to die of the cancer. They thought maybe the cancer would go away and then they'd have an old lady addicted to morphine to deal with. That doesn't happen anymore.

My brother has just "accident," which freaks him out. It freaked us all out. Usually the machine is pretty specific. Car accident, household accident, whatever kind of accident. Just plain accident is pretty rare. For a while he went through what everyone goes through—the whole avoidy thing. He put grab bars in our shower. He walked to school, instead of riding the bus or his bike or driving. He was really worried that it would keep him from becoming a pilot, which is what he really wants to do, but then he talked to a recruiter and the guy said they don't really pay attention to that so much. He said so many pilots actually have "plane crash" that he knows ten guys, personally, who are nicknamed "Crash." It's like a macho thing, to get in that plane every day knowing you're going to die in a crash. Of course most of them crash flying their own personal miniplanes, not the jets.

My grandmas are both dead; one died before the machine, just had an aneurysm. The other grandma, my dad's mom...she was one of the first ones to use the machine in their town. Her ticket said suicide. My dad said she didn't tell anyone she was having the test. She just waited for all of them—my dad, his sister, his dad—to leave the house the next day, and then she took two bottles of sleeping pills. They didn't even know she had them; she got the prescription in another town and had been saving them. She didn't leave a real note. She just wrote "I'm sorry, I knew it" on her machine report and left it on the table. My grandpa—her husband—he's never taken the test. He says that it's wrong to know, and that the whole human race is going to descend into mediocrity because of it. (He talks like that a lot.) He says that the fear of death, coupled with its unpredictability, is what drives humanity to achieve. He likes to talk about how there haven't been any real scientific advances since the machine. He says everyone is too busy spending time with their families and enjoying life to do any real work. Then he laughs and lights another cigarette. He's the only person I know who smokes. It's crazy old-fashioned, like wearing a monocle or having a gas-powered car. He can't even buy them in town anymore, he has to have them imported from India. Once they shipped him the wrong brand and he had to smoke bright pink ones for a week until he got more. The pack played this loud Bollywood song whenever he opened it. That was even funnier.

My other grandpa, my mom's dad, is going to die from pneumonia. He says his goal is to put it off as long as possible. He always gets a flu shot, he drinks all this horrible green vitamin juice powder stuff, and he exercises more than anyone I know. We all tease him about it, but he says he's going to be the world's oldest pneumonia victim.

I don't really know too much about other people's tickets. Most people don't talk about it. It's hard to know what to say, when you find out someone's going to be shot, or hit by a car, or fall from a height. You either find yourself saying "that's not so bad" or you just talk about something else. It's kind of rude to ask someone that you don't know well. And since it's so vague, sometimes it's hard to know what to do. I heard that there was this girl in Charlotte, one of the first people to get the test, and her ticket said she'd die at graduation. So she wore black all through high school, really gothed-out. She was like, queen of the goths. And her graduation came and went, and nothing happened. College, too. She went to law school: nothing. I heard she finally died driving across a totally different campus and the crane that was putting up the graduation reception tent backed into her car. I know this is probably an urban legend but I don't want to snope it and find out.

Some people you do know how they'll die. Like, if they're famous. Famous people's tickets always get out. Someone they told will tell the tabloid pages—I've heard they pay a lot of money for famous tickets. Politicians have to disclose it. One guy who was running for governor in Tennessee faked his—his really said "shot by a hooker" and he got it to read "stroke." Of course someone sold that story. Now the politicians have to have their tests taken in public and read right there. That one movie actress, the really pretty one, what's her name—her ticket actually says "broken heart." I've never heard of anyone else having that one. Of course people didn't believe her so she went on TV and had the test retaken, and there it was. She is always being paired with her costars in the tabloids, like, she'll be in a movie with some guy and the headline will read "WILL HE BE THE ONE TO KILL HER???" She just laughs it off, but I'd be afraid. You can't help falling in love, right? It's not like you can have a grab bar for going on dates.

The day you get your results back there aren't any classes; you just show up for homeroom. They call you in one by one to another room to get your ticket, and then you just go home. Lots of people's parents take the day off. If they're really dorky they meet you at school. You can't really hang around after, although everyone's texting each other on their phones. Not asking, outright, just "U OK?" Lots of people don't talk about theirs, and that's cool. The teachers discourage it, for the most part, and sometimes your parents get mad if you tell somebody. There was this girl, Julia, in my brother's class and hers said AIDS. She told just one person, her best friend, and then they had a fight and that girl spread it all over school. They wrote "SLUT" on her locker and stuffed it full of condoms. It was awful. Her folks didn't know what to do. Finally they just moved. I think they live in Asheville now. Maybe she even changed her name.

When they called me I felt a little nervous. Like, everyone knows they're going to die, but it's still a wobbly feeling to find out exactly how. My knees felt like they wanted to bend the wrong way, and I almost tripped getting out of my chair. I grabbed my bag and waved to Kells. She mouthed "old age!" at me and gave me a thumbs-up. I smiled back.

I went into the room and sat down, and the counselor made me go through the whole routine. I had to tell him my social, twice. I had to do the iris-scanner, both eyes. I had to show him the waiver from my parents that allowed him to tell me without them present, and I had to sign a form allowing him to tell me, period, and releasing the test people from liability. Then I had to do the breathalyzer; a couple of years ago kids would show up wasted or high for their tests, so now you can't get the results unless you're sober.

Finally he brought out my ticket. It wasn't in an envelope or anything, it was just the top one in his folder. The folder was black, which I thought was kind of weird. Like, why make the folder black?

He was dressed in just regular clothes, tan pants and a blue shirt, no tie or anything, so the black folder just seemed kinda pretentious.

"You have a slightly unusual result," he said. That wasn't good. Unusual meant stuff like mauled by a bear, or electric-mixer accident, or choked on a pickle. Stupid stuff. Not dramatic or cool.

"Let me see." I really didn't want to wait. He pushed the ticket over to me.

In block letters, it said NOT WAVING BUT DROWNING.

The man said, "It's a line from a poem." He held his pen like he didn't know what it was for.

"But it still means I'm drowning, right? It's not so bad."

"We'd like you to have the test retaken. It's unusual to get something like this. Something so…allusive."

I looked at him. He hadn't done a good job shaving that morning; it looked like he used a real razor and not a depilatory laser. Maybe his ticket said he'd be killed by a laser?

"I don't know. I like this one. What if it changed to something worse?"

"That doesn't really happen. They don't change. Sometimes they get more specific—we think yours would get more specific."

"I think I'm good with vague, thanks. Vague and poetic is okay with me."

"Are you sure? You could retake now…" I noticed that he had a test kit, too, next to his chair.

"Nah. I'm okay." I put my ticket in my bag, careful not to fold it. Some people framed theirs, and kept it somewhere safe, especially if it was a cool one, like "saving a child." Mine was totally frameable.

"If you change your mind, here's a number to call." He beamed a number to my phone from his pen. "And we'd like your permission to keep a tracer on you, so that our department will be alerted when you die."

Wow—I was important enough to have a tracer? That was also

cool. I couldn't decide if I'd tell anyone about the ticket, but I could definitely tell people I had a tracer.

"Sure, okay." He pushed another form to me.

"We have to let you think about this one for twenty-four hours, and your parents have to sign it, too. I have to disclose to you that tracer information is subpoenable, which means that if you are accused of a crime the data from the tracer can be used by the prosecution and the defense. It cannot be requested for civil matters in this state, but it can in New York, California, New Mexico, and Mississippi. You can drop off the form in homeroom tomorrow, or you can ping us if you sign it earlier and someone will come by to get it from you and your parents."

He stood up, so I got up, too. He shook my hand. "I think you are a remarkable young woman," he said, like he didn't say that to everyone. "Please use this knowledge to focus and direct your life, and to live while you can." Then he recited the machine motto, *Dum vivimus vivamus*. Although nobody really knows Latin anymore, everyone knows that bit. It means "while we live, let us live."

On my way home, Kells texted me. "OLD AGE OMG YAY!!!" was her whole text, so I just sent back a smiley and an "IM OK" and another smiley. Mine really wasn't something you could text. I was glad for her, though. I bet she was going to be the great-grandma-in-the-room-full-of-flowers kind of old age dying.

My folks were home, and I think they had been crying. It's hard to think of people you love dying. Like they thought if they didn't know, I'd live forever or something. My dad gave me a big hug and kind of sniffled, before I even showed him the ticket, which was weird.

I didn't really know what to say about the ticket, so I just pulled it out and showed it to them. "The guy said it was from a poem." My folks looked a little shocked, but then my mom just googled up the poem on the living room screen. We just stood there and read it, and clicked through to read about the poet. It was by somebody named

Stevie Smith, who I first thought was a guy but who turned out to be a woman. The poem was kind of famous, but pretty old, older than my parents. Stevie died of a brain tumor, which was as close as you could get back then to knowing for sure how you were going to die. Not a lot of people survived brain tumors. I kind of liked that she died that way. Not that she died, of course, but that she probably knew.

My grandpa, for all he talks about how he hates the machine, came in while we were clicking around. My dad hates that he just walks in, but my grandpa always forgets to use the bell, or even to set his phone to ping us when he's close, and of course the house is set to let him in. My dad didn't notice him until he was right there, close, and then he said "Jesus, Pops!" in a kind of shaky voice.

Grandpa didn't even ask, he just looked at my ticket. "Ho ho!" he said. (He's the only person outside of the vids who ever says "ho ho!" in that old-timey way, instead of in the "ho ho ho" Santa way.) "Now that's a poetic death. I could almost warm up to a machine that spits that out."

Anyway, that's when my mom and dad and grandpa started arguing about whether it was good or awful, and my dad started in again telling my grandpa he should get tested, so I kind of sneaked away and went up to my room. I didn't know myself, but I kind of liked the not-knowing. The fact that it was a line of a poem: cool. The fact that I could get a tracer: cool. Drowning: not so bad. I'd heard it was peaceful, and I really hate swimming anyway (it messes up my hair) so that was good to have an excuse not to swim.

I pulled up the poem again and made it the background on my screen. I think I'll leave it there for a little while.

Story by Erin McKean
Illustration by Carly Monardo

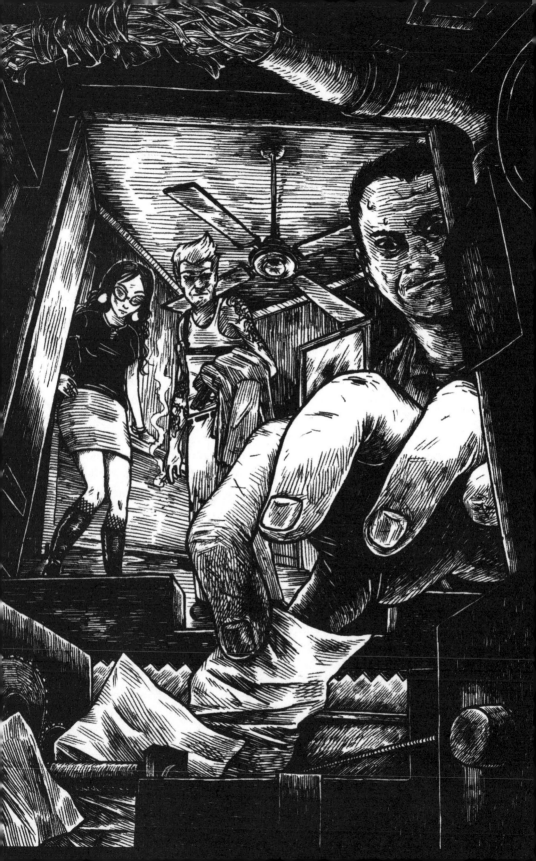

IMPROPERLY PREPARED BLOWFISH

ISHIKAWA TSUENO AND HIS JUNIOR, KIMU MAKOTO, SAT HUNCHED
IN THEIR CHAIRS, PANTING IN THE HUMID, DARK RECEPTION OFFICE.
Kimu removed his suit jacket and plaintively massage-punched himself in the arms, while Tsueno just cracked his neck and upper back
with a slight tilt of his head, sat back, and breathed deeply. The air
in the little upstairs room was faintly curdled by the persistent scents
of ancient sweat and menthol cigarettes. The ceiling fan did nothing
to banish those odors, nor to dissipate the heat in the room that had
built up all day.

Relaxing, Tsueno slipped off his shoes, and looked down at them.
He noticed a wide smear of gooey blood on the left one. Shaking his
head, he tugged a handkerchief out of his pants pocket and wiped
it off. As he was leaning forward, he noticed that there were bits of
brain and clotted blood spattered on his pant leg, too. He cussed
to himself: *stupid bastards*. Why couldn't they have just handed the
damned machine over? It would have saved him a trip to the dry
cleaners.

As he finished wiping his shoe and picking bits off his pant leg,

and crumpled the handkerchief in one hand, Itō's woman Yukie
entered the room through the back door. Yukie was not Itō's wife,
but his 22-year-old lover. She was young enough to be his daughter, and looked sexy as ever: miniskirt, skintight black t-shirt, big
amber-
tinted sunglasses, all kinds of jewelry, heavy makeup. She was carrying
a tray of some kind, though it was too dark to see what was on it from
across the room. She shut the door behind her with a high-heeled
foot, closing off the inner sanctum of the mens' boss, "Father" Itō.

Yukie walked right up to the machine, bent forward a little, and
gave it a close look.

"Heavy," she mumbled.

Tsueno nodded, shoving the bloodied handkerchief into his
pocket. Kimu nodded, too, and smiled toothily at her. It was indeed
a heavy machine, about the size of a small photocopier but apparently densely solid inside. Carrying it up three flights of stairs at a
leisurely pace would have been bad enough, but hurrying the thing
up to Itō's office had just about killed Tsueno. Once again, he regretted that the smaller models Kimu had found online had not been
released in Japan before the machines had been banned. Yukie
smiled as she looked at them, still trying to catch their breaths, and
then turned back to the machine. She started sounding out some of
the English labels on the buttons.

Tsueno turned and saw Kimu staring at Yukie's backside, and
sighed. Damn undisciplined *Zainichi*. Yes, he thought to himself
as his eyes brushed her long bare legs, her body was perfect—not
that his own wife's was anything to sneeze at—but you don't stare at
your *Oyabun*'s woman like that. He'd worked with Korean-blooded
Japanese before, and had been reluctant to take Kimu on because of
his experience with crap like this. Tsueno wondered just how foolish
Kimu was. The guy was young, and fit. There were thousands of girls
in Fukuoka alone who'd sleep with him, many of them almost as sexy

as Yukie. Was the chip on his shoulder *that* big? Tsueno wondered whether Kimu's father hadn't perhaps been killed for the same exact behaviour, leaving his son orphaned over a momentary leer.

"Here," Yukie said, turning and setting her tray out on the table. On it were some paper cups and a few glistening bottles of iced green tea.

"*Arigato gozaimasu,*" Tsueno said, conspicuously polite without even thinking about it. Yukie was the boss's woman. The last man who'd spoken to her too familiarly had, rather famously, been chopped up and fed to one of Itō's pet crocodiles. Tsueno reached for one of the bottles. It was ice-cold, and the droplets of condensation on the plastic felt wonderful in his hand, against his forehead as he raised it to his skin to cool himself. He felt like shoving the bottle down his shirt-front. Why the hell hadn't Itō ever installed an air conditioner in the reception room?

Yukie just smiled, and sat down to wait. She turned her head, and looked at the machine some more.

She doesn't usually serve drinks, Tsueno observed. She must've been sent to fill time. Was their *Oyabun*—their boss—stalling? But why? Itō had always had a predilection for old things: An old sword hung on the wall behind his desk, and he was always reading old novels. Perhaps he was even old-fashioned enough to be terrified of tempting fate, by actually using the Machine of Death? Some kind of Kawabata-type dramatic crap? Tsueno had read a book by that guy. He much preferred manga. Especially vampire manga.

After a few long minutes, Yukie said, almost sang, "It's very big." Her voice was high-pitched, melodious. Tsueno quipped silently to himself about how her conviction was very well-practiced on this familiar line.

"Yeah. It's an older model, ya know," Kimu said, and retrieved a pack of cigarettes from his shirt pocket. He was slouching noticeably, where Tsueno had sat up a little.

Tsueno wrinkled his nose, scratched it with the tip of a finger, looked at Kimu and Yukie.

"Do the older ones work as well?" she asked, mellifluous.

"Sure, they're all the same inside. Like men," Kimu blurted, with a smirk. "The newer machines are lighter, but there still aren't many of them around. They've been banned." Kimu flicked his lighter, and lit the cigarette. After a few puffs, he sighed in obvious satisfaction.

She nodded again. Tsueno watched the two of them talking. He felt hungry. He slid his chair toward the wall, away from the other two. He wished softly to himself that she would go back into their *Oyabun*'s office.

"Does it plug in?" Yukie inquired, suddenly.

"Yes, ma'am," Kimu said, and winked.

"Where's the cable?"

Tsueno sat up, alarmed, and looked at the box on the table. He cussed mildly at Kimu. "Hey, where *is* the cable?"

"Probably in the trunk," Kimu said with a shrug.

"Go get it," Tsueno said, suddenly speaking with all the authority of a proper *senpai*, an elder whose orders were to be respected without question. "Now."

A defeated look crossed Kimu's face, but he nodded and rose to his feet. A bottle of iced green tea in one hand, he left the room. That, at least, Kimu seemed to understand: *senpai* orders, and *kōhai* obeys. The relationship between junior and senior was something even a depraved, orphaned *Zainichi* like Kimu understood to the bone.

Tsueno looked at the machine some more.

"It's a lucky thing I asked," Yukie said, after a few moments.

"Yes, miss." Tsueno took a swig of the iced tea, and then held the bottle to his face. The chill moisture on the surface of the bottle moistened his skin, cooled him a little.

"Very hot today," Yukie said stiffly.

Tsueno didn't respond except to nod. She didn't really expect him to. They just sat there in silence awhile, and then Yukie turned and picked up the remote control for the TV on the far counter. She turned the TV on, and laughter filled the room.

It was a sitcom about a salaryman and an alien and a licensed chef and a talking dog. The dog was a real one, a German shepherd with its voice dubbed on; it spoke Japanese with a funny accent that was supposed to be canine but sounded more Chinese than anything. It was fed caramel toffee or chewing gum or something to make it move its mouth like it was talking.

Tsueno had seen the show before and wasn't really interested, but he found himself watching just the same, counting the passage of time by the explosions of laughter that emerged from the tinny speaker on the front of the old TV. The alien was trying to buy the dog a business suit so it could get a job like the salaryman's. The dog was complaining that it didn't want to have to go to an office and work like stupid humans have to do.

Kimu came back, cautiously, the cable coiled in his hand, and shut the door behind himself. A slow snaking trail of smoke rose from the cigarette that was still hanging from his mouth.

"Has he come yet?" he asked.

"No," Tsueno mumbled, and sipped his iced green tea. "Hurry up and plug it in."

Kimu hurried around the table, and jammed one end of the cable into the back of the machine. Then he bent down, his cheap black pinstriped slacks wrinkling around the bend in his knees, and he plugged the other end into the wall.

"It's got an adapter," he said. "Foreign plug."

"Mmm. Black market." Tsueno watched him carefully, and Yukie muted the volume on the TV, suddenly banishing all laughter from the room. The sudden silence drew Tsueno's attention back to the screen. The dog was wearing a business suit now, and speech bubbles showed it moping and whining about its ill luck in actually getting a job at its first interview ever. The poor animal was being hired straight into middle management, because it couldn't read or write or do math.

That last bit made Tsueno grin.

Kimu pushed a button on the main display, and lights started flickering on the side of the machine as it came to life. A strange whirring sound filled the room, and then a slow, rhythmic clicking.

"Did you drop that thing on the way up?" Yukie asked, a little leery.

"No," Kimu said, conspicuously not calling her *ma'am*. "I think this is just how it boots itself up. We'll see in a bit."

Tsueno cleared his throat. "Kimu. Maybe we should test it?"

"Do you think so?" Kimu asked. "Elder brother," he added a moment later, a gesture of respect.

"I don't see why not," Yukie said. "I won't tell him if you won't," she smiled. Tsueno could see how a man could get into serious trouble with this woman.

"What if he walks in, right now?"

"He won't," she said, and made a pained face, and pointed at her groin. "Pissing," she whispered. "It's his prostate..."

Kimu turned to Tsueno and chuckled out loud. Tsueno's only response was to frown at him and say to Yukie, "I don't think you ought to tell us that, miss. He's our *Oyabun*."

"It's okay," she smiled, and her eyes went to Kimu. "Why don't you try it out?"

Tsueno followed her gaze to Kimu and gave him one of those *don't do it* looks, but the younger *yakuza* took the bait. *Boldness and intelligence rarely roost together,* Tsueno reflected.

"Okay," Kimu said loudly, and stuck his finger into a hole in the side of the machine. With his free hand, he searched around the buttons slowly, until he found the one he was looking for. He pronounced the word aloud, a foreign word that Tsueno had never heard before, and then he pushed the button and held it down.

A sudden hiss and a mechanical clanking sound emerged from the machine. Kimu cursed, and his cigarette fell to the floor as he yanked his finger out of the machine's blood sampler.

"Are you okay?" Yukie asked immediately, moving toward him. Tsueno remained seated, looking annoyed.

"Yeah, yeah, I'm okay, Yukie," he said, and cursed again. He held up his finger. It was bleeding, more of a small cut than a puncture. "I don't think it's supposed to cut me like that."

Tsueno looked on as Yukie examined the finger, and then stuck it into her mouth. She sucked the blood right off it. Tsueno inhaled sharply, and by reflex glanced over to the door to Itō's inner sanctum. He could almost *swear* he saw a shadow move across the glass, just for a moment, and his stomach fluttered.

"What does the paper say?" he asked, hoping to break up the scene.

"Paper?" Kimu asked, his eyes still locked with Yukie's, and then his attention returned to the machine. "Oh. Yes, yes, the paper. It should come out of this slot."

But nothing did. The machine whined a little, as if some internal feed were broken. It whirred, and whirred, and whirred. A green light was blinking as it whirred.

Kimu bent down to read the label under the button. "I can't read it," he said.

Yukie leaned toward the machine, and sounded out the label for the light. "Processing." She clapped. *So she can speak English*, Tsueno thought. *Maybe she is a college girl, after all.* "It works! Now, you, Tsueno. You should try."

"I don't think..."

"Try it," she said, her voice suddenly low.

"But..."

"Itō told me to tell you to try it."

Shit. Tsueno's heart sank, and he wondered what the hell Itō was planning.

Tsueno nodded, and went over to the machine. He stuck his finger into the same hole that Kimu had, and Yukie pushed down on the same button. A nasty little flash of pain stabbed at his finger—worse than a nurse drawing a sample of blood—and he yanked his hand back, squeezing his thumb against the pricked spot.

The machine began whirring louder, and the blinking light kept going, but only for a minute or so. Then the whirring stopped completely, and a humming sound started up. The hum was followed by a kind of mechanical cough, and then silence. Then a red light began blinking.

Yukie leaned toward the display, and sounded out the button. "Paper jam," she translated it aloud immediately. "The paper is stuck inside."

"Shit," Tsueno said. "We broke it."

"No, no," Kimu said. "I used to work in an office, when I was a teenager. Machines do this all the time. I just need to clear the jam, and..."

Itō's door swung open into the room, just then, and he entered. He was an imposing man, though physically small. He was shorter than Kimu, and only a little taller than Tsueno. But he was solid, thick and bull-faced. A scar ran across his face, from one eyebrow down his nose to the corner of his mouth.

The two gangsters bowed deeply to their employer, as Yukie stepped ever so slightly back, away from Kimu.

"Kimu," Itō said. "Tsueno," he added. That was out of order. Tsueno's name always came first, as he was the senior. Both men, still bowing deeply at the waist, tensed slightly because of the change. It *meant* something, and they both sensed it, but neither knew exactly *what*. The air buzzed with their almost-palpable guesses and imaginings.

Itō did not greet Yukie, of course.

"Sir," the men answered in unison.

"You got the machine, I see," he said, strolling toward it with his hands behind his back, as an office manager might do.

"Yes, sir," Tsueno answered. "From a black market dealer's hide-away. It's an older model, but that's all that ever made it to Fukuoka before these things were outlawed altogether. It was functioning, as of a week ago. This was the machine that correctly predicted the death of Watanabe Yoshiro."

Watanabe had been an enemy of Itō's, and rumor had it that this machine had told him, months before the fact, that he would get a knife in the windpipe, just as he had done Sunday last. It was whispered that someone—the names given varied in each telling—had been waiting for the local *yakuza* bosses to die of old age, but had lost his patience and had started taking them out, one by one. That was why Watanabe had gone to such great lengths to get his death foretold in the first place.

Not that it had helped.

Perhaps it was because of Watanabe's fate that Itō had even considered getting a Death Prediction Machine of his own. He was sure that, unlike Watanabe, he could avoid doom if he knew it was coming. It would take a certain kind of rare intelligence, of course, but Itō was used to feeling smarter than everyone around him.

"Very good work. Today we will find out how we are all going to die," he said, smiling. He did not look at Kimu.

"Thank you, sir."

Yukie was visibly uncomfortable. She looked, in fact, a lot like the way Tsueno imagined a woman would if she'd been carrying on with one man behind another's back, and suddenly found herself in the same room with the two men, standing in between them. Itō hadn't congratulated Kimu on a job well done, though he'd obviously been involved in getting the machine. Yukie frowned. Tsueno wondered where her real sympathies lay at that exact moment.

"I can give this machine a blood sample, now?" Itō asked.

"Yes, sir," Kimu replied, and he began to explain it, hurriedly: "There's some kind of internal sterilizer. It's totally safe. Why don't you give it a blood sample, and while it's processing that, we can clear the paper jam?"

"Hmmmm," Itō said, and nodded. He stuck his middle finger into the opening. "Now what?"

"Allow me, sir," Tsueno said. He rose and went over to the machine, and pushed the same button he'd seen Kimu push earlier.

Again, the hiss, the clanking, and then a new sound: a slow, steady humming that got louder with each passing moment.

"It stings," Itō said, withdrawing his finger from the machine and looking at it. Yukie held out a pale blue handkerchief, patterned with images of children at play. Itō looked at the handkerchief, and shook his head. "What a waste that would be," he muttered. Then he stuck the bleeding finger into his mouth and sucked off his own blood, his eyes still locked with hers, and asked, "How long will it take?"

"We're not sure," Tsueno said. "For some people, it only takes a few seconds. For others, longer. Maybe twenty minutes, even."

"In that case, I have other things to attend to. Cleaning house, for example. Mr. Kimu," Boss Itō turned his attention to the younger thug. "I know that you've been working hard...working overtime, on projects I haven't even assigned you. I fear you've been working way too hard, lately. Too much overtime." Itō put one arm around Kimu's shoulder, and the other around Yukie's waist. "I would like to discuss this problem with both of you."

He led them towards the exit, leaving Tsueno standing by the machine. When they reached the door, Itō turned and said to Tsueno, "Get that machine working, will you? Fix the paper problem, or whatever it is. We're going for a drive in my car."

"Yes, sir," Tsueno said, and bowed as he flooded with relief. In a few minutes, it would all be over, he thought, holding the deep bow as long as he could. As he finally straightened up again, he saw Kimu looking back over his shoulder, a grin on his face. Gallows humor?

Or did that idiot Kimu have something planned? Tsueno wondered, and shook his head. *He's going to screw up everything.*

He focused on opening the lid of the machine. At least, at first it had seemed like a simple lid. He discovered that it was more complicated than the hood of a car, or the latch on a suitcase, however. He fiddled and jiggered with knobs and levels until, finally, he got something right and a crack above the feed slot opened enough for him to see the slips inside.

Outside, it was still quiet.

The papers were jammed in deep, and a little ripped up, but he tried his best to extract the two little cream-colored strips without damaging them further. The problem was, his fingers were too big to reach all the way in. For a moment, he wished that Yukie had been left behind. She could have reached them, easily, with her long, slender fingers.

He pushed and shoved until his fingers were touching the papers, but by then they were so tightly wedged that he couldn't actually grasp the little sheets, much less pull them free. Just then, the machine stopped humming, and after a mechanical cough, a third slip of paper slid into the jammed slot.

Yanking his hand out, he cursed mildly to himself. He could rob rival gangsters, misdirect cops, talk a board of shareholders into paying him protection money, and assassinate enemies without getting caught. Would he let a mere *paper jam* hold him back? Ridiculous. Especially now that his plan was about to bear fruit.

But try as he might, nothing helped. Digging at the slips with a pen just ripped one of them in half. Turning the machine on its side had no effect. Shaking it didn't do anything at all. He was staring at the damned thing, thinking hateful thoughts of broken plastic and metal, when something caught his eye. It was a button with a blinking light underneath.

It was labeled, he discerned with some difficulty, "Form Feed." A half-formed memory from high school, of a dodgy dot-matrix printer (and a caning delivered unto him by the middle-aged computer lab supervisor) bubbled to the surface. He realized this was the very thing he needed. Tsueno jabbed at the button with his thumb.

A soft whirring sound started up again. Moments later, three slips of paper were spat out of the front slot, like a trio of tongues sliding out of a single expressionless mouth. They dropped to the ground.

Tsueno reached out to catch them, but they slipped past his fingers to the floor. As he bent to pick them up, he looked carefully at them.

Damn.

They were written in English. Of course they were. This machine hadn't been made in Japan, had never been properly adapted to the Japanese market, since it had become illegal so early on…so of course, it was all-English. Unlike Kimu, Tsueno had never worked in an office. He had slept with a blond American cram-school teacher for a while, back in his twenties. Busty; he remembered her cleavage better than he could remember her face. He certainly hadn't picked up any words or phrases from her that were of any use outside of a bedroom, though. (Though he had once laughingly hollered, "Harder, harder," while another of Itō's thugs had kicked some drunken, disrespectful American jerk's teeth in.)

He stared at the first slip of paper, and then the second. One of them had only one word. Another had two, and the third had three words. Which was which? They were all mixed, and Tsueno had to figure out which was Itō's. The one with three words? It made sense on a hierarchical level: a boss should have three words on his deathslip, as opposed to underlings, who only warranted one or two. Yes, the slip with three words would be Itō's. Unless, of course, terseness was a sign of respect, and a boss's paper ought to only have one word. Tsueno sighed. That was stupid bullshit. He was just looking for a shortcut, but he knew that he'd have to translate them all.

There was a computer on a desk in the corner of the room, near the window overlooking the street, that was always left on. Sometimes, while on lookout, he played computer games on it-multiplayer games, online adventures full of swords and blood and scantily-clad anime Valkyries. He sat down in front of the computer and wiggled the mouse. The screen lit up.

He searched for an automated translator, and in a few seconds, he found one. Scrolling down to select the "English to Japanese" language pair, and switching the language input to English he painstakingly typed in the three words on Itō's paper.

I-M-P-R-O-P-E-R-L-Y–P-R-E-P-A-R-E-D–B-L-O-W-F-I-S-H

As he scanned the results, he realized that he could hear his boss and Kimu yelling at one another, outside. It was an industrial neighborhood, so probably nobody would hear. But it was a little worrying. He stood up and looked out the window, and saw Yukie was off to the side, shrieking. Kimu and Itō were shoving one another. It was a prelude, of course, to death. As he watched, Itō stepped back from the *Zainichi* and gestured toward his car.

Good, Tsueno thought to himself, and felt a grin spread across his face. *Go for a drive*. He felt giddy with his impending success, and sat down to read the results onscreen.

"Badly cooked *fugu*?" Tsueno shook his head, and hurriedly typed the phrase from the second slip—

C-A-R–B-O-M-B

—and hit ENTER. As the results loaded, Tsueno's attention wandered back to the slip with the weird message about the *fugu*. His eyes widened. *Wait*, he thought. *If Itō and Kimu are getting in the car, then that has to be* my *slip*. He resolved never to eat any kind of fish ever again, *fugu* or otherwise, and smiled. He was going to cheat death after all.

A horrific sound erupted outside. He leapt to his feet just in time to see an enormous ball of orange flame burst out through the exploding windows of Itō's car. The blast shook the office, sent pens and books falling to the floor.

He grabbed the slips and ran to the door. Throwing it open, he stood still and stared for a moment, as a second and then a third explosion went off. It was awful, like something out of a gory movie. Yukie's slim arms flailed wildly against the front windshield, inside the car, and a hand on the windshield on the driver's side, melted onto the plastic-coated glass. It was just like he'd planned. Maybe a *touch* more horrific.

But Tsueno's smile melted away. He felt a little bad, now that it was done. Kimu wasn't supposed to have been in the car when it went off. Tsueno scanned the area for anyone who might be watching, when suddenly his eyes traveled to the bottom of the stairs, where what he saw sent a shock through his body.

Itō stood alone, gun in hand, staring up at him.

"The slips?" his *Oyabun* asked flatly.

"Boss!" Tsueno answered, still shocked, his mind racing.

Maybe he doesn't know.

"I *know*."

"Know what?"

"I know how Inoue got you to plant that bomb."

"*Oyabun*..."

"Shut the fuck up! I want to tell you how I know."

Tsueno nodded, but didn't lower his head.

"Yes, boss."

"You thought I didn't know about Kimu and Yukie. Any shit-dripping idiot could see what was going on. But you think I'm the only one who's been cuckolded?"

Tsueno stared at Itō. "You slept with my wife?"

Itō shook his head, and gestured at the car. "Kimu told me your plan. She told him a few days ago, after one of their 'meetings.' I thought you might enjoy this being your last sight."

Bitch, Tsueno thought. *That cheating slut.* Suddenly he felt sympathy for Itō, and could understand why Yukie was in the car, dying with Kimu.

"Thank you, boss," Tsueno said.

"The slips." Itō said again. "Where are they?"

"Beside the computer, *Oyabun*," Tsueno said.

"Good. Thank you, Tsueno. Now, come down here and show your boss some respect."

Tsueno breathed deeply. He'd already scanned the stairway, thought out his chances of getting back into the office alive. Itō probably had a couple of thugs in his inner sanctum, waiting. He went down the stairs slowly, and before his *Oyabun* whom he had so shamelessly betrayed, Tsueno bowed his dizzy head.

And then Itō put a bullet in it.

Story by Gord Sellar
Illustration by Jeffrey Brown

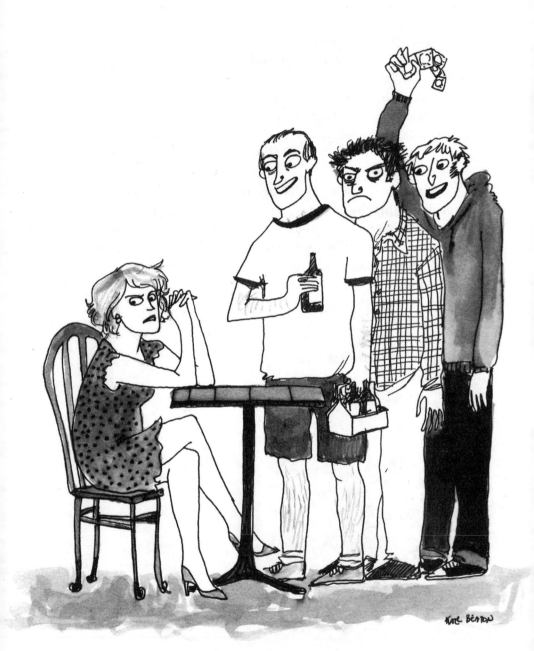

LOVE AD NAUSEUM

The Times, 5/18/04 A.M. (After Machine)
SWF, 35, seeks SM 25–50. Must love
outdoors, adventure, fun! Box 1876.

The Times, 7/21/05 A.M.
SWF, 36, seeks SM 25–50. Must be
employed, love outdoor hobbies. No
OVERDOSE, ALCOHOLISM, similar
readings, please. Box 1876.

The Times, 11/1/07 A.M.
Health-minded SWF, 38, seeks same,
SM 21–55. Steady employment a must,
like outdoors. No OVERDOSE,
ALCOHOLISM or INFECTIOUS
DISEASE readings please. Send
photo. Box 1876.

The Times, 3/12/08 A.M.
Health-minded SWF, 38, seeks same,
never married SM 21–60. Steady
employment a must. No OVERDOSE,
ALCOHOLISM, INFECTIOUS
DISEASE, or JEALOUS EX-WIFEs.
Send photo and copy of reading. Box
1876.

The Times, 10/4/10 A.M.
SWF, 41, seeks SM 18–65. Send photo,
resumé, health records and notarized

Story by Sherri Jacobsen
Illustration by Kate Beaton

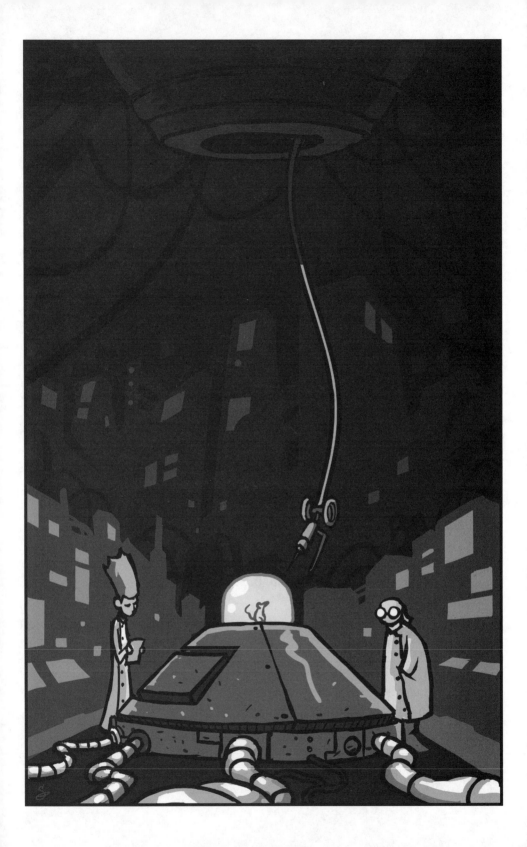

MURDER AND SUICIDE, RESPECTIVELY

SCENE: Two scientists, Dr. Rosch and Dr. Nelson, are discussing experimental results in a lab. A machine is at the centre of the room, wires leading from it to various terminals at the edge of the room. A hand-made label affixed to the machine by one of the technicians identifies the machine as "The Machine of Death."

DR. ROSCH: So the machine works. Given a sample of blood, it tells you how you're going to die.

DR. NELSON: Yes.

DR. ROSCH: And we know this because we've done experiments on lab mice and on ourselves. Once the mice started to die, we started to get 100% accuracy. And with the passing of Dr. Chomyn last week, it seems it works on humans just as well.

DR. NELSON: Yes—we need more data points, of course, but there's no technical reason why it won't work just as well on any mammal.

DR. ROSCH: Okay. This being the case, I have a question.

SCENE: Outdoors, Dr. Rosch and Dr. Nelson are strolling outside, walking and chatting.

DR. ROSCH: So, I know I'm new here, and I wasn't around for the invention of the Machine. I'm necessarily approaching this from an outsider's perspective.

DR. NELSON: Yes, but that's fine.

DR. ROSCH: Right. So, here's a thought experiment. We're going to assume that we're ignoring the animal cruelty laws, we're getting around them somehow.

DR. NELSON: Without jail time.

DR. ROSCH: Yeah. So, given that, we pick out a rat—let's call him Timmy.

DR. NELSON: Okay.

DR. ROSCH: So we take Timmy the Rat and we decide that we're going to kill Timmy by braining him with a hammer.

DR. NELSON: *(surprised noises)*

DR. ROSCH: Okay, so stay with me. We decide, we promise to ourselves, that as soon as the test is done, we're going to kill Timmy the Rat by smashing in his skull with a hammer. We run Timmy through the machine and it comes out "KILLED BY BEING BRAINED WITH A HAMMER."

DR. NELSON: Well, not necessarily. It could be any number of things. It might say "KILLED BY SCIENTIST" or "GOT HAMMERED" or what have you. We don't know why there's such variability, but there is.

DR. ROSCH: Right. But what all those predictions have in common is that they all fit with being hit on the head with a hammer.

DR. NELSON: Correct.

DR. ROSCH: Okay, so we take this prediction, read it, and then we kill Timmy by smashing his head in with a hammer. Everything's fine, right?

DR. NELSON: Right. Of course, if we decided to spare Timmy, then the paper would reflect that. It wouldn't have said "KILLED BY BEING BRAINED WITH A HAMMER," it would have said something like "DIED OF OLD AGE," or whatever.

DR. ROSCH: That's fine. It's crazy and creepy, but it's fine. The predictions are infallible. Sometimes they're unclear or ironic, but they always always come true.

DR. NELSON: That's correct.

DR. ROSCH: Okay. So what if we decide we're going to kill Timmy by smashing his skull in, but we're not going to do it right away. We run him through the machine and then put him in a box, where he'll have food and water and be cared for, and we leave him there for a few months, and then we brain him. The prediction's still going to be hammer-related, yes?

DR. NELSON: Most likely. Of course, the longer we try to keep him alive, the greater the chance that the rat might die from some other cause, a heart attack or something else we can't control.

DR. ROSCH: But we can know that by the prediction: if it says something like "HEART ATTACK"—something that's inconsistent with being killed by us with a blow to the head—then we know the rat isn't going to live long enough for us to kill it.

DR. NELSON: I suppose.

DR. ROSCH: So let's, say, take a sample of blood from Timmy and we put him in this box, this life-support box. Then, we take this box and we ship it overseas. Overnight. We ship it to Fred, say.

DR. NELSON: Dr. Merry?

DR. ROSCH: Yeah. And we tell Dr. Merry that it's coming, and then when he gets the box, let's say Timmy's survived. We've instructed Dr. Merry to open it up and kill the rat inside with a hammer at precisely 11:59 p.m., which he does without hesistation.

DR. NELSON: A stroke before midnight?

DR. ROSCH: Sure! For drama's sake. Then, one minute later, at midnight, we actually run the blood sample we took earlier through the machine. What do you suppose it'll say?

DR. NELSON: Something about being killed with a hammer, of course. It's already done.

DR. ROSCH: Precisely.

(A beat.)

DR. NELSON: So?

DR. ROSCH: You don't see it? What if we could ship this box further away? What if Dr. Merry lived thousands of light-years away, and we could somehow get the box to him? If we set a time for him to do the killing, and for us to run the blood through the machine shortly afterward, then as soon as we read the machine's prediction, we've sent information faster than the speed of light.

(Dr. Nelson thinks for a second.)

DR. NELSON: Well, it's an interesting thought experiment, but we can't send things thousands of light years away, much less with precise timing. The rat would be long-dead by the time it arrived.

DR. ROSCH: Sure. But if we could—

DR. NELSON *(interrupting)*: Even if we could, no information is actually being transmitted. If Merry's good at following our orders, he's going to kill the rat, yes? And we could expect this when we sent the rat in the first place. Besides, we could run the test as soon as we take the first blood sample, and we'd already know how it's going to turn out. So yeah, we're getting information about the future, but it's not breaking any universal speed limits. The information was always there, encoded in the rat's blood.

DR. ROSCH: Hmm.

DR. NELSON: But...but...

(He trails off, lost in thought. Dr. Rosch stares at him for a moment.)

DR. NELSON: You're just using one rat in your example.

DR. ROSCH: Yes. Just to make things easy to imagine. We could send lots of rats—we probably would, in case some of them died for whatever reason.

DR. NELSON: Okay. Okay. What if we made, say, 100 of these life-support boxes, and put a few rats in each.

DR. ROSCH: So, about 300 rats.

DR. NELSON: Yes. And we don't send these rats light years away or overseas, we just...put them in storage.

DR. ROSCH: Each collection of rats in their own life support box...

DR. NELSON: Right! We number each box. *(excitedly)* And a lab rat, properly taken care of, lives for, what, 2–3 years?

DR. ROSCH *(slowly catching on)*: On average.

DR. NELSON: So we put these rats in storage and then, 2 years later, or sooner, if need be...

(Dr. Nelson looks at Dr. Rosch, eyes wide with the idea.)

DR. NELSON: ...We take them out.

DR. ROSCH *(understanding)*: And we kill them.

DR. NELSON: But we don't kill them all with a hammer to the head. We have a code.

DR. ROSCH: Each death means something different.

DR. NELSON: It'll be noisy—we can't trust the machine to make it clear exactly how each rat dies. But we've got more than one rat for each letter. And if we choose the deaths carefully...we should be able to minimize the overlap between predictions.

DR. ROSCH: A different death for each letter of the alphabet. Each box equals one letter.

DR. NELSON: We could send a message back in time to the point when we first took blood samples from the rats.

(Dr. Rosch and Dr. Nelson stare at each other.)

DR. ROSCH: We've got to get to the lab.

Story by Ryan North
Illustration by Aaron Diaz

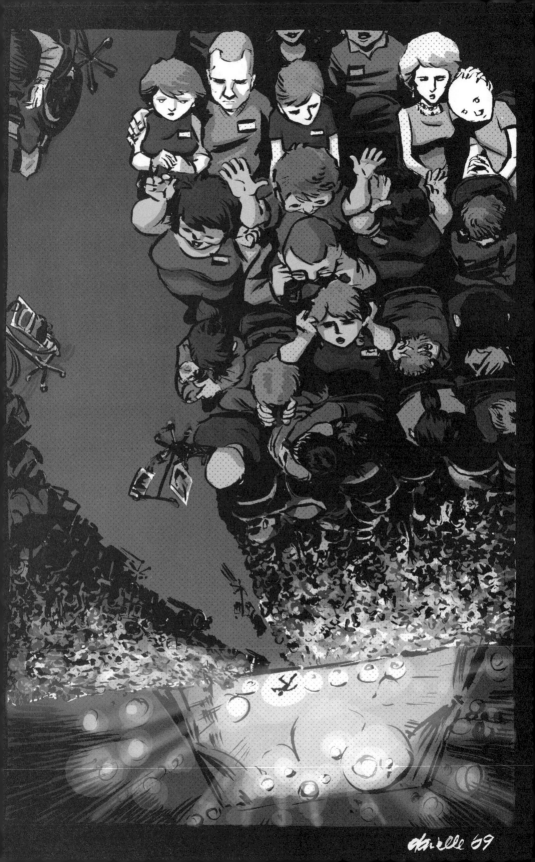

CANCER

James spoke up as soon as he heard the door close. "You went to that kid's house again, didn't you?"

His father sighed; his mother dropped her purse on the long stone table. "It's late," she said. "Go to bed."

"You didn't give him any *money*, did you?" James stood up, following his parents up the stairs. "I don't care if you sat there and nodded, or sang songs, or *whatever* you do there, but tell me—*please* tell me when that basket came around you just passed it down the line."

"James, I'm tired," his father said, and James heard in his voice that he was telling the truth.

It had started with the doctor's visit a year ago. Dad had complained of trouble swallowing. The doctor had clucked disapprovingly at Dad's lymph glands. He had taken some blood and scheduled some tests. He had not been surprised by the results.

"If there's anything you want to do, anyplace you want to travel, anyone you want to see," he had said, "I would do it now."

James had seen the brightly-colored flyer in the mailbox, but hadn't given it much thought and had thrown it away with the supermarket coupons. So he was surprised to see it later, rescued from the trash can, its glossy color beaming from the fridge beneath a smiley-face magnet.

He plucked it down and had already begun to crumple it when Mom stopped him.

"Doesn't that look fun?" she said. "We're going to the one next week."

In garish red and yellow, the flyer announced that You, Too, could "Defeat the Machine!" A colorful cartoon hammer smashed a predictor box, starbursts flying out zanily. A beaming man in a tie beckoned to his new best friend, You. Bright blue type advertised an (800) number. Seats for the seminar were limited.

"Are you *joking*?" James sputtered to Mom, deeply afraid that she wasn't.

She hadn't been, and she and Dad had gone to the seminar, returning with bulging plastic bags crammed with flyers and hand-outs and brochures promising intensive weekend workshops and personal counselors and private consultations with Dr. Gene Eli himself. Dr. Eli (who, as far as James could tell, seemed to have a doctorate purely in smiling broadly) called himself an "indus-try-leading expert in recovery medicine," which meant that his literature was peppered with positive, boisterous terms about *mankind's potential for self-healing* and how the *psychic capacity of the human spirit* could surpass the limitations of current medical science.

Dr. Eli's follow-along lecture notes—carefully annotated in Mom's looping script—claimed that according to the laws of nature, ancient man should have become extinct. But mankind had, instead, *evolved*. According to Dr. Eli, the same impossible power that had allowed cavemen to conquer their murderous world already existed in *you*. With this power at your disposal, a slip of paper from a predictor box was no more a guarantor of death than chicken pox or diabetes —a thing to be conquered, a thing a person could overcome.

By now James had forgotten his skepticism, engrossed in Dr. Eli's argument. He sat with his eyes unfocused for a time, suddenly certain of a raw, innate strength that lay latent in his blood, in his father's blood.

When he finally turned the page, he realized with a start that he couldn't make out the words: The sun had set, and the room was dark.

He reached up and snapped on the lamp. Blinking through the brightness on the page, he was suddenly angry at his own belief: *There* were the prices for the weekend retreats, the private consultations, the intensive one-on-one counseling. Clearly, Dr. Eli and his team of "recovery therapists" were not altruists. James felt a knot of revulsion catch in his throat. His blood bellowed betrayal.

When his parents returned from an afternoon doctor's appointment—with another set of new pills for Dad, these with side effects that could damage his heart—James waited until Mom had eased Dad into his recliner and turned on the TV before pulling her into the kitchen.

"These guys, this Dr. Eli, they're just taking your money," he said. She shook her head, like she'd already considered the thought and dismissed it.

"All the meetings are free," she said. "We're not going on the weekend retreats or anything; we can't afford them anyway. We're not giving them any money. And it brightens him up—it brightens both of us, a little. What's so wrong with that? After these depressing appointments every day, what's wrong with a little *hope* for a change?"

James clenched his jaw before his mouth could spit out, *But it's false hope*. He stared at the cupboard door, willing his breathing to slow, willing his eyes to focus. When he turned back, Mom was halfway up the stairs.

Dad still sat on his recliner, head leaning to one shoulder, eyes pointed at the TV but not really watching. James took a few steps into the living room, then sat on the couch. Dad rolled his head around, lifted a hand. James grasped it—grip still strong; skin thick and calloused from decades of labor. His own hand felt thin and smooth in comparison. He felt young.

"How's it going?" Dad asked him. "How's that car doing? You still checking the oil every day? Oil and water?"

"Yeah," James lied. Dad always bugged him about this, and James always forgot. "Looks good."

"Keep checking it, every day, every day," Dad said. "If your oil gets too low you'll blow that engine, and then it's a headache."

They sat in silence for a few minutes, watching an antacid commercial, which was followed by a drug commercial that mainly consisted of old people pushing their grandchildren in swings and a long list of quickly-read side effects.

"These pills," Dad said suddenly, sitting forward in his chair, "these pills they give me, new pills all the time, new ones, new ones, the pills are worse than the disease! Heart problems, they said today, this one has risk of heart problems. I *never* had heart problems! Never in my life. What *is* this, when the medicine is more problem than the...than the first problem? I never *heard* of this!"

He settled back, and released James' hand to fidget with the pillow beneath his lower back. The news came back on; the screen filled with sports scores.

James looked up the stairway, up where his mother had disappeared, and then leaned closer to Dad, trying to think of something to say, anything. He finally settled on, "So, you've been going to those meetings, huh?"

Dad looked over. "Yeah, this Dr. Elo, Oli, whatever his name is. I think he's Egyptian—he looks like an Egyptian."

"What kind of stuff does he say?"

"Oh, I don't know, bunch of baloney mostly," Dad said, and James breathed a sigh of relief, leaning back.

Dad continued. "He says all kinds of junk, about evolution, I don't know what he's saying. He wants to sell you a weekend retreat, they call it. With his fancy doctors, you go up in the mountains for a weekend, they take a look at you."

"Yeah, I read the brochure."

"It's a bunch of baloney," Dad said. "Your mom, she likes to go, so we go. I don't know what it's about. But I tell you"—here he looked over at James, and leaned in close, and lowered his voice—"I tell you, some of the people at those meetings—old people, sick people, these people look like they died *already*."

—‡—

"It's the last day before the seminar leaves town," Mom said. "You know how much it would mean to your dad."

"I don't think those meetings mean as much to him as you think they do," James yawned, rolling over in bed, trying to pull the blankets from Mom's grip. With a single yank, she pulled them off, and James curled tightly into himself.

"We're going," she said, and they did, all three of them.

Dr. Eli's seminars were held in the banquet hall at the Hilton. By the time James and his parents arrived, the place was already packed. Wheelchairs crowded the aisles; near the front, a few gurneys lined the walls, attended to by nurses monitoring IV trees. As soon as he passed through the doors, James was hit by the smell of Mineral Ice and sweat.

Dad handed him a paper name tag. "Here," he said, and James saw that his own name had been pre-printed on the tag by a computer. Mom and Dad already wore theirs.

They elbowed their way through the crowd, moving past sad-eyed old men and heather-haired old women, past fat men in sweatpants and sickly women with track marks. There weren't three seats together anywhere but the very back, in the corner. Dad carved a passage between a huge woman in a muumuu and a quivering girl holding a very young infant. James saw that the girl was trembling so hard that her baby was becoming dizzy.

They sat on folding chairs next to a delicately poised middle-aged woman with elaborately sprayed hair. Her teenaged son sat next to her, his bald, chemo'd head resting on her shoulder. James watched her idly stroke the boy's neck and shoulders with her painted fingernails. The kid's bare scalp was textured with goose-flesh. He shivered.

Suddenly the room came alive with pounding music, and lights overhead began to flash, and smoke poured onto the far-off stage, and a swell of cheering began to rumble the walls, and James closed his eyes and sighed.

—✦—

"I'm moving on to other cities, other states, full of people like you," Dr. Eli said, pacing frantically back and forth on the stage, microphone clenched in one hand, the other hand circling like he was launching airplanes off a carrier. "I'm meeting thousands of folks, telling them they don't have to be afraid, just like *you're* not afraid. Telling them what *you* already know. Telling them they don't have be *shackled* to that little black machine in their doctor's office." Here he paused to allow raucous applause, taking a sip from a bottle of water on a stool. "Telling them they can tap into that *power* that's in all of us. That power that's in *you*, and *you*, and *yes* ma'am, it's in you too."

The room burned with cheering. As soon as Dr. Eli had taken the stage, awash in strobe lights and sparklers, the entire massive family sitting in front of James had climbed onto their chairs, flailing their arms and shouting, and forty minutes later, they hadn't come down yet. James noticed that the bald boy and his mother were not clapping, or standing on their seats, or swaying with their eyes closed, or even paying much attention at all. The hair-sprayed lady next to James wasn't so much as craning her neck, although she did occasionally check her watch. The boy's head now rested in her lap.

The aisles were crammed with people eager to be a part of Dr. Eli's last seminar in town. More kept trying to shove their way into the room, pleading with the black-shirted security guards, rattling the locked doors elsewhere in the hallway. James watched his parents: Mom held her purse on her lap with both hands, and Dad sat slumped in his chair, occasionally shifting uncomfortably. Was *this* what he'd been so worried about?

Dr. Eli welcomed a line of people onto the stage to share their experiences. A tearful young woman clutched Dr. Eli's microphone with both hands; he wrapped his arm around her shoulder.

"My—my paper said 'airplane,'" she said, to a loud chorus of boos from the audience. Dr. Eli quieted them with a look, nodding to the woman to continue.

"My paper said 'airplane,'" she went on, "and I was scared to go anywhere *near* a plane after that." Laughter. "No plane rides, no airports. I couldn't pick up my brother from his trip. I couldn't visit my Grandma out in Chicago. We had to move because our house was too close to the, to the flight path. I couldn't get no other job, I had to ride the bus every morning back to the same old neighborhood. I was scared every morning to get too close to the airport, but I had no other job, I had no other place to go."

The crowd was quiet now, watching as she blotted her eyes with a mascara-stained tissue. Dr. Eli squeezed her shoulder.

"But Dr. Eli told me, you don't got to be afraid, you don't got to live your life that way," she said. A few scattered cheers from the back of the room. "He told me, we have control. We don't live our lives because of what some box says, what some piece of paper tells us. We are human beings. We are free. We are alive."

The room erupted with approval. The family in front of James screamed their lungs out. James looked over and realized that his mother was pressing her hand to her eyes. He met her look with his own, and she laughed, embarrassed, and turned away.

Dr. Eli's staff brought a small metal box out onto the stage. It was shiny black, with vents along both sides and a small control panel on the front. Its lights were dim and its LCD screen was dark. The circular receptacle on the right side was empty—no thin glass vial of blood—and the printer had no inch-long strip of paper protruding like a tongue from its serrated mouth. But all the same—it was a predictor box.

The black square loomed huge on the video projection screen, and when Dr. Eli's assistant handed a sledgehammer to the sniffling woman, the crowd went nuts. She heaved it up and brought it down on the box, sending plastic knobs and circuit-board fragments whirling into the audience. James saw that a stack of predictor boxes waited at the rear of the stage, one for each person in line for the microphone.

They kept coming, one after the other:

"My wife will tell you: I'm a new man. I stay up late. I leave the house."

"Yesterday I did it. I drove to the store for the first time in five years."

"Finally, I took my grandchildren to the zoo. Thank you, Dr. Eli."

"Thank you, Dr. Eli. For giving me my life back."

"God bless you, Dr. Eli. Thank you."

James was speechless.

Mom and James kept their hands on either side of Dad, helping him step down from the curb and into the Hilton parking lot. They passed through the knot of people at the weekend-retreat sign-up tables, seeking out the night air, finding it cool and calming.

"I think that was really interesting," James said. Mom gave Dad a knowing look, then smiled at the sidewalk.

"It's just a lot of junk," Dad said. "They don't cure you. This Egyptian, he doesn't heal you. It's a bunch of baloney."

"Well, it seems like he helps a lot of people get over their hangups," James said. "I mean, those predictor boxes really mess up a lot of people."

"These predictors, schmedictors, they are a hazard," Dad said. "People don't realize this, scientists, idiots. They are a real hazard."

The lady with the bald son stood underneath a lamppost, a stack of bright paper in her hand, shoving pages into the stream of people. Mom took one.

The bald boy watched them walk away, twisting his fingers around each other as if he were kneading clay.

James watched the boy until he grew uncomfortable. The boy never looked away.

—✦—

The new flyer was bold black text from a home printer, photocopied onto yellow paper: "TIRED OF DR. ELI'S LIES?"

James picked the paper from the floor, where it had fallen as they entered the house last night. "No more cheap theatrics. Ready for REAL HEALING?" it read.

Dad called him from the other room. James put the flyer on the table by the door and ran into the kitchen, where Dad was struggling with the juicer.

"Mom makes me some of that carrot juice," he said, holding a bundle of carrots in his hand. James took the carrots and fed them into the juicer, one by one, until he had filled a glass with carrot juice. When he turned around with the glass in his hand, his father was sprawled on the floor.

"There he is," Dad slurred, his eyes slowly focusing, urging the doctor to look to the doorway. "This is my son. This is my son, James."

James shook the doctor's hand and hugged his father, his hands recoiling at the spine thin beneath the paper gown, the shoulder blade jutting into his palm, the ribs, each one distinct. Dad's face was swollen; he worked his jaw like he was chewing taffy. He took a sip of water, and it took him three tries to swallow.

"I'd like to watch him here for a few days," the doctor said. "He had another episode last night that required the shock paddles. I think this is some cause for concern."

"My...my heart is acting up now," Dad said, fighting to get the words out. "I never had problems with my heart, never."

"It's possible the medication he's been taking for the lymphoma may have adversely affected the cardiac system," the doctor said. "I'm really worried that there is a potential for arrhythmia. I'm going to prescribe some treatment that will hopefully keep his heart running smoothly."

"Pills, pills, more pills," Dad said. "Everywhere you go, they give you pills. One pill for this, one pill for that."

The doctor wrote on his prescription pad. "Does he have any history of respiratory or kidney problems?"

After Mom arrived, James began to wander the hospital's halls, trying not to glance into open doors as he walked. When he did, he saw the same thing, over and over: death on hold, waiting, biding its time, typically with its mouth open, breathing shallowly, its eyes either closed or open staring at nothing.

He realized for the first time that he was scared; he did not know if he would have the opportunity to complete his relationship with his father, and it worried him. He didn't know if he would trust himself to seize the opportunity, even if it presented itself.

He wondered how long it would be before he would no longer be able to recognize his father in the figure that lay in the bed down the hall, the father that had once hoisted him onto his shoulders, or balanced his tiny body on the palm of his hand. The man in James' memory was strong and robust, and did not have the dim, sallow eyes that the man down the hall seemed to have.

James wondered, not for the first time, why his father had read the slip of paper from the predictor box in the first place, and if it would have even mattered had he not.

"Who *is* this kid? What makes him qualified to do anything?" James asked, perhaps more bitterly than he meant to. His mother glanced over at the living room where Dad lay sideways on the couch, and gestured for James to keep his voice down.

"His website says—"

"His *website*," James sneered.

Mom sucked in her breath, held it for a second. "A lot of people say he's helped them feel better."

"People. What people? People we know?"

"Sick people. I don't know. They're on the website."

"*His* website, of course it's gonna tell you—"

"We already went to see him."

James stopped short, and closed his mouth.

His mother turned toward the living room and put a hand on her cheek, and then leaned backward, so that James caught her by the shoulders. She leaned into her son, and James wrapped his arms around his mother, and she sighed, and she spoke softly:

"We saw him at Dr. Eli's seminar—the kid sitting with his mother. The, you know, bald head?" James nodded. Mom went on: "His name is Tim and he's just the sweetest little guy."

She leaned her head on James' shoulder. His own mother was smaller than he was, more frail, tired from shuffling her husband to doctor's appointments every day, tired from administering pills and treatments and praying late into the night, tired from waking up early to make sure he woke up at all.

"Tim said he could...reach inside you," she continued, as she and James watched the softly heaving body that lay on the couch a room, a world away. "He said he could close his eyes and feel inside you, and feel what was wrong, and move his fingers around and fix it, just like running his fingers through your hair, just like untying a tangled knot."

"Mmm," James said, because he didn't know what else to say, and also because he felt so sad for the woman that he held in his arms, and wished that she wouldn't believe in things that would just disappoint her, and also wished that maybe it were true.

"He said he could feel the atoms in your body," she said, whispering now, still looking away, still watching her husband sleep. "He said he could reach into your dad's throat and feel the tumors and pluck them off like strawberries."

"Did he?" James said.

"No," Mom said.

—‡—

James' parents went back to see Tim and his mother with the painted fingernails, even though they didn't bring up the subject with James again. James found Dr. Eli's brightly-colored flyer under a stack of unread magazines, and looked it over again and laughed and shook his head and thought of all the people who'd read that tiny, fortune-cookie slip of paper torn from a predictor box and who had never again gone near buses or bathtubs or microwaves. People who'd stopped smoking or drinking or started smoking or drinking, people who knew there'd be no risk in skydiving and so sat there stone-faced as they fell ten thousand feet through the air, never having any fun at all.

Most of all he thought of Tim, the skinny, bald kid lying curled in his mother's lap in the back row of the Hilton's banquet hall. Did he have leukemia or something? What was his game, and what did he want with James' parents?

And why couldn't he heal himself?

So one night, James stayed up late and confronted his parents as they came home from Tim's house, and made sure they hadn't given him any money, and watched his father take slow steps up the stairs. And after they disappeared upstairs, James sat alone on the couch, and exhaled and admitted to himself, well, really, when it came right down to it, what's the harm?

The ambulance woke James up. The siren grew louder and then stopped, deadly close, and James was on his feet instantly.

Mom let the paramedics in the front door and James stood in the hallway as strange men shouted to one another, 100 cc's of this and that and finally they eased him down the narrow stairs on a backboard and slid him onto a gurney, and James took his father's hand for a brief second before the red doors slammed and he was gone.

—✝—

"It's his heart," the doctor said. "He hasn't been taking his medication."

James stared at his mother, who looked quickly away down the hall. "He was worried about the side effects," she finally said.

The doctor took a few moments to choose his words. "At this point, I'm not too concerned about the side effects," he said.

She looked up at him, and got his meaning, and James felt her weight press into him again.

"Dad, you have to take your pills."

His father looked up from his prone position on the pull-out couch bed, his throat swollen like a bullfrog, his breathing thick and labored, his face drizzled with a week's worth of downy beard. "Get that junk away from me," he managed.

James sucked his breath and leaned back on the recliner, drumming his fingers on the leather arm, and sighed. "I don't know what to tell you. The doctor says the pills are going to keep your heart strong. You don't want that to happen again, like the other night."

"That doctor is a crook," Dad gasped. "Those pills are what's a killer. Worse than that lymph, whatever you call it, lymphoma. The pills are the killer."

"Dad—"

"I *never* had heart problems," Dad cried, suddenly strong, fidgeting to get an elbow underneath himself. James leaned over, but Dad struggled, righting himself on the couch. "I never had any heart problems whatsoever. Until that crook gave me those pills. And now look at me. Now look at me."

"That's why you have to take them. Yeah, call him a crook, maybe he is—but your heart will get worse unless you take the pills, and there's nothing you can do about that."

"Nothing I can do," Dad said, shaking his head, trying to laugh, but it came out a choke. He eased himself back down onto the couch. "Nothing I can do until it wrecks my lungs, my kidneys, right? Same old story. Nothing I can do."

James handed him the glass of water, rattling the pills in his hand, but Dad didn't take it.

"At least I know this heart won't kill me," Dad said. "Whatever that mickeymouse box is good for, at least the heart won't kill me."

"That's not necessarily true," James said. "It—it's kind of vague, I think."

Dad looked at him, chewing his words, forcing them out. "So what, then? Every day I wake up it's worse. I can't talk, I can't swallow! Now you want me to take pills so I can't breathe, I can't take a piss? Isn't this bad enough?"

"Okay, Dad," James said, setting the glass on the coffee table hard enough that it sloshed onto the magazines. "Go and see that kid, Tim, then. Go and see him, is that going to make you feel better?"

"At least *he* has some hope for me," Dad said, and James bit his lip.

Tim's house was one-half of a duplex on Brightwood Avenue, a wrongly-named street in a part of town without sidewalks. Brown front lawns ran straight into the cracked asphalt of the road, or at least they would if they were visible: Cars choked the sides of the road, and Mom had to park a block and a half away.

The people at Tim's were sadder than at Dr. Eli's, and some were sicker. Tim's mother welcomed everyone inside with polite, weak handshakes. James stood in the corner, trying to shuffle as close to the wall as possible, so that everyone had room to sit.

The air was fogged with incense and something that sounded like Enya being played on a cheap boombox. Everyone kept quietly to themselves, occasionally shuffling one family at a time down a narrow hallway. The CD was on its second repeat when Tim's mother called James' parents to Tim's bedroom.

Tim's bed had Snoopy sheets on it, and model spaceships dangled from the ceiling, but there were no video games, no books, no other toys that would suggest that a child lived here. Tim sat cross-legged on his bed, thin and tired in the dimness of a single overhead lamp, and James almost gagged on the incense as he walked through the door.

He and Mom helped Dad to sit on a mound of pillows, then sat beside him. Tim was quiet, praying perhaps, his eyes closed, and he sat that way for some time before Dad started to moan loudly with discomfort.

"Thank you for coming back," Tim said softly, and when he opened his eyes and saw James he froze for a moment, looking caught, looking terrified. Then he recovered, and extended his hands; Mom took one, and James, with some reluctance, the other, warm and wet. They both took Dad's hands.

"Do you believe that you have the power to be healed," Tim said. Dad said nothing until Mom nudged him, and even then he just murmured.

"Do you believe in the power that God has given to every man of his creation," Tim said, louder, and Dad said, "Yes."

"Do you believe that the power within you is strong enough to move mountains, because it is from God," Tim said, his voice strong now, and Dad said, "Yes," and Mom moaned.

"Remember to keep the flame of faith strong, for there is nothing I can do for you if you do not believe," Tim said, softer now, and handed Mom's hand and James' hand to each other. He rose to his knees on the bed, his eyes closed, and started to flex his hands, as if preparing to play the piano, breathing sharply, quickly.

"It is your belief that allows the power to grow," Tim said, "and opens a channel for me to reach into you."

James watched his father closely, watching his head bob heavily on his neck as he slumped more deeply into the pillows. Tim's hands moved deftly around one another, tracing intricate patterns that might have been tying bows with string, and Dad coughed and made a noise and spoke in syllables but not words.

After ten minutes of this Dad was not healed, but it was time to bring in the next family, so James helped his parents to their feet and nodded to Tim's mother with a tight smile and concentrated on helping Dad into the car before he said anything.

"I think that kid is dangerous," he finally said.

They drove home in silence. Dad was sleeping downstairs now, on the pull-out couch bed, and James helped him out of his shoes and socks. His feet were swollen, but his legs were as thin as James' arms. James lifted Dad's feet onto the bed and covered them with the blanket.

"How you doing," he said to his father, because he had so much to say but didn't know how to say any of it.

"What should I say," Dad said. "Should I lie?"

James asked his mother not to go back to Tim's.

"What exactly are you afraid of?" Mom said, brushing her hair in the darkness of her bedroom, as James leaned on the full-length mirror behind her. "That he'll get better? That he'll *feel* better, if nothing else? Like he's trying to *do* something, instead of sitting around the house feeling awful, waiting—waiting to—waiting around?"

"I'm afraid he'll think it's his fault," James said, and his mother stopped brushing.

When she didn't say anything he spoke again. "I'm afraid he'll feel like he didn't believe enough. Like if only he could have more faith, or something, like if only he'd tried harder then Tim could heal him, and it's *his* fault if he doesn't get better."

"I don't think that," Mom said, putting the brush away.

"I know, but does he?" James followed her down the hall, where she took a towel from the hall cupboard.

"I don't think so."

"How do you know?"

She whirled and faced him, and her voice was strong but he saw that her eyes were very wet. "Because I know him," she said, and walked back to her room and closed the door and he heard the water come on in the shower.

"So do I," he said.

"Bless this food to the nourishment of our bodies," Dad said, slowly, "and thank You for all the blessings You give us. And I believe that You have the power to heal me, if it is Your will, and I ask that I be allowed to continue in Your service."

They sat on the back porch, the sun a red ball on the horizon.

"I guess this is the end of my rope," Dad said.

James thought of lots of things to say.

But nothing sounded right, so he put his arm around his father, and they watched the sun set together.

Dad was buried on a tall hill, overlooking the valley where their house rested, and James stayed around his mother all the time for as long as he could, while she took the chance to sleep in late and rest and recuperate.

The few days before the funeral had been distressing for him, because he found that the truth of *Dad is gone* had begun to usurp his memories, retroactively erasing his father from his recollections—so he'd had to fight that, with photographs, reconstructing a skeleton in his mind of who his father had been, finding it sometimes not aligning perfectly with what he thought he remembered.

And he hated that the sharpest picture he had of Dad was of a weak animal in a hospital bed, and he fought to recall the vigorous, looming figure of his youth. Sometimes, he succeeded.

The last few days had been the hardest. Mom never left his side in the hospital room, sleeping in the hard wooden chair. After a few days Dad started talking about things that weren't there, and staring off into the distance, and then he would call your name and squeeze your hand and you wouldn't be able to understand the words through the thickness in his voice.

On the last day he hadn't spoken at all, and by the time James arrived in the morning Mom said that he'd stopped squeezing her hand back, and he lay there in the soft white bed sucking air like a fish on land, then lying deathly still; gasping, sucking, wrenching the oxygen from the atmosphere by force, then slumping, spent from the effort.

After a few hours of this, the gasping became less pronounced, and the hills and valleys of the heart monitor became an undulating stream, and the shrill sound of the monitor's alarm became annoying, and they turned it off.

Then there was nothing left to do but watch his face turn yellow and his jaw stop moving and the man who was James' father become something *other* than a human being, something that was diseased meat and bone and cloth that there was nothing of Dad in at all. And they cried and held each other and sat very still for a very long time, weeping into each other's arms.

And that night, when they came outside to the parking lot, they found that Mom's car was dead, that its battery had been drained from the lights being left on, and without any further tears they left it in the parking lot, an empty machine, a shell without a driver.

James wondered if his father had heard him on that last day, whether his unresponsive hand and closed eyes belied some deep consciousness that had survived buried inside the ceasing functions of his body, and if the echoes of his voice had carried all the way to it. For whatever it was worth, he'd told the mute Dad not to be ashamed or guilty; that it wasn't his fault; that he'd done everything he could. That he was loved.

He wondered if Dad had been disappointed in him, for not believing in Tim, or for not attending the meetings, or for continuing to push the medication that he so despised. Dad hadn't taken any pills at all, the last month or so, but his lymphoma by then had spread to the stomach and lungs and bones and so there wasn't really any point and James felt bad for arguing, for making a big deal about the pills, for causing his father stress about that and Tim and everything, for refusing to just go along.

He stood on that new patch of grass, where he could very easily picture the long oaken box a man's height under his feet, and recalled his reluctance to view the body, to have his recollections of the strong man of his childhood contradicted by physical reality. But it hadn't been bad—the figure in the box was just a thing of tissue and skin, and posed no threat to the memories that were now the only thing that James had left.

But even still it was *something*, it was *physical*, it was better than ether and void and thought and dreamstuff, and so he stayed there on the green hill overlooking the valley as the wind blew heavenward.

And in that lonely moment he thought about Tim, and wondered if he would call Tim to ask him to untie the knot he felt deep in his guts. And then James wondered if there wasn't something of his father in him after all.

Story by David Malki !
Illustration by Danielle Corsetto

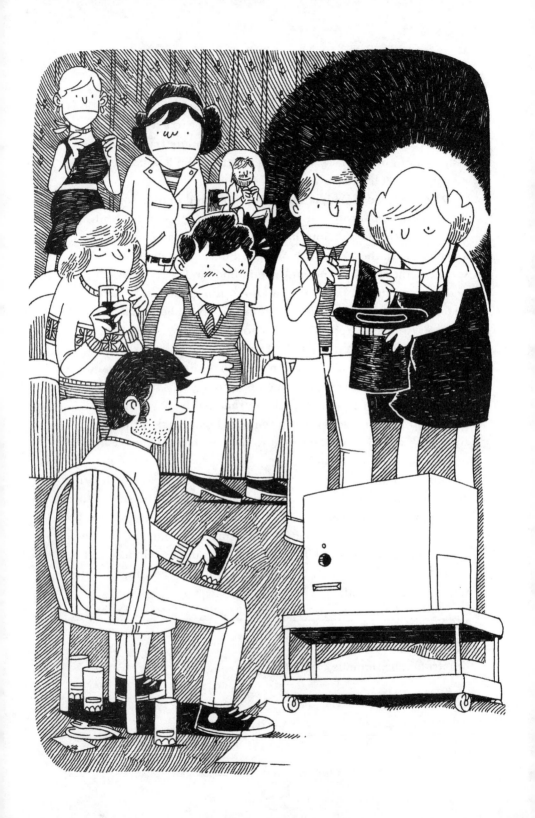

ANEURYSM

"It's a new party game," said Norma, as she pushed a small cart into the living room. A white sheet draped over the top hid the cart's burden—something boxy, no larger than a microwave oven. The guests all turned to watch as the little mystery was wheeled into the room, squeaking slightly, leaving a visible groove in the carpet. Norma stopped and stood; she made no move to uncover her secret, only smiled at the seven faces around her. Every guest had a fresh drink in hand and a hot *hors d'oeuvre* on a toothpick. Music played loudly enough to keep the room cheerful, but not so loud as to hinder conversation. And now she had piqued everyone's curiosity by wheeling out this odd little cart. Norma was an excellent hostess.

"And it's called 'Death Match?'" one of the guests asked—a florist with the unfortunate name of Melvin. "That sounds awfully violent," said another.

Sid said nothing, just watched quietly as the other guests responded to Norma's little show. Her entrance wasn't a huge spectacle—not like in the old days of birds and smoke. She just enhanced the presentation a bit with her dashes of secrecy and drama. Norma still had a sense of staging, Sid had to give her that. She appreciated the way a hint of anticipation can make any event even more memorable than it might have been.

Sid already knew what was under the sheet. Norma had warned him of what she had planned because she knew how much he would hate it. He had tried to dissuade her, of course, but she insisted on proceeding, just as she insisted that he be there as always. They'd been divorced for three years, but he still couldn't bring himself to say "no" to her. He never could: That's why he was thirty-eight years old and on his third career. His second career had lasted exactly as long as his marriage, and had been entirely her idea. He missed it almost as much as he missed her.

"Oh, it's not violent," Norma was saying now. "Well, a little violent, sort of. You'll feel a little pinch, but it's nothing to get worked up over."

The truth was, Sid adored Norma, he really did. He adored Norma, and he adored her parties, and he adored her taste in music, and her *hors d'oeuvres*, and all the witty conversationalists she routinely assembled for her Saturday night gatherings. And even though the romance between them had ended long ago, he still loved being in her life and having her in his.

But he loathed party games. Really and truly.

Oh, he liked games in general. He wasn't opposed to fun and frivolity. He'd participated in a murder mystery party once, and thought that was just splendid; he'd even played the role of the villain without complaint. If she had brought out boxes of Scrabble or Trivial Pursuit, he'd have been all for it. But "party game" invariably meant some sort of getting-to-know-you game: truth or dare, I never, packing your desert island luggage. The sorts of games that had only two outcomes—either they stayed entirely superficial (boring) or they probed into deeply intimate information (humiliating). Knowing that Melvin's three favorite CDs included David Hasslehoff's greatest hits didn't make Sid feel like he really knew Melvin any better. Neither did knowing that Melvin had once had sex with his cousin's boyfriend's sister in a glass elevator. But Sid had learned both these facts about Melvin at a previous gathering.

And as much as Sid hated these games, Norma loved them. So here he was, getting ready to play again.

"So," Norma taunted, "isn't anyone going to guess?"

"Stop teasing," said Vince, Norma's latest boyfriend. "Let us see what you've got under there. It's no fun staring at a bed sheet." Vince was a banker with no appreciation for showmanship. Living with Norma meant living in suspense. Always and forever. Sid suspected Vince wouldn't be around much longer.

Sid, of course, was perfectly happy to keep staring at the bed sheet, absently thumbing the thin slip of paper in his pocket. He had no interest in playing the game, but he very much enjoyed seeing an audience toyed with. He enjoyed the show. So he was disappointed when Norma gave in easily, rather than drawing out the suspense. "You're such a poop, Vince," she said as she did what he asked, taking the corners of the sheet between her fingers. At least she still put a flourish into the process, whipping the sheet dramatically from the cart and snapping it over her head, nearly overturning a vase of tulips on top of the TV.

The audience let out a satisfactory gasp.

They all recognized the machine, of course. They'd seen it on television and in movies. They'd seen it in doctor's offices and pharmacies. Some of them had even used one. But still, it was strange to see it sitting on a rolling cart in their friend's living room.

"Is that what I think it is?" Melvin asked, refusing to believe what was already obvious.

"That depends," said Norma. "Do you think it's a Machine of Death?"

"Yes?"

"Then yes, it's exactly what you think it is." She grinned devilishly in her satisfaction at having so befuddled her guests.

"You paid for that?" Vince appeared horrified at the very concept, his eyes bugging out like an old cartoon.

"Well, I certainly didn't steal it."

"But those must go for thousands of dollars!"

"I have a friend in the company. He let me buy it at cost."

"That still couldn't have been cheap…"

"Oh, Vince," she said, cutting off the line of conversation, "stop being dull. Don't you realize how much *fun* we're going to have? It'll be worth it, I promise!"

With that, she began unwinding the power cord that hung from the back of the machine, pulling it toward a free outlet near the TV. Once it was plugged in, she flipped the switch to turn it on. A small fan revved up to full speed. The internal workings clicked and popped as a fresh needle was loaded. A little red light turned into a little green light.

The machine was ready to dispense party time fun and pithy little visions of the future.

Norma giggled her delight.

"So you're just going to give us our death readings?" asked the same woman who had questioned the game's name earlier. Lottie. That was her name—Sid had only met her once before, but he was sure her name was Lottie. "I've already done that."

"Well, don't tell what your reading was yet. That comes later. Getting the reading is just the first part; the real game is guessing whose death is whose. Can you guess how I'm going to die? Can I guess how you're going to die? That's the game. That's Death Match. Isn't that a *gas*?"

"I love it," said Melvin.

"Yeah, okay," said Lottie. "I'd do that."

"I'm not playing," said Marie. Like Sid, Marie was a restaurant critic, though this provided precious little common ground. For instance, Sid held that Norma served consistently excellent *hors d'oeuvres* at her cocktail parties, and even better food at her dinner parties. She made everything from scratch, never once served frozen wieners or potato puffs. He had shopped with her; she knew quality, knew her ingredients, paired the right cheeses with the right fruits with the right wines. He offered input where he could, but he wasn't actually needed. He found no fault at all. Whereas he had more than once overheard Marie belittling Norma's culinary talents to other guests. The cheeses were too sharp, the fruits overripe, the wines improperly poured. She had even once tried to include Sid in her conspiratorial condescension. Sid and Marie hadn't spoken much since then.

Tonight, though, Marie's was precisely the reaction Sid was hoping for. If enough people objected to the machine's morbid prognostications, then Norma would have to give up and the evening could pass without a party game. This one time at least.

"You know there's nothing to be afraid of, Marie," Vince said. "These machines are so cryptic, they don't really mean anything."

"Well, they sort of do," said Jorge, Norma's oldest friend from her college days. "But only in hindsight. By then, who cares?"

"No, I know," said Marie. "It's not that. I just don't like needles."

"Oh, please," Vince chided. "I can't stand when people say that. You realize *nobody* actually *likes* needles, right?"

"Well, yes, of course…"

"And you don't want people to think you're antisocial, do you?"

"I'm not anti…"

"I'm not playing either," broke in Bettany, the last of the evening's guests, and a new face in the group. According to Norma, Bettany was a professional mountain climber; Sid had no idea how she'd fallen in with this crowd of devout indoorsmen.

Vince sighed ostentatiously. "And what's your excuse?"

"Well, mostly I'd just like for everyone to think I'm antisocial. I can't help it—it's my natural response to juvenile peer pressure. You know how it is, high school flashbacks and all."

Sid stifled a chuckle; it seemed Bettany didn't like Vince any more than Sid did.

"Marie, you don't have to play," Norma said. "But if you do decide to play, I promise, you won't even see the needle. It's hidden away inside the machine. You just put your finger in, and it feels like barely more than a mosquito bite. And that's it. But you don't have to play, really."

Marie sighed. Norma meant it when she said Marie didn't have to play. Marie knew it. And Sid knew it, and everyone else knew it. But still, nobody liked to disappoint Norma. It broke her heart when her guests didn't like her games.

"How about this," Marie said finally. "I'll play if Sid plays."

Sid snorted. Oh, it was a clever tactic on Marie's part: It put the onus of disappointing Norma on Sid instead of Marie. And she knew how Sid felt about party games, too. She knew he'd be hard-pressed to resist an opportunity to derail his least favorite pastime. Clever tactic or not, though, it was a bad play this time.

"Sid's playing," Norma said with a triumphant grin. "He already promised."

Marie gave Sid a desperate look.

"It's true," he said. "She cornered me last week and twisted my arm. What could I do?"

"You could have said 'no.'"

If only.

"Sorry," he said. "I have weak arms."

And with that, all resistance died, and everyone agreed to play.

"I'll go first," said Melvin as he popped out of his chair and approached the machine. With no hesitation at all, he stuck his finger into the machine's orifice, punched the button, and gave a little laugh when the needle stuck him—"It kind of tickles"—then waited as the machine processed his blood and loaded a new needle. It spat out a slip of paper just like an ATM receipt.

"You can read your own if you want," Norma instructed, "but don't tell anyone else what it says. Then fold it in half and drop it in the hat."

Somehow Sid hadn't noticed the hat. It was on a second shelf on the cart, underneath the machine. It was a black felt top hat, a perfect gimmick for a game like this. But Sid recognized it immediately—it had once been his. It was just a straight hat with no hidden pockets or secret compartments, but still, it gave him a pang of nostalgia for their time on the stage. He hadn't known she still had it. But he was glad. It was encouraging, in a way. He put one hand in his pocket, touched the paper he had hidden there.

Melvin dropped his death into the hat.

Vince went next, making a show of what a good sport he was, and how *not* afraid of needles he was, but winced visibly when the needle stuck him. Sid rolled his eyes for Bettany's benefit, and she stuck out her tongue in agreement.

Marie was third, eager to have the unpleasantness done with. She closed her eyes and inserted her finger into the machine. The color left her face when she pushed the button, and for a moment Sid thought she might faint. But she stayed upright as she hurriedly tossed her death into the hat and returned to the couch, where she sat sucking the injured finger.

Sid went next. The needle really did feel like a mosquito bite, though he wouldn't have said it tickled. When the machine spat out his death, he didn't bother to read it; he already knew how he was going to die. He had all the documentation. He'd seen the CT scan. He folded his death in half and dropped the slip of paper into the hat.

"Thank you," said Norma.

"No," he replied. "Thank you."

She looked at him quizzically, but he said nothing else. Just put his hands in his pockets and returned to the other side of the room.

The remaining partygoers all took their turns, until there were eight folded slips of paper in the hat. Norma was delighted and favored everyone with a big smile.

"Okay," she said. "Here are the rules:

"One. One death will be drawn from the hat at a time.

"Two. We'll all debate whose death we think it is and why.

"Three. Debate ends once everyone has officially cast a vote.

"Four. Players earn one point for each correct vote. No points for guessing your own.

"Five. No death's owner will be revealed until all deaths have been voted on.

"Is everyone clear? Any questions?" There were no questions. So she reached into the hat and drew the first death.

"Oh, good, we're off to an interesting start! The first death is: LANDSLIDE."

"That's easy," Melvin chirped without hesitation. "It's Bettany. Mountain climbers get killed in avalanches all the time."

"Not *all* the time. And besides, it was 'landslide,' not 'avalanche.'"

"Same thing."

"No they're not," Jorge said. "Avalanches are snow and ice. Landslides require, obviously, land. That means dirt and rock."

"So then it's probably you," said Vince, gesturing in Jorge's direction.

"How do you figure?"

"You do construction. Construction means excavation, and excavation leads to landslides."

Jorge frowned. "I'm not a construction worker."

"Aren't you?"

"I'm an architect, Vince. I design buildings. I don't build them myself. I work in an office. I even wear a tie sometimes, if that helps your mental image."

Vince held Jorge's gaze, but said nothing.

"But don't you ever inspect a construction site," Lottie asked. "Or go to watch something you designed getting built? How can you resist?"

Vince finally shrugged and looked back at the rest of the group, though Sid caught his petulant eye-roll.

"Okay, I do visit sites sometimes," Jorge said, returning to the game. "But that's not where I work."

"But the risk is there," said Marie. "More than on a mountain top, anyway."

"Sure, I guess."

"Any other theories?" Norma asked after debate dropped for a few moments. "Okay, then it's time to lodge your votes."

Vince, Bettany, and Marie voted for Jorge. Jorge, Melvin, Lottie, and Norma voted for Bettany. Sid voted for Vince.

"You were supposed to argue your theory before the voting," Norma scolded.

"I don't have a theory," Sid replied. "I just think it'd be funny."

"Ha," said Vince flatly. Norma scowled at Sid, but he just shrugged—"I'm playing your game, aren't I? What do you want?"

"Okay," she said as she reached into the hat again, "our next death is: HUNTING ACCIDENT."

"Oh, that one's Lottie," Sid said without hesitation.

"But I'm a vegetarian!"

"So?"

"So I wouldn't go hunting in the first place!"

"Which is precisely why it would be so satisfyingly ironic."

Jorge raised an eyebrow at Sid. "So, what you're saying is that the less likely it is that a person will die in a particular way, then the more likely it is that that's precisely how they'll die?"

"Well, not so much 'more likely' as 'more entertaining.'"

"That sounds about right to me," said Bettany. "Put my vote down for Lottie."

"Hey!"

"Seriously, though," Marie asked, "Does anyone here hunt?"

All heads shook in the negative. "I went once when I was a kid," said Jorge. "But I hated it."

"Then it's obvious," said Melvin. "Bettany spends the most time out in the wild. She's the one most likely to get shot accidentally."

"You already voted for me to get killed in a landslide! I can't die twice."

"No, but I can vote for you twice. One of them has to be right."

"You can do that," said Norma. "But we all get to make fun of you for being wishy-washy. Agreed?"

"Agreed," said Melvin. "So long as I get my points, I'm happy."

"I'm voting for Vince," said Marie. "He's the person most likely to have to do something stupid to appease a rich client."

"I'll buy that," said Jorge.

Norma took count of votes again, with two votes going to Lottie, two to Bettany, and four to Vince, including Norma's.

"Actually," she said with a wink to Melvin, "I think Bettany is more likely. But I already gave her 'landslide,' and I wouldn't want to be wishy-washy."

After HUNTING ACCIDENT came TAINTED BEEF. Debate was brief and the votes divided evenly between Sid and Marie, the two restaurant critics. After TAINTED BEEF came DRUNK DRIVER. This was followed by an awkward silence as everyone avoided looking at Jorge, except for Vince, who said, "Well, obviously that's Jorge." Norma gave Vince her most lethal scowl, but Jorge just shrugged.

"You can vote for me if you want to. I don't care. I'm sober. I've *been* sober for three years, and I don't even own a car. I promise you, that's not how I die. Besides, it says 'DRUNK DRIVER' not 'DRUNK DRIVING.' Whoever it is is the victim, not the culprit."

Ultimately, three votes went to Jorge, three to Marie, and two to Vince.

After DRUNK DRIVER came RADIATION.

"But we all live so close together," said Lottie, "if there's some sort of nuclear accident, shouldn't we *all* die of radiation?"

"Maybe it doesn't happen for a long time," Melvin suggested. "Maybe only the last of us is still alive when the meltdown happens."

"Or someone could go on vacation to someplace that has a reactor," Norma offered.

Jorge disagreed. "There's no reactor, there's no bomb. It's nothing nuclear at all. The machine's just being coy. There's always radiation. Solar radiation, electromagnetic radiation, microwaves, radio waves, whatever. A lot of them cause cancer. That's the death here. It's just cancer."

"So then it's Bettany," said Melvin. "She spends the most time outside, so she probably gets skin cancer."

"Geez, you sure are eager to kill me off, aren't you?"

"It's not my fault you lead a conspicuously dangerous life."

"I don't see how any of us is more likely to die of cancer than the others," said Jorge. "I say we each just vote for the person on our left, and then we all get an equal number of votes."

"In that case, I say we all vote for Jorge," said Sid.

"Seconded," said Bettany.

So everyone voted for Jorge. Including Jorge, just to be a good sport.

"You should be careful, Sid," Norma said. "You almost seem like you're enjoying yourself."

"Maybe just this once," he said. And he actually sort of was. Just this once.

Norma reached into the hat once more and pulled out the next death.

She unfolded the paper and read it.

She opened her mouth, but said nothing.

"Norma, what's wrong?" Vince asked.

"What does it say?" asked Melvin.

She looked up again. She looked at Sid. She pressed her lips tightly together, in a look that most of the guests would confuse for worry, but Sid knew it was pure irritation.

"It says 'PARTY GAME MISHAP.'"

Everyone was silent.

Then, Lottie: "I don't get it."

Melvin: "It means someone could die right now. Playing this game."

Marie: "How?"

Melvin: "I don't think I want to know."

Lottie: "Right now?"

Jorge: "But that doesn't even make sense."

Vince: "It never makes sense."

Melvin: "Maybe the machine electrocutes one of us…"

Lottie: "I don't want anyone to die."

Bettany: "Whose is it?

Melvin: "Or maybe…I don't know. It could be anything!"

Jorge: "I know the machine likes to be vague and cryptic."

Bettany: "It's Sid, isn't it?"

Lottie: "I don't want to see it happen."

Vince: "Nobody's going to die."

Jorge: "But they always at least sound lethal. What's lethal about a party game mishap? That's not cryptic. That's the machine actively thumbing its nose at us."

Melvin: "The machine can do what it wants. I'm done."

Bettany: "It must be Sid. He hates these games."

Lottie: "I don't want to play anymore."

And finally, Norma: "I think the game is over."

She folded up the slip of paper and dropped it back in the hat. The hat went back onto its shelf under the machine. The machine was turned off. And unplugged.

All through this process, Norma never took her eyes off Sid.

She understood what he'd done, of course. That was obvious. And it was a stupidly simple trick, just a bit of palming. The only challenge was forging the death prediction—fortunately, she had warned him about the game days beforehand. She'd be kicking herself for paying him that kindness for a long time, he suspected. But she wouldn't tell the others. She wouldn't reveal what he'd done or how he'd done it. She'd been a magician's assistant for too many years, at least until she broke up the act and they'd both retired. But she still knew the code. She still believed in the code.

Sid's real death was safely hidden in his pocket. When he arrived home, he would take it out and read the single word printed there. But it held no surprises, just confirmed what he already knew.

He could die that very night.

Or he could live another ten years.

You never could tell with these sorts of things.

But he'd never have to play another stupid party game for as long as he lived. However brief that might be.

Story by Alexander Danner
Illustration by Dorothy Gambrell

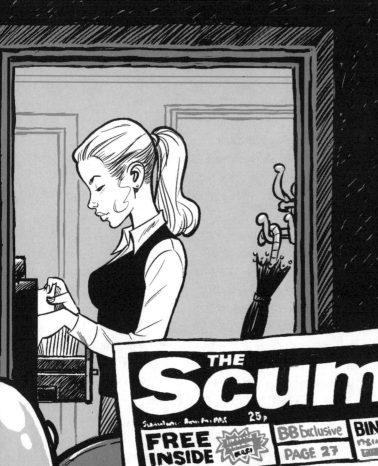

THE Scum

25p

FREE INSIDE

BB Exclusive PAGE 27

BINGO

SAVE £15 TECSO VOUCHERS INSIDE

Fortham due
auto accider

WHAT'S HE HIDING?

...mere's death secret

EXHAUSTION FROM HAVING SEX WITH A MINOR

"The job of Prime Minister is no job for a weakling," said Derek Fortham MP, eyes shining in the TV spotlight. "Centuries of British politics have shown us that. It's a job that calls upon all of a man's strength. It's a job for men who know their limitations. Men with perspective. With drive."

The audience was utterly silent, staring with goggle-eyed hero-worship as Fortham reached into his inside pocket and produced a white slip of paper, which he held between his first and second fingers and waved in time with his speech.

"I always keep my death prediction close to my heart. At the age of fifty-seven I will be knocked down by a car; that's what it says. I don't fear it. I'll never run from it. When I see that car coming, I will stand with feet firm. That's the kind of strong leadership this country needs."

Pander, the interviewer, coughed meekly to signal his next question. "Mr. Fortham, how old are you now?" He was a man who knew his allegiances, and it was the most softball question he could have possibly asked.

"Fifty-three," came the reply instantly. "And yes, I understand perfectly that I have only four years at most, and could only possibly serve Britain as Prime Minister for that long. I see that as my greatest strength. Who wants to vote for some self-serving bureaucrat with one eye constantly on his retirement fund? I have only four years to make my country great and leave a legacy for which I will be fondly remembered."

A quiet, lovestruck sigh ran through the audience, as Fortham concentrated on keeping his face toward the camera at the best angle to show wisdom and dignity.

"If I could just turn to you, now, Mr. Dunmere," said Pander, turning to Fortham's opponent in the polls. "Do you have anything to say to that?"

"Yes, I do," said Dunmere, shifting in his seat. "While I am in total agreement with my honourable friend concerning the importance of strength and courage in a Prime Minister, one should not play down the equal importance of optimism." He paused to let it sink in and re-steeple his fingers. "I think it's naïve to think a Prime Minister would only be a good one if he knew he wasn't going to last. Rather, it would lend a certain...fatalistic approach to policy. A sense of not having to care about long-term issues because you won't be around to face them."

No one seemed moved. Someone in the audience coughed loudly, mingling it with the word 'wanker.'

"Mr. Dunmere," wheedled Pander, "how are you, yourself, fated to die?"

Inwardly Dunmere rolled his eyes. This was exactly what he didn't want to be asked. "I have not received my prediction. I don't believe in letting yourself get bogged down with that sort of thing."

There was a murmuring in the audience, and it definitely wasn't on Dunmere's side. "To be frank," said Fortham. "I have enormous respect for my honourable friend and his achievements in the House of Commons, but his stance clearly shows he just hasn't the belly for the job of Prime Minister."

"Now look—"

"Sorry, I'm going to have to stop you there," said Pander, now addressing his autocue. "We've run out of time. Remember to tune in next week for our election special, and we'll see with whom the nation lies. Next tonight on BBC2: the new series of *Crotch Rocketeers.*"

"You have to admit, he's won everyone over," said Volger, staring out of Dunmere's office window. Volger was Dunmere's campaign manager, a man born, in Dunmere's opinion, from a long line of evolutionary descendants of rats, lizards, and slimy fish. "Ten points ahead of us and rising."

"That interview was a sham," said Dunmere, sitting at his desk with his head buried in his arms. "Not a single question on party policy. Nothing about political experience, nothing about past achievements. Everyone's. I don't know. Fixated on his damn death."

"Well, it's the crux of his campaign." Volger plucked one of Fortham's campaign leaflets from the dartboard. "'Four courageous years,'" he read aloud. "I wouldn't be surprised if he believes it himself. I thought you did as well as could be expected. That bit where you talked down fatalism was shooting us in the foot, though. Maybe you haven't noticed, but 90% of the country's voters know how they're going to die. Fatalism is very much the 'in' thing right now."

At that point, there was a cheerful knock on the door and a head and shoulders peered around it. It was Carol, the work experience girl. "Just dropping off the newspapers," she reported cheerfully, tossing a pile of newsprint onto a nearby chair. "Anything I can get for you, sirs?"

"No, nothing," snapped Dunmere. "Just leave us alone."

"Rightosie." She left.

"I don't know why you have to be so hard on her all the time," said Volger. "She only wants to learn from you."

"She's seventeen."

"So what? Youth isn't the handicap it used to be. The MP of Rugby and Kenilworth is barely into high school. Everyone grows up so much faster these days. Everyone rushing to reach their ambitions. Nothing motivates people better than a glimpse of their own mortality. I guess you know that."

"I'm sorry. I just get edgy around young girls."

Volger went over to the newly-delivered papers and flipped through the headlines. "Not good at all. The media's one hundred percent behind Fortham. 'Dunmere Fears Truth,' Jesus Christ."

He glanced over at the party leader, who had sunk down into a visible despair. For a moment, the unfamiliar feeling of pity sparked in Volger's mind. He sidled over to the desk, perched upon it, and injected what he felt was a fatherly tone into his voice. "Look, Fred. You're a good politician. Everyone sees that. Frankly we should probably be a hell of a lot further behind than we are, but you're just about keeping our heads above water. And you could turn this race around in a second. All you have to do is go to the nearest death machine and find out—"

"I've already had my prediction."

"You—what?"

Dunmere looked up. There was a deep sadness in his eyes. "For Christ's sake, Volger, I said I've had my prediction. I had it done years ago like everyone else. I just don't want people to know about it."

"Fred, that little slip of paper is the one thing that could still get you elected. What the hell is your problem? How bad could it be?"

Dunmere looked his campaign director square in the eye, and spoke each word in a quiet monotone, as if each one could set off an earthquake. "I am going to die of exhaustion from having sex with a minor."

Close to a minute of silence passed between the two men. Volger's face remained frozen throughout.

"Oh," he said, finally. He glanced to the door where Carol had been, then back to Dunmere. "So that's why—oh."

"When I was nine, my father was arrested for molesting a little girl who lived next door to us," said Dunmere. "He'd never done anything like that to me, we never suspected a thing, but he was caught red-handed. He was one of them, one of those they'd always warned us about. I hated him for that. And for years now I've known that I am destined to do the same thing."

"Well...the machine can play tricks," thought Volger aloud, while inwardly making a mental note to jump ship at the earliest opportunity. "Are you sure it wasn't, like, a coal miner..."

"Minor. With an O. And I'm pretty sure it wasn't talking about music." He sighed. "Volger...it makes me wonder if I deserve to be Prime Minister. Knowing that I'm going to do that, I mean."

"Oh, come on. That's just the depression talking, you'd never have pushed yourself this far if you really thought that. Look, Prime Ministers have done much worse. You're not going to let one little future mistake destroy your whole career, are you?"

"It doesn't matter, does it? Fortham's going to win."

It said something about the change of tone in the room that Volger made no effort to contradict him, or make comforting noises. For the rest of the day they spoke of minor business details, scheduled meetings and appearances, neither daring to return to the issue of the death notes or the possibility of overtaking Fortham. Finally, when Dunmere could not stand the stuffiness of his office any longer, he made his excuses and left.

He wandered the streets of London in something of a daze, with no particular destination in mind. Revealing his secret had brought on a strange new perspective. All those concerns he had kept secret and bottled up had finally been revealed. Only to Volger, but even that had been draining. Dunmere stopped dead on a darkened street corner as he realised that he no longer had any wish to be Prime Minister at all. Perhaps it really was just the despair talking, or rationalising the hopelessness of beating Fortham. But he couldn't shake the bristling hot sense of shame that now ruled his world.

Two days later, Derek Fortham died.

"Run that by me again," said Dunmere, at his desk.

"He's been killed," said Volger, fighting to keep the morose expression on his face. "Stone dead."

"How?"

"Knocked down by a car, obviously."

"No, I mean...how? He's not fifty-seven yet!"

Volger tossed the morning's newspaper onto the desk. "Turns out Fortham never gave the exact wording of his prediction. Turns out the phrase was 'knocked down by a car aged fifty-seven.'"

It took Dunmere a few seconds to figure it out, but when he had, he placed his hand over his eyes. "The car was aged fifty-seven."

"It was a photo-op at a classic car rally. Wanted to show he wasn't afraid of cars, I guess."

"Who's running in his place?"

"That's the beauty of it. It's Winslow. Old Fatty Winslow, old Simon 'you'll never get me onto one of those machines' Winslow. He's about as popular with the proles as a Christmas tax increase and now the death notes aren't a campaign issue anymore!" He had now abandoned all pretence of solemnity and was grinning like a man with a coathanger stuck in his mouth. "We can still make it. You can still make it!"

"Oh."

"Well, don't sound too pleased."

"Volger, I—"

He was interrupted by a knock at the door, and Carol appeared, she having temporarily taken over from Dunmere's secretary. "Er, Mr. Dunmere? Sir Richard Merryn is waiting. He's the owner of—"

"—International Media, yes, I know who Richard Merryn is. What's he doing here?"

"Jumping ship," predicted Volger smugly. "Don't keep him waiting any longer. Bring him in. I was expecting something like this." Carol glanced to Dunmere for confirmation, who nodded.

Merryn was an imposing figure, as could be expected from the man who ran every mainstream newspaper in the hemisphere. His suit was at least twice as expensive as Dunmere's and he knew it, judging by the way he walked. He was very tall and very stout, and one could almost feel the floorboards shake as he dropped himself into the chair in front of Dunmere's desk.

"I'd like to speak to you in private," he said, pointedly making a gesture toward Volger as if swatting a fly. Volger, ever the diplomat, bowed low and left the room, but Dunmere picked up on the noticeable increase of pressure on the door that meant he was still listening in.

"How can I help you, Sir Richard?"

"Terrible shame about Fortham," he said, tutting loudly three times. "Terrible, terrible shame."

"Yes, it was pretty terrible," replied Dunmere, thinking that, if Volger was slime, then Merryn was the primordial soup from which all slime originated.

"Shame about his party, too. Can't possibly introduce a credible new candidate in the time they have left. They'll never get in now."

"And since your newspapers have been backing them from the start, it's kind of embarrassing for you. Yes, I know where this is leading."

Merryn smiled thinly. "I wonder if you do. Of course my papers are going to back you. Even this close to the election our support will guarantee your election as Prime Minister. And in return..."

"Let me stop you there," said Dunmere, bored. "In return, you want to have my ear. You want to be able to call in favours. I know how this works. Well, forget it. I don't need your support and I won't be controlled. Sorry."

"Don't apologise, I wasn't expecting you to go for it. You're one of those boring, predictable, idealistic sorts." He crossed his legs and leaned back, sighing luxuriously. "Off the record, you're pretty relieved about Fortham, right?" It was only barely phrased as a question. "Gets you off the hook with the whole death note thing. So you don't want to know how you die. Makes sense to me. I mean, I know how I'm going to die, yachting mishap, but I can understand your point of view. Just don't want to admit that you're afraid to know, right? Nothing wrong with that."

Dunmere just nodded. "Perhaps. If there's nothing else…"

Merryn silenced him by rapidly pulling a slip of paper from his breast pocket. A slip of paper with very familiar dimensions. "Something not many people know about the death machines," he said, wiggling the slip between his fingers. "Everything they output they also record. The manufacturers keep archives of everything. And you'd be surprised what a few bribes in the right place can get you."

Dunmere remained silent, his face expressionless.

"See, I couldn't think of any reason why you wouldn't get your prediction, not while it was costing you the vote and all. So, out of curiosity, I had a look for myself. And when I did, suddenly it all fell into place."

He got up. "My papers will start talking you up first thing tomorrow. You'll become Prime Minister and everyone will be happy. You just remember who your friends are and no embarrassing personal destinies will have to be revealed. I'll see myself out."

Dunmere took a deep breath and stood up. "I don't want to be Prime Minister!"

"Well, not everyone gets what they want, you know," said Merryn, not turning around. Then he was gone.

Volger came back in, all seriousness returned and practically oozing his way up to the desk. "Do you really not want to be Prime Minister, Fred?"

"God, that's all you care about, isn't it. No, since you ask, I don't particularly want to be Prime Minister anymore. And I definitely don't want to be a corporate puppet."

"Look, don't you worry about Merryn," said Volger, effortlessly side-stepping the issue. "We'll dig something up on him. There're bound to be all sorts to choose from. You just play nice doggie for as long as that takes and then we can assert ourselves. He publishes, we publish. You know how it goes. The old scandal cold war."

"I'm not happy with any of this. All this…backroom dealing."

"Well, you've always been an idealist, Fred, and no offence, but it's always been your weakest feature." He pretended to notice the documents in his hand for the first time. "Oh, the BBC want you in for another interview tonight, just in time for the election. They're probably sensing the tide turning as well, so it should go easier on you than before. We should go over the issues that need addressing."

Volger was still going over the issues during the ride to the TV studio that evening, and Dunmere had learned to block him out. He was trying to think. If he stepped down from the race, Merryn would publish, and his political career would be ruined. On the other hand, if he became Prime Minister, he turned the country over to corporate rule: a dangerous slope. And even if that could be avoided, was it fair to let a country be ruled by someone who didn't want to? It would be like an unwanted child, growing up without getting the love it needed...

The only possibility that Dunmere liked was to continue running, but to lose. Merryn couldn't blame him for that. But that seemed the least realistic scenario of them all. The opposition was in turmoil after Fortham's death and no one would ever go for a third party. Like it or not, Dunmere was ahead in the polls. It would take something drastic to change that...

By the time he had dragged himself from his reverie, he was already seated in the studio, baking under the spotlights and the layer of makeup, fidgeting with his hands as the programme's theme tune heralded the interview. Before he even knew what was happening, Pander was turning to him with questions in hand.

"So, Frederick Dunmere MP," he said. "How would you say Fortham's death has affected the possible outcome of the general election?"

"Well, of course the death of my honourable friend was an unqualified tragedy and I was deeply saddened," said Dunmere, going into automatic. "I have great sympathy for his family and his colleagues at the party, and can only hope they will be able to continue working hard for the values Derek held dear. But having said that, I believe that the cornerstone of a new government is stability, stability that I fear the opposition currently lacks. We're living in a new age, and it's time for a new kind of government. Open, accepting, and...honest."

From the emphasis he had placed on that last word, Volger figured out what Dunmere was planning. Out of the corner of his eye, Dunmere could see him frantically waving his hands and mouthing 'no.' He ignored him.

"Yes, honest. And in the interests of this philosophy, and partly in honour of my late friend Mr. Fortham, I have decided to reveal the manner in which I will die. I am to die of exhaustion while having sex with a minor. An underaged person. I apologise for not having been open about it sooner, but I think under the circumstances you could understand why I would wish to conceal it. What has also been concealed from public eye is the fact that my father was himself imprisoned for a paedophilic act, and in the name of our new commitment to honesty, I feel these things must be aired. Frankly I'm glad to have gotten them off my chest, and I can only hope the British public will see these trivialities for what they are and vote for what they know is right."

As he left the stage in silence, the audience not applauding, he wondered if he had overdone it.

Two days later, Frederick Dunmere became the Prime Minister of Great Britain.

"Run that by me again," he said.

"You won," said Volger, leaning on the desk, his smile tight and forced. "Landslide."

"But I thought I killed myself up there."

"So did I. So did a lot of people. But the reactions of the general public have been impossible to predict since the death machines started messing with their heads, and even more so since the voting age was lowered to 14. You of all people should know that, now you're the youngest Prime Minister in British history."

"But...I told everyone about my death. I told them I was going to..."

"Yes, Fred, and I'm telling you that no one seems to care. Probably because you, yourself, are still technically a minor."

"I turn 18 in a month," argued Dunmere sulkily.

Volger consulted the papers in his hands. "You already had the teenage vote, of course. The adults, well...half of them didn't trust you because you were clammed up on the death note thing, and the other half didn't think you were mature enough for the position. That interview pretty much made all of them about-face."

"Oh, Jesus..."

Volger injected that fatherly tone into his voice again. "They were impressed by the way you confronted your past like that. The whole stuff with your father. Seen the papers? They're saying how that one event combined with the knowledge of your future is what sparked your unstoppable drive, what made you become an MP at 14. It's an inspiring story."

"No," wailed Dunmere, clasping his hands to his face. "I wanted to fail. I don't want to be Prime Minister. I don't deserve to run the country."

Volger sniffed with disapproval. "Maybe, but you were elected anyway," he said, dropping his papers on the desk with a loud slap. "So maybe it's the country that deserves you."

Story by Ben "Yahtzee" Croshaw
Illustration by Cameron Stewart

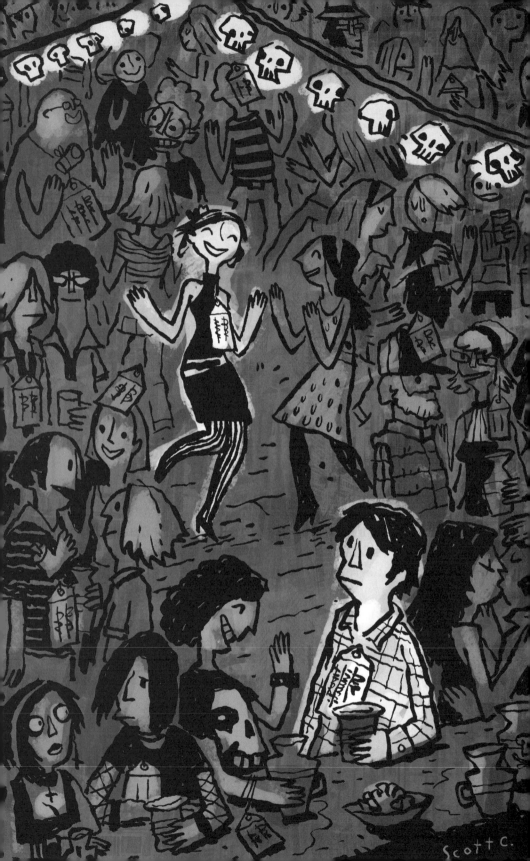

AFTER MANY YEARS, STOPS BREATHING, WHILE ASLEEP, WITH SMILE ON FACE

"No way!" She laughs. "You're shitting me!"

Jill's seated on the edge of my desk, in my cubicle. Picture Lady Day. Atop a grand piano. She has that effect on a room. Or a cubicle. I am not shitting her. "*Really?*" she says, wide-eyed. "Did you have it certified?"

I roll my eyes. "My mom did. Drove straight from the doc's to the nearest Memento Mori office. Hung a big ol' framed copy on the wall as soon as we got home." I smile. "On the fridge too."

"I bet!" Jill says, laughing harder now. Her nose wrinkles when she laughs. Eyes crinkle. It's a real laugh, the kind you wish you could see every day of your life.

"And she had this bumper sticker: My Child Is Going to Die WAY BETTER Than Your Honor Student."

Now this time I *am* shitting her, and she knows it. It earns another wrinkled nose. "Well, hell," she says, laughing, "all I got was 'Brain Aneurysm.' Borr-ring!" She grins, and then suddenly her eyes go wide again.

"Hey, Ricky, you know what? You should *totally* go with us to Toe Tag Night at Club Congress this Thursday. You'll be a huge hit!"

To recap: Jill Harrah is currently seated on my desk. Her leg, below the skirt, is covering my memo pad. She's smiling and, evidently, making plans. With me.

"Well—I guess I have always wanted to be a huge hit…"

"*Yessss*," she says, triumphant, and holds up her hand for a high-five. But with Jill you don't just get a high-five; what you get is some kind of complicated "secret" "urban" handshake she's invented on the spot. Or, maybe, like now, just some additional dap.

"Thursday," she says, scooting off my desk. A memo slides to the floor, and immediately looks abandoned and forlorn.

And then, because I just *have* to push it, I ask, way too casually, "So is Brian going, too?"

When she looks at me, her eyes are neither wide nor crinkled with amusement. "No he is not," she tells me, and walks away.

Brian is her fiancé. I am an idiot who will apparently die in his sleep someday.

—‡—

"You gotta be fucking kidding me!" says one of Jill's friends, leaning forward to get a better look at my shirt.

On Toe Tag Night no one wears tags on their toes. What we do is use a template on our PCs and print a *graphic* of a toe tag, which we then wear attached to our clothing somewhere, like on a t-shirt. The graphic looks like the toe tags you see on dead bodies—or at least on dead bodies in movies—and yes, sometimes people also include a cartoony image of a toe, or a even a whole foot. Often bloody. Printed on the tag is your Name, and How You Are Going to Die. For mine, I had to use a smaller font size.

Jill's friends gather around, squinting. Jill's friends. Three of them came with Jill to pick me up at my apartment. Guy from upstairs, Leonard, an older, also single man, happened to be in the lobby when the cab pulled up. "Daymn!" Leonard said, pronouncing the "y." "Big pimpin'!" The truth was, stepping out to the curb, I didn't feel much like a pimp. More like the pimp's tagalong little brother, who had not himself gone into the family pimping business, but chose coding instead. Plus, to be fair, these women all had legit jobs. Smart too. They just happened to be dressed strikingly. I really don't know how they do it, pull off these transformations. Jill was something in the office, but tonight she was something else again. Shiny, exotic, her hair, braided, streaked red, held with these little butterfly clips. The effect was multiplicitous: as if you were used to seeing this already fantastic creature, one of those supernaturally good-looking people straight out of classical mythology, and then one day she shows up with wings. And offers you a ride. I might've stood there all night, staring at Jill, stunned, but luckily she gave me a high-five followed by a vigorous chest bump, which basically got me moving again.

"Is he for real?" Jill's friend says now, under the club lights, gesturing with her thumb at my tag. Her name, according to her own tag, is "LIZA." Liza will die from "A COLLISION"—one of the vaguer predictions. She and the others are all standing around me in a way that feels great and incredibly awkward at the same time. Jill tells them I'm for real, all right. The club is starting to fill up, getting hotter. Karen, with the long black hair, leans forward, reads, leans back. "Huh," she says. "Not my type." She flips her hair over her bare shoulder. "I'm more into the whole 'Gunshot Wound, Fiery

Motorcycle Crash' thing, y'know?" On her tag, Karen has written "O.D." The "O" is drawn like a skull with little x's for eyes. One thing I learned right away upon entering the club is that not everyone prints their toe tags on a laptop at home. Most just use the Sharpies and blank tags you can get for free at the door.

The club is really filling up now, people pouring in, and Jill's friends start to drift with the incoming flow, Liza turning away, Karen already gone, and the last friend, Aimee, as if an afterthought, turns to me and says, "Well, *I* think it's cute." Which I'm then left to interpret on my own.

Aimee had written "NEVER" on her tag.

As a joke.

I feel a hand on my shoulder. Jill. "You coming?" She tips her head toward the crowded center of the club. It's hot there, pulsing. A bare-chested man beneath a strobe light is performing a dance that appears to somehow involve kung fu. Lots of kicking. I tell her I'm good.

Jill smiles, studying me. "Relax," she says after awhile. "Have a drink. Hang out. People-watch." She pats my shoulder, lightly, once.

─┼─

The bar is strung with skeleton lights. They're already out of the urn-shaped mugs when I get there, so I settle for a plastic cup. The girl ordering next to me reads my tag and laughs. Another guy slides up on her right and says, "Hey, what's your sign? Mine's CANCER!" Grins. My whole generation stands on the gallows, sharing the same humor. And because this is Toe Tag Night and not a certified dating service, people are free to write pretty much whatever the hell they want about how they're going to die. Which can be confusing. Right away, I count no fewer than five people who've each written "ALCOHOL POISONING" under their name, and you can't say for sure, looking at their sweaty, shouting faces, who is just being funny and who is actually on the way. Over there by the winking Coors sign, a guy named "STEVE" has stuck a tag on his trucker hat that reads "AFTER MULTIPLE ORGASMS." That's another popular one, but considering it from the perspective of Steve's partner, maybe not so much fun?

Then again, like the bumper sticker says: "We're All Necrophiliacs Now." Not quite accurate, but oddly appropriate, I think, to our absurd condition. I lift my beer. In the corner by the bathroom, a man is groping a woman who's painted her face and lips blue, his face is smeared blue now too; his eyes, squeezed shut, have pennies tattooed on the lids.

Cheers.

—⸎—

"Seriously?" the guy in the Misfits shirt asks. "Dude, that rocks." He leans forward, slaps my tag. "You take that shit to a real dating service," he says, swaying toward me slightly. "Fuck amateur hour. You know?" I nod. Smile. Swaying a little myself. I know what he's trying to say. I've been told before that from a matchmaking perspective— particularly to those looking for an LTR—how I am going to die is considered extremely desirable. "Pussy magnet" as Leonard put it. Then he went back upstairs to watch his *Battlestar Caligula* internet porn and eat a single-serving microwave dinner.

The guy in the Misfits shirt stumbles back into the crowd. On the far wall they are projecting footage from last year's *Dia De Los Muertos* parade, a festival that has become increasingly popular in recent years. The images of the parade revelers in full costume superimposed on the club-goers creates a blurred, surreal effect, and I realize I have been drinking too fast. I turn away, toward the stage. The flyers posted everywhere said that tonight would feature the shock-punk band, Anna Nicole's Death Fridge. Instead there's an all-woman three-piece called Violet who play straight ahead rock-

and-roll refreshingly free of irony.

I'm bobbing my head, not a thought in it, when suddenly there's Jill. She gives me a high-five, and then, still clasping my hand, manages to snap her fingers three times in a row without letting go. "What's the haps?" she says jokingly, her nose crinkled and perfect. Her face is flushed from dancing. She looks wholly alive.

A group of goth kids push their way up to the bar. Jill peeks at me over the tops of their heads and smiles. Or maybe they're just dressed like goth kids. If you're a real goth kid, every night is basically a kind of Toe Tag Night. And words like "SUICIDE" make for extremely stylish tattoos. I lean toward Jill and shout over the music. "Hey!" I shout, cupping my mouth with my hand, "I read that in England they don't have Toe Tag Nights! It's Headstone Night!"

"Really?" Jill scoots down the bar, closer to me. She tilts her head, tucking her hair delicately behind one ear. Our knees touch. "Yeah," I continue, my face hot, "you know: 'Here Lies So-and-So,' died of 'Shingles' or whatever..." I want to say something else, about how their graphics are probably much better, all graveyards and moonlight, but I stop myself because I don't want to sound like a dork.

"I bet their graphics are killer!" Jill says. "Hey!" She squeezes my arm. "We should do a shot!" She orders and the bartender brings out a cardboard box painted to look like the machine and we reach inside and get our cards. Mine says "BOURBON." Jill gets "SAMBUCA." "Trade ya!" she shouts. Her eyes are ablaze, reflecting neon. She winks. We don't trade. We share. One of each.

— ‡ —

The band is taking a break and Jill has just finished showing me a new handshake that somehow ended up with both of us locking elbows and wiggling our open hands above our heads like antlers or antennae, laughing helplessly, and for no reason I can name I ask her why Brian doesn't come to these things. Jill stares at me, pop-eyed, for a full second. Then gives me the finger. Only it's the finger next to the middle one, which I'm guessing is kind of like the variation she gives to her handshakes, and I'm just glad she's still smiling.

A guy immediately slumps onto the stool next to hers. "Hey, what's your sign?" he says through a loose grin. "Mine's—"

"Cancer. Got it." Jill turns on her seat back to me.

Liza arrives with a guy dressed in Spandex and a cape. He's made his tag into a giant crest, emblazoned with the word "HEROICALLY." He has a gym-built body; the wide chest and shoulders and comparatively small legs make him look, fittingly, like a Bruce Timm cartoon character. Except for the hair gel. Liza makes no introductions. She whispers something in Jill's ear, and I'm thinking of the people you sometimes read about, who learn that they're going to die from "A BULLET" or "FLAMES," but rather than spending their lives hiding or trying to avoid their fate, go on to join the police department or become firefighters. Aimee and then Karen slowly walk up to the bar and nod to Liza and Jill, but not the guy. Aimee heads immediately to the front of the drink line and returns almost as quickly, a sweating death's head cocktail in hand. Karen smokes a cigarette and looks at nothing.

There passes several moments when no one speaks, which I can only describe as uncomfortable. The Spandex guy suddenly remembers the friends he left at the other end of the bar, and returns to them in a single bound or so. Aimee, I notice, has scratched out "NEVER" on her tag and written in "BOREDOM." I am glad to have a drink because it gives me something to do with my hands.

Later, I am taking a deep breath, preparing to say something, anything, when the band starts up again—incredibly loud. Which is how I know Jill's phone was probably on vibrate. She leans forward on the barstool, holding the phone to one ear and plugging the other with a finger. A deep crease begins to form between her eyebrows. Suddenly, still bent forward in that same position, she bolts. "Don't—!" I hear her yelling into the phone as she darts headlong through the crowd.

I look to the other girls. "What an asshole," Liza says, turning to Aimee. "Brian's tag should read, 'Crushed Under Own Ego.'"

"'Being a Total Dickweed,'" Aimee replies.

Karen exhales a cloud of grey smoke. "'Cock Suckery.'"

I have been trying to follow this exchange arcing back and forth over my head like a lethal volleyball. *Really?* I say at last, with a look of what I can only imagine is total astonishment on my face. "Why is she going to marry him, then?"

All three turn to me, silent.

"Hey, Dies-In-Sleep," Liza finally says, after what feels like a long time, "you've got a good life ahead of you, why don't you go buy us a round?"

I am hustling back from the bar, a glass in each hand and one balanced between them on the tips of my outstretched fingers, forming a kind of drink triangle—Liza's non-sequitur having seemed somehow perfectly reasonable coming from her—when an entirely different thought finally occurs to me: The finger that Jill gave me earlier was the ring finger. Without the ring.

—‡—

I find her by the bathrooms, wiping her eyes with toilet paper. "He wasn't always like this," she says without preamble, sniffing. "He got one of those fucked up predictions. You know? Like Liza?" She wipes the corner of her eye. "'Attacked.' I mean, how fucked up is that?

But instead of just dealing, it made him all paranoid and mean. And he never wanted to go out, and when we did stay in he was always—" She stops and blows her nose. Laughs. "Fuck it," she says, her wet eyes shining. "He probably was always like that, and is just using it as an excuse for being a shitty person." She sniffs again and tosses the wadded tissue into her purse. "That's what I've been telling Aimee, anyway."

From the stage, the bass player begins an elaborate, extended solo.

"Um, listen," I say, lamely. "Aimee and everyone, they want to leave. Go to this party they heard about." I attempt a wry smile: "Karen says this place is dead."

Jill looks at me seriously, and doesn't break eye contact. "I'm really tired," she says at last. "Can I just stay at your place?"

—‡—

I am standing outside in the warm Arizona night air, waiting for a cab. I am a little drunk maybe, and trying to make things fit together in my mind. Me. Jill. Jill and me. When the cab pulls up, we get in, sliding to the center on the hard vinyl seat. The door handle on my side is made almost entirely of duct tape. Jill smells like flowers and other people's cigarettes. Her presence fills the cab. Jill. I give the driver the address to my apartment and I'm trying to remember, is there still a dirty cereal bowl on my living room table? Clothing balled on the floor? Underwear? The driver's accent has a recognizable musicality which I think places him from India. The air conditioner in the cab is not strong, but Jill and I stay huddled together in the back. It seems like the most natural thing in the world to put my arm around her. My arm lies stiffly across the back of the seat. "I don't understand those dating services," she says to me. "All those 'Heart Attacks' and 'Tumors' getting together. It all seems so grim."

I nod but it's dark in the back of the cab.

"I like yours, though," she says. "It's sweet."

"Sweet like, 'That-baby-is-so-sweet?'" I say, smiling nervously. "Or sweet like, '*Dude. Sweeet.*'"

She doesn't answer but moves her body right underneath my arm, and then it is, it's the most natural thing in the world to let my arm fall across her shoulders. We cross seven intersections under green lights and all I can feel or hear is my own heartbeat. I want to blurt out something to the driver, to ask him if it's true that in India everyone who goes to the machine gets card after card after card, thereby proving reincarnation, but I know that some cultures are much more private and reverent about these things. They don't wear tags.

There is a new weight to Jill's body now, and her breathing has become heavier, more even—she is asleep. I look down at the hair on the top of her head, braided and clipped with tiny butterflies. Someday a blood vessel will rupture inside her brain and end it. Someday. But who knows, maybe "AFTER MANY YEARS." Maybe "WITH SMILE ON FACE." It happens.

We pass an apartment complex, not mine but like it, Saguaro cacti planted out front and spot-lit, their limbs held stiffly at attention, like sentinels on guard, row upon row.

I tell people I don't, but the truth is, I do think about it sometimes. My death. And yes, it does bring me comfort—but not as much as you'd think. Like just knowing a story has a happy ending alone doesn't make it a good story. All you have is the effect without the cause. The "then" without the "if." And life, I think, doesn't work like that. You can't just plot it out on a line graph, point to point, straight through to the end. It operates in many dimensions—each action, each decision, branching out in complex, often unexpected, directions.

We pass the turn that would take us to my street; the cab driver taking the long way around, the meter running, my arm around Jill, tingling slightly, and I don't say anything yet because I know where we're headed, and when we get there and step out of the cab and into my apartment and her eyes are open and anything is possible, do I make the right decision then, do things begin, or do they end, do we, for example, kiss?

Story by William Grallo
Illustration by Scott C.

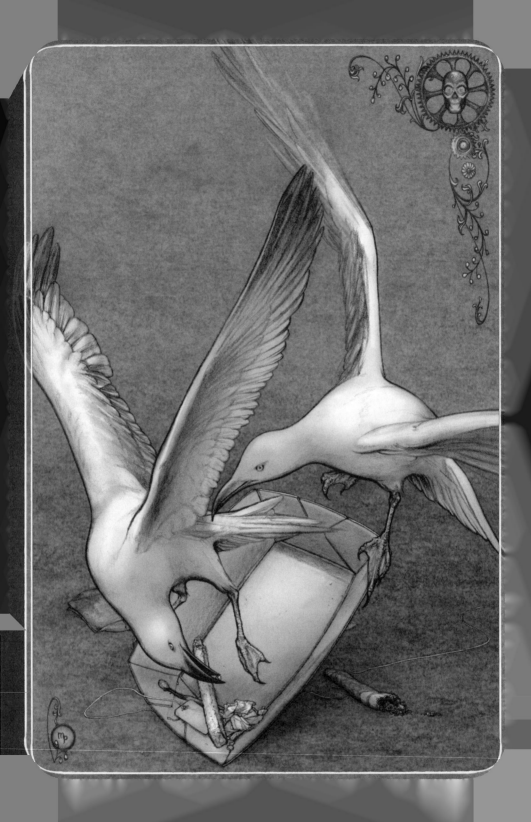

KILLED BY DANIEL

He got the results in April, and his first thought was that he had no idea what to do with them. For a while, he kept the little slip of paper hidden at the back of a desk drawer at work, still inside its official envelope. He didn't want it in the house—Phil was bound to ferret it out. Phil wouldn't even have to try, bless him; he was just one of those people who found things.

He'd thrown away all the other stuff that had been in there, all the leaflets about counselling and help-lines and support groups and whatnot. Everything seemed to be full of leaflets these days. It was like the Sunday papers: you always had to give them a proper shaking over the coffee table before you read them, otherwise hundreds of shiny advertisements would be likely to slither out and attack you.

After three weeks, Robin took the slip of paper out of his desk drawer and burnt it in the wastepaper bin.

"Morning, sunshine."

Robin groaned, reluctantly dragging himself out of sleep as the familiar scent dug its little caffeine hooks into him. He hauled himself ungracefully into a sitting position and took the mug from Phil.

"I hate you," he said, blinking resentfully at the bright spring morning filtering through the curtains.

"Oh, cheers, sweetie!"

"Why do you always have to look so *shiny* at this time of day? You're like a scout leader or something."

"Well, that's what I am. Sort of."

Phil ran team-building holidays and survival courses for groups of business people, teenagers, anyone really; people looking to find themselves or each other. He and Robin had actually met on one of these excursions, five years ago come July. Badgered into it by his then-boss, Robin had hated every second but slogged through it valiantly, getting stuck in bogs and out of breath on mountains. One damp morning, after Robin had spent a nightmarish hour trying to light a campfire with two sticks, Phil had quietly slipped him a cigarette lighter and winked. "It wasn't favouritism," he said later. "It was a reward. I admired your persevering spirit."

He was doing well these days, Phil. The survival business had never been so popular.

"Here you go. Read this and stop whinging." Phil thrust a copy of the Guardian in front of Robin and continued to bustle around the bedroom, tidying things that, as far as Robin was concerned, didn't really need tidying. It was an annoying, yet comforting habit. Phil sometimes reminded Robin of Mrs. Tiggywinkle, the hedgehog from the Beatrix Potter books. There was something small and neat and prickly about him. He'd told Phil that once, and wasn't allowed to bring it up ever again, on pain of death.

"I think you're very cruel, waking me up," he called over the sound of Phil rummaging through the cupboard on the landing. "It's the weekend."

Phil's head poked round the bedroom door. "It is also Child Day." The head grinned at him and disappeared again.

"Oh, yeah."

Robin put his coffee down on the bedside cabinet. It didn't seem to be agreeing with him this morning. He carefully folded the newspaper and put it to one side. That little printed slip, long gone to ashes, floated unbidden into his mind. It might not mean that, he thought. It probably means something quite...

"Can you stop by Sainsbury's on the way back?" Phil called from downstairs. "Fresh basil is needed, I fear."

Robin realised he'd been holding his breath. He let it go in a sigh, and got out of bed.

Driving to Angela's felt strange today, as though he'd never done it before. He ended up missing a turn and found himself on the wrong street, where fat, tracksuit-clad women glared at him from their front gardens as he passed. Outside a chip shop, a group of hooded youths stood around smoking, their shoulders hunched. One of them caught his eye and made as if to run in front of the car, jumping back at the last minute. The other kids grinned, spilling out into the road as the car went past, reclaiming their territory. Robin saw the boy's face for a second in the rear-view mirror. The hood had fallen back onto his shoulders and he was laughing, running a hand through his hair, the sun in his eyes. Only a kid.

When he finally reached Angela's house, he found himself unwilling to walk up the path and ring the bell. He sat there in his seat with his heart thudding wildly, feeling as though he couldn't quite catch his breath.

"I don't know whether you want tea," said Angela distractedly. "I don't think there is any, anyway."

She went to the foot of the stairs and called up, "Love, did you get teabags?" Her cigarette was dangling heavy-ashed over the carpet. Robin winced and forced himself to look away.

The answer floated faintly down from an upstairs room. "It wasn't on the list."

"Sorry," she said to Robin, and shrugged. "What can you do?"

"Doesn't matter, honestly." Robin smiled. "I'll pick some up for you if you like, I've got to stop at Sainsbury's anyway. How've you been?"

"Oh, you know..." She stood awkwardly next to the sofa, thin arms folded across her chest, cigarette still dangling.

Robin knew. Even in the long-ago days of their marriage, Angela had had a strange, aimless quality to her, as though she needed something heavy to anchor her down. When she was happy it could be a lovely thing. They'd drifted together, the two of them. Drifting along the seafront on windy days, into the country for makeshift picnics where neither of them remembered to bring any food. She'd had such a nice laugh, like music, he'd thought fancifully. Neither of them had known where they were going, really. Not then. And Angela never had found out. Sometimes, even in those days, her aimlessness had made him want to kick her or shake her. Anything to get a reaction.

Now she drifted from room to room inside her little house, leaving traces of cigarette-ash on all the surfaces, living in a dressing gown. She hadn't stepped out of that house for two years, give or take. She had a counsellor she thought the world of, and a certificate from the doctor saying she was unable to work. And her son. Their son. Not much else.

A tree, the test had told her. A tree would kill her.

It was best not to risk it, she always said, peering out mistily from behind the net curtains. Not today, anyway.

There were footsteps on the stairs. Robin hesitated for a second before he turned around. Be normal, he thought. Be the same.

"We ready to go, then?" said Daniel.

Daniel. His hair flopping in his eyes, like it always did. Those ridiculous jeans and the battered army bag with all the badges on it. Just Daniel. Robin smiled. He couldn't help it. Daniel made him smile.

"Hiya, mate. You all right?"

"Yep. See you, Mum." Daniel was halfway out the door already, Angela plucking nervously at his sleeve, cautioning both of them against this, that, and the other. Robin reassured her, escaped, and followed his son out to the car, the way he did every Saturday. It was easy, he found, to pretend that things were normal. Daniel made everything easy.

As he walked down the path, Robin smiled up at the blue sky.

The spring sunshine was warm on his face, and it felt like an unexpected gift.

"So..." he said, sneaking a sideways look at Daniel as they waited at the lights. Needs a haircut, he thought automatically. He wondered whether that was just something that came with parenthood, the desire for everyone to have a decent haircut. He couldn't remember ever looking at someone before Daniel was born and thinking 'needs a haircut.' Now he found himself doing it all the time. That girl at the newsagents, for instance. He always wondered how she could see to count the change through that ridiculous fringe. He shook his head.

"Lunch!" he declared. "Then...I don't know, we could wander down to the seafront. Anything you fancy doing, Danny-boy?"

Daniel rolled his eyes at the nickname and shrugged. "Dunno really."

"You staying over?"

He shook his head. "Nah. Got Club tonight. Is Phil cooking?"

"Obviously. Unless you've got a real yen for beans on toast, that is."

Daniel laughed. Absurdly, Robin thought 'Score!' Then, remembering, a sickness rose up into his throat.

The lights changed. He swallowed and concentrated on the traffic.

"How's your mum doing?" he asked, using the deliberately light tone that always went with that question. He felt rather than saw Daniel's shrug.

"Same."

"Right."

"She got Katherine out in the middle of the night, Wednesday. The nightmares again—thought she was having a heart attack."

Robin frowned. Poor Angela. She could stay indoors as long as she liked, hiding from real trees—it couldn't stop imaginary ones from getting into her head. Poor Angela...

But he'd joined that club now, hadn't he? Perhaps he should be feeling sorry for himself. Poor Robin.

"You know what we said still stands, don't you? You can always—"

"Dad..."

"There'll always be a room for you at ours. Whenever you want. No problem."

"Yeah? And what about Mum? She's a problem, isn't she?"

Robin sighed. They went through this every week. "We can get care for her...we can help more. You'd still see her, as much as you wanted. Everything doesn't have to be down to you, you know."

"It's fine! I can handle it, okay? I like things the way they are."

"But—"

"Dad!"

"Yes, yes, all right." He sighed. "Just so long as you know, that's all. We're only at the end of the phone. Anyway... How's school?"

"All right."

It was just an ordinary drive. An ordinary sunny Saturday. How strange, thought Robin, that it should be so.

When they got back, the kitchen smelled appealingly of Phil's lasagne.

"I knew you'd forget the basil," he said. "So I made do. On your own head be it." He pointed a wooden spoon accusingly at Robin.

"Shit," said Robin. "Sorry, sorry..."

"Luckily for you, my darling," said Phil, kissing his cheek, "I am a culinary genius. Hi, Daniel."

"All right?" said Daniel by way of a greeting, and threw his bag down on a chair. "That smells brilliant, I'm starving."

"Gratified to hear it." Phil blinked at them both, then turned back to the stove. He was funny in the kitchen, Robin thought— almost shy, as though he'd been caught doing something embarrassing. It was stupidly endearing. Daniel sat down at the table and started flicking through the Guardian, discarding the various sections, looking for the music reviews. "Jesus," he said. "Why do they have to put so much crap in this thing?"

Watching them, Robin suddenly felt terribly separate, as though he were observing through a pane of glass, or a screen. He wondered for a second whether he should leave. Just sneak out the back door, quietly; he knew how to work the latch so that it wouldn't squeak. Probably, neither of them would notice. In a minute or two, one or the other of them would look up, and...he wouldn't be there.

Stupid thing to think. Running away never solved anything. And where would he go? To his parents? Hardly. He'd have to go far enough away... He'd have to leave everyone and everything. Except that nowhere he went would ever be far enough, would it? You couldn't run away from death, even if you could from life. He felt his eyes begin to prickle, and covered his mouth with his hand.

"All right, people," said Phil. "Prepare yourselves, please. Lunch is imminent."

A sharp breeze blew off the sea, whipping Daniel's curly locks back and out of his face. That's better, thought Robin in his mum's voice. Can see your eyes now. Then his dad: That ought to blow the cobwebs away, right, son?

I'm getting old, Robin thought.

"Do you want to go on the pier?" he asked Daniel, who shrugged. "Don't mind."

Robin pushed his hands deeper into the pockets of his jacket. Anorak, he thought. There's no other word for it. I'm the sort of dad who wears an anorak. He'd never quite realised before, how much he loved being that person.

"Sorry," he said. "Probably a bit boring for you really, coming over here every weekend. Nothing much to do."

Daniel looked at him scornfully. "Don't be an idiot, Dad. It's fine."

He did seem fine, Robin thought, underneath all that teenage scowling. He allowed himself to admit, with a touch of pride, that Daniel looked happier when he was here. He was a good kid, but he had an overdeveloped sense of responsibility, and it frightened Robin sometimes. The world on his shoulders, that was Daniel. When he was with them it was as if he could relax in a way he couldn't around Angela. He seemed to frown a little less, smile a little more.

We *should* be proud, he thought, defiantly. We've done everything right, Phil and I. What the hell have we ever done wrong?

Daniel darted forward suddenly, picked up a stone and skimmed it into the waves. "Phil said he's going to show me how to skin a rabbit next weekend," he said.

"And where does Phil plan to get a rabbit from, exactly?"

"I dunno."

"Hmm. That's what worries me."

They did wander up to the pier in the end. Daniel had a half-hearted go on the amusements, before pronouncing them "a bit rubbish, really." He's too cool for that now, Robin thought fondly, and bought him a Coke.

"Don't tell Phil," he said. "He'll have my guts for garters."

"You don't have to do everything he says, you know."

"I don't!" said Robin, stung. "I was joking. You get on with Phil, don't you?"

"Course," said Daniel. "He's cool. But, you know. You're my dad and all that." He shrugged and leant further forward over the railing, frowning down at the grey sea.

Robin smiled around the lump in his throat. Behind them, a commotion started up as two seagulls had a scrap over an abandoned cardboard chip-tray.

Later, on the drive back to Angela's, Daniel started telling him about the club.

"We're organising this gig night," he said. "You know, for fundraising. It's gonna be really cool, we've got the Labrats down already. And the January Architects, even though they're crap, but the girls like them 'cos they all fancy that Oliver bloke. Jimmy reckons he can book King Prawn, but I dunno. They're getting pretty big now."

"Right, good...you realise I have very little idea what you're talking about."

Daniel rolled his eyes. "They're *bands*, Dad."

"Yeah, I got that part."

"It's gonna be cool," Daniel said again. "They all want to support the cause."

Robin winced at the phrase.

"What?"

"No, nothing."

"I dunno why you're so against me actually having something to believe in," said Daniel defensively.

"I'm not! It's just...you're still young, aren't you? You should be out enjoying yourself. Girlfriends, whatever..."

"I know you agree with me, though. You do, don't you? What we stand for, being against the machine and the test, all that. You believe in it, too."

"It's not a question of that," said Robin tiredly. "In principle, yes, of course. I'm glad you're thinking about this stuff. It's just—"

"It's *wrong!*" Daniel said passionately. "No one should ever know how they're going to die. *You* said that! Look at Mum, what it's done to her. It's just—it's fucked up and it's wrong!"

Robin could feel Daniel's eyes on him even while he watched the road. He knew, without having to turn round, what Daniel looked like right now. A certain light in the eyes. That note in his voice. It was this part of Daniel that he could imagine fearing. He tried not to imagine it, but he could, and he knew this because it was something that was part of him, too. It was a deeply buried something, very deep, but it was there.

"Things have got to change, Dad," continued Daniel. "What if I went out and got that test? I'm nearly old enough. You wouldn't want that, would you? You wouldn't want me to know."

"No!" said Robin, and shuddered. "No, God forbid."

"We're just trying to make a difference," said Daniel. He sighed, and his voice changed, went small and muffled. "Thought you'd think that was good."

"I do. Honestly." Robin gripped the steering wheel. His head throbbed with a dull ache, as it had done all day, and all yesterday, too. He wondered vaguely when the headache had started, and realised he couldn't remember.

"I just...don't want you to get hurt. Don't want you doing something you might regret. That's all."

It was dusk by the time they reached Angela's house. He saw a curtain twitch in the living room as they drew up outside. Daniel, grabbing his bag and opening the passenger door almost as soon as Robin stopped the car, seemed as eager to get back to Angela as he had been earlier to get away. Robin never took it personally. It was just the way Daniel approached everything—the same intense concentration and restlessness. It'll be the death of him, said Robin's mum's voice in his head. He wished she would just be quiet.

"See you, Dad."

"Bye. Love you."

An eye-roll and a smile, and then he was gone. Robin sat in his car and watched the night slowly deepen to black around the haloes of street-lamps. In Daniel's bedroom, a light went on.

On the way home, Robin drove past the street he'd accidentally turned down earlier in the day. The chip shop glowed brightly at him from the corner, but he couldn't see any of the kids. He wondered whether they'd moved on to new haunts for the night, or whether they were still there somewhere, lurking in the shadows. Instinctively, he checked to make sure his doors were locked.

Lots of people are called Daniel.

He'd been having bad dreams lately about dark alleyways,

muggings, blood. Men with knives and baseball bats. Thugs and queer-bashers. There was this boy who kept turning up, night after night. Hooded, his face in shadow. And dog-tags on a chain around his neck. Every time, Robin twisted in the boy's grip, struggling not to get away, but to see the name he knew was marked on those tags. Because he had to know. Before...before what?

There were other dreams, too, and those dreams were worse.

He stood at the back door for a full ten minutes when he got home, his hand frozen on the latch. Through the kitchen window he could see Phil sitting at the table, tapping away at his laptop with a cup of coffee next to him, the steam rising from it in faint wisps. As Robin watched, he looked up and their eyes met. Phil hurried over and pulled open the door, concern on his face.

"Love? What's the matter? What's happened?"

He was reaching out for Robin, trying to pull him inside, out of the dark. The brightness and warmth of their kitchen spilled in a little pool from the open doorway, as though the house, too, were trying to embrace him. Robin tried to answer, but felt himself paralysed. Even the smallest of decisions—to move, or not to move—seemed far beyond him. When he looked down at his hands, though, he saw that they were moving, just a little. Shaking, as though with cold. They looked like someone else's hands, he thought, not his. Someone who was very old, and very tired.

He made an effort and cleared his throat. "I've got to tell you something," he said, and stepped forward into the light.

Story by Julia Wainwright
Illustration by Marcus Thiele

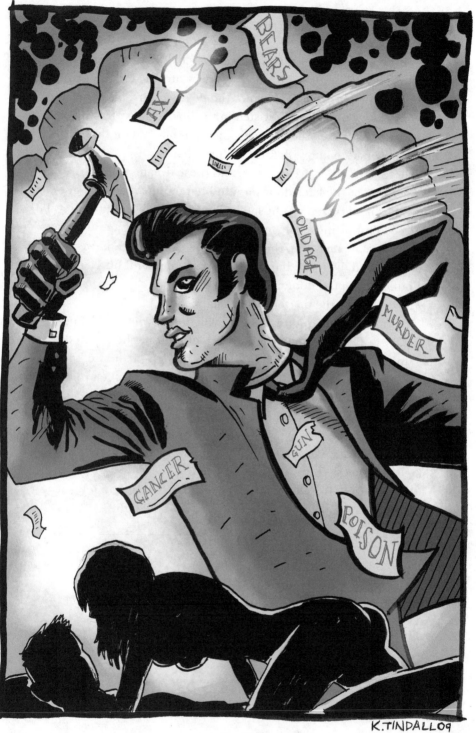

FRIENDLY FIRE

THEY PULLED THE WOMAN FROM THE PADDED SEAT WITH CARE. She wasn't the enemy. Ignorant, a buyer of the big lie, but not the root of the problem. She was somewhere north of forty. Her dark hair showed silver strands, and the beginnings of crow's feet bracketed chestnut-colored eyes. Tommy noticed her fingertips, purple and tender. She was a Repeater. It touched a nerve.

Confusion and fear mingled on her face. "Don't hurt me!" She wrapped an arm around herself, a reflex of protection. "Take my purse. I don't have much."

"We don't want your crap," Mitch said from behind the rubber face of Elvis Presley. He pushed past her. The silver head of a hammer, produced from inside Mitch's overcoat, reflected a hundred mall lights. He ripped the curtain off the booth and went to work.

The hammer found its mark again and again, denting and bending and breaking the shell and guts of the machine. Pieces clattered to the floor of the booth. Slivers of paper fluttered loose, the world's smallest victory parade.

"Run," Tommy told the Repeater. She was transfixed by the spectacle.

"I needed to know," she said, empty. "If it would change. If I could change it." She rubbed a thumb over the tip of her index finger.

Tommy, hidden behind the John Lennon mask, positioned himself between her and the booth. "Go. NOW!"

The woman retreated into the mall. Tommy watched for uniforms from the same direction, waited, counted in his head. "Let's go, Elvis!"

Mitch gave the device a final blow. It popped from its mounting and fell in a shower of sparks. A crowd of shoppers had become gawkers, but Tommy saw no heroes among them. Not for the machine.

"KNOWLEDGE IS SLAVERY!" he shouted as he and Mitch retreated. "DEATH TO THE MACHINE!"

He heard the first cry from mall security as he crossed the threshold. Outside, Barb idled the Impala in the drop-off zone, disguised as Frank Sinatra. Ol' Blue Eyes bobbed behind the wheel, impatient. Mitch climbed in front. Tommy jumped head-first into the back through the open window. Tires squealed as he pulled his feet inside.

They drove down side roads and doubled back on their path twice. Mitch called the other teams on his cell. No one had been apprehended. Tommy scanned for signs of pursuit.

"We're clear," he told Barb.

"How did we do?" she asked Mitch.

"Including ours, we knocked out fifteen of them."

It was better than they'd hoped. Tommy had expected twelve demolitions and at least one arrest. They'd all made it through unscathed, fifteen mechanical soothsayers laid low in their wake. It was a solid night's work.

Barb dropped Mitch at the corner of Watson and Fifth. He left his mask in the glove compartment, ceded the front seat to Tommy, and was swallowed up by the night. Tommy grabbed the fake tags from over top the real ones. He stowed them under the front seat. He kissed Barb, relishing the response of her warm lips to his before she pulled back into traffic.

"Stay with me tonight?" she asked.

Tommy nodded. It had taken some getting used to, the casualness of their relationship. They had no commitment to each other outside their common cause against the machine. He was nineteen, a stew of hormones and adrenaline, and at times he wanted more than an itch-scratching lay. But while Barb would wreak havoc with him, and sleep with him, there was no romantic patter, no disposition for roses. She kept that part locked away, saying it was better that way. He didn't debate her wisdom. Sex on a regular basis was a strong dissuader of upsetting the apple cart.

Barb rented an apartment over a detached garage. It was a cozy fit for the Impala, beside the owner's moldering boxes and stray furniture, but the door locked and the landlord, who lived up the street, stayed out of her business. The wooden stairs up to the door creaked under their ascent. The apartment was small, well-kept. Barb liked order. It carried over to her planning of their hit-and-run attacks.

Tommy had noticed her in his Anthropology class, but they met for the first time in conversation on a website. Called "Deathics: The Ethics of the Death Machine," it hosted an endless and often bitter debate about what the machine's combination of technology and magic had wrought on mankind. Tommy and Barb were fellow travelers. Each had their reason to hate the device and its uncanny ability.

Tommy studied her as she undressed, tracing her delicate curves with his eyes, following the cascade of long hair about her shoulders when she undid her pony tail. The dark strands flirted with the tops of her breasts. She should have been subverting society from the pages of a fashion magazine instead of driving getaway cars. Tommy doubted that many revolutionaries looked the way she did, moved with her grace.

She glanced over her shoulder at him and smiled, as if she could peer inside his head the way the machine did into blood. It was a wicked grin, a silent invitation. She took mock pains to hide her body from his view as she slid under the covers in the lamplight. She patted the bed beside her. Her skin was warm and velvety against his when he joined her. She doused the light and wrapped her legs around him.

They cuddled for a time after the sex, which had made him tingle and drained him of the remaining adrenaline from the evening, and he fell asleep to the whisper of suggestive words in his ear.

He slept and dreamed of Davey.

When Tommy was eight, his parents had sat him down in the living room and told him they were having another baby. His memories of Davey's arrival were faint, blurred together at the edges—a lingering sense of his mother's absence, spending the night at Aunt Ruth's with his cousins Melanie and Sara, and then the sound of crying and the stink of dirty diapers.

By the time he turned eleven, Tommy had noticed the protective bubble his parents wrapped around Davey. Things that hadn't been an issue for Tommy at Davey's age were withheld from his younger brother—toys with small or moving parts; puzzles; board games. He wasn't allowed to pick up change, or stones that fit in the palm of his hand. His parents were phobic about Davey putting things in his mouth, about him not chewing his food, about any cold that produced a cough.

One event haunted Tommy. When Davey was three, their mother flew into a frenzy of motion and sound when she noticed Davey playing with a plastic grocery bag. He was bothering no one, piling his blocks in the bag and taking them out, over and over. Ma tore the bag from Davey's hands, sending blocks tumbling through the air. Shaking, she stood over him, screaming "NO!" as if he'd soiled the rug. A lone block clutched in his quivering hand, Davey cried with a lack of comprehension that cut Tommy to the bone.

Articulate, bright, Davey was always looking over his shoulder, petrified of running afoul of rules he couldn't predict. The sole time he tried to explain it to Tommy ended with a long sigh and a question. "Tommy, could they love me too much?"

A week after he turned five, Davey died in his room, alone, a victim of his own curiosity. Out of sight for a few minutes, he'd taken it upon himself to explore forbidden fruit, denied him for so long and snatched from a kitchen cabinet with everyone unawares: a handful of peanuts. Anaphylactic shock was the official cause. Much later, when Tommy was in high school, his father added the missing colors to the picture. Tommy's parents had consented to a machine test of Davey's blood at birth. The doctor had promoted it to them as a "preventive measure." The little slip of paper spit out as result read "SUFFOCATION".

"We started out worrying he'd get strangled in his blankets," his father said. "Then we focused on the size of things. We even considered allergies. He never had a problem with peanuts before." Dad, a man of small stature bowed even lower by his younger son's death, shrugged as if trying to loosen an unseen grip on his neck. "What good is knowing the future if you can't do anything with the knowledge?"

They'd swallowed the poisoned punch and Davey had died from it. Even if the machine was infallible and Davey was meant to die young, it enraged Tommy that his brother's brief life could have been measures better if his parents hadn't tried to second-guess the future.

Tommy had refused testing at every juncture from that day. He didn't want to know what waited for him.

Barb's story was as senseless in its tragedy, trading an innocent brother for a pragmatic father. Her dad had given up living when the machine looked into his blood and foretold "CANCER." Even when his doctor confirmed the disease and declared it treatable, survivable for decades, Barb's father surrendered. He didn't want anyone to bear the burden or the uncertainty of a protracted fight. When the cancer consumed him in months, rather than the years it might have taken, Barb was galvanized against the machine's unholy test.

After long discussions online, and the discovery that they were classmates, Tommy and Barb began to meet in the real world. More like-minded souls joined them over the course of a year. What began as a support group evolved into something else. They discovered in themselves the spirit of Berkeley, of Kent State—radicals

standing against the powers that be, taking back something stolen from them, reclaiming it in ways impossible through endless
debate in a chat room.

Tommy awoke to Barb shaking his shoulder. Pale pink light from
the streetlamp outside gave the shadowy room a spectral glow. Tommy
rubbed his eyes and groaned. Phantoms of Davey, three-year-old
hand still clutching a block and quivering, receded into the corners.

"You were whimpering," Barb said.

Tommy nodded. "Sorry. Dreams. Davey."

He was quiet for a long time, listening to his own breathing.
Barb laid a hand on his chest. "Where are you?"

"Thinking about tonight. The Repeater at the mall."

"What about her?" Barb wrapped her arms around him and eased
his head to her chest. He snuggled against her, sought solace in the
sift of her fingers through his hair.

"All her life, she's been taught how to increase her chances of
living a long life. Then one day, she learns she's going to die in
some fashion she's always been told can be prevented. Maybe 'heart
attack.' She makes changes—quits smoking, improves her diet, joins
the gym—and she keeps going back to see if she's tipped some cosmic scale, to no avail. She might die of a heart attack when she's
a hundred years old, except she's crippled inside by waiting for it.
She's stopped living her life. She's devoted it to her death."

Barb kissed the top of his head. "We did well today. We'll never
know whose lives we may have changed just by breaking the right
machine at the right time. For all we know, we may have shaped
the opinion of a future leader who will finally outlaw the damned
things."

"It still doesn't feel like enough," Tommy said. "Half of what we
trashed today will be back in action in a week or two. It's like trying
to empty the ocean with a soup can." He stopped, sighed. "We need
something bigger. More effective. A statement."

Barb reached out and turned on the bedside lamp. For a few

moments, Tommy's field of vision was a bright blot. As it cleared, he saw Barb, still beautiful and pale and very naked, rooting around in the night table. She pulled a gray file folder from under a stack of notebooks and papers. "I didn't want to say anything until I thought we were ready."

She set the folder on the bed. Tommy leafed through it—diagrams, floor plans, handwritten notes of conversations.

"What is this?" he asked, fascinated by the photos of long hallways and large rooms filled with equipment. Barb slipped back under the covers beside him.

"This," Barb said, "is as big a statement as we can make."

Klemm Fabrication Incorporated, located in Caruthers, fifty minutes down Route 171 from Barb's apartment, was the largest manufacturer of Death Predictive Devices in the Midwest. They'd come to Barb's attention via a Newsweek article discussing the company's efforts to meet the rising global demand for the devices. She'd done a lot of social engineering to gather information from workers, county engineers, technicians who made service calls at the plant. She used her smile and charm, taking pieces from every encounter to form a complete picture of a vulnerable site.

"We take out the key points in the assembly line," Barb told the group when they met to discuss their next action, four days later. They were all still wired from the success of their blitz, and Tommy could see everyone was hungry for more. They'd gathered in Penny's suite on campus because it was the largest, plus it was in the Brewer dorms, where a large gathering would go unnoticed among the louder, more obvious frat parties. "Belts. Motors. The computers that control the operation. We destroy power conduits. We destroy the swing-arms that do the detailed work on the guts of the machine. We put them out of commission for weeks. Months."

"How do you propose we do all this?" Roger asked. He ran a pro-machine Web site as a cover for his lesser-known affiliations. He was also a campus radio personality. "A hammer's good one at a time, but it's balls for heavy work. Too time consuming."

"We use localized, shaped explosives," Barry said, with a nod from Barb. He was a chemical engineering student who blamed the machine's predictions for hastening the suicides of two friends. "Small, hot, hard blast, localized within a few feet. Like a cutting charge. You could snap the rear axle on a car and only nudge the engine." As if the words were insufficiently shocking, Barry pulled a sample out of his backpack. Non-lethal and inert, he assured them, but it drove Mitch from his chair.

"I signed on for small public disruptions, not bombs," Mitch said. "The malls, the one-off drugstore machine, fine. Explosives are crazy. We should step it up on larger medical testing locations instead. Doctor's offices, clinics, hospitals. If people think they're at risk, they'll stay away."

"That makes us look like terrorists," Tommy said.

"Isn't that what we are?" Mitch persisted. "Let's not kid ourselves. You think people in malls aren't scared of a guy in a mask with a hammer?"

"Right now, we're stirring debate about the machine and what it does, not about ourselves," Barb said. "The first time we threaten the safety of people with no interest in the machine, in a place of trust like a hospital, we become the bad guys."

"I understand that, Barb," Mitch said. For the first time, Tommy noticed the kid of seventeen inside him. Tommy was accustomed to a Mitch who was calm, decisive, old beyond his years. Before him now was a boy, nervous and uncertain. "I just think moving on to bombs is asking to get someone killed."

"It will be after hours," she said. "Clean. Surgical. We cripple the infrastructure, sting the corporation, make a statement to the press. We open peoples' eyes wide to the issue."

They debated a while longer. In the end, Barb required a

unanimous decision. Mitch held out until he knew he was standing alone. He went on record that it was a bad idea before voting to go forward with the action.

Once they were in agreement, they sat around the coffee table in Penny's living room and began walking through Barb's plan.

They rehearsed for two weeks. They went over timings and variables until they could navigate the factory building with their eyes closed. Penny wrote the manifesto for mailing to the Tribune, the New York papers, the Post in Washington, and the L.A. Times. They called themselves the Unknown Future Liberation Front, "proud architects of last night's targeted strike."

They took the evening before the operation to relax.
Barb invited Tommy over to her place to blow off steam. Despite the sparkle in her eye and the excited ache he felt, he declined. Saying no didn't come easily, but he wanted some space, though he couldn't articulate why. Beyond her disappointment, he thought he saw hurt in her eyes, but dismissed the notion. That wasn't who they were.

His roommate out of town for the weekend, Tommy stayed on campus. He ordered Chinese take-out to his room, hung out with a couple of girls from the East wing of the dorm and watched anime until he fell asleep. His dreams were crowded with massive steel machines that towered over him, sharp teeth trying to draw his blood, ribbons of paper blotting out the sky and inscribed with the words "MISADVENTURE."

His cell phone rang, piercing his sleep and dragging him up to consciousness. The room was bright with daylight. Sounds of student life filtered in from beyond the door. Tommy answered on the last ring before voicemail. He expected Barb or Mitch with bad news, a call to flee the dorm one step ahead of the police, the fate of all dozing rebels. Instead, it was his mother.

His mother never called.

She made small talk about the weather and his father's job and her current book club selection, while Tommy stretched and threw on a layer of day-old clothing. When she finally ran out of stalls, she said "They're voting on a draft bill Monday for soldiers for the Middle East."

"I know, Ma," he said. "It's college. We keep an eye on these things." They had been talking about it for weeks, in and out of class. Had he not been involved in disrupting the machine, Tommy would have joined one of the protests. He had friends who would vanish on a straight line to the sand in the wake of such a bill. "It'll be fine. These things get voted down every year. This one will, too. And even if it doesn't, I'm protected by the deferments."

"No you're not," she interrupted.

"I'm an only child. Plus, there are very specific criteria for selection of college students. Believe me, I've looked into this. Don't make yourself crazy."

"Tommy, I had you tested when you were three years old."

It was a graceless blurt, but it hit his chest like a finely tossed grenade. "You did *what?*"

"I always planned to tell you when the time seemed right," she said, and fell silent. Tommy could hear her ragged breathing into the receiver.

"Why are you doing this, Ma? Why now?" He stopped. He didn't want to know, hadn't wanted to, so long as no one else did. And here was his mother, the woman who overcompensated his brother into misery, the unknowable known to her, not for a day, or a year, but for sixteen years.

"I wouldn't mention it if I didn't think it was important."

"How?" he asked, even as a voice inside told him to hang up the phone and walk away. "What does the fucking contraption have to say about it?"

"I don't want you to worry. That wasn't my intent—"

"Just tell me," he said. "You wouldn't have called unless you wanted to say it, so say it." There was silence by way of response. "God damn it, tell me!"

"It says 'FRIENDLY FIRE.'" Tommy heard her begin to cry. "You were three. Your father and I ignored it. When you have a little boy, combat is putting on a birthday party. You never showed any interest in the military. We saw no reason to worry until now."

Tommy had always left room for the possibility that some day, he would be tested, with his consent or against his will. He hadn't expected ambivalence as a response, but his immediate sense of it was akin to a shrug. It couldn't be changed. Why would it matter?

He heard his mother swallow, half a continent away. "Tommy, we made mistakes with Davey. Everything we tried to do, we couldn't— didn't—see it coming. We failed him. I think sometimes if we'd talked to him, explained it, we could have avoided it, or at least put it off. I thought about telling you what your slip said after he died, but I didn't want to fail you, too."

Tommy was glad she was on the phone and not standing before him. The contemplation of violence had a twisted, calming effect. "You don't get it, even after all this time. You didn't fail Davey because you couldn't save him. You failed him because you never let him live." He paused, numb. "At least you gave me that much."

His mother started to speak, but Tommy buried it with a thumb of the button. She'd said enough. He didn't want to say too much.

He turned the phone off and crawled back into bed. He considered calling Barb to talk through his newfound knowledge, and decided it could wait until after their visit to the factory. He grappled with daylight, the prediction rattling around in his head, until he abandoned sleep in favor of a late breakfast.

Zero hour arrived in desperate darkness.

Barb, Tommy and the rest infiltrated the grounds in two places where the fence all but invited them, according to plan and unaware that prying eyes were following their movements. Soft radio calls and infrared scopes tracked them from the shadows.

Barb led Tommy and Mitch to the Assembly 2 building and through an easily-jimmied loading-dock side door. The line inside was silent, populated with machines left mid-motion when the line was stopped for the weekend. The trio walked the length of the conveyor, identifying strike points from the packaging queue all the way back to the head of the line. The room smelled of metal, solvents and sweat. Pallets of petrochemicals in drums lined the back wall. Tommy saw more of them, all part of a fresh delivery, through the doors that led to Assembly 3 in the adjacent room.

Mitch went to work on the main motor drive for the line. Tommy wired a charge further down the line, on the computer control center that coordinated activity for the length of the belts. Barb sought the thickest bundle of cabling that fed the equipment. By Tommy's measure, they had seven minutes to finish wiring and fall back to the yard.

The authorities waited for them to begin arming explosives before moving in. The head of the government's operation, a former Marine turned Homeland Security tactical consultant, wanted a bloodless take-down and an open-and-shut case. He envisioned a large and very public trial, something to quash grassroots protests and power his career forward.

The first shot was fired by accident in Assembly 3. Penny, caught in the beam of a flashlight, reached for her ID. She thought she'd been caught by a watchman they'd overlooked in their planning. Instead, the man was a soldier no older than Penny herself, hyped up, overstimulated in his first anti-terror deployment. He was certain she was reaching for a gun.

Roger, seeing Penny shot at close range for no reason, *did* have a gun, and brought it to bear. The kid soldier died hard and fast. A second one, older by ten years, put out the call that he had a man down, that the terrorists were heavily armed. He was silenced when Roger shot him in the chest.

It pivoted toward hell with jackrabbit speed.

The bark of a gunshot made Tommy jump. The report echoed through the room, seeming to return from a half-dozen directions. He had a gun, one of several they had obtained through back-alley channels, but Barb had been specific: weapons were a last resort. If caught, surrender, with a polite warning about the explosives. "No fatalities," was her order.

Next door, Assembly 3 erupted in a firefight, driving Tommy to a crouch. He was moving up the line, towards the door, when hands grabbed his ankles from under the line, tripped him, dragged him down. A bullet tore into the sheet metal behind where he'd been standing. He was still fumbling for the gun when Barb put a hand over his.

"Come on," she whispered.

They scuttled under the line and towards cover. Several more shots echoed. Roger screamed somewhere in the darkness. The pair found Mitch crouched behind a skid of shipping boxes and joined him.

"We're screwed," Barb said. "They're everywhere, and they're not asking questions."

"How did they know?" Tommy asked. "How could they?"

Mitch shook his head. "It wasn't supposed to be this way."

"Thanks for the headline," Tommy said and cocked his pistol.

"No," Mitch said. "They said they were going to scare us. That's what they said. Homeland Security would arrest us and scare us straight." He looked at Barb and Tommy. He was terrified. "That's what the guy told me. No one was supposed to have guns. They were just going to scare us. They swore to me."

A voice called from the darkness, demanded they throw out their weapons. Tommy stared at Mitch. The kid's recent nervousness began to make sense. Oh, did it make sense.

"What did you do?" Barb asked.

Mitch's face twisted, anguished. "I needed money. My kid sister got into some trouble, and had no one else to go to. My parents would've killed her." His voice faltered. "They just wanted to know what we were up to. The guy who called me, he was hanging around the Deathics board. He said they figured out who we were, wanted to keep us from screwing up. They made it like a job, and I needed the extra money. There weren't supposed to be guns." He craned his head up from behind the stacked boxes. "You weren't supposed to have guns!" he shouted.

A shot crashed and Mitch ducked down, right into Tommy's grip. Tommy shook him.

"Stupid shit! They used you!" he shouted, shoving Mitch back into the boxes. He had to stop himself from doing more. He looked at Barb. Her composure helped him focus.

"We need to give up," Barb said.

Tommy realized his desire to run, to fight his way out, was naked in his expression. Barb saw and read it and shook her head. "We'd never make it," she assured him.

He stared. Nodded. That's why she was the boss.

"We're coming out!" Tommy shouted. "Don't shoot!"

He rose with care, gun hanging by the trigger guard around the thumb of his wide open hand, arms stretched overhead. Barb followed suit. Tommy heard Mitch slip away in the darkness and found it didn't trouble him. Mitch was already dead to him.

Tommy and Barb stepped from behind the boxes, frozen. They could hear footfalls in the darkness, glimpsed the passing of silhouettes across distant windows. They waited. A quiet, hard voice startled them from the left.

"This is for Dawes," the voice said, and Tommy heard a gun being cocked. He turned and saw the soldier in shadow. Tommy pivoted, gun back in his grip.

Three shots overlapped in a hellish firecracker pop. The soldier fired a round that struck Barb in the arm. In turn, he received a bullet in the face from Tommy's pistol. As Tommy's gun barked, he felt a punch in his left shoulder. He twisted as he fell, saw the still-smoking automatic in Barb's hand.

Tommy landed on his wound, the pain blinding. His arm went numb.

Barb scrambled over to him, grimacing, issuing apologies under her breath. She examined him with frantic hands.

"It looks like it passed right through your shoulder," she said. "Who's your angel?"

"Wish I knew," he said, ignoring his mother's voice fighting to be heard above the din of his thoughts.

Tommy's eyes picked Mitch out in the darkness, sandwiched between two of the nearby pallets of chemical drums, shouting obscenities, crying. He was no longer a revolutionary, instead reduced by his sins to a wounded youth. "No one uses me! I'm nobody's Judas!" The silver detonator shimmered in his hand. Tommy saw one of their charges stuck to a 55-gallon drum. Tommy felt Barb's gasp. They heard nearby footfalls, soldiers unawares.

Tommy rolled, shoved Barb to the floor and draped himself over her. There was nowhere to go, and no way for them to get there if there was. He had no idea if shielding her would make a difference. He didn't care.

There was a new light in her eyes, admiration and sadness and warmth mingled in a single gaze that told him here, at the end, she wished for something different for them.

As the room transformed into thunder and flame, Tommy was glad he'd lived to see that look.

Story by Douglas J. Lane

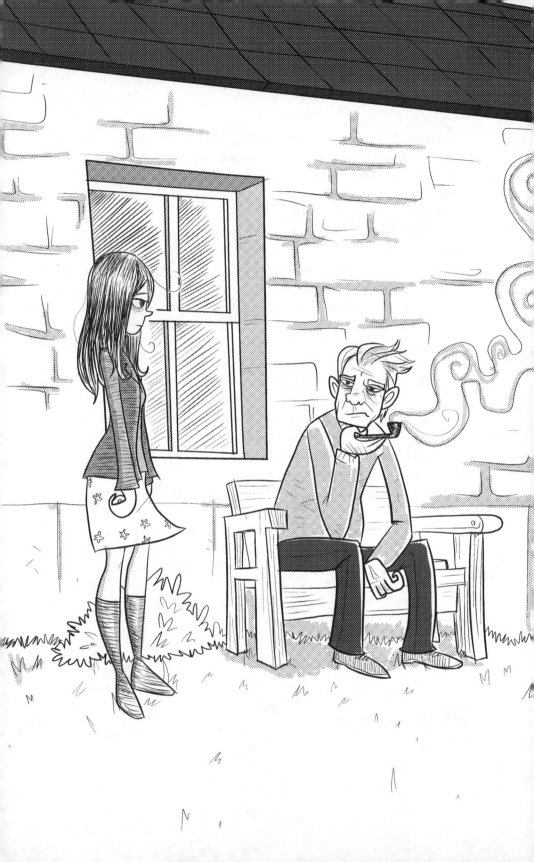

NOTHING

She had started to pant several hundred yards earlier; now a small trickle of sweat was beginning to make its way down her back. She stopped, turned around. The view was majestic: meadows and hedges made a chequered pattern toward the horizon; chimneys puffed out small, dark grey clouds over farms and villages; and as always, the grass was a certain vivid, dark, and slightly translucent green, which she had associated with a particular smell since child-hood—a smell of sea, of fields, and of burning coal.

The grass really is greener here, she thought. *The greener grass of Ireland.*

She waited until she had caught her breath, then turned again and continued up the hill. The footpath wound 'round crags and rocks, but had now taken her almost all the way to the little house. It had been invisible from the road, appearing to be just another patch of grey rocks. Now it had taken on the familiar appearance of Grandpa's house: stone walls, a roof of reddish brick tiles, and the door painted in a bright colour—she recalled it as green from her last visit; today, it was a clear blue.

The door opened when she was still a few yards from the house. An old man made his way out, standing on the three steps leading down to the yard, straightening his back. He looked exactly the same as last time—five years ago, or maybe seven? She couldn't quite remember—thin, tall, with a wisp of nearly white hair that blew whichever way the wind fancied.

She smiled at him. "Hi, Grandpa."

He nodded at her, smiled as she came closer. "Hello, Christine. I see you're keeping well." His voice was clear, but not altogether strong: It sounded as if his words were going to be blown away in the wind.

"You too, Grandpa." She hugged him, carefully: He still felt strong, but since she was twelve, she had always been afraid that one day, he would become frail and be crushed by her embrace.

"It's been some time now. Years." Not reproachfully, simply a statement of fact.

"I did write."

"But now you wanted to see the old man."

"Yes." She looked around, saw that the wooden bench was still there—most of it grey, weathered wood, but one armrest was a dull yellow, some plastic material. She sat down on it, gingerly: Not only didn't it creak, it felt like sitting down on a rock.

"You're grown now. A woman."

She laughed, briefly. "Twenty-six. Not much more than a child, to many."

He sat down beside her, folded his hands in his lap. He was quiet, but looking at her expectantly, waiting for her to tell him why she had chosen to come.

"Grandpa James died last week. On Friday."

He sighed, slowly. "So it goes. What of?"

"Cancer, just like it said on his slip. Nothing unusual about it. Painless, he was asleep toward the end."

Again, a sigh. "He was a dear one, that child."

Christine nodded. "He did tell me, the day before he fell asleep, about you, and when he was a child."

He nodded, lost in thought. "A dear one. I'm glad you came to tell me. It's not a thing you'd want to read about in a letter."

She looked at him. *He knows now, doesn't he? He knows. He knows that I know.* "Grandpa, how old are you?"

He seemed to come back into focus. His voice was stronger, less an old man's: "Older than I care to remember. I don't count the years anymore. No one does, after a while. You're just grateful you saw another one."

"I always knew you were older than Grandpa James. I always thought you were my great-grandpa. I thought everyone had just got into the habit of calling you Grandpa, that you became everyone's Grandpa. But he said that he'd been calling you Grandpa even when he grew up."

"The years pass by, Christine. One by one. One day at a time. You get up in the morning, you stay awake, the sun sets. I don't count them."

She rose, abruptly. "I still do." She turned, opened the door into the cottage. He sat still on the bench as she went in.

The smell was the same, after all those years. A hint of coal, a hint of food cooked slowly and lovingly, a hint of damp that wouldn't go away even in a heatwave in summer. And a lot of old paper. Old books, old letters in a desk, old newspapers in a pile by the fireplace. She had lain awake at night, when they had come visiting, and felt the smell. It felt like they did it all summer, every summer, but when she looked it up and did the sums, it couldn't have been more than five or six summers, and probably only two weeks, possibly three. But that is the way childhoods are constructed, long afterward: you remember scattered parts, some chosen at random, some that affected you deeply, and you string them together and say "this was me growing up." Your parents say something else, your grandparents something different still, but you stay by the story you've told yourself.

She looked around, in a way she never had before. There had to be some clue in here. He had been born across the sea, only returning to Ireland and what he called "the land of my ancestors" as he was becoming an old widower. Surely, there was some sort of paper, some record of it.

It didn't take long. There was only one desk, only a few drawers, and she ignored those holding mementoes and the various odds and ends. But at the back of one drawer, with some plastic cards—probably long defunct—and various receipts, she found what she was

looking for. A passport, an old-fashioned passport, possibly undis-
turbed since he had first settled in this house. With a birth date.

He was puffing on his pipe, peering through the smoke at her
when she came out again. It floated near his face for a moment, protected from the constant wind by the walls of the house, until it gently
drifted into the wind and was torn apart, dispersed faster than the
eye could follow.

She sat down again, and picked up the small lump that had been
weighing down her right jacket pocket on her way up the hill.

He nodded knowingly. "That's one of the latest models, isn't it?
A Predictor."

She put her head to one side, looked at him thoughtfully.
"You've seen them? This is the new pocket-size."

"No. Well, in the papers. The man from the village usually brings
me an old newspaper or two with the groceries. But you didn't have
to bring it, you know. You're family. I'd tell you if you asked."

A moment of silence stretched out. Finally, she said the words
that were so rarely said, even among family: "What does yours say?"

He puffed on his pipe again, took it out of his mouth, picked up
a burnt-out match from the bench beside him, and poked carefully
at the glow. "You know, I had it figured out as soon as I saw the slip.
Both what it really meant, and that I had to go."

"Why? Grandpa, what does your slip say?"

"Why, nothing. It was empty. I never showed it to anyone, of
course. There would be no end of trouble, wouldn't there? But I
figured that if I went here, back to what my parents always called the
Old Country, and settled somewhere I wouldn't be noticed, everyone
would just think it said 'Car Accident' or some similar. No cars here,
see?" He gestured with the pipe, indicating the entire hillside. "This
place had stayed the same for many years. It has stayed the same
since I came. Nothing much changes."

"What sort of trouble?" She knew it well enough—she had had all the time the trip took to work it out—but she really wanted to hear the full story.

"The manufacturers and operators would go mad about it, of course. They'd drag me to court, or something. Then there would be all sorts of religions wanting to have a look at me. Some of them would probably try to burn me at a stake, or say I was an abomination or a heresy. Others might make me their Saviour. Some would try to lay their hands on me, lock me up, and pretend I was never here. Of course, I reckon the Jehovah's Witnesses would be the worst. They'd say I was the first of their one hundred and forty-four thousand, and I'd never see the back of them." He chuckled slowly. "I think I actually moved too far away even for them. I certainly haven't seen one since I came here." A puff at his pipe. "But I had it all worked out. You know, the slips are accurate, they're just not always truthful."

She nodded. Sometimes it was in the news, but more often it wasn't. Some of the stories she had heard were urban legends, naturally, but a sizeable proportion of them were true, as far as anyone could check them.

"So, what does a blank slip mean? Nothing, of course. I'll die of nothing. And there's one kind of nothing that's all over the place. Literally." He looked at her, with a twinkle in the eye as if to see whether she was with him. "Vacuum." Again the waving with the pipe, but this time toward the sky. "Most of the universe is nothing. So they tell me, not that I'm an educated man, but I've read it enough times to believe that they know what they're talking about. So if I ever went out in a spaceship, I'd be darned if it didn't spring a leak, and the vacuum would kill me. And that's where the real trouble comes in, of course."

"How?" She suspected she knew where this was going, but she wasn't going to trust herself to guess his next leap.

"The scientists. They'd be next in line after the priests and prophets. And they'd run all their tests on me, and one day the brightest of them would come up with the idea that if they put me in a test tube and removed the air, that'd be the 'nothing' that'd kill me. And when it did, they'd just say, "QED," clean out the test tube, and go to collect their Nobel Prize. So I just figured I'd stay here, at the back of everything. It'll come after me one day, not that I'm in a particular hurry, but I've lived for a long time now and even if I don't want to go, I did better than I'd hoped for." He smiled, puffed again at his pipe.

She sighed. "Grandpa, I found your passport. You're a hundred and seventy years old."

He seemed to shrink, as if he felt the weight of all those years. He chewed the pipe, took it out of his mouth, and looked at it thoughtfully. "That many, is it. Well, that's a lot." He paused for a moment. "I've buried my children and my grandchildren. And your Grandpa James was the last of their children. All gone now. All gone."

"But you kept in touch with us. Why, Grandpa? You knew some-one would figure it out one day. The world would come back. There are still prophets and scientists."

He looked up at her. His eyes were watery, as if they were about to burst with tears. "You get lonely, Christine. You get so very lonely. All your friends are gone. And then your wife and sisters and cous-ins and uncles. And then, one day, everyone in your generation. One day, you're the only one alive to remember the days when you were a child. All the things you used to say and do, and all the places you used to go. And then the only one to remember the days when you had become an adult. What the politicians were like, what the news was about, the foods and smells and worries and music and all the small things that tell you that this is *now*, the time you moved with when you were young, the jargon and idols and the excitement of what has become ancient history. You're a refugee in time, living on after your world has turned to dust. And the family, Christine, your own descendants, are the only link you have with everything you've lost. They are the only way you have of still being attached to the world."

She found her eyes starting to water, as in response to his. Her hand moved toward the Predictor, as it lay on the bench.

"I don't think we have to do that," he said slowly. "If you say it's a hundred and seventy, I say you're right. I might have missed a dozen, but that would really make no difference. And I'd really not like the world to come stampeding here to look at me, if it's all the same to you. Not at my time of life."

Christine shook her head. A strand of hair was caught by the wind, and settled across her face. "I believe you, Grandpa. I figured it out, more or less." She kept her eyes fixed on him, while her index finger found the hole in the Predictor. "I brought this here to show you." A click, a quick sting in her finger, and a whirr as the Predictor ejected the small slip of paper. "I thought you wouldn't believe me if you didn't see this." Still without letting her eyes leave his, she picked up the slip and gave it to him. The slip that—just like last time, just like always—had no text on it.

He looked at it. He looked at her. After a moment, the tears started to roll down his face. And slowly, and still silent, he turned and looked out over the landscape.

She sighed, and relaxed. And as he had done, she turned and looked out over the landscape, illuminated and painted in red and gold by the setting sun.

Story by Pelotard
Illustration by John Allison

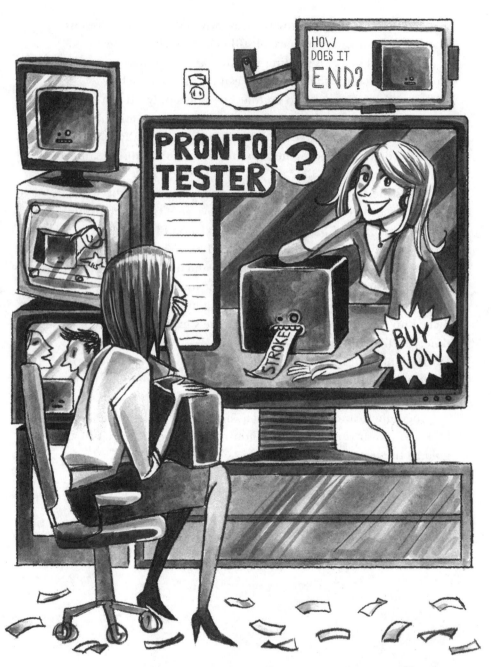

COCAINE AND PAINKILLERS

At nine o'clock on a Tuesday morning, the parking lot in front of Jack Bogg Enterprises was somehow already full. Kelly didn't know quite what to do. It had never happened before, not once in the year she'd been working for JBE. Especially troubling was that her favorite spot—right by the planter, the only spot in the office park guaranteed to be in the shade at six P.M.—was taken by some cruddy old Volvo. But three circuits of the lot only served to make her late, so she sighed, pulled around to the other side of the long metal building, and reluctantly parked by the O-ring wholesaler. She doubted she'd be leaving work before sunset anyway, if the last six weeks were any indication.

A wave of heat rolled over her as she pushed open the driver's door. Today was a summer scorcher, and knowing Big-Spender Jack, he'd have an oscillating fan going in his office while everyone else broiled like breakfast sausage. She checked her makeup in the mirror, grabbed her computer bag, gathered her courage, and went for it.

After three minutes crossing asphalt that threatened to melt her from the shoes up, Kelly pushed through the door with the white vinyl letters and gasped. It was *cold* in here—against all odds, Jack was actually running the air conditioning. A breeze from the vent ruffled her hair, and she blew a loose strand away from her face. She didn't even know the office *had* air conditioning.

The next thing that struck her was the *noise*. Ringing phones, voices chattering—she glanced over at the phone bank as she walked to her cubicle, and was surprised to find two extra folding tables crammed into the corner of the room, manned by a dozen unfamiliar faces haltingly reading from scripts and tapping into computers that hadn't been there when she'd left at two o'clock Saturday morning. Something was going on—something big.

"Great news!" Jack grabbed her from behind, sweeping her up in a powerful hug. His sweaty bulk pressed into her, his round face over her shoulder glowing red with the exertion of walking around the corner. Kelly gently extricated herself and slipped into her best professional good-morning face, turning to face him—but he was five feet away now, pacing in a tight circle, his eyes darting like bumblebees, flitting around and then landing on Kelly for long, uncomfortable seconds. "Fat-It-Out is huge. *Huge,* so huge I can't even *tell* you! You did great, babe, *great.* Look at this place!"

His sweeping gesture included the new bank of computers, the chattering kids, the cold wind blasting musty odors through long-dormant ductwork, even the too-bright fluorescent lights that were making Kelly's head hurt already. She'd slept through most of the weekend plus Monday trying to *recover* from this place. It was clear her body didn't want to be back.

Jack grabbed her wrist and headed off down the hallway, Kelly stumbling to keep her balance. "Whole new phone-response staff," he explained. "Orders are through the roof. We made back our airtime costs in 80% of markets within *six hours* of broadcast. It's a whole new era for JBE, and it's all thanks to Fat-It-Out." Her computer bag slipped from her shoulder as Jack pulled her into his office. She snagged the strap with an inch to spare.

Fat-It-Out was Jack Bogg Enterprises' latest premium offering to the direct-response television market. The product (essentially a skillet with a spit-valve) was fighting fiercely for attention in a crowded field of similar junky crap that seemed to exist solely so that third-tier cable channels wouldn't go completely off air when everyone stopped watching at one in the morning. And apparently, it was winning that fight—for the moment at least.

Jack sifted through papers on his desk, pulling one from a pile and shoving it at Kelly. "Look at these numbers!" She couldn't make heads or tails of it, but got the gist when he grabbed her shoulders and shook her like she was in an earthquake. "This is record-setting, Kel. *Record-setting!* Ron Popeil never saw numbers like this. George Foreman would shit a *brick* if he saw numbers like this!"

"Sounds pretty good," she managed through the quaking, turning away from Jack to grab his file cabinet for balance. She held fast to the squarish metal, wary of aftershocks.

"Pretty good?" He grabbed his chest and sank into his creaky leather chair, sweating through his shirt. He looked like he was going to have a heart attack right there on the spot. "Kel, you're killing me with 'pretty good.' This is the sort of response that you normally have to *hone* over time. You have to run focus groups and market research. You have to massage price points and premiums and giveaways in market after market, trying to find that perfect balance—you remember Ab-Mazing? We couldn't *give* that piece of crap away." He shook his head with a rueful sigh. "I can't explain it, Kel. To do this right, it's like landing a jumbo jet. It doesn't just *happen*. But somehow you *did it*. People *want* this thing—it's selling *everywhere* now. Sunday morning I had to call China in a panic. Lucked out—those guys work seven days. Not like *this* country. Those guys don't go to church. *I'm* their church. The American businessman."

She stood there, not quite sure how to react, afraid that maybe he'd jump out of his chair and grab her again—it was the sort of thing he did all the time. Jack Bogg was a tactile individual, always placing a hand on her shoulder, or tapping her on the head when he walked by her cubicle, or doling out high-fives at random times, then claiming she'd been "way too off-center" and insisting on doing it over and over until they'd achieved the perfect synergistic clap.

But he was her boss, and he paid her well, and he'd apparently done a great job mentoring her for her first campaign to be such a super slam-dunk. The least she could do was be professional.

She used to wonder if Jack misrepresented her polite friend-liness as flirtation. She had long ago stopped wondering. He was hard-core in love with her, she was pretty sure.

"So what happens now?" she asked.

"What happens? We rake in the *dough,* is what happens," he said, kicking a stack of papers off his desk to make room for his feet. Kelly stared at the worn soles of his shoes and wondered if perhaps she should have taken today off, as well.

"But seriously," Jack said, suddenly swinging his feet back down to the floor and assuming a Serious Tone, "you did a really great job on the Fat-It-Out campaign. I know I gave you a bit of a hard time along the way, your first big DRTV campaign and all. But in the end, I bit my tongue and trusted you, and you broke out of the box with some great new ideas. You deserve every bit of this success."

"Th-thank you," Kelly said, feeling momentarily bad for cursing his name every waking moment for the last six weeks straight.

"With that settled," he said, breaking into a huge, sweaty grin— "now we put that patented Kelly Craig brain to work on the next big JBE blockbuster!"

From beneath his desk he produced a cardboard box plastered with customs forms and shipping labels. Flicking Styrofoam dust from his fingers, he handed Kelly a red plastic device about the size of a shoe box, covered with smudgy fingerprints and basking in a distinctive Tupperware smell. "I got this on a hot tip from one of my sources overseas," he said. "He's thinking *big,* talking about a pan-Asia launch next month, and he *was* gonna pass up North America completely, got no distributors out here. Then he heard about Fat-It-Out, and *I* get an email asking if we could match that day-and-date domestically. I said 'of course,' had him send me a demo unit right away." He shrugged. "It's a tall order—but it's a big opportunity. We're going to the next level. And I know you can knock it dead."

The red device had no name, no branding, no cheap, colorful decal. An unplugged cord trailed out of the rear; a power switch was the only button. She turned it over in her hands. On the front, a darkened LED was inset next to a hole about the size and apparent depth of a lipstick. Beneath them both was a thin slit edged with tiny plastic teeth.

She frowned. "What *is* it?"

"I'll admit, the details are sketchy," Jack said. "English is not my guy's main language, maybe not even in his top five. But here's what I've got so far." He gestured for her to come around to his side of the desk. He could have turned his computer monitor around, but she knew that he wanted her near him, hovering at his side, maybe brushing his shoulder. She held her collar closed as she leaned over.

From his email he opened a photo of a big metal machine—wheeled base, dials, and gauges galore. It looked like a drill press, or something from a metalworking shop. *"This* is basically *that,"* Jack said, pointing to the red device in Kelly's hands. "Some brainiacs made this big monster for the medical market, tried to sell it at trade shows for a hundred grand a unit. It's some kinda blood analysis thing, checks your sugar, your cholesterol, all these diseases, all this battery of tests. It's got a computer chip, it gives you instant results for everything. No more waiting for lab results." He shrugged, flicking a sideways glance to Kelly's shirt, then up to her face. "They built the prototype, but couldn't find the cash to go to market."

Kelly walked back around the desk. "No kidding, it's huge. That would take a ton of capital."

"Then the guy died," Jack said. "Lead guy, scientist guy up and died—plane crash, boom. So our client, this investor friend of mine, bought out one of the patents."

"This plastic piece of junk can't be the same as that whole big thing," Kelly said. "Nobody'll believe that, no matter how fancy your graphics."

"No, no, let me finish. Now as I understand it, the big thing is mostly one-stop-shopping for tests already available separately—you can get a blood sugar thing at the drugstore, you can get cholesterol at the, whatever, at the doctor's office I guess. But the patent my guy bought was specifically for something called a 'C-18 algorithm,' some little circuit board in the middle—some new discovery. So he says, anyway. Who knows. My guy puts that piece in a red box, and *voila.*" He pronounced it *voyla.* "He thinks it's gonna go big—he's got half a million units on the assembly line already. Chinese versions, English versions, Japanese, Spanish, all of 'em."

Kelly put the red device back on Jack's desk. "So what's the pitch? What does it *do?* Sing, dance, change the baby?" She fished in her computer bag for her notebook, and jotted down *proprietary C-18 algorithm.*

Jack shrugged. "That's just the thing, I'm not totally sure—like I said, my guy's got trouble with the language. As far as I can figure out, it's a drug tester, prints out a little slip of paper says 'pot' or whatever. It really is a good business-to-business angle, there's a lot you can do with it."

She made rapid notes. "It's literally a blood test? Or do you pee in that little hole—'cause I don't have to tell you, unless it comes with a funnel, to half the audience that's a real tough sell."

A second later she regretted putting the image in his mind. He seemed to take a full five seconds to collect himself, before heaving a deep breath, blinking a few times, and picking up the device. "You stick your finger in here, there's a little needle inside takes a blood sample, and it prints in like ten seconds." His hands were quaking, and the device rattled. "With the previous version, the big clunky one, they tried to go the whole health-care route—I'll forward this email to you. They had some Chicago ad agency involved, whole direct-to-trade promo campaign with a bunch of cheeseball doctors in lab coats yapping away about this and that, blah blah blah. Soft-sell crapola." Jack was fond of pointing out the differences between traditional, more restrained methods of marketing and intensive half-hour blocks of full-volume paid programming. His method sold more products over the phone, for one.

"Doctors see right through a staged testiomnial," Kelly said. "Point of pride when they do."

Jack nodded. "Screw 'em. Our folks are the working folks, just givin' 'em a break from all that Hollywood, Madison Avenue B.S. No one with a medical degree is buying Fat-It-Out, you know? You know?" He laughed. "Oh, speaking of Fat-It-Out, I got some choice letters from doctors. It's starting already. Here, let me read you this—"

"That's okay," she said quickly. If people were complaining about Fat-It-Out, she didn't want to hear about it. It would make killing herself for months on that campaign even harder to justify.

"You sure? It's hilarious! They take it so seriously! But hey..." He knocked on the drug-tester's red plastic shell. "At least this is pretty straightforward: finger in, paper out. Idiot-proof! You can use that if you want. What do you think—is 'idiot' too harsh? They got those *Dummies* books."

"I'll come up with a few concepts," she said. "I'll have scripts for you this week."

He waved the offer away with a thick hand. "Run with it," he said. "I trust you. You can take this, yeah? 'Cause I got skillets to ship."

Kelly shrugged. "Whatever you need."

"You're the star of the show now, babe."

She named it the ProntoTester, and within a few days she'd filled an outline with glowing ad-copy hyperbole. The infomercial would have to be pretty elaborate if they wanted to hit Jack's sales expectations. In addition to the usual staged presentation, they'd have to shoot some testimonials—meaning they'd have to get some people to actually *use* the product. That meant orchestrating trial events, recruiting participants, working through the whole process of weeding out non-photogenic faces and people who couldn't string a sentence together on camera. They'd have to get trial units shipped in from China, plus because of the needles they'd have to get a whole health-and-safety inspection—Kelly felt her fingertips begin to shake. This was going to be a big job. And Jack wanted it to air *when?* Within a *month?*

"C'mon, superstar," she muttered to herself. "That's non-superstar thinking. Get to work!"

She tapped at her laptop, writing snippets of dialogue for the presenters and then erasing them, letting her fingers bounce on the keys, whittling key selling words out of phrases and concepts. "Patented detection-control mechanism." "The proprietary C-18 algorithm delivers instant results." "One poke finds one toke." She deleted the last one immediately. It wasn't *all* gold.

The next thing to do, she decided, was to test it out. She called in Julio, the company's A/V guy—editor, cameraman, and all-around technical whiz. They probably wouldn't use any footage of the initial test in the infomercial, but she'd learned to shoot everything, just in case. Besides, she'd spent hours upon hours in the editing bay with Julio working on Fat-It-Out, and enjoyed his companionship—he was the anti-Jack, low-key and calm, and didn't take the job too seriously. After all, it wasn't *his* money on the line.

She had the college kids take short breaks from manning the phones to sign waivers and get their fingers pricked on JBE's standing set. She was expecting the test to unearth a few potheads, maybe one kid on something harder—she'd had to repeatedly promise that the test results wouldn't affect their jobs. Besides, they'd reshoot everything later, with auditioned participants and makeup and applause and everything—for now she just wanted to make sure the thing *worked.*

It didn't.

It pricked fingers, and spat out pieces of paper, but none of it made any sense. Most of the test results weren't drug-related at all, and the few that were—ALCOHOL and MORPHINE—were lacking the level of detail she expected a drug-tester to provide. In the rest of the cases, the thing spat out arbitrary dictionary words like IMPALE and XYLOPHONE and LAOS and HEMATOMA, and she knew for a fact that the XYLOPHONE kid had been high as a kite the whole time. Was it a translation issue? Bugs in the software? Some function she didn't understand? Or was this unit just broken?

The ProntoTester's failure wasn't a huge deterrent to Kelly—after all, Fat-It-Out didn't work that well either—but it was an inconvenience. It meant they would have to fabricate test results for the sake of the infomercial, thus walking that fine line between "dramatization" and "false advertising." Kelly knew that walking the line was part of their business, but she still couldn't totally silence the voice that told her she spent every day suckering innocent idiots out of their hard-earned disability money. Most days, though, her work ethic drowned out that voice with shouts of "DO YOUR JOB."

Julio had no such moral qualms. He'd clocked a lot of overtime hours by simply doing his own job well, disconnecting his higher brain and working the editing computer like a maestro at a piano. "Sure, I have questions about my job," he'd once told Kelly. "Like what should I spend my paycheck on this week? New TV or new stereo?"

If the thing even worked *poorly,* she'd have had no problem. An instant drug-tester would be an immediate and huge seller—every business in the country would want one, if it really were cheap, easy, and even half as accurate as her infomercial might suggest it was. But the ProntoTester didn't seem to work at *all*.

She'd even, with some reluctance, administered the test to herself and to Julio—but the results, STROKE and OVERTIME respectively, only confirmed her belief that the stupid thing was nothing but a random-word generator.

"But that *can't* be it," she complained to Julio. So they racked up four hours of time-and-a-half, getting tipsy and giggling on Jack's dime, coming up with increasingly-silly explanations for what the device actually *did*. She started with "psychic label-maker," to which Julio suggested "masochistic Scrabble dictionary," which didn't make a ton of sense but by then it was eleven o'clock and they were buzzed. Kelly came back with "circumstances of one's conception," and Julio countered with the equally-ridiculous "circumstances of one's demise," with a rueful glance at both the clock and his eerie result slip.

Kelly laughed (slowly, given the hour), closed her laptop, gathered her coat, and went home. Even by the awful standards of the late-night-consumer-products industry, the very same folks that had gleefully sold the public on Hair-B-Gone and Gyno-Paste and the MuffinMagic X-Treme, she had to admit that the ProntoTester was a big red plastic stinky turd of a product.

As a function of the type of neighborhood that Jack Bogg Enterprises was located in, there was a Wal-Mart right across the street. Kelly felt guilty in principle for shopping at Wal-Mart, for some vague liberal reason—but there was literally nothing else but office parks for miles, and it just so happened that the megastore stocked a brand of yogurt she'd been unable to find anywhere else. So when the college kids' sales chatter down the hall became too much to ignore, she closed her laptop, grabbed her sunglasses, and headed across the street.

She tried not to look around the store as she marched toward the dairy case, conveniently located on the back wall past just about everything else imaginable. She averted her eyes from $4.99 DVDs and 3-for-$8 T-shirts. She was mostly successful at avoiding glances into the overflowing carts of people with poor impulse control, and felt guilty for the smug sense of superiority that crept in to reward the effort.

Halfway between Home Electronics and Furniture, she rounded a corner and was blindsided by Housewares. Brightly-colored boxes of the Fat-It-Out Advanced Nutritional System crowded an entire endcap. She'd only *just* pushed that ridiculous-looking skillet-with-a-spit-valve image out of her mind but *here it was again*, the packaging blasting Healthful Advantages™ at her in 100-point yellow type. She whirled away and hid by the food-storage bins to catch her breath. She felt chased by a monster.

She'd tried hard, *really* hard, to do a good job producing her first big campaign for JBE. And Fat-It-Out had repaid her by taking over every waking hour of her life.

Six months ago, when she was burning out working for Jack as an associate producer, she'd tried taking her portfolio to Rockefeller+King, the big ad agency—the one with the athletic shoe account and the soda account and the three competing insurance accounts. But they'd laughed her out of the office, and told her to take her weight-loss cream and her hair-removal spray and her leather-repair paste with her. (Well, they hadn't said that *exactly*, but she'd gotten a distinct vibe of contempt from their trendy glasses and carefully tousled haircuts—and they hadn't called back, so what did it matter what they'd actually said?)

And then Fat-It-Out had come along, and Jack had handed her the reins, and she'd buckled down and tried her best to do a good job—the only thing she knew *how* to do—and she'd knocked the ball out of the park.

So this was it, now. She was an infomercial producer.

She gathered herself. She straightened, and took a breath. She tried to picture the ProntoTester on the shelf here in six months, but stalled trying to imagine what the box copy could legally say: "Inaccurate drug test!" maybe, or perhaps "Random word generator!"

"Ooh, Dolores, have you seen this one?" The voice filtered from around the corner, back by the Fat-It-Out boxes— Kelly heard the squeak of shopping-cart wheels, the wheeze of labored breath, the rustle of hands on a cardboard box; the clank of pans shifting inside.

Then, another woman's voice: "Look, it's got a valve for draining the oil out! Isn't that clever? I'll bet Lacey would love this for her new apartment. She needs to start eating healthier."

"What a great idea!" came the chirping response.

Kelly wanted to round the corner and scream, *No! It's just cheap pans that one Chinese company couldn't sell on their own married with cheap valves that another Chinese company couldn't sell on their own.* As the unseen women read each other the hyperbolic statements from the back of the box—statements that Kelly herself had written and revised and erased and re-written and ultimately approved for the packaging—Kelly felt her cheeks begin to burn. She wanted to shout: *I wasn't being* serious *when I implied it would change your life; it's just something you* say *in marketing!*

But instead, she said nothing.

"How's it coming?" Jack asked, grabbing Kelly's shoulders and squeezing.

Kelly jumped in her plastic chair, startled—then shrugged his hands away. "Slow," she said, standing and crossing the breakroom to retrieve a mug of hot water from the microwave, opening the door with ten seconds left to go. "But it's coming along." She didn't mention that in the last two weeks, the only progress she'd made at all had been in her level of anxiety.

She'd stalled creatively. Without consistent results, she had no sales angle; without a sales angle, she had no campaign. The Pronto-

Tester seemed to mock her; its LED, finger divot, and serrated mouth formed a leering face that watched her pace a furrow into the carpet. Periodically it stuck its tongue out to mock her—in the form of another cryptic slip of paper that raised more questions than it answered. As the slips began to accumulate into a terrible mountain of frustration, each new theory dashed by the next result, its blank expression seemed to her absurdly, maddeningly calm.

And other pressing matters had come up for her—health insurance paperwork, renewing magazine subscriptions, getting a new cell phone and transferring her whole phonebook. Days had rolled by unmarked, save by her nightly resolution that tomorrow would be more productive.

Still, she knew she'd get it done eventually. After all, she was the genius behind Fat-It-Out.

"I bet it's gonna be great," Jack grinned. He turned to retrieve a stack of papers from the printer, paging through them, throwing a few away. "I could get used to this whole hands-off kinda deal. I mean, don't get me wrong, shipping out skillets takes up most the day. But I'm working on courting some new clients, drumming up some business. I even got a new slogan, check it out—'J-B-E is going up, up, up!'" He spread his hands like a presenter on one of his infomercials, his showman instincts kicking in. "Came to me in the shower! I'm thinking of having new cards printed. Orange is hot, right? You want an orange business card?"

"Absolutely," Kelly said, fumbling with a tea bag, splashing it into the mug, spilling hot water on the counter. How long were you supposed to steep it? Did it get bitter if you left it in too long? She was bad at tea.

"I *knew* it! I *knew* you'd love it!" Jack rubbed his meaty hands together. "And here's a little incentive for you. Let me take you *behind the scenes*." He shuffled through the stack of printouts and produced what looked like an invoice, written entirely in Chinese.

"Take a look at this!"

"I have no idea what that says."

"Say hello to the proud new owner of two hundred thousand ProntoTesters," Jack said smugly.

Kelly suddenly felt her vision swim. She tried to talk, but her mouth was dry. Reflexively she sipped her tea, nearly scalding her tongue. Through a haze of steam she choked, "You bought out the factory?"

"Every English one they made!" Jack beamed. "Did I tell you before? How those idiots tried to screw me on the Fat-It-Out? Cheap bastards quoted me three-eighteen American per unit, something like that—then, all of a sudden, when I have to fill ten thousand orders in a week, the price *mysteriously* jumps to five-oh-one! Trying to screw me over!"

"That's a big difference," she acknowledged.

"They blamed it on the exchange rate," Jack said, tossing the invoice onto the counter atop the other printouts. "The dollar sucks, but not *that* bad *that* fast. In the end I paid the bill, I mean, I had to, or else that's it for our sales—and *we* were charging thirty-nine-ninety-five-plus-S&H. But still." Kelly cringed as he popped his knuckles, one after the other. "ProntoTester is gonna do *great*. I *know* it will. This"—he tapped the Chinese invoice—"this is me *believing* in you, Kel. Two hundred thousand now, two million tomorrow, twenty million next week! Who knows? This could real easily be our *careers*."

Kelly felt a knot settle in her stomach. The possibility of spending an entire career with Jack made her queasy. She took a cautious sip of the tea, and thought she felt the steam cloud up inside her skull.

"Oh, and one other thing, no big deal," he said. Kelly noted a sudden change in his tone—forced casual, now. "In case you get a call from some lawyer. There's some B.S. class-action out there building against Fat-It-Out. It's nothing—gold-diggers, trying to get a

piece. It's always the way when you make it big." He waved his hand
dismissively, as if he were all too familiar with the trappings of success. Kelly watched a bead of sweat roll down the back of his neck.
"They're going after the non-stick coating. Toxic something-or-other.
It's totally baseless, but in case you hear from someone—which you
shouldn't, because I've been keeping your name away from this—I
want to make sure we all know the story." He began to tick off
points on his fingers. Kelly suddenly had the odd feeling that he'd
had to recite this particular list before. "JBE has no role in manufacturing our products, we are simply marketers and distributors.
JBE makes no warranty claims as to the condition or durability of its
products. JBE relies on its customers to make determinations of quality prior to purchase. Many thousands of customers have reported no
complaints with JBE products in the past."

He jerked up to look her in the eye, his red-rimmed gaze belying
a deep, sudden intensity that gave Kelly a chill. "You got all that?"

"Okay, show me this amazing idea of yours," she told Julio, slumping
into the uncomfortable chair behind his editing workstation. Four
weeks now, and she was maddeningly no closer to a finished product than before—even though Julio always seemed to be working on
something. He told her it was just how he filled his days, scrolling
through the hours of useless footage they'd shot, looking for funny
outtakes and re-cutting words and phrases into bizarre non sequi-
turs. He did this a lot, during downtime. He said it was how he kept
his perspective.

She'd even seen glimpses of other projects on his monitor, stuff
they'd shot for Fat-It-Out or even older material predating her ten-
ure—raw footage from campaigns like HairGlo-5, the hair-sculpting
wax made with "real bee proteins," or the TradeCenter, a kids' bank
that had unfortunately hit the market in September 2001.

And she had to admit that Julio had his fake-busy work down to a science. Jack could burst in the door at any given time, and Julio would look every bit as productive as his timecard claimed he was.

"Tell me what you think," Julio said, tapping his spacebar to start the video playing.

Sappy music swelled. On the monitor, handsome parents played with beautiful children. (Kelly recognized shots from the "Contemporary Family" stock-footage collection.) Julio's voice, lively and bright, rang from the speakers: "Do you suffer from anxiety about the future? Concerned about what tomorrow may bring? Are you *afraid of dying?*"

"This is hilarious," Kelly grinned.

The ProntoTester appeared on the screen with a flash. "Now, the solution to all of life's uncertainty! *The Machine of Death.*" One of the phone-response kids stuck his finger into the device, then held it up with a cheesy smile. A close-up revealed that his test result was SKYDIVING ACCIDENT. Julio's voice continued: "It tells you exactly how you'll leave this earth!"

Kelly burst out laughing. "You sound so *serious!*"

"We're gonna run this on air, right?" Julio deadpanned, stopping the playback with a keystroke.

"Totally. You just made my job a lot easier," Kelly said. "Oh, man. Early lunch for everyone!"

Julio spun in his chair. "Awesome! But I'm still billing the hours."

"Go for it. It's not my money." Kelly motioned to the computer. "Keep playing! How long is it?"

"So far I've got, like, thirty-two minutes." Julio laughed at Kelly's gaping expression. "Been a slow couple of weeks!"

He moved his mouse and cued footage on the video moni-tor. "See, here we've got outtakes from Fat-It-Out—these guys are dying from CHOLESTEROL. And check this out." He pressed the spacebar, and they watched a woman in Spandex do a series of awk-ward crunches inside a spring-like contraption. A big red graphic slammed onto the footage: SHODDY EXERCISER.

Kelly doubled over with laughter. The Ab-Mazing had certainly been the shoddiest exerciser she'd ever seen, though it hadn't stopped JBE from peddling them in no less than three successive infomercials as Jack tried desperately to sell his back stock. "Jack's brain would go nuclear if he saw this. You have no *idea* how much money he lost on that piece of crap."

"Oh, I have an idea." Julio half-twisted to glance back at Kelly. He seemed to consider adding something else—but a sharp rap on the door silenced him. He whirled back to the computer and cued footage of the ProntoTester onto the monitor.

Jack burst into the room officiously. "Kel, quick question—you haven't heard from that lawyer I talked about, have you? About Fat-It-Out?"

Kelly shook her head. "No. Should I have?"

"No! No, it's fine. But if you do get a call, don't say anything, okay? Let me know right away." He glanced at the monitor and beamed. "Looks great! Coming right along! When do I get to see a cut?"

Kelly swallowed. Luckily, Julio's complicated timeline on the computer screen gave the impression of progress. "Soon," she said. "Still tweaking."

"That's why you're gonna go far," Jack said, leaning his bulk on the creaking desk. "Never satisfied!" He thumped the desk twice for emphasis, clapped Kelly heavily on the shoulder, and slammed the door viciously behind him.

Kelly and Julio sat shell-shocked as the echoes of his presence faded. Julio was the first to speak: "I am so glad that guy is dumber than I am."

Kelly drummed her fingers on the desk nervously. Suddenly she felt stupid, wasteful. "How soon do you think we could have a *real* cut?"

Julio's new laugh was bitter. "You're not serious. Give me a script! Shoot us some footage!" He looked at his watch. "When is this thing supposed to air? If I cared about that sort of thing, I would be freaking out right about now."

Kelly nodded slowly. "Yeah. Unfortunately, I *do* care about that sort of thing. The airtime's been bought for weeks." She stood and paced in a tight circle, trying desperately to make all the problems go away by waving her hands around—after all, nothing *else* was working. "I just can't wrap my head around this stupid thing! All Jack can say is, he thinks it's a drug test. Well, guess what! It's clearly *not*. I *can't* sell it as a drug test because he's going to get us sued and we'll all be out of a job! Why the hell does he think it's a drug test?" She blew loose hair from her face and slumped back into the chair. The whole thing was asinine. She'd even begged him to hire a translation firm and get the schematics translated from Chinese, but he was paranoid about information leaking to competitors. So she banged her head aginst the wall for four weeks, and the result was that they were nowhere.

But she was the superstar. This was the type of problem superstars were supposed to *solve*.

"Well, you *know* why he's on about the drug-testing," Julio said, working his chair's pneumatic lift in spurts, becoming shorter inch by hissing inch. "The thing *does* work, as far as that goes. It's just—only for him, is the problem." He twirled in a circle. "Well, and for me too."

Kelly looked up slowly. He'd lost her completely. "Back up like ten steps."

Julio spoke seriously, confessingly. "I...I'm addicted to overtime, Kelly." He buried his head in his hands. "I got my eyes on some new rims. They're shiny—*so* shiny."

"No, what did you mean, 'it worked for Jack'?"

"Oh, man, you know he tested positive, right?" Julio spun back towards his computer, clacking keys like a machine gun. An overflowing email inbox appeared on his screen. "Tested himself the first day. COCAINE AND PAINKILLERS."

"Oh my God," Kelly said, leaning towards the screen. "That

makes so much sense. That explains so much." And then she realized what it was that she was looking at. "You hacked Jack's email?"

Julio turned to her with a shrug. "Not so much 'hacked' as 'guessed a ridiculously obvious password,'" he said. "I mean, *jackis-great*? Seriously, it was my first try."

That night, she spent six hours drinking beer and reading through Jack's email.

She discovered all kinds of stuff in that ill-sorted inbox. He was "involved" with half-a-dozen airheaded bimbos from a handful of sleazy dating sites, but that was par for the course. He was continually buying Vicodin from Mexican pharmacies, which was like a puzzle piece fitting firmly into place. And he seemed to have written to everyone he could think of who might shed light on his "hypothetical" ProntoTester result: several people from China, plus a bunch of people at various university email addresses.

Running a search on the addresses popped up a series of file attachments sent from the Chinese client. She couldn't make much of the actual messages because they largely seemed to refer to phone conversations he'd had with Jack (and were written with a command of English best described as "good try"), but the attachments were English-language research papers, apparently from the American team that had originally developed the C-18 algorithm.

She clicked the first one open, eager for any clue as to what the device was actually meant to *do*. Unfortunately, the papers weren't much easier to read than the manufacturer's fractured English; all the scientific charts and technical jargon left her lost. She did, however, read with interest the list of initial results the C-18 had generated for the research scientists themselves: WATER, STROKE (like her own result), ASLEEP—and, disturbingly, HOMICIDE.

For an alcohol-addled second, she forgot that Julio's "Machine of Death" infomercial had been a joke. She sat very still in the darkness of her living room, letting the implications settle around her like ash from a distant volcano. STROKE sounded like it could be a way to die. HOMICIDE was *definitely* a way to die.

But then she remembered Jack saying that the lead scientist (who'd drawn WATER) had gone on to die in a plane crash, and with that realization came the reassuring reminder that the ProntoTester's slips were simply, maddeningly, just random words. Nothing in the research seemed to indicate anything different— although she had to admit that she didn't understand much of what it did say.

Even still, Jack had clearly gotten *really* agitated about COCAINE AND PAINKILLERS.

And Julio *did* put in a lot of OVERTIME.

And she had been on the crew team in college.

Creepy coincidence, right? It *had* to be. Just...just *logically*.

To set her third-beer, one-A.M. mind at ease, she scrolled through file after file of lab notes until she found a mention of the plane crash. It was a brief note on the very last page, describing how the Cessna returning the scientist from a meeting in New Mexico had suffered engine failure over the desert.

Following that, she read some sketchy notes about a sudden loss of investment capital, and the subsequent termination of the research. Nothing at all about WATER.

She closed the files and paced around the room awhile, telling her hands to stop shaking. She popped open another beer before returning to Jack's inbox, and was just starting to feel better when she read about the lawsuit.

Forget "building"—the class-action suit was *built*, over a hundred people claiming that the non-stick coating on the Fat-It-Out pans had flaked apart above 150°F. Which wouldn't have been so bad by itself, except that the coating was also, apparently, highly toxic.

She felt her gut constrict as she read a message from Jack to his attorney, idly suggesting that *she,* as producer on the campaign, should have conducted "scientific trials or something" on the pans to determine their safety. The logic being, if it were Kelly's fault that JBE sold shoddy pans, then—conveniently—it couldn't have been Jack's fault.

Luckily for Kelly, the attorney seemed to think that the excuse would stick about as well as the coating on the pans. Jack was pissed.

She sat frozen for several minutes, unable to stop her mind from reeling. He was even more of an ass than she'd thought. Who knew what else she'd still find, lurking in that digital Pandora's box of malice and despair? More plots to undermine her that she should know about?

She kept digging, and found a message from two weeks ago in which *marty@rockefeller-king.com* had written: "Dear Mr. Bogg, I would love to speak to you about the creative team involved in the Fat-It-Out campaign, which I understand has been very successful for your company."

Jack had responded, in his typical idiom, "thanks! home-grown here at JBE. that's why they pay me the big bux!! just kidding."

Rockefeller+King had come *looking* for her. Jack hadn't told her, and true to his word, hadn't even mentioned her name to them.

She ran out of beer.

When she woke up, her first thought was about her pounding headache. The second was about Rockefeller+King, a potential life-line out of JBE. And she had to get word to them before the news broke about the Fat-It-Out lawsuit.

She tried to remember if Marty was one of the tousle-haired hipsters who'd scoffed at her in her interview—but that was so long ago she couldn't remember any of their names.

She called R+K. A receptionist answered. Marty was out. Would she like to leave a message? Yes, that would be great. Her heartbeat drowned out the ringing.

A youthful recorded voice informed her that he was on vacation for the next two weeks.

Damn. *Damn.* The beep caught her off guard. She licked her lips and launched in. When she hung up she walked in a circle and repeated everything she'd said. Then she revised it. Mentally backspaced over it and made it better. For herself.

She almost called back, but what would she say? Who would she talk to? She couldn't think. Too much to consider. Too much to manage. The ProntoTester. Damn it!

She drove to JBE with so many things rattling in her mind that by the time she arrived, she'd already forgotten the trip itself. She parked by the planter without noticing that the lot was mostly empty. The college kids had been laid off, one by one, as Fat-It-Out sales had slowed.

No blast of cold air greeted her at the front door. A far-off buzz betrayed a fan oscillating in Jack's office. The folding tables where the college kids had worked were empty; the rows of computers were dark.

She found a cardboard box in the breakroom, and methodically emptied her cubicle. It took her awhile. She was surprised to find that it was difficult to do.

She gently pulled a thumbtack from the carpeted wall and took down her calendar. This Thursday had been circled in red for weeks now. "Ship to network affiliates," it said.

Her conscience screamed at itself to get to work, then screamed back to burn this place to the ground. She closed her eyes, and tipped the scales with a mental slide-show of Jack's constant *awfulness,* trying to recall every leering touch, every shady business deal, every pointless hour of weekend overtime selling junk to idiots. The lawsuit. Trying to sell her out. Her hatred frothed and roiled. Every muscle in her body wanted to strike something.

"Hey!" Julio's voice almost threw her into the cubicle wall. She snapped her head up and nearly knocked over a standing lamp. Julio ducked back around the corner, lifting his hands in mock surrender.

"Sorry! Didn't mean to scare you."

"It's...it's all right." Kelly plucked a soft black rubber band from her desk, the last refugee of her belongings. She pulled her hair back, tugging it tight, unable to do it any other way.

"Moving to a new office?" Julio asked slowly, looking around, reluctant to voice the other, more awful possibility.

"Something like that," she said. She struggled for something to say but couldn't think of anything appropriate, so she turned to the desk behind her, weighing the advantages of taking the stapler home with her.

He shrugged. "Look, I've been reading his email for years," he said. "I know it hits you hard at first. Getting the rock-hard truth of how crappy this business really is." He glanced down the hall, not meeting her eyes. "Then I look at my time card, you know?"

"I'm happy for you," she choked, and rushed past him, down the hall and into the office's one small bathroom, hearing his half-apology echo out behind her before she closed the door and lost it.

It came out all at once: the long hours, the awful products, the constant harassment, the lies and manipulations and good-ole-boy attitude that she thought she'd been too smart to fall for. Jack had played her, she knew—giving her rope to hang herself, then reaping the benefits when she hadn't, taking the praise and the profits for himself. She wanted to storm into his office and...and...and what? Staple him to death?

She knew she couldn't face him. He'd launch into some buttery, enthusiastic monologue and she'd walk out of there an hour later having signed a five-year contract or something. If nothing else, he was good at what he did. He was a salesman, through and through.

If she could just crawl out to her car and leave this place behind, she decided, that would be victory enough for her. Leave his Pronto-Tester campaign high and dry. Leave him wondering. It wasn't brave. It wasn't cathartic. But it would get her out of here.

She reached for the knob, but before she touched it, the door crashed open and Jack almost bowled her over.

"Oh! Door wasn't locked! Didn't know you were in here!" he squeaked through a faceful of red tissues. His bloodshot eyes widened around the clumped mass, a crimson ribbon suddenly tracing a line down his chin and spotting onto his rumpled shirt.

"Eep," she gulped, ducking out into the hallway as he slammed the door. She heard the water turn on; then he hacked, blew his nose, coughed, then blew his nose again.

She realized she was staring at the closed door. Then she realized that this was her chance to escape.

Julio was waiting by the front door with her box of stuff in hand. Without a word, he held the door open for her and they walked across the parking lot side by side.

"You sure everything's in here?" he said. "Sorry, I just grabbed it."

"Thanks," she said.

Once the box was in her car's back seat, they stood still for a few seconds, knowing this was goodbye.

"I know you need to do this," Julio said. She nodded, but realized there was more he wanted to say.

He seemed to chew on the words for a while, eventually coming up with "ProntoTester is still due on Thursday."

"So run your spot," she said. "The Machine of Death. Cut it down to twenty-eight thirty, put the blue-card on the back. Heck, record a narrator. Make it look good. Make it look serious."

He looked up at her. "You really want to put me out of a job?"

"It's nothing personal," she said. "Not with you, anyway. You'd find another gig."

Julio shook his head. "Look, I understand you're mad. I read those emails. I know how he screwed you over."

"You knew? Great," she spat. "Thanks for telling me about it." She opened the car door and slung herself into the driver's seat. The faster she could leave this place behind, the better.

"Wait," he said. "I'm sorry. It's not—I mean, look, a *lot* of vile stuff goes on. After awhile you just stop noticing. It was nothing personal."

She started the car. "So do it," she said. "Run the spot. Say it was my idea. I don't care, I'll take the blame if it means..." There it was. There was the thought she'd been dancing around. "If it means it brings him down. Brings the whole company down."

It was said. It was out loud. It was real.

Suddenly it even seemed *possible.*

"I got a good thing going here," Julio said lamely.

She felt something weird. She glanced up at the rearview mirror and realized that she was smiling. It would be malicious to air the joke spot. It would be *fun.*

"You know you want to," she said. "Just make sure you cash your check first."

It had been so long since she'd had this kind of time to herself that she felt paralyzed.

She paced her living room, waiting for anything. A text message from Julio. A call from Rockefeller+King. Any indication that she'd done the right thing, that her decision had made *any* sort of difference at all to anyone.

Jack called. She didn't answer. He called again. She sent him to voicemail.

She had trouble sleeping, so she bought more beer and spent the night sending press releases to every news outlet she could think of, promoting the Machine of Death—"new, from the makers of Fat-It-Out."

When she didn't come back to JBE the next day, or the day after that, or the day after that, Jack eventually stopped calling. She tried accessing Jack's email again, but the password didn't work anymore. Her heart seized in her chest at the thought that he had discovered her intrusion.

She called Rockefeller+King three times, but each time hung up before the receptionist answered.

The weekend passed in fitful bursts of anxiety, and she heard nothing from any quarter. She presumed that Julio had either improbably grown a pair and shipped the spot as-is to the affiliates, burning the place down, as it were; or that Jack and Julio had spent a frantic, sleepless 72 hours preparing an all-new, twenty-eight-minute infomercial.

Either way, she felt guilty.

She went to Wal-Mart to buy yogurt and saw Fat-It-Out still on the shelf, toxic coating and all, and it renewed her fervent hope that Jack would burn in hell.

Her phone woke her up, and she answered it groggily without looking at the caller ID.

"Kel, can you please come in today, please," Jack said. There was something different about his voice—he wasn't demanding, pleading, or shouting; he was just *asking politely*. It threw her off guard.

She thought about asking how things were, but didn't. She tried to think of an excuse, but couldn't. Then the call was over and her conscience had said "okay" before the rest of her had even woken up yet.

"Moron! You are a moron!" she shouted at herself in the shower.

"'Can you *please* come in today, *please*,' oh, you son of a bitch," she chanted mockingly to her shoes.

"Damn it damn it damn it," she told her mirror as she pulled out of her driveway.

She turned on the radio, and the voice that greeted her almost made her wipe out her mailbox. For a moment she thought she was still asleep, and dreaming.

"Get the *ultimate* peace of mind—from one *tiny* machine that fits *anywhere*," a jaunty voice told her. It was Mark, the announcer they used for every infomercial. He could sound excited about *anything*.

"Order now and *we'll* pay the first payment of $29.97. *You* only pay shipping!"

Then, a studio full of laughter. "We're going to get one for the studio right away," the morning-zoo deejay said. His dimwit partner chimed in with an old-man voice. "Maaake sure to get the ruuuush delivery," he squeaked. "I don't know how loooong I haaaave."

When she got to JBE, the parking lot was full. Inside the office, college kids chattered into headsets.

She tried to walk to Jack's office, but her feet led her the other way, towards Julio's edit bay. Towards a friendly face.

Julio wasn't in yet, but something weird was definitely going on. After a second of nervous fidgeting in the hall, she ducked into Julio's room, closed the door, and woke up his computer.

Blogs were buzzing. Clips from Julio's joke spot were Featured Videos on YouTube and littered the Reddit front page. The AP had cribbed from her press release, which meant that major outlets and networks would pick up the story in the coming week. Everyone had an opinion—was the Machine of Death just a hilariously bad commercial, or a subversive viral marketing gimmick?

Or maybe—just maybe—something more?

"A spot-on satire of infomercial idiocy, made better by the fact that there apparently *is* an actual product you can buy," wrote a columnist at AdWeek magazine.

"rofl i'd totally buy one," a YouTube commenter added.

And then this, from an article on Slashdot:

> According to patent records, this JBE product (from the folks who brought you Gyno-Paste!) is actually a repackaging of a genuine medical device developed by a UCLA team who never found an investor. It's one of those "who knows what REALLY happened" scenarios—the head of the project died in a plane crash (allegedly after a meeting with the Defense Department), just before he was set to unveil the device at MD&M East, the big medical-equipment trade show in NY. It doesn't sound too far-fetched to think that

> this is a case of sabotage that nobody cares enough to investigate
> (or is being prevented from investigating), because according to
> the NTSB report the cause of the plane crash was "water contami-
> nation of the fuel system"—something every pilot is trained to
> check for during preflight.

Kelly's eyes froze on the word *water*. She felt the blood drain from her face. She could still see that research paper hidden away in Jack's email, the one that contained the lead scientist's C-18 result.

WATER.

This was nuts. The ProntoTester—the Machine of Death—was a stupid cheap device that didn't work, just like Hair-B-Gon didn't *actually* remove hair, just like Gyno-Paste didn't *actually* rejuvenate genital skin, just like Fat-It-Out didn't *actually* replace eating healthy and exercising, no matter what Mark assured the consumer in calm, earnest tones.

They couldn't actually *believe* the spot. They must think the spoof infomercial was a joke, postmodern geek-humor. The radio dee-jays and the kids on YouTube wanted ProntoTesters to go with their Ninja Turtle toys and Super Mario-emblazoned hoodies.

But if Julio had somehow been *right*—if those little paper slips could say WATER and *somehow* mean water contamination in an airplane's fuel tank—then someday, maybe soon, those blogs would go into overtime, and Jack's Chinese warehouse would sell out in a day and a half, and the box would be reverse-engineered by everybody, everywhere, and there would be lawsuits and govern-ment inquiries and everything would go to hell and nobody would be laughing.

A machine to predict death. The most ludicrous idea in the world.

But people had bought Fat-It-Out.

She stood up and closed her eyes and could picture bright red boxes lined up at Wal-Mart, crammed into a million shopping carts. "Machine of Death," the boxes would say, "now with potassium." And everyone would buy ten of them.

She opened her eyes, and turned around, and Jack was standing in the doorway.

"Are you hot?" he asked. "You're sweating. Here, let me hit the A/C." He walked into the room and brushed past her on his way to the thermostat. She felt her skin prickle.

He turned back to her, standing closer than normal conversation required, searching her face for any indication—of what?

After a long moment of silence, he spoke in a dramatic whisper. "I was right to trust you," he said. "You've made me a lot of money. You've made *us* a lot of money."

She burst into tears, and of course, he swept her into his arms.

She hated it—she hated him touching her, making her flush, making her tense—but at the moment she really did need a hug.

Story by David Malki !
Illustration by Jess Fink

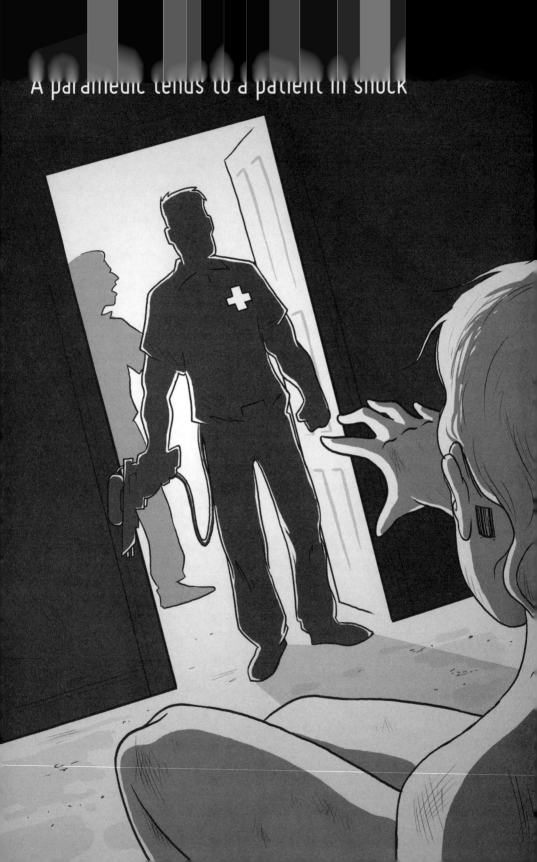

LOSS OF BLOOD

I'VE GOT THREE MONTHS LEFT TO LIVE, AND I'M IN AN APARTMENT BUILDING ON FIGUEROA, KICKING DOWN SOMEONE'S DOOR.

"Paramedics," I shout. "We're coming in."

No response. Sweat rolls down my back, and the hallway stinks like the inside of a fish. I'm a scheduled man, the living dead, but here I am: tagging and bagging in the slums of Angel City like it's any other Tuesday.

Titus, my partner, leans against the wall behind me and scrubs his fingernails through his goatee. "Hundred credits says it's a scag overdose."

I give the door another kick and plaster dust trickles down from the ceiling. All we know are the facts that came in with the ping: black female, early twenties, unconscious and unresponsive. No name or class registered, no datafeed on her at all.

"Come on, a hundred credits," Titus says. "Class J-8, overdose. I bet you." He puts out his hand for me to shake, but I'm in no mood for this shit. My head's full of sand and my eyes won't focus. I slap his hand away from me.

"What crawled up your ass today?" Titus asks.

I haven't told him I'm scheduled. I think about how it feels to be wrapped in my body, the speck of my soul floating in all this meat. Everything I know will end in eighty-six days.

I give the door another kick and the whole thing splinters off its hinges.

We head into the apartment, back toward the bedroom. The floor plan's typical thirties construction, slapped together in the years after the Separation, when the upper classes all evacuated to the Garden. On the kitchen table, empty beer bottles huddle together with cigarette butts in their bellies: the wreckage of others' lives.

Last night, Helene and I had cried into each other's cheeks, then made love with our teeth knocking together in the dark. This morning she'd hung on my shoulders as I stood at the door in my uniform. Her round stomach, our unborn baby, pressed against my belt.

"Let's stay home," she had said. "Otherwise I'll think myself crazy."

"Titus needs me. The grid's lit up with calls."

"I'll scream if you go."

I put my hand over her mouth and she bit my palm.

Sometimes at night when I touch my forehead to Helene's, I can feel her thoughts turning inside her. They brush my skin like whispers and I imagine the two of us melting together.

But now, in the scummy one-bedroom on Figueroa, I'm frozen in my own blood and the apartment's armchairs slump in the corners, nightmares on casters.

Titus and I find the victim sprawled on the bedroom floor with her skirt knotted around her thighs and her feet bare and one arm stretched out across the stained carpet. The window's open behind her. Whoever called this one in must have climbed out and run off. I kneel down over the woman and I feel her strong steady breath on my cheek.

"Can't smell scag on her," I say. "You lost the bet."

"Not like we shook on it," Titus says. I turn the victim's head and brush her hair back to expose the barcode tattooed behind her left ear. Titus leans in and scans her.

"Miss Pepper Dawson," he says, then flicks the LCD on his tagger. "No class listed, though. It's drawing a blank."

"Fake tags?" I ask.

"Looks like. Encryption's misaligned."

I can't find a thing wrong with her: no bleeding, no bruises, no breaks, and she's not liquored up or sludged-out on drugs. Looks peaceful, like she's sleeping. I touch the line of Pepper's jawbone and I think about Helene. I think about our baby. I think about freefall from thirty thousand feet, the cold gray ocean rushing up to meet us. My stomach flips.

Pepper coughs and her eyes snap open. Then she yelps and recoils from me, my white uniform and blue gloves, my belt blinking with electronics.

"No, I'm fine," she says. "Just fainted, is all." She scrambles backward across the floor.

Everyone tries to do this, soon as they recognize who we are and what we're there for. It never does any good. We already have our hands around Pepper's arms and I'm trying to shush her, keep her calm while Titus does the blood sample. He presses the tagger's piston to the inside of her left elbow.

"Don't," she says. "I can explain."

"Heard that one before," Titus says. His cheeks are pale gray, his face a chisel. He pulls the trigger and the piston snaps and the tagger's lights go blue as it uploads the blood sample. Pepper thrashes, pounds her heels on the floor. I fight to hold onto her.

It goes like this: We check the victim's tags and run their blood; if their fate matches their symptoms, we cart them off to St. Michael's Hospice so the priests can euthanize them. But if their symptoms don't match, we don't do a whole lot—just slap some bandages on, give them some pills, that sort of thing. Patch and release. We can't afford to waste too many Hospice supplies on the non-dying.

We shouldn't even call ourselves paramedics. We're bus-boys. We ship bodies and clean up messes, that's all.

"What'd you bet her blood's fake, too?" Titus asks me. He wipes sweat from his forehead.

Black-market blood isn't unheard of, especially in this part of Angel City. In the fate-scrubbing shops, they'll alter your tags, mod your fingerprints, scramble your retinas, and swap out your slumlander blood for some nice, clean Garden-class blood. None of it actually changes your fate, as far as anyone can tell. But slumlanders are desperate bastards.

"Please," Pepper says. Her voice has become small, like a child's, and I can feel her pulse jumping in her arm. I want to tell her that I know what it's like. I know how it feels to look at death, to have its teeth on your neck.

Two weeks ago, Helene and I had argued with our death counselor about our Notice of Scheduling.

We're too young, we had said. This whole thing had to be a mistake, a clerical fuck-up somewhere. The counselor had folded his arms. He looked like a typical Ministry fob: bad haircut, high collar, face pocked like sandstone. He took off his skullcap and tucked it under one arm and crossed himself. I wanted to spit in his face.

"What you're feeling is natural," he'd said. "Your denial, your questioning. All very natural at this stage."

He licked his thumb and flipped through our files. His voice oozed like motor oil. "You're R-4s. Plane crashes, both of you. The longer we wait to schedule you, the more likely your fate will be expressed in, ah, *unexpected* ways. Last time that happened, an airliner hit Denali Microchip. $8.2 billion in damage."

Damage, sure. But when I looked around at our apartment, a mildewing hole in a neighborhood full of garbage and rotting linoleum and blowflies and broken glass, all of us skeletons shuffling around down here in the ruins, I wondered what the difference was between this life and wreckage. When something blows up in the slumlands, you're just moving rubble around.

Helene picked at the frayed edges of her bathrobe and tried to smile at the counselor, but it wound up looking cruel. The lack of sleep had turned us into marionettes.

I asked about the appeals process, and the counselor shoved a thick stack of paperwork at me. FORM 1678-ATF: REQUEST FOR EXTENSION OF FATE APPLICATION. It was crowded with dotted lines and small type, layers of sub-forms, bricks of legal jargon. Helene's knee pressed against mine under the table.

The counselor explained that it'd take two weeks for the Ministry's office to process our request. At that point, our case would be passed to a higher court in the Orthodoxy, where a panel of clerks and lay-priests would review it. If all went well, the counselor said, they'd contact us for interviews, background checks, and then they'd give us an application.

"I thought this was the application," Helene said.

"No," the counselor said. "It's a request for the application."

I felt hollow. Outside the window, searchlights swept the edge of the slums and a siren wailed. The Ministry, hunting for someone. I imagined beastly slack-jawed men with guns patrolling the ruins.

The counselor mumbled on about the beauty of sacrifice. He talked about the strength of our nation, how scheduling deaths prevented wars, famines, natural disasters. It was all so much bullshit. But we crossed ourselves, mechanically, as he led us in prayer.

"Providence," the counselor recited, "help Kelvin and Helene to meet their fates with grace."

"I'm pregnant," Helene told the counselor. She'd twisted the sash of her robe around her hands and her breath came in quick, shallow gulps. "You'll kill our baby."

"I know," the counselor told us. "And for that we are truly sorry."

"Motherfucks," Helene said. She swept her arm across the table and our paperwork cascaded to the floor. The counselor didn't flinch.

"I prayed," she said, her voice shaking. "We made tithes. I anointed myself and used the rosaries. Our baby's not supposed to come with us."

Helene had always had a stubborn sense of justice. Once, when we'd been in high school, a rainstorm had soaked the ruins for days and scads of earthworms had crawled from the dirt to drown on the sidewalks. Helene spent hours on hands and knees, rescuing the squirming things. Her jeans soaked through. Her hair plastered to her forehead.

The counselor shook his head and tapped a few notes into his palmtop. "Mrs. Hayashi," he said, "I'm a little dismayed at your progress to date."

"Piss off," I told him.

The counselor raised his eyebrows. "The Ministry won't be pleased with my report," he said.

"The Ministry can go to hell," I said.

The counselor glared, set his skullcap atop his damp hair, and got up to leave. He pointed at the paperwork scattered across our kitchen floor.

"Don't even bother with the forms," he said.

—✠—

In the apartment on Figueroa, the sample's come back with a read-out of Pepper's fate.

"Whoa," Titus says. "'Loss of Blood.' Definite Class X. Ambiguity's off the charts. Possible group-risk, possibly violent circumstances."

Pepper flails her arms and arches her back and just about pulls my arms from their sockets. Titus plants his knee on Pepper's chest, pinning her to the floor. His tagger starts beeping and its lights flash red.

"Her blood's not in the system at all," Titus says.

"What's that mean?"

"An Untagged," he says.

Holy shit.

I look at Pepper. An Untagged. A traitor, a terrorist, a ticking time-bomb.

The Ministry makes a big show of hunting down the Untagged, weeding them out. They haven't been tested at birth like the rest of us, so they don't have classes, don't know how their lives end. I wonder what it's like for them, not knowing.

Well, I thought. She sure as hell knows now.

"What's the reward up to these days? Ten mil?" Titus asks. "Hold her for a second."

I take both Pepper's hands and she tries to twist them away from me. My gloves are wet now, sweat covering everything. Ten million credits for turning in an Untagged. Ten million credits for killing someone. Titus pulls the plastic zip-ties from his belt and wraps them around Pepper's wrists.

"No police," he says. "They'll just want a cut of the money. We take her straight to the Ministry."

"They'll kill me," Pepper says. "I haven't done anything and they'll kill me."

They'll kill me, too. On September thirteenth, the Ministry men will take Helene and I to the airfield in their black cars, they'll pack us onto a plane with the other R-4s, and then the pilot will fly us out over the Pacific and kill us all.

"Can't run from our fates, honey," Titus says.

Last week, I'd tried a new tactic. I'd slipped my credstick into the counselor's palm as he left our apartment, told him I'd do whatever it took to get this straightened out. I told him there should be enough in that account to keep him happy, keep him quiet. He'd just snarled at me and let the credstick clatter to the floor.

"Don't think for a second that you're the first person who tried to bribe me," he'd said. His eyes narrowed.

I shuddered. A few choice words from the counselor, and they'd toss Helene and I into a holding cell. The Ministry excelled at torture: Once they knew how someone died, they knew how to inflict pain without killing him. They knew exactly what he'd be most afraid of.

"We're in the business of reducing ambiguities," the counselor hissed at me. "What do you think would happen if everyone sidestepped their fate?"

After the counselor left, Helene and I had lain in our sour sheets, listening to the sirens and clatter of our neighborhood. Trash fires crackled somewhere down the block, aerosol cans exploding in the flames. Kids shouted and tossed rocks at each other.

Helene pressed her toes against my leg and stretched her arm across my chest. She slept on her side these days—on her back, she felt like the baby was crushing her, and on her front she felt like she'd been draped over a bowling ball.

"We're zombies," I told her. I cupped my palm over her cheek.

"We've always been zombies," she said. "Just now we've got a date for it."

For years, I'd had the same nightmares. Sterile white plasticine and a seatbelt tight across my lap. Cold wind rushing past me. In the dream, I would look out the window of the plane to see the ocean at a sickening tilt. When we hit the whitecaps there'd always be a shriek of metal and then static. Death sounded like static. And the dream kept going after that. A black canvas stretched across my mind. No eyes to see or skin to feel, and the static kept churning like an engine in the dark, on and on.

"Feel this," Helene said, and guided my hand across the taut skin of her stomach. "Feels like his spine."

We wanted what every parent in the slumlands wanted. We wanted our baby to come out healthy, and we wanted the priests to tag him and smile and tell us our son was a class A, a Cancer or a Heart Disease and not a squib like we are. We wanted the priests to hustle our precious baby away, evac him out of Angel City on black Ministry helicopters, take him across the fifty miles of desert to the Garden.

The archbishop and the rest of the orthodoxy lived in the Garden. So did the financial district, the nation's politico-corporate headquarters. Towers of glass and steel, beautiful people in clean houses. Only the upper-classes could live there: people with slow deaths, or predictable ones, or fates with low violence ratings. Low-classes weren't allowed to come close. Too much risk to the government, to the economy.

All of us gunshot wounds, shrapnel deaths, stabbings, poisonings, industrial accidents, we'd been pinned down here in the slums with the factories and pollutants. Better for society that way.

Helene and I stared at the ceiling. The air smelled thick with gypsum dust.

"What if we'd never been tested?" I asked her.

She laughed. "We'd live in the desert with the Untagged. Starve to death out there."

Helene and I both lay silent for a while, breathing across each others' lips, thinking about the sun-blasted wastes, the yucca and brush in the open countryside. If we were Untagged, I thought, we'd disappear into the arroyos and the Ministry would never find us.

I tried to sleep, but I'd barely shut my eyes before sunlight trickled in through the holes in our curtains.

We strap Pepper onto the gurney and carry her outside.

The heat's like an oven. In front of the apartment complex, a statue of an angel glowers, its wings casting scythes of shadow. The engraving on the statue's pedestal reads: "Your sacrifice benefits humanity," but someone's crossed out "benefits," and spraypainted "derails" in its place.

All around us, the slumlands spread out in a geometric sludge and aerials scrape the afternoon shit from the sky. Titus pops open the back of the ambulance.

"Ten million credits, Kelvin," he says, and he shows me teeth. He opens the driver's side door and climbs inside. "Load her in and let's go."

I look down at Pepper. She quivers, jerking against the leather straps, her skin goosebumped.

Our baby won't ever have a name. They'll fly Helene and I out over the ocean and put the plane into a spiral. The scream of the engines will swallow us and our baby will never have a name.

Before I can think about what I'm doing, my hands move over Pepper's restraints, unfastening them. She sits up and blinks.

"Me and my wife," I tell her. "We're scheduled. Our baby." I'm shaking. "You must know people. Someplace we can hide."

Pepper nods and cranes her neck to look back at Titus. He's fiddling with the radio in the cab, and isn't paying attention to us. My breath rasps in my mouth, my tongue feels suddenly heavy.

"There are safehouses," Pepper says. Her wrists and ankles are still zip-tied together, and she holds them up. "We have a whole network of them. Cut me loose."

"We'll need a blood swap," I tell her. "We need someone to lead us into the desert."

"We will," she says.

I can already picture the lone highway stretching out through the cholla. Helene and I will raise our baby in the cacti, away from the smog, away from the Ministry. I pull out my knife and I slice through Pepper's zip-ties. She rubs her wrists and scrambles to her feet.

Then she rears back and spits in my face. "Fucking pig," she says.

She shoves past me and ducks into an alley filled with garbage bags and oil slicks. She sprints out into the maze of the sprawl.

Titus slams the door of the ambulance. "The hell's wrong with you?" he asks.

I open my mouth, but no sound comes out.

Story by Jeff Stautz
Illustration by Kris Straub

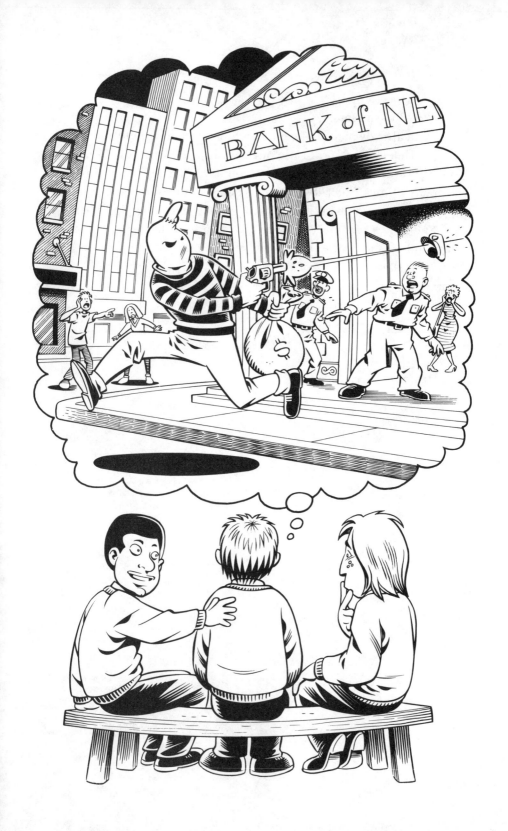

PRISON KNIFE FIGHT

VERY EXPENSIVE NANNY. VERY EXPENSIVE TUTOR. Montessori nursery school priced competitively with Yale. Phonics, piano lessons from age four, one edifying vacation in a major European city per year, a diet of both organic *and* local produce cooked to order from a menu drawn up by a personal nutrition coach, and a white-noise machine. A portfolio of coloring-book samples. What was missing? Oh, yes...

Mr. Slocombe peered over the thick sheaf of paperwork. "We'll have to see his medical records, of course."

"His medical records?" said Mrs. Weathington-Beech, a little too innocently.

"That's confidential information," said Mr. Weathington-Beech, with studied huffiness.

"Nonetheless," sighed Mr. Slocombe, "Saint Maxwell's requires it, as you should be aware from our brochures, website, and application forms. We do ask that you come prepared," he added coldly, hoping that a touch of Stern Headmaster would snap them to attention.

It didn't. "I don't see why you'd need that kind of thing," Mrs. Weathington-Beech lilted. "I mean, really, why would you, unless you're planning to discriminate against—"

"Against a five-year-old," Mr. Weathington-Beech hrrumphed. "It's just kindergarten," he added.

"Saint Maxwell's, sir, is hardly 'just' a kindergarten. That's why you're trying to convince us to admit little Cotton, correct? His medical records, please."

After a long and wounded pause, Mr. Weathington-Beech produced another set of papers from his briefcase. Mr. Slocombe skimmed them. There was only one line that mattered. Not everyone had their children scanned, of course, but the parents who applied to Saint Maxwell's wanted their offspring to win the great footrace of life, and they missed no opportunity to equip the towheaded sprites with life's metaphorical jet packs and rocket shoes. A death machine readout cost money, and that meant it must be an advantage. Q.E.D.

Ah, there it was...

Mr. Slocombe pulled out the familiar certificate, signed by a licensed technician and stamped with a golden death's head seal. His gaze dropped automatically to the six neatly typed words at the bottom. And stayed there. For a good minute.

"Cotton Remington Weathington-Beech," he said at last. "Prison knife fight."

Mr. Weathington-Beech turned very red. Mrs. Weathington-Beech turned very white. Both Weathington-Beeches squirmed.

Mr. Slocombe gazed evenly at them from across his polished mahogany desk. "Prison knife fight?"

There was another, longer silence. Finally, Mrs. Weathington-Beech said, "Well, you know, it might be the good kind of prison."

"*The good kind of prison?*"

Mr. Weathington-Beech leapt in gallantly. "Minimum-security."

"Exactly." Mrs. Weathington-Beech nodded energetically. "For tax evasion or something. Tax evasion's not so bad."

"I think," said Mr. Slocombe, the temperature of his voice dropping several degrees, "that the type of prison to which, say, a corporate CFO is sent for tax evasion is very unlikely to play host to lots of knife fights."

"It *could*," said Mrs. Weathington-Beech, sounding like a child who's had her favorite binky taken away and stomped on.

"Look," said Mr. Weathington-Beech, "surely you've gotten this before."

"No. No, we haven't." At the sight of the Weathington-Beeches' fallen faces, Mr. Slocombe relented. "We get some suicides."

"There!" Mr. Weathington-Beech jabbed a manicured finger across the desk. "If you ask me, knife fight shows a lot more character than suicide. Suicide…suicide's cowardly." Mrs. Weathington-Beech nodded.

"I've got a nephew scheduled for suicide," snapped Mr. Slocombe. "Fine boy. A little tense."

In fact, Saint Maxwell's received, and often accepted, applications from preschoolers slated to die criminal deaths. It was just a question of, well, the quality of the crime. You let in the cocaine overdoses; you kept out the crack overdoses. But this was so obvious it was hardly worth mentioning.

"I don't see why you people even care," Mr. Weathington-Beech was saying. "It's not like he's going to die in a prison knife fight while he's at kindergarten."

"Prep school, maybe," said Mrs. Weathington-Beech vaguely. She seemed to have abandoned all hope of Saint Maxwell's and drifted into a soft pink private world of her own, a world blissfully devoid of knives, fights, or prisons to contain them.

"It's a matter of reputation," said Mr. Slocombe, gathering up Cotton's paperwork. "In seventy-eight years, Saint Maxwell's has never had an alumnus die in a prison knife fight."

"But you're our last hope!" cried Mr. Weathington-Beech, his final layer of expensive psychic armor falling to reveal naked, lower-class desperation. "We've tried every decent school in the county!"

"So we're your last choice, are we?"

"You know how it works! If Cotton goes to a sub-par kindergarten, he'll go to a sub-par elementary school. If he goes to a sub-par elementary school, he'll have no choice but a sub-par high school. And if he goes to a sub-par high school..." Mr. Weathington-Beech shuddered.

"Brown," said Mr. Slocombe sympathetically.

"There's always public school," said Mrs. Weathington-Beech, gazing off into the middle distance. This was such a tasteless joke that the men had no choice but to ignore it.

"We've done everything right," moaned Mr. Weathington-Beech. "Sarah stepped down at Berkshire Hathaway to do full-time attachment parenting. I switched consulting firms so we could move to a town with a lower level of mercury in the water. We've already got breeders working on the puppy for Cotton's seventh birthday and the pony for his tenth. Everything. Everything right." He looked up at Mr. Slocombe with haunted eyes.

Mr. Slocombe felt too tired to be diplomatic any longer. "Then how do you explain the shiv in his gut?"

"Well, maybe the machine is wr—" To Mr. Weathington-Beech's

credit, he stopped himself. The death machine was never wrong.
They'd done tests.

"We shouldn't have named him Cotton," sighed Mrs.
Weathington-Beech to no one in particular.

"I'm sorry," said Mr. Slocombe, and he really was. "But this is why
we check, you know."

"Have a heart," said Mr. Weathington-Beech, defeated. "Sarah
and I both got 'car accident.' That could be tomorrow."

Mr. Slocombe gave him a long, sad look. Deep in his plushly-lined
heart, he knew he was liable to succumb to cheap sentimentality.

Mrs. Weathington-Beech suddenly fluttered back to Planet Earth.
"Maybe a donation to the school would help?"

Well. Perhaps not *too* cheap.

Cotton Remington Weathington-Beech did acceptably at Saint
Maxwell's. He excelled at music and fingerpainting, and his best
friends were Akiva Smythe-Button (prostate cancer), McGregor
Rigsdale (chronic lower respiratory disease), and Resolved
Stutzman (botched coronary bypass operation). The four of them
went on together to the Tinker Hill School, and then—minus
McGregor, whose parents moved to Hawaii for his asthma—to
William H. Howland Prep.

Cotton officially learned about the prison knife fight at age
twelve, when he came across a copy of his own school records in his
father's study, but he'd more or less always known. He'd noticed the
special disapproving, pitying, and/or terrified gazes he got from
teachers when he acted up in class. He'd been pulled aside on the
playground by any number of authority figures and warned about
roughhousing, even when he was just standing around with a kick-
ball. And his parents insisted on watching *The Shawshank Redemption*
whenever it was on TV.

His friends knew theirs, too, of course. Akiva's parents had sat
down with him over freshly-baked chocolate cake, told him very

solemnly while patting his hand, then stiffly hugged him, exactly as the family therapist had suggested. The whole performance had scarred Akiva for life, ensuring years of future business for the therapist—and—Akiva often thought darkly, if illogically—probably causing his prostate to act up. Resolved had heard it from his big sister, who, incidentally, was going to drown, one of those inconveniently vague forecasts that were impossible to prepare for. They hadn't believed Cotton until he'd shown them the certificate, but from that point on they'd had to acknowledge that he was their king.

"How do you think it'll happen?" Resolved whispered one day during free period. "You don't even know how to use a knife, do you?"

"Yeah, well, that's why he dies, right?" said Akiva.

Cotton shrugged. They'd had this discussion before. "They say you shouldn't try to guess. There's basically no way to know until the big day."

Resolved pressed on. "Yeah, but why're you in prison in the first place? Are you going to kill someone? Rob a bank?" A few students at the neighboring tables glanced disapprovingly at them. Raised voices were not encouraged during free period, or in general.

"Maybe I don't do anything," whispered Cotton, warming to the subject despite himself. "Maybe I'm wrongly convicted of a crime I didn't commit." This scenario was one of several current personal favorites, although there were times when the idea of a brutal crime spree held more satisfaction for a growing boy.

"Maybe you're not a prisoner," said Akiva. "Maybe you're a guard who tries to break up the fight. Or one of those guys, you know, who goes in to teach the prisoners how to weave baskets or something."

"Or a priest," suggested Resolved.

"Maybe," said Cotton. They were sixteen, and supposedly their futures still lay shrouded in glowing promise, but Cotton was pretty sure he could make out the dim but unmistakable outline of an upper-echelon position at one of the major accounting firms. He was doing very well in pre-calc and statistics that year. Whether he liked it or not, some things didn't need to be printed out on a magic machine to be inevitable.

"Mine's not so bad, you know," said Resolved, hoping against hope to talk about his own death for once. "Killed on the operating table. I'll just go in my sleep."

"If you think about it, though," said Akiva slowly, "that one's really the worst. I mean, you already know it's going to happen."

"So?"

"So that means one of these days, you're going to go in for a coronary bypass, and you'll have to let them put you under and everything...*knowing that you'll never come out.*"

Resolved stared, his lips parting silently. He was not an imaginative boy, and he'd never thought too vividly about the final reward that fate and the death machine had reserved for him. Now unpleasantly precise details were suggesting themselves. From the back of his throat emerged a faint whimper.

"Probably still beats prostate cancer," said Cotton brightly, which didn't make anyone feel better.

"I wish we all had prison knife fight," said Resolved. It was a thought they'd all shared many times over the past few years, but this was the first time one of them had come out and said it.

"It'll really hurt, though," said Cotton, in a last-ditch effort to patch things up. "I mean, even before the stab that kills me, I bet I'll get cut pretty badly."

"Yeah," said Akiva, "but at least we'd all be headed for the same place. We've been together since kindergarten, and now you're on your way to prison."

"We'd all go out together," said Resolved dreamily, the rusty gears within his skull grinding slowly to life.

Cotton looked at him. "Stabbing each other?"

"Yeah."

"Yeah," sighed Akiva.

The bell rang. They didn't move. One of the monitors gave them a meaningful look, which they ignored.

"I dunno," said Cotton. "I mean, my parents are probably dying in a car crash together, and they don't seem too happy about it."

Akiva brightened. "Hey, maybe that's what you go to prison for!"

"Huh?"

"Involuntary manslaughter." Unlike Resolved, Akiva had a healthy and active imagination. He'd won creative-writing prizes. "You're drunk behind the wheel, and your parents are in the back seat, and then you drive the car off a bridge and kill them."

Cotton rolled his eyes. "Yeah, and maybe Resolved's sister's riding shotgun and that's how she gets it, too."

"It could happen!"

"What's that about my sister?" said Resolved, the eternal bronze medallist of the trio.

"That's not going to happen," said Cotton, gathering his books. A mood had been shattered.

"How do you…" Akiva frowned. "Don't tell me your parents already thought of it."

Cotton slung his backpack over his shoulder. "They won't get in the car if I'm driving."

College admissions rolled around, and Cotton started getting a lot of thin envelopes and not many fat envelopes. His parents glowered at the world. "It's his medical records," said Mr. Weathington-Beech. "The school passes them on."

"Can we discuss this later?" snipped Mrs. Weathington-Beech. "We just had a nice dinner."

"You don't have to talk in code, you know," said Cotton. "I know I'm dying in a prison knife fight."

Both parents shot him poisonous looks. They knew he knew, and he knew they knew he knew. They just would have been happier if he'd done the polite thing and pretended he had no idea what they were talking about. Usually he did. Cotton was vaguely uncomfortable about discussing the death machine with his parents; it was almost as icky as the sex talk, and probably for similar reasons.

"It's a self-fulfilling prophecy, is what it is," muttered Mr. Weathington-Beech.

"Jim…" said Mrs. Weathington-Beech in warning tones. She turned away and started fiercely rearranging the magazines on the coffee table.

Mr. Weathington-Beech slapped down his newspaper. "Well, it's true. They ostracize a boy like that, how do they expect him to end up?"

Cotton gave up on his Latin homework. "Dad, I've gotten three acceptances so far, plus my safety school. It's not like I'm gonna land in the gutter. I'm just not going to Yale."

Mrs. Weathington-Beech stifled a sob.

"We have not," growled Mr. Weathington-Beech, "heard back from Yale."

"Anyway, you don't even know that's what's going on. Maybe my application just wasn't that great. I don't have a lot of extracurriculars."

"I know what's going on," said Mr. Weathington-Beech.

Cotton had to admit he had a point. Even Resolved had managed Cornell.

"So what?" he said. "So I go to one of those little liberal-arts schools. They're still good schools. Probably a lot more fun than the Ivy League anyway. Akiva's brother says Harvard sucks, everybody's stressed out all the time and the freshman classes are all taught by TAs in big—"

"The point," said Mr. Weathington-Beech, "is that we sent you to Saint Maxwell's to get you into Tinker Hill. We sent you to Tinker Hill to get you into Howland. And we sent you to Howland to get you into the Big Three, and now the whole damn thing with the—the—"

"The PKF," suggested Cotton, who thought it had earned an acronym.

"...this *thing* is screwing up the whole system again." Mr. Weathington-Beech looked suddenly very sad and tired. "We had everything planned out for you, son. We've spent a lot of time and a lot of money. It just doesn't seem fair."

"Aw, geez. Dad..."

Mrs. Weathington-Beech spun around, moisture sparkling in the corners of her eyes.

"Cotton," she said, "when we're killed, promise you won't seek revenge on the driver."

"Oh, god." Cotton slammed his Latin book shut. "I'm going out."

Cotton's car was new and expensive. It was fast but there was nowhere to take it, so he drove slowly. Besides, his parents were big on safe driving. He drove out the gates of his neighborhood and past the gates of countless other neighborhoods, all tidy and mani-cured, all dead at night except for the guards reading magazines in their glowing guardhouses. The scenery repeated itself, like a Flintstones cartoon, for miles. The spring air was moist and sugary.

Maybe there was a party somewhere. Maybe there was a football game. Maybe there were guys drinking down at Akiva's parents' boat shed. It all melted into the same flat, dark quiet.

After a while, Cotton pulled over and sat on the hood of his car. It was as good a place to stop as any. A dozen yards away, a guard leaned out of a gatehouse window to look him up and down. Cotton felt like a criminal. It wasn't so bad.

He leaned back and looked up at the stars. He really hoped Yale was going to say no. Some of those little schools looked really good, and if he didn't go there, he'd do something else. Something bet-ter, maybe. Poor Akiva was going to Harvard like his brother, and Resolved...well, to be fair, Resolved probably would've been screwed anywhere. But Cotton was going to go where he wanted and do what he liked. That was the funny thing about the death machine. When it cut your future down to that one steel inevitability, it seemed to open up more possibilities than you ever could have imagined.

Cotton smiled shyly at the stars. He was looking forward to prison. It was going to be fun to be free.

Story by Shaenon K. Garrity
Illustration by Roger Langridge

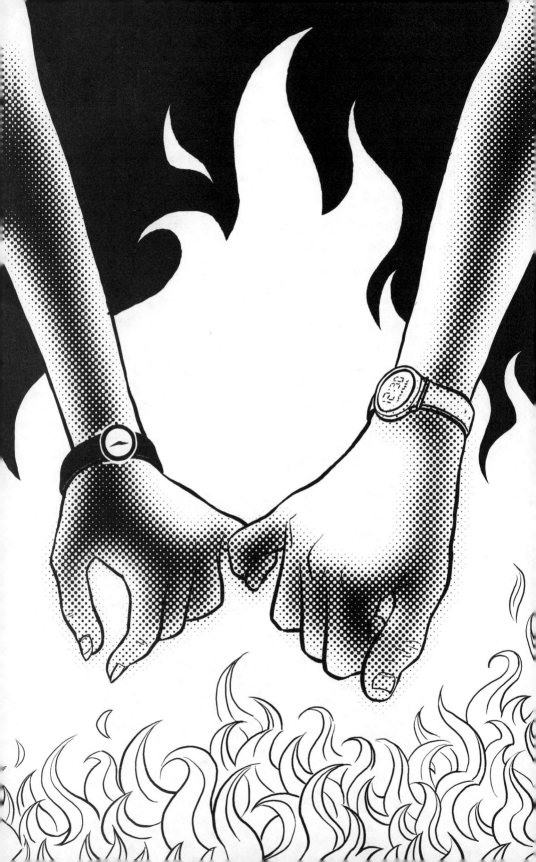

WHILE TRYING TO SAVE ANOTHER

101

IT WAS ONE OF THOSE DAYS AGAIN. The eight of them travelled by
bus, car, or walked to the church. They left coats on hooks and
made their way to the basement where coffee, tea, cookies, and
Reverend Shamus Brooker waited for them. The underweight
clergyman shook Raymond and Krishna's hands. He hugged Julie.
Annabel got a kiss on both cheeks, Hanna a kiss on one cheek.
Timothy, Nqobile and Benito were late so they got a nod. The
Reverend frowned upon lateness.

"There'll be one more today," he warned them. "I told her to
come at half past so we'd be able to talk."

"Couldn't she join another group?" Timothy objected. It had
taken him over a year to get comfortable with the people in the
room.

"She's Iranian."

"She'll be more than welcome," Krishna said firmly. Of course he
did. In a few years he'd be killed by a group of skinheads with knives
and baseball bats. Racism was a soft spot to say the least. He gave
Timothy a challenging glare.

"I was just asking." Timothy gulped down his coffee and poured
a refill.

"Don't be confrontational," the Reverend interrupted. "Discomfort any of us feel with the introduction of a new member should be discussed."

"I don't have a problem," Timothy replied.

"I do," said Julie.

Krishna lashed out at her, assuming her reason was race. She shouted back. Raymond, who had a crush on Julie, joined in. Soon there was lots of yelling and Timothy's mind wandered. He couldn't be arsed to join in. He was staring at the doorway thinking about what movie he'd see on the weekend when she arrived. She was head to toe in Goth getup: leather boots with thick soles, a black velvet corset, silver chains, and bracelets dripping off her.

Timothy smiled. "Here comes an awkward silence."

His prediction turned out to be as accurate as any of the Death Machine's. Ten seconds later the others realized they were being watched.

"Isma…" Reverend Shamus Brooker's lips kept moving but no more words came out.

Benito, class clown, came to the rescue. "Whatever your old ED group used to do, forget it. We communicate here by insulting each other."

"OK. You're ugly and you smell bad."

Everyone laughed. Some of them were faking. Timothy wasn't.

Isma took some tea and cookies and then the real session began.

"My name is Reverend Shamus Brooker and I have two hundred and seventy days left. I'm going to be hit by a car."

"I am Annabel, cancer, four hundred and ten days."

"Nqobile. I'm the record holder. Some cunt's going to shoot me in the head in forty nine days."

Timothy got up. "One hundred and one here; just like the Dalmatians. I'm going to die in a fire while trying to save another."

"What?" Isma exclaimed.

"What's wrong?" asked the Reverend.

She spoke slowly; she was visibly trembling. "I'm going to die in one hundred and one days as well. In a fire."

100

Later Timothy and Isma sat outside on a bench. Isma's hands clenched and unclenched, clenched and unclenched.

"Meeting you, it makes me feel like a puppet on strings."

"It suddenly feels more real, doesn't it?"

She looked up at the crucifix above the doorway. "He has a sense of humor doesn't he?"

"When did you find out you were an ED?" Timothy popped a cookie (stolen booty) into his mouth.

"Six years ago after hearing a war hero talk on television. He said to the press that he wasn't courageous; he admitted he had used a Death Machine and he knew he was going to freeze to death on a mountain. As long as he was posted in a desert, jungle, or urban warzone he felt no fear. When watching that broadcast, I realized for the first time that a forecast could be a gift. I arranged a session. I thought that if I knew how I was going to die I could stop being afraid of everything. I didn't expect to find out *when*."

"ED's a bitch isn't it?"

For years many had been sure the only reason no one had changed their fate was Death Machine forecasts were too vague. They were proved wrong when the first Exact Date spat out. For the first time, a man knew not only how he would die, but knew when it would happen. The first ED knew he would die in a bus crash on the 6th of March 2032. He prepared for that day. No matter what happened he would go nowhere near a bus on the 6th. He booked himself on a yacht cruise; no way could a bus crash happen while at sea. A week before his predicted death he was hit by a car and put into a coma. On the 6th the hospital was forced to transfer him to a private clinic. En route, a bus slammed into the side of the ambulance.

"How about you, how did you find out?"

"British Airways has all prospective pilots do a compulsory forecast just in case the Death Machine spits out 'plane crash.' They told me I couldn't get the job because I was an ED and I had seven hundred and eight days left. I wish they hadn't told me. Ignorance was bliss." Timothy reached into his pocket and retrieved another cookie. "You want one?"

"No thanks. I'm on a diet."

Timothy's right eyebrow rose.

"I know. I'll be dead in a hundred and one days. Why the fuck am I dieting?"

Timothy glanced at his watch. "A hundred days now."

"I just thought of something. You're not going to die in a plane crash. Why didn't you get the British Airways job?"

"No one would insure me because I only had two years of life left."

"Isn't that illegal?"

"Of course it is; prejudice is just a reality."

Isma stuck her hand into Timothy's jacket pocket, an action that struck him as surprisingly intimate. She fished out a cookie and took a tiny nibble, a bird bite. "I was part of an Arab student association in Uni," she said. "Every week we met and complained about the way we were discriminated against and treated like we weren't real British citizens. That made it hurt all the more when they found out I was an ED and started treating me differently. Not that they called me names or anything like that. They just started tip-toeing around me."

No one knew why exactly, but for every thousand people who used a Death Machine, it only spat out an Exact Date for two or three.

"I hate the bloody pity," Timothy said.

"I had an abortion last year," Isma said suddenly. "I wouldn't have lived to see my child's first birthday."

"I...I don't know what to say."

"I wanted to mention it in there but the reverend...I wanted him to like me."

"Shamus isn't a cliché. He doesn't judge."

"I'm glad I didn't. It feels easier to just tell you. It's weird, but I feel connected to you."

Timothy smiled humorlessly, "Linked by fate and all that."

"How can you be cynical about fate, knowing what you do? Isn't that proof enough?"

"I don't believe in fate, God or anything. It's all random. Sure, the Death Machine can punch a hole through time and can predict the result of the randomness. That doesn't make it any less random."

"So there's no God, no life after death?"

"Zip."

"How can you stand living like that?"

"Same as you, one day at a time. One hundred now, ninety-nine tomorrow."

"Look at me," Isma said.

He turned and their faces were only a few inches apart. "Do you think we'll be together?"

He shrugged.

"Don't do that." She sounded angry. "I can tell your 'I don't care' stuff is an act."

He almost lashed out with a "fuck you" but it was harder to do so while staring into her eyes. It was too dark to see their colour. "I don't want to die alone."

"Me neither."

97

"Do you ever think we're trying to force something into existence," Timothy said to her three days later. They were on the grass at Piccadilly Gardens. It was loud so they were speaking with raised voices.

"What do you mean?"

"The only reason we've seen each other the last two days is because there's a chance we could die together. I kind of feel like we're trying to create a meaningful relationship because…well, the alternative is dying alone. I look back at my life and it's been forgettable. Instead of a pilot, I'm someone who does data entry. I go to work at a place where my contribution makes no difference. I've left no legacy or accomplishments. I doubt anyone will miss me. Meeting you… there's so much pressure to make this work. It's like a last chance to have some semblance of—it's ridiculous and cheesy to say it-true love. If fate had somehow guided us to that, it would somehow validate everything else."

Isma was quiet at first. "You're looking for true love? I just thought we were going to be really good friends?"

"Oh." Timothy's cheeks burnt. He wanted to crawl into a hole.

Isma leant forward and captured his lips with hers.

90

Isma hated her body. She thought her bones were big and awkward and her face was boring. Timothy told her she was beautiful over and over again. Eventually he stopped trying. She insisted they make love in the dark. His fingers traced her figure, reading her contours like Braille. On the inside of wrists that were usually concealed beneath bracelets, he felt the raised ridges of twin scars.

"Yeah," she said, offhandedly. "I tried to kill myself."

"When?"

"Four months ago. Paul had just left me. Nothing was the same between us after my abortion. The situation was so fucked up. I wanted to keep the baby but I'd die right after she was born so what did my opinion matter. Even so, I still could never forgive him for making me…"

Timothy kissed Isma gently and she recoiled. "Not right now."

"I'm sorry."

Isma rose and went to the bathroom.

Waiting for her to come out was torture. He was reminded that he knew nothing about her. She might step out of the bathroom and tell him to leave, or she might come out bawling and throw herself in his arms.

When she did come out she apologized. "Sorry. This is the first time I've talked about Paul leaving. We were together for three years. We were so happy. He never knew I was an ED until near the end."

Three years. Timothy felt suddenly inadequate.

"My father found me before it was too late..." Isma was saying. She was looking down at the scars on her wrists. "I had passed out."

"Do you wish you were still with Paul?" Timothy asked. He wished he could take back the words immediately. How selfish of him to say that when she was telling him something so personal.

"I don't."

"We only have ninety days, no time to lie to each other."

"All right then, I wish I were still with Paul." Isma came back to the bed. The springs creaked as she sat. "Don't you wish I were someone else?"

"No. There is no one else. There never has been." In a Harlequin bodice-ripper, that line might have been romantic, but in this room, in this place, it was an admission of how pathetic a person he was.

She began to speak but Timothy interrupted. "No lies, no matter how much you think it might be what I want to hear."

"OK." She took hold of his hand and pressed it against her cheek, right where he had kissed, when she flinched. "I remember when I had the shaving razor against my wrist, I thought I was cheating the Death Machine by choosing what day I would die—but I didn't really have a choice. Right now though, this, between you and me, it is my choice. I know we're both going to die on the same day, but it could be in different fires on different sides of town. I am choosing you to be by my side at the end. I choose you. Being able to have some control, however small, is precious to me. Maybe I can't be that 'true love' that would make it all worth it, but…"

"Isma," Timothy said. His palm had descended from her cheek, down the curve of her neck and to her right shoulder. "It's enough."

53

Nqobile spent her last night in the house she grew up in. It was a large three-bedroom in Didsbury. The carpets, chandeliers, paintings, and curios were all African. Her parents were immigrants who had fled South Africa and always dreamt of going back. Every object was an altar to their longing.

Everyone came. Reverend Shamus Brooker brought a tiny bag with white powder in it. Krishna brought a plate of roast pork, wrapped up tight with cling film. Julie brought her guitar. Annabel brought a cell phone. Hanna brought nothing. Benito brought a photo album. Timothy brought a piece of paper he'd paid 700 pounds for. Isma brought a bag full of clothes.

"So the star-crossed lovers have seen fit to make an appearance," said Raymond, who had brought a set of car keys. He was joking but there was an aggressive undercurrent to his intonation.

"Star-crossed?" Isma asked.

"Well, he's going to die trying to save you."

"What?"

"Not necessarily," said Timothy. "We might both die trying to save someone else. I like to think we'll succeed. Then our deaths will be more worth it."

"You considered this?" Isma looked betrayed.

"Of course I thought it might be an option. Didn't you?"

"If it is me, don't try. Just leave me."

"The Death Machine is always right."

"So far, maybe, or maybe it's been wrong and nobody knows."

"You know that's not true."

"Please, if it's me, promise you'll leave me."

Nqobile made her entrance. She looked even more beautiful than usual. Her hair was braided into long cascades falling in a torrent halfway down her back, and the patterned kikoi she wore was a mesmerizing corolla. Her smile was radiant, akin to a child's. "What's all this fuss about?"

Raymond sneered. "Isma just realized she could be the one Timothy dies trying to save. I never thought she was dumb until now."

"Enough of that," ordered Nqobile. "Today, it's all about me. If you want to act jealous and petulant, Raymond, be jealous of me. If you want to argue, argue over who will get the privilege of sitting next to me. And tonight you two are not lovers. I am the only one you adore. If I decide to have my way with Timothy in the attic, there'll be no complaints, okay." Nqobile smiled devilishly and walked into the living room where the others were finishing up the preparations.

"It's exactly how I dreamed it would be. No, scratch that, it is better."

They had extrapolated the decorations for the living room from the first painting Nqobile had sold. In the painting, the Queen of Spiders presided over an intricate multicolored skein of webs. They had used dyed mosquito netting, gauze, and silk stretches of fabric to recreate the queen's lair.

"I love you all," said Nqobile and the festivities began.

As always, the Reverend led the way. Shamus tipped some cocaine onto an ash tray and shaped it into a line with his thumb. "I don't know how to do this properly." His hands were trembling.

"Are you sure about this?" Nqobile asked.

"For you, my queen," He knelt and took a deep snort.

Julie went next. She began to strum chords on her guitar. "I'm sorry I'm out of practice but…"

"No excuses," said Nqobile.

After one false start, Julie began to sing and her untrained grav-elly voice spilt over them all. Five men and five women, Timothy noticed their symmetry for the first time. It made him wonder about fate. Was this all preordained? Julie was a stockbroker through and through, yet the song she was singing gave him chills. And its lyr-ics suited the night perfectly. Why had the only song Julie wrote as a naïve sophomore with rock-star dreams been about farewells? Coincidence? Fate? Or maybe she had cheated? Maybe this was actu-ally a song she had just written?

By the end of the song, Nqobile was crying. "I meant to store them all up for one big cry at the end of the night. Damn it." She pointed at Krishna. "Get on with it."

"For you my queen," he said and he stabbed a fork into a hunk of roast pork. He took a large bite and chewed. He winced as he ate.

"Allah be praised," said Nqobile, sniffling.

Annabel dialed her mother's number and waited. "Answering machine. I'll try again later."

Timothy stepped forward and knelt dramatically before Nqobile. He held out the proof of his purchase.

"Tomorrow afternoon, at two P.M., I'll be in the air for two hours flying an ATR 42. Not a Boeing, but close enough."

"Thank you dear," said Nqobile. "Now it's your lover's turn."

Isma laid the bag on the floor and unzipped it. She took a deep breath. She pulled out a pair of baby sized ballet shoes. "I dreamt she would be a dancer so I bought her these. She would have been so graceful." She laid the shoes beside the bag and pulled out a blanket with a dragon embroidered into the fabric. "To keep her safe from monsters, her own personal, misunderstood mon-ster." She pulled out a tiny jacket. "To fight Manchester's icy weather. She would have thrown snowballs at passersby." One by one she pulled out the clothes and told the "what if" story. She was surprised she did not cry. The last item of clothing in the bag was a cloth cap with flaps to cover her ears.

Annabel tried again to get through to her mother's phone. Again she didn't get through.

Raymond tossed Nqobile the key to his BMW. Timothy wanted to smack him. They'd all put in such thought and bared their souls. His big gesture was a car. Why the fuck was he in the group anyway? He clearly didn't care about anyone but himself.

"Thanks," said Nqobile. "I'll take it out for a spin tomorrow. Now Hanna."

Hanna got up, a forty-one year old as nervous as a debutante. She approached Nqobile with her arms open.

"For you my queen," said Hanna.

"No, not this one," said Nqobile. "This one's for your daughter, Helen, and that lover of hers whom you refused to meet, what was her name?"

"Bea." Hanna had not even gone to their wedding. "For Helen and Bea."

"Yes, for Helen and Bea."

Nqobile took Hanna in her arms and kissed her hard on the mouth.

Afterwards, the still shaky Hanna said "thank you" to Nqobile.

After her third attempt, Annabel realized what must have happened. "I think my mother's blocked my number."

"Don't sweat it," said Nqobile. "Just make me a promise. Swear you'll go visit her in person. If she doesn't let you in, smash the window and climb in."

"Can't I just snog you like Hanna did?"

"No."

Benito groaned with simulated pain. "Please...snog her anyway. And rub her tits."

"Okay, perv, your turn."

Benito leered lasciviously at Annabel and Nqobile one more

time and then he opened his photo album. Benito the clown, the rubber-face, pointed at a photo of a boy, a girl, and a woman with horn-rimmed glasses.

"They never found who did it," he said. "They just found the bodies piled up with four others on the beach..."

He talked without pause for forty minutes.

52

The shooter was a seventeen-year-old. He was being chased by two men in a red Corvette. He shot at them three times. One of the bullets missed and killed Nqobile.

While she lay dying, Timothy and Isma were in a plane, soaring through the clouds.

"This is wonderful," said Isma, staring out from the cockpit. "Though, it would be better if you could do some flips."

"Aerobatics are overrated. They just make you feel nauseous. Besides, I wanted to be a commercial airline pilot, not a stunt pilot."

"What little kid would rather fly an Airbus than an Air Force jet?"

"Guilty as charged."

"Sexy uniform," Isma teased. "Can you keep it?"

47

"I went to her funeral anyway," Shamus admitted at their next meeting. Nqobile had made them all promise not to go. She wanted their last memory of her to be the party.

"I thought about going, too," said Timothy.

Isma gave him a questioning look. He hadn't said a word. He had been different though—he'd been more withdrawn and irritable over the last two days. She wasn't sure Nqobile was the only reason.

They went round the group. Everybody said a few things about how Nqobile's death made them feel. Benito's words hit the group sentiment most accurately. "I feel like the countdown's officially begun. Next will be Isma and Tim, then me. One by one like in that nursery rhyme. Ten green bottles standing on the wall, and then there're nine. On and on until in two years, it'll just be Krishna sitting in this basement alone."

"Unless he finds replacements," Raymond suggested.

"You think we should just find a replacement for Nqobile," said Hanna. She wasn't shouting, but her anger was obvious.

"That's not what I meant."

"Did you do it?" Shamus asked Annabel, eager to change the subject. "Did you go to see your mother?"

"It was an anticlimax. I expected tears or shouting or some other kind of fireworks. We just talked cordially. Makes me feel like an idiot for waiting so long. If not for Nqobile I might have died without talking to her."

"Thank God for Nqobile," said Shamus. He closed his eyes and whispered a prayer. It was the first time he had done anything during a session that called attention to the fact that he was a reverend.

Afterwards, on their way to Isma's apartment, she shared one of her sillier insecurities. "After Nqobile's final night was so perfect, I feel like whatever we do for ours will be a letdown. Hers was so beautiful. She came up with something that was for her but also a gift for every one of us. I have this recurring image of them meeting after we're dead and one of them saying, 'so, that last meeting, total shit, eh?'"

"Probably Raymond saying it, right?"

"Bang on."

"You shouldn't worry about it. Our last night will be for us—they will all be there to support us. Also, we'll only have a few hours of life left. We could decide to hold hands and sing songs by Abba and it would be profound and meaningful."

"Do you have any ideas about what you want to do?"

"Well..." Timothy hesitated.

"Do tell."

"I..."

"Spit it out."

"I was thinking of asking them if we could have our final meeting as a group two days before our last. I kind of just wanted to do something with you on our last night."

Timothy's arm was around Isma when he said this and he felt her muscles knot. "I think we owe it to them to share our last night with them."

"What difference would it make if it were one day earlier?"

Isma stopped walking and faced Timothy.

"No lies," he reminded her.

She did a double take. She had been readying to pacify him. "I want to be with them on my last night."

"You haven't even known them that long."

"I've known you just as long," she replied, which was the wrong thing to say.

"You still don't love me," he said, which pissed her off.

"Why is it always about that with you? Stop being so fucking insecure. We'll be with each other day in day out for the next forty-seven days. You'll die by my side. I want you to. And it's not like I'm saying I want to go off with some strangers on my last night. I want to be with the group, which you are part of."

"You're right, you're right," Timothy replied, too quickly.

"Don't just say that. Listen to what I'm saying."

"I think I'll go to my apartment tonight."

He disengaged from her and started walking away.

"Don't be a child, Timothy."

He kept going.

"Fine," said Isma. She waited a few moments to see if he would turn around and come back. He didn't.

44

Timothy opened the door. He looked a mess. He was unkempt, unshaven, and looked like he needed sleep. "I didn't think you wanted to see me again."

"You're an idiot." Isma walked passed him into his chaotic apartment. "You know what we just did? We wasted three days. I didn't enjoy them. Did you?"

"No."

"Then let's not do it again."

"Agreed."

"The time we spend together is wonderful. Isn't that enough? Can't you just enjoy what it is? Do you have to compare it with ideal movie notions?"

"What we have is enough," said Timothy.

Isma wasn't sure she believed him but she didn't want to fight. "Go shower," she said. "You need to get out of here."

31

"I should have just lied to him," Isma said to Hanna at her house. Hanna had invited her to come and take a look at two paintings of Nqobile's that she had bought from an art gallery in Edinburgh. "I should have pretended that it was some big epic love from the beginning."

"You wouldn't have hated that?" Hanna said.

"I really wouldn't have. I don't have any qualms about lying. I can do it well. I can cry at will, hesitate, and do whatever else it takes to sell it."

"He would have known. On some level he would have known."

"That's what people always say. I never knew with Paul. I believed every word the bastard said."

"Are you going to contact him, before the end?"

Isma shook her head. "No. Maybe. I want to...I just..."

"You don't want to hurt Timothy."

"That's not it. Nothing I could do can hurt Timothy. He does that all by himself. He loves torturing himself. I'm just an excuse."

"Then why don't you want to see Paul?"

"He left me when I needed him most."

"Pride aside, you want to see him. You should or you'll regret it. When you die, wouldn't it be great to have no regrets?"

"Don't be all worldly wise earth-mother all of a sudden. It doesn't suit you."

One of Nqobile's paintings was of a robotic fisherman seated by a riverside. In the water, a strange three-eyed creature was approaching the hook. The other was a self-portrait, but she had given herself purple skin.

25

"Hello. This is Paul Durocher. Who's calling? Hello? Hello?"

22

They had spent the day at the races. It was one of those things Timothy had never done. Between the two of them they'd made a list. They were ticking them off one by one. Timothy was in a tux and he was wearing a top hat, a ridiculous insistence of his. "I don't care if I look like I'm from the wrong century; I'm going to do this posh pompous ass thing right no matter what you say."

Going there was fun, but the actual races were boring. Nothing about watching horses run in circles remotely exhilarated Timothy or Isma.

Afterwards, Isma gave Timothy an envelope.

"What's this?"

"You'll see."

It was a birthday card. "Today's not my birthday. We'll be dead before I turn twenty-eight."

"They didn't have a special card for what I wanted to say."

"The message?" He flipped the card open. "Happy 528. What is 528?"

"You're always saying how many days we have left. I don't think that's a healthy way of looking at it. We have 528 hours. Or if you like, on the back page I've written how much time we have in *minutes*."

"31680."

"Sounds like a lot of time, doesn't it."

"I guess."

10080

"Now, now is when you call me, when I've got one week left." Isma wanted to be angrier than she was. It was good to hear Paul's voice. She'd missed his soothing baritone and his French-tinged accent. She had resigned herself to never hearing it again.

"I'm calling now. I wanted to before; I just couldn't mount up the courage."

"Lame excuse."

"How have things been?"

Isma brushed aside his attempt at small talk. "Are we going to meet?"

"Wow, that's very direct."

"The 'dying in a few days' thing omits the need for bullshit."

"I'm out of town right now."

"Classic. Why do I bother?"

"I'll be back next week Tuesday."

"And after all this time, you think I'd want to spend my last night with you. You're as arrogant as ever."

"I'm sorry...I just...I booked a flight to come back then because I knew it was your last day. If you don't want to see me..."

"You're a bastard, you know. I should just tell you to fuck off. The sick thing is that, asshole that you are, I want to see you before I die.

Maybe just so I can stab you in the eye with a fork."

"Take it easy."

"Not my last day. I have plans. Not Monday either. I've promised that night to someone."

"Someone?"

Isma laughed. "What? You thought I'd be a celibate nun pining over you ever since you left."

"Isma, if I had stayed with you, do you really think we would have been happy? Every conversation was a fight. It would have kept going. I regret leaving all the time, but I think back and..."

"I won't have this conversation on the phone. I refuse to. Sunday. Can you make it for Sunday?"

"I can."

5760

Isma wasn't as good a liar as she thought. Timothy knew immediately. He wasn't sure whether it was her body language or inflection, but something told him. He wanted to call her on it, remind her about the "no lying" rule, but he didn't.

She wasn't looking at him. She, the big "eye contact" lady, wasn't looking at him. "I know it's last-minute, but Hanna and I have gotten to know each other much better than I would have expected. Maybe it's because I never really knew either of my parents, but having an older woman friend—it just makes me feel something intangible. Comfort maybe, but it's more than that."

This part wasn't a lie. Timothy had noticed at the last few meetings that Isma and Hanna had become as close as family. It was just the "I'll be meeting Hanna tomorrow" part.

"I hope you don't mind," Isma said.

"Of course I don't."

Why is she lying? Maybe she's planning me a surprise? he thought suddenly. He could see that. Hanna and Isma conspiring to create something that would make him laugh until it hurt.

4320

Nothing good could come of this, Timothy knew. Secretly following someone you were supposed to love and trust was always a stupid idea. It was like opening her diary. Whatever he read would be out of context and it would hurt no matter what it said.

He should have just told her, "I know you're lying, tell me the truth; no matter what it is." He hadn't because he knew it was something bad. In fact, he was pretty sure he knew exactly where she was headed. *You're paranoid,* he told himself at first. Then he remembered the old joke: "Just because I'm paranoid doesn't mean they're not out to get me."

He followed her through the streets, one hundred yards behind her. He was ready to duck behind something if she turned. She didn't. She was too focused on where she was going. It was too important to her. *If I walked right in front of her,* he thought, *she probably wouldn't even notice me.*

She turned into Oldham Street and he dashed forward so he wouldn't lose her.

Why am I following her? he thought again. *I know where she's going.* All pretense in his mind that he wasn't sure was gone. *I know, but I'm heading after her anyway.*

Isma turned into a café and Timothy crossed the street. He knew what he would see, but he crossed anyway. Unless…maybe it would be something else? There was always the possibility that he was exactly as paranoid and childish as she said. That's why he'd followed in the end. Because there was a hairbreadth of a chance he was wrong.

He walked down the street until he was adjacent to the café. Isma was seated opposite a handsome, curly-haired man in a business suit. Timothy recognized him from the digital photos she had stored on her computer.

Timothy turned and walked away.

1440

"What? You knew you were an ED when you decided to join the clergy?"

Julie's total shock made Shamus laugh. "It was one of the main reasons I joined the church."

"To make sure you go to heaven?"

"No, no, no." That was what his father had thought, too. *Throwing what little life you have left away*, his father had accused. "Knowing I had very little time made me want to make a difference in the time I had."

"I understand that," Julie replied. "Since I started writing songs again I've been wishing more and more that I never stopped. It would've been nice to leave behind something that people could play in the future. Some sort of proof that I was alive."

Shamus nodded. "Everyone wants to leave a legacy."

The two of them were the first ones there. The basement of the church had been freezing when they arrived, but it was heating up. The church heaters wouldn't be able to make the basement truly warm but that's what the alcohol was for.

Benito came next, smiling like an idiot. With the exuberance of a child he told them about a woman he had met.

"Does she know?" Shamus asked.

"No."

"You should tell her. She deserves to know."

"Would you stop being a reverend for five minutes and just be a guy?"

"I'm with you," Julie said. "Better she never finds out."

"She has lovely tits," he boasted.

Krishna came in next and commented on how when he went, this is how he wanted his last night to be. "None of that New Age stuff Nqobile did. Just some friends and some laughs."

"And booze," Benito piped in. "The booze is important."

Hanna came in next and the mood changed instantly. Her pallid face screamed that something was wrong. "Have any of you seen Timothy the last two days?"

"No. Why?"

"He was meant to meet Isma yesterday. He didn't show."

Shamus clutched the crucifix dangling around his neck. "Something bad must have happened. Did you call the police?"

"Two days have to go by before you can report someone missing. And by then...he'll be dead."

They asked Raymond and Annabel when they arrived, but they hadn't seen or heard from Timothy either. Isma arrived at nine and she looked worn down. Looking at the seven of them sitting there, the last flicker of hope she had harbored faded.

"Maybe he was in an accident?" Shamus wondered.

"No," Isma said. "He decided not to come. Him not coming yesterday, I understand. But I still thought he would come today..."

"Don't think like that," Shamus insisted. "If Timothy could be here, he would be."

"No." Isma hadn't admitted it even to Hanna. She had just told Hanna he was missing, not the reason she suspected he had left. "I did something, I did something that hurt him. I don't know how he found out, but he did. That's the only explanation. He's somewhere alone and hurt because of me."

"You really shouldn't blame yourself." Hanna cut in.

"I saw Paul," Isma admitted, and the admission made her tongue feel like it was rotting. It was a chore to get the words out but she forced them out. She told them and she felt the self-righteous ones (Shamus, Raymond, Annabel) judging her.

Hanna took her side. "You were with Paul for years. Of course you saw him. You're dying tomorrow. If Timothy was angry he should have faced you, not run off like a coward."

Isma just shook her head and nothing anyone said could make her feel better. Benito suggested she try and make the best of it, but she replied "I just want to leave. I'm going to go home and have an early night."

Hanna put her arms around Isma. "You shouldn't let him make you feel like this on your last night. Stay and we'll cheer you up."

"No," she said, forcefully. "I'm going."

She said her goodbyes to the ED group and none of the goodbyes were what she had imagined. They all felt flat, even with Hanna. Hanna was crying but Isma's eyes were dry. "How did this happen?" Isma asked Hanna before she left. "I've only known him three months. I shouldn't feel this. One week ago, if you told me this would happen, I wouldn't have thought it would affect me."

"Should I walk you home?" Hanna asked.

"No. Thanks, but I'd rather be by myself." She stepped out into the rain.

When Timothy got to the church, only Shamus was still there, putting things away. He told Timothy that Isma had already left, so Timothy drove to her apartment. What would he say when he got there? He had no idea. A part of him wanted to confront her about Paul and ask for specifics. Why did she lie? Did she sleep with him? Did she still love him? Another part of him just wanted to be with her and not to bring up Paul in any way whatsoever.

The traffic was dense, which was unexpected for a Sunday. The cars moved at a crawl. Timothy wondered where everybody was going to or coming from. Yesterday he'd been driving out, no particular destination in mind, just getting far far away. He'd planned to go to another city, to get a hotel room, a lot of alcohol, a thousand-a-night escort and whatever else he needed to make sure his last day was perfect even without Isma. That had been the theory. In practice, he'd felt miserable and had not been able to stop thinking about her.

So here he was, driving to apologize? Grovel? Scream at her? Well, something. "I've got one day left and I want to spend it with you," he whispered to himself. "That's real romantic. Who could say no to that?"

Timothy turned round the corner to Isma's apartment block and he saw the fire. The top three floors of Isma's building were ablaze. Timothy looked down at his watch. 00:27. Half past midnight.

"No," he breathed as the realization hit him.

This was it. This was how it was going to happen. Isma was in her apartment right now trapped and she would die in there, if she wasn't already dead. If he went into the building to try and save her, he would die too. That was the prediction. This was how it was going to happen.

The Death Machine had always been right but that was because everyone had always known too little information. Even EDs. But this time, Timothy knew everything. This was how it would happen. There wouldn't be two fires. This was the only one. All he needed to do to survive was to stand by and watch. That's how simple it would be to prove the Machine wrong. All he needed to do was do nothing. It's not like he could save her anyway.

Timothy stopped his car just outside the building. He heard screaming from within.

He stared up at the billowing flames and looked at the window he knew to be hers. She was in there, pinned under something or unable to run for some other reason. She must be so scared because she knew this was the end. She was in there, about to die. Waiting to die. Alone.

Timothy got out of his car and ran toward the fire at a full sprint.

Story by Daliso Chaponda
Illustration by Dylan Meconis

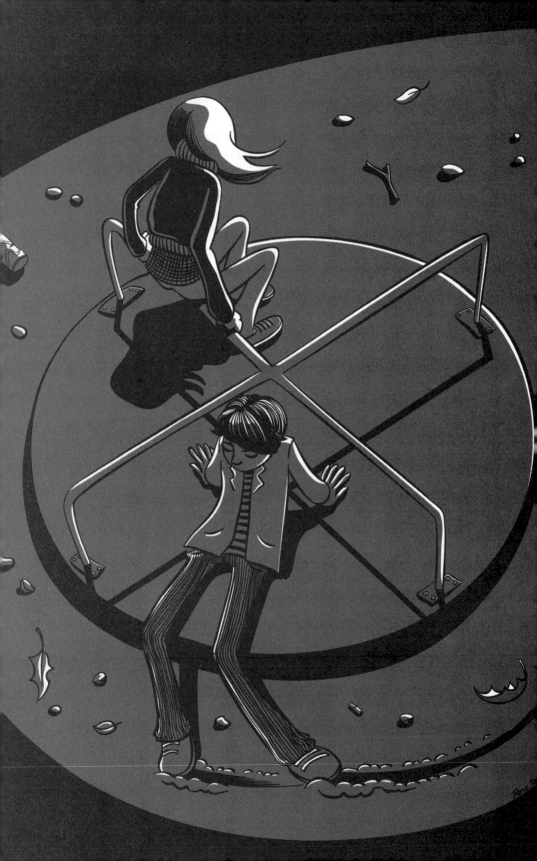

MISCARRIAGE

THE CITY IS BEAUTIFUL AT NIGHT. Long after the sun goes down, when the last rays have left the horizon scorched and aching, the buildings show their true shapes, silhouettes against the black with lights that twinkle orange and red. These are not the buildings, not anymore—rather, they're the buildings' ideas of themselves, the barest sketches. The burned-in after-image of a skyline put to bed.

With the fall of dusk, things simultaneously expand and contract. The streets open up, and familiar drivers can run them like rabbits in a warren, every turn practiced a thousand times and unimpeded by hesitant outsiders. It's a delicate dance. The people thin out, and suddenly the extra interactions—the vacant smiles and nods that mean nothing—are stripped out as well, and every meeting becomes one of significance. You see only who you want to see, and if you see someone else, it's because you wanted to see them and just didn't know it. Or they wanted to see you.

At the same time that the streets are opening up, they're also closing in. The city is a city during the day—people coming and going on business, tourists waltzing through and then back out, leaving snapshots and traveler's checks in their wake—but at night it becomes a home. Everyone acts a little different—after all, we're all roommates on a grander scale. This is my home, but it's yours, too. *Mi casa es su casa. Mi ciudad es su ciudad.* We're all in this together.

Those smiles to passersby that seem forced in the light become smirks at three in the morning. The raised eyebrow that says, "How was she?" or "I bet you could use a drink, too." People's walls start to come down. Masks are for daylight—once dusk hits, it's the moon's turf, and she likes us naked, naked, naked, just the way she made us.

Or at least some of us. The poets. The dreamers. The dancers and weavers. Sure, there are children of the sun out there—hardworking proponents of duty and righteousness—but not at night. We are the merrymakers, the children of the moon. And the moon, she takes care of her own.

She was taking care of Ryan as he ran across the bridge, her light following him as he took in the skyline, the radio towers and bedroom windows that lit his way home, offering nothing but asking nothing in return. It was a sight that had taken his breath away the first time, and every subsequent viewing was a chance to return to that original moment—who he was with, what he was doing.

Ryan wasn't interested in going back tonight, nor home. The globes on the streetlamps glowed soft as he turned down the footpath, hedges forming a tunnel before opening up into the park proper. Here it was dark enough that the moon washed away the colors, leaving only stark whites and grays. And black. Lots of black.

Annie was waiting on the merry-go-round, one foot dragging in the dust. The contrast of blonde hair over heavy black peacoat was enough to fry the rods in his eyes and blind him to more subtle distinctions, but he knew they were there. The tiny triangle where her nose met her lips. The scar on her cheek that made her hate cats. The ears that poked through the sides of her hair in a way that only she found awkward. She stood up, and the diminishing momentum of the merry-go-round carried her up to him, then stopped.

"Hey," he said.

"Hey," she replied.

They stood awkwardly for a moment, then she sat and he followed, close but separated by the toy's dully reflective steel rail.

"How was the hospital?" she asked.

"Not too bad. Long." He sighed and pulled his jacket closer around him. She knew it was a loaded question—it was every time. How could he explain that working in the ER was simultaneously exhilarating and crushing? That in any given day, he worked miracles and failed miserably, complete strangers giving up and expiring beneath his hands? He couldn't, and once upon a time he'd told her so. So now she asked how his day was, and he said fine, and both of them knew that the exchange was one of affection, not information.

The machine didn't make his job any easier, either. You'd think it would warn people, let them know what was coming, or at the very least aid in diagnosis and emergency room triage, but somehow it rarely did. Every day he saw people making good on their little certificates, and every day it took all but a select few by surprise. Some were straightforward—the middle-aged man with the steering column in his chest and DRUNK DRIVER on the laminated slip in his pocket, or the kid who quit breathing on Sloppy Joe Day and hadn't yet been informed by his parents that CHOKE ON CAFETERIA FOOD was the last entry in his abbreviated biography. Others were more complex—the third-degree burn victim who tried to cheat death by never smoking a pack in his life, only to be done in by the upstairs neighbor who fell asleep with a lit cigarette near the drapes. Or the woman with SAILBOAT ACCIDENT in her wallet, crushed by a towed yacht in a five-car pileup. The list went on. One way or another, things always worked out in the end.

Though the residents and long-time nurses did their best to combat complacency—after all, you could never know if the heart attack implied on the slip was this one, or another in thirty years— you could still see the knowing look in the doctors' eyes when someone crashed. If you were lucky, the advance warning made things a little less traumatic for both patient and doctor. More dignified.

Annie pushed off from the ground and the merry-go-round spun hesitantly, their weight throwing it off balance and making it squeal against its steel and rubber fittings. Ryan realized he'd trailed off and snapped back to the present, turning toward her.

"Did you talk to your mom?" he asked.

"Yeah."

"How did it go?"

"About how we expected." She reached up with one hand and tucked a lock of severely cropped white-blond hair behind her ear. "She doesn't really trust it, and has all sorts of philosophical mis- givings, but in the end she knows it's our decision and supports us without question. She'd like us to come out and see the new house whenever we can—she's trying to hold it back, but I can tell she's already gearing up to play the doting grandmother. She's probably already got the shower half-planned. I told her you're booked solid, but that we might be able to make it out in a month or so. What do you think?"

Ryan grunted noncommittally, feigning reluctance. She shoved his shoulder hard, tipping him off balance.

"Oh, come on," she said. "You know you love it. You don't even have to help cook—you just get to read and ride the horses and hang out with William. I'm the one who's going to have to go visit eighty- year-old great-aunts and listen to stories about people who died in 1967." She stood and grabbed his hand. "Come on, let's go sit on the swings."

Ryan stood and let her pull him along. In the dark, her tiny hands glowed against her sleeves, and he marveled at the boundless energy contained in something so small and delicate.

The park was nothing extravagant—a gravel-covered box edged with trees on one side, with the merry-go-round, a few big climbing toys, and a swing set. Nothing like the expansive playgrounds both of them had grown up with, but that was the price they paid for living in the city. During the day, every square foot was covered in running, yelling children, offering local mothers a few minutes to read their books on the surrounding benches. But at night it stood empty, save for the occasional drug deal or sleepy hobo.

Annie had exploded into Ryan's life like a mortar round, with only the faintest whistle to warn him. A smile across a crowded party, and suddenly she was right in front of him, introducing herself with a confidence that made him sweat. The rest of the party had suddenly paled in comparison, fading to a dull buzz, and the two had quietly excused themselves, drifting out into the silent streets.

Something about each of them opened a vein in the other, and the conversation flowed in great torrents, both of them pushing further and faster, daring each other to greater depths of intimacy. In a heartbeat Ryan found himself offering up his deepest secrets, astonished and enraptured by the care with which she picked each one up, examined it carefully from all sides, and then replaced it. They'd walked for hours, finally stopping in this park to rest on the swing set. When they eventually left, he'd gone home alone, but something had changed. It was a new sort of alone, relaxed and refreshed.

He'd invited her out again, and once more they'd walked until they dropped, taking a different path but still ending at the park. He'd repeated the date three times, reluctant to risk changing any variables, before she finally suggested that they might want to try going out to dinner or a movie once in a while. The fact that she said it while lying in his bed, hair tousled and one pink-tipped breast peeking out from beneath the threadbare cotton sheets, had taken any sting out of her words. They'd built a life together, but the park had always maintained a special place in their relationship. It was there that he'd asked her to marry him—not the most creative choice, but she'd still said yes. Even once they lived together, it had still been a place of significance. Neutral ground. Holy ground.

Annie sat down in the lower of the two swings and leaned back, toes barely dragging in the gravel. In the one beside it, Ryan's feet were flat on the ground, weight pulling down on the rubber until the chain pinched his sides.

"How was it?" he asked.

"Pretty easy," she said, slowly beginning to pump. "It's pretty much the same as amniocentesis—there was more than just the pinch they tell you to expect, but not much. It was over in like thirty seconds."

"I'm sorry I couldn't be there."

She reached over and twined her fingers in his, making his arm sway in time with her.

"I know," she replied. "You had to work."

He stiffened, but her eyes held none of the old resentment. It was true—she really did know. And it was okay.

They'd conceived before. The first was a surprise, when they'd been married only a few months, and the tears of joy had been tinged with shock and a vague sense of panic. When she'd miscarried two months in, they'd been heartbroken, of course, but eventually both admitted to pangs of guilty relief.

The second time the stick turned blue, it was intentional—they had good jobs, a car, a house, and a strong desire to take the next step. They'd surprised their parents with it on Mother's Day, and were immediately enveloped in a whirlwind of blue and pink, both grandmothers good-naturedly attempting to outdo each other with baby preparation. Ryan's father, the paragon of stoicism, had cried and hugged him, tears leaking out from behind Coke-bottle glasses. Annie glowed.

When the baby spontaneously aborted in the eighth month, the pain was unlike anything Ryan or Annie had ever known. The doctors explained that there was nothing they could have done, that sometimes these things just happened, but their words fell on deaf ears. Annie blamed herself. Ryan felt helpless. In their sadness, they turned away from each other. Conversations became arguments became battles. Annie, the picture of brazen self-confidence for as long as Ryan had known her, became weepy and dependent. She resented his long hours at the hospital. He resented her resentment. They'd separated for several months, her flying back to her parents' place in Maine, him staying in Seattle and picking up as many extra shifts as he could. But in the end, neither could stay away, and one Saturday she'd showed up on his doorstep with tears and a suitcase. Together, they'd worked through their grief. When it was done, they were a little bit harder, a few more wrinkles in their faces, but the love that had been soft and warm and all-pervasive was now iron-hard, a steel cable that suspended them above the dark pit they'd both stared into. Their love had been tested. It had passed.

There followed a long stretch where neither mentioned trying again, both of them reluctant to reopen old wounds. But all around them friends began having children, and both watched the way the other smiled when they saw small children running, the way their faces lit up when they cradled a newborn in their arms. And finally, after careful consideration and numerous late-night discussions, they had tossed out the box of condoms. Three months later, Annie was pregnant.

They'd gone back and forth on whether they wanted to test the fetus with the machine. These days, most adults went ahead and got tested, with the exception of the religious nuts and the staunch free-will atheists, who finally had a common cause to rally around. Both Annie and Ryan knew how they would go, and had shared that knowledge with each other early on. Yet the decision of whether to test a child, let alone an unborn one, was difficult, and raised a bevy of uncomfortable questions: would you abort a child that had a horribly painful death in store for it, or one that might die young? Sudden Infant Death Syndrome made frequent appearances on the machine's little slips of paper. Was it better to die at six weeks or to never be born in the first place? And suppose your child survived to adulthood. When did you inform them of the method of their eventual demise? Some parents advocated raising children with the knowledge from birth, in the hope that never knowing a life without a prescribed death would make it easier. Others waited until the child asked, or graduated from college, or got married. Whatever the call, knowledge of the means of death quickly wrenched the title of "the Talk" from comparatively paltry topics like "where babies came from" and "you're adopted."

Pundits on both sides raged, but in the end, for Annie and Ryan, there was no question—if this child was going to miscarry as well, they needed to know as soon as possible so that they could induce it themselves. Abortion was far safer for Annie, and though neither of them said it, both knew that it would be easier to end things if they had less time to get attached.

Annie put her feet down, stopping herself, and squeezed his hand once before letting go. Reaching inside her jacket, she pulled out a small envelope, turning it over and over in her hands. The service she'd used had embossed it with pastel blue angels and clouds. She wedged a finger under the flap and looked up at him.

"Ready?" she asked.

A sudden lump in Ryan's throat kept him from speaking. He nodded and reached over, placing jittery hands over hers. She broke the seal and pulled out the small, plain white card. On it, in large block letters, were printed three words:

CONGESTIVE HEART FAILURE.

Ryan let out a breath. The world was spinning, sparkling at the corners. His stomach felt like he was falling.

"Do you know what this means?" he asked, voice husky and strained.

Annie turned toward him, tears glistening on cheeks pulled tight by a shaky smile.

"We're going to have a baby," she whispered.

Story by James L. Sutter
Illustration by Rene Engström

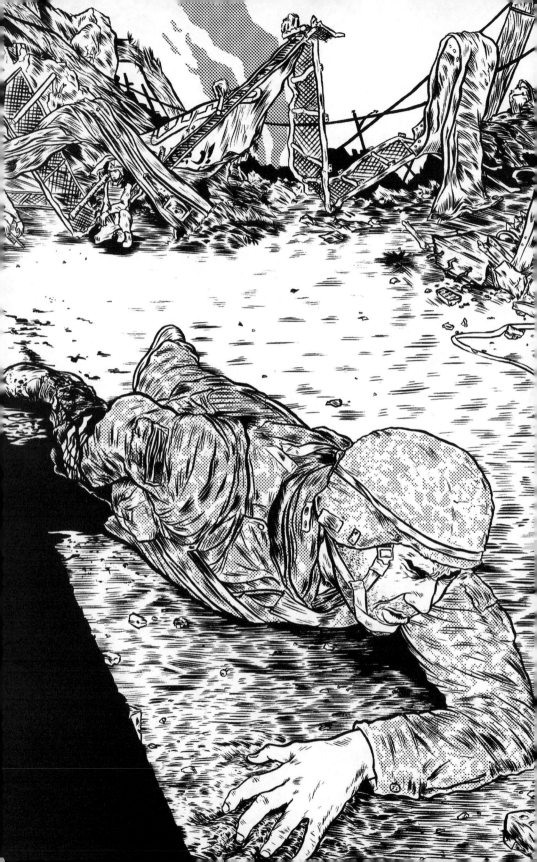

SHOT BY SNIPER

LIEUTENANT GRALE CRAWLED THROUGH THE ASHEN SLOP BENEATH AND BEHIND THE SLANTED BILLBOARD THAT'D HALF-FALLEN FROM THE ROOF ABOVE, its Arabic advert made all but illegible, even to the locals. The machinegun fire crackling through the air was background and indistinct. If one were careless, the sound would become ambient, like the bustling traffic in New York or the steady hum of a computer.

A shot kicked up dirt in front of Grale's face. He pulled himself backward, back to the dubious protection of the fallen sign.

A sniper. "Shit."

He looked across the road. His men hadn't noticed yet.
"Sniper!"

Everyone moved at once, except for Paula. She was green, and waited just a second too long. She turned to face Grale, and as she did, she staggered backward, blood flying from her arm. Gearhead leapt out, grabbed her, and pulled her behind the cover of the still-standing wall of a long-destroyed hotel.

The sniper waited, silent.

Across the street from the fallen billboard, Grale's men looked at him, pasty-faced and wide-eyed. One of the men—Simmons—signed for him to stay put.

"No shit, Simmons."

A panic swept through the men as they crouched behind the wall. They were reacting, damn it, not thinking, and Paula's cries of pain were rattling loose what little cohesion they had. Grale needed to cross the street and reach them, and he needed to do so before the SNAFU became FUBAR.

But those three little words on that tiny slip of paper kept him from dashing across.

The focus of the panic shifted from Paula to Grale. They knew she'd be fine, after all. But the eyes on Grale hadn't the slightest shimmer of hope. No. They all knew Grale would die here. God damn that machine.

It'd been a week ago, back when the insurgency seemed stoppable. A couple of rookie privates had found the machine in the wreckage of a casino. (Well, Grale called it a casino. The locals insisted it wasn't. The locals insisted a lot of things.) The machine still worked.

Grale had said to throw the damn thing out, but most of the platoon kicked up a fuss. "It's one of the newer models," Gearhead had said, looking at it. "Forty different languages. Takes a pinprick of blood—less than most blood-sugar machines—and it's supposed to be the wittiest model yet. Come on, Lieutenant? What harm will it do?"

Machines weren't infallible. That was Grale's sole understanding of computers, and even Gearhead (reluctantly, at times) agreed with him. So let the boys (and girls, Grale, you can't forget them) have their fun. Right?

"Says I'm going to drown."

"That blows."

"Paula—What's yours?"

"Uh—car accident."

"Oh, what the hell? Mine says 'Killed by cow.'"

"A cow?"

"Always knew you'd amount to great things, Simmons."

"Blow me. Hey, Lieutenant!"

"Lt. Grale! You gotta try this."

"I really don't," Grale said.

"He just doesn't want to see the words 'old age' in print."

Everyone laughed. An explosion and the sound of wrenching metal pealed through the open windows, a distant and painful reality check.

"Gearhead," Grale said, "Take ten men and go see who killed who."

"Yes, sir!" the skinny youngster said, snapping gum that'd been in his mouth since morning.

The rest of the men kept joking about the machine's one-line fortunes, and Simmons, with a half-smile plastered on his face, said, "Come on, Lieutenant. It won't hurt you to see what it says."

"Yeah, Lieutenant, come on."

A chorus of "come ons" and "yeahs" broke out, and Grale couldn't see the harm in a little fun.

He stepped up to the machine—it was such a humble thing— and Paula showed him how it worked. It reminded Grale of a slot machine. Maybe that was why it'd been in a casino.

A tiny slip of paper curled out.

Grale ripped it free, read it, stared at it for a moment, and then let it fall to the floor with a shrug. Like jackals, Grale's men fell on the scrap and gaped at it, horror-struck. By nightfall, everyone on base knew how Lieutenant Grale was going to die.

The change came the next morning. Some of the men wouldn't talk to Grale unless they had to. Overnight, he'd become the most beloved and still (somehow) least-popular man on base. And anyone with something bad to say about Lt. Grale: Watch out!

Everywhere Grale went, his soldiers looked at him with wide, wet eyes and the color would swirl out of their faces. They'd utter "yes, sir," as if the post had arrived with a thousand pounds of Dear John letters.

What harm could a little fun be? Grale snorted at the thought. Aside from bringing morale to an all-time low? Not a goddamned thing.

"I want that damn machine turned into scrap."

"Yes, sir."

"You hear me? If it stays on this base, it'll be reincarnated as a locker."

"Yes, sir."

"Now! I want to see you do it, Marine!"

That caused some grumbling. Word went out that ol' Grale was afraid of the death machine. "And who can blame him?" they'd say.

What the hell did they know?

Grale crouched behind the billboard and watched the disaster unfold across the street. His boys (and girl), the whole lot of them, in an instant, decided that they were going to defy fate, to prove Grale's slip of paper wrong. He couldn't hear what they were saying over the gunfire, and they weren't signaling anything.

A bullet sliced through the sign and sent bits of brick from the building behind Grale into the air. The damn thing almost parted his hair. He pressed himself against the ground.

He saw Gearhead on the radio. Calling an air strike. Good boy.

Simmons put a new mag in his gun and shifted his legs.

No, damn you, Simmons, stay put. Grale gestured for him to stay down. He didn't.

"No!"

But Simmons charged around the corner. Gearhead looked across the ruined street at Grale and Grale shook his head. Gearhead stopped the others from following. Good boy.

Grale ground his teeth. Once, his daughter had left at seventeen hundred hours, back at the base in Germany, and never reported for dinner. She'd come home at oh-one hundred, drunk and battered. Grale knocked a few heads in that night, that was for sure. But the time between seventeen and oh-one hundred hours? That excruciating wait? That was how Grale felt when Simmons turned the corner and charged toward the ruins of the office building.

A crack shattered the other sounds of the urban fighting and Grale knew what'd happened, even before he heard Simmons cry out. Just like he knew what happened that night, so long ago, before his daughter had opened her mouth to start crying.

Grale peered over the sign. Simmons was down, hard. The sniper had shot his leg. The bastard was hoping to draw out more.

Grale made a gesture at Gearhead.

Gearhead shook his head.

Grale made ready to spring, putting his back against the sign and shouldering his rifle. This was his job, damn it, these were his children. Screw that miserable machine and its miserable opinion.

"Covering fire!" Gearhead screamed. NATO rounds poured upward toward the office building. Grale turned at the edge of the sign and dashed into the street. Throughout, the sniper was silent. Good boy, Gearhead.

Grale reached Simmons, and winced. The boy's leg was mangled badly—he'd be lucky to keep it. *Have to carry him,* Grale thought.

"Lieutenant?"

"Shut up. You gotta live so that cow can kill ya."

Grale squatted and hefted Simmons up. Boy could use a meal or two extra. Damn, it was hot out.

Grale's eyes were glued up to the building.

He saw the sniper.

He could see into the sniper's eyes, all the way from the ground. They were like brown glass, and the man behind them—the man behind the rifle—hated Grale, hated Simmons, and he'd hate anyone else that stepped into the street. The NATO rounds weren't keeping him down anymore.

Grale knew what was going to happen. He always did. He turned away from the sniper, Simmons curled on his shoulders, and started running back to cover. If the bastard was going to shoot Grale, he'd have to do it from behind.

A puff of dirt flashed up between Grale's legs, as if to say, "I don't mind that."

But Grale was almost there.

Gearhead and the others were still firing, trying to keep the sniper down. But the man behind the rifle had a pair made of brass. Another round zipped past Grale's ear.

Ten yards to go. Not even that.

But Grale could feel it. The muzzle of the rifle may as well have been pressed against his back. The sniper, he knew, wouldn't miss a third time.

A rocket streaked through the heavens. Half of the sniper's building caved in. As Grale turned the corner and set Simmons down, he heard Gearhead yelling into the radio.

"Kill confirmed. Repeat, kill confirmed. You got the bastard!"

Simmons looked up at Grale, his eyes beaming with gratitude and admiration.

"But, sir, your paper said—"

"Some other sniper, son. Some other war."

Story by Bartholomew von Klick
Illustration by John Keogh

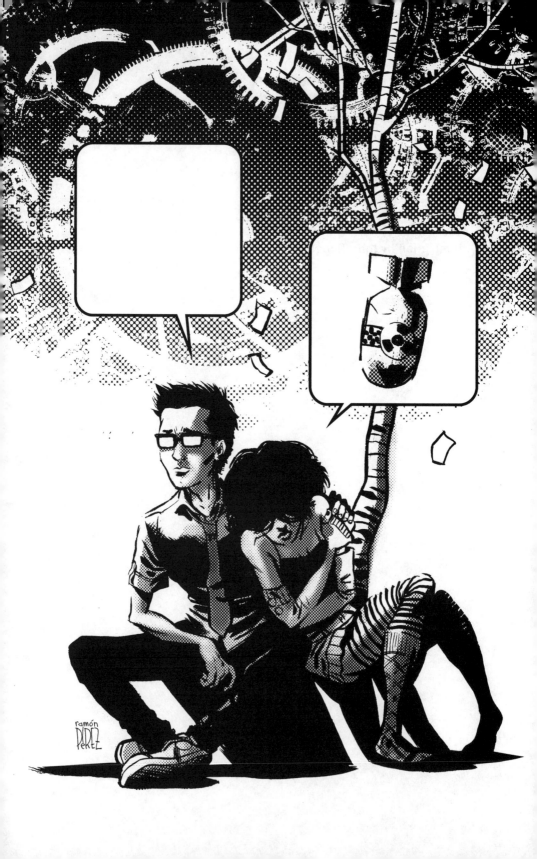

HEAT DEATH OF THE UNIVERSE

I MET MAGGIE AT A KEG PARTY IN THE BACK YARD OF THE HEAD
CHEERLEADER'S HOUSE. The cheerleader didn't know I was there, and
probably would have objected to my presence. I was a nerd. I didn't
earn acceptance from my peers until we were too old and too jaded
about high school cliques to care.

Maggie and I had been at the same school since junior high,
but we had never really met each other before. She was a name on
a roster, another face in the background noise. She was tall for her
age, and had knobby knees and a flat chest, and a nose that was
a little too big, but I thought she was beautiful. Seeing her at the
party again, in different and unusual circumstances, was like waking up and everything seeming smaller than it was before. I had seen

Maggie every day for years, but suddenly she was the most wonderful girl I had ever seen. Before that moment, before I saw her laughing over the rim of a red plastic cup, I don't think I even noticed girls.

We got off to a good start. We talked awhile, and shared a drink or two in the freshly-cut grass, giggling. Later, I held her hair back while she puked in the kitchen sink. Maggie had too much Jagermeister, drawn by its sweet smell and licorice taste. She had always liked licorice. Between bouts of gut-twisting heaves, Maggie cursed the liquor companies for making the stuff taste exactly like her favorite candy. Childhood to adulthood, things don't change as much as they used to. Maggie blames commercialism and the corporations. I think I agree with Stephen Hawking.

I read his book during my sophomore year. The other kids would have made fun of me if they hadn't gotten that out of their collective system in junior high. They were too busy getting laid and trying to get laid, and trying to get into good colleges. I had already been accepted with a big scholarship because I'd discovered a new kind of algae in the stream near my grandparents' house. It was just a science project to me, but to college admissions departments, it was as if I had rushed for a million yards last football season.

I had scholarship offers, and ended up going to the school that Maggie was going to. I told my parents that I had picked the state university because I had read that graduate programs matter much more than undergraduate programs, and that I should go to a big state school for undergrad because I needed the social acculturation that happens at those kinds of places. They agreed with me, or at least let me have my way, because that new kind of algae made them think I was smarter than they were.

I'm not as smart as everybody thinks I am. When I tell people that I'm not as smart as they think I am, they think I'm being modest. I keep expecting to wake up one day and know that I'm that smart and be comfortable with it, and be able to think my way through any problem and come to the right conclusion every time, like there's a door locked in my mind and if I could unlock it, everything would be fine, and I would be a modern-day Mozart. I'll never be Mozart, though. I played the baritone tuba in junior high band, and faked my way through it. I never even learned how to key or read the music. I just pretended. I wonder if Stephen Hawking tells people that he's not as smart as people think he is.

According to Hawking, all this certainty is going to be bad for us. We spent the first few billion years of our collective existence scrabbling through a random universe full of uncertainty, pain, suffering, and unpredictability. Hawking thought that if you put a little bit of order in the chaotic soup of human existence, then the order will crystallize and spread itself throughout the whole human experience. Life will either get very boring or very interesting, in the Chinese sense. There's some debate about what this would look like, because nothing like it has ever happened. Some people think Hawking is wrong and that a little bit of order in a whole lot of chaos is no more effective than an ice cube dropped in a lava flow. Others believe that it's going to be the social equivalent of metal fatigue, simultaneous across the whole planet. Civilization will shatter like an icicle. Too much order is worse than too much chaos. We evolved in chaos. We survived chaos. Life thrives in chaos.

I thought about that a lot during our senior year. The chaos of high school and all the politics of it and the cliques sort of dissolved and became more permeable. Nobody cared about that stuff anymore. They cared about college, and their new lives: High School 2.0. It was a kind of order of its own, though I thought it was kind of temporary. Maggie and I visited a few colleges together and it seemed pretty chaotic to me.

Maggie and I had sex for the first time right before our birth-days, on December 31st. No liquor for us, no wine, no champagne. We hung out in the treehouse in her back yard, which had over-grown with spidery ivy and creeping, snaking tree branches. Her father was a contractor, so while it was in a tree, it was pretty well insulated, and two bodies in it warmed the place up pretty well, especially if those bodies were humping. I had heard that sex for the first time was always messy and weird and gross, but it wasn't for us. I had researched it a lot on the Internet, but Maggie wasn't interested in the technicalities. She just wanted to be close to me.

"I'm scared," she said, after we did it, and we were spooning on the floor of the treehouse, wrapped in the blanket I had brought from my house. It was blue and white, in a pattern like a summer sky with clouds on it. It was wool, and scratchy and soft at the same time.

"I don't want to get my blood read."

"We don't have to," I said.

"Yes we do," she said. "My mom won't stop talking about it."

"Moms suck sometimes," I said.

"Especially mine," she said. "It's worse than when I had my period for the first time. She kept telling me it was going to happen soon. She bought me six kinds of maxi pads. I was afraid she was going to demonstrate how to use a tampon."

"Ew."

"Yeah. Boys are lucky." She sighed and grabbed my hand and squeezed. "I hope we get the same reading."

"Me too," I said. "But it's okay if we don't."

"I guess so," she said. "But what if I get CAR ACCIDENT and you get DROWNING? Or what if I get CANCER and you get OLD AGE?"

"Nobody gets OLD AGE," I said.

"Sometimes they do," she said.

"It's an urban legend," I said. "Because nobody actually dies of

OLD AGE. They die of cancer or something."

"That's not what my uncle says," she said. "His friend in college pulled OLD AGE. And he was killed by an old guy driving a car."

"I don't think that's true," I said. "It's too weird."

"Just because it's weird doesn't mean it doesn't happen," she said. "Things like that happen all the time. Like those people who pull STABBED, and they fall on some broken glass, or that lady who pulled HANGED, and got wrapped up in telephone wires when she jumped off her roof. That stuff happens."

"Yeah, I guess it does," I said. "But it's rare. If that were always true then nobody would get their blood read at all. People wouldn't be so secretive about their certs. There wouldn't be laws against having your blood read before you're eighteen. It would just be a joke, you know? Like a horoscope."

She didn't have an answer for that. I was the smart kid. People always thought my logic was perfect, even if they knew it wasn't, because I was smarter.

"I don't want to know how I'm going to die," she said, finally. "It doesn't seem fair."

"Everybody does it. They still live their lives."

"Some of them," she said, a reference to her uncle, the black sheep of her family. He had pulled GUNSHOT, and got scared and moved to the wilderness out west somewhere. He didn't live his life. He started living someone else's.

"We'll live ours," I said. "Together." I squeezed her tight, for emphasis.

"Yeah," she said. "Together."

If order really were crystallizing across the whole quantum stratum of human existence, then Maggie would have turned out to be my sister or something.

But that didn't happen. We had blood drawn at the doctor's

office. Our families let us go by ourselves. I drove us in my mom's Taurus. The salt-stained tires ploughed twin canals through the chunky, gray slush. The snow unspooled from the roof in loose, white ribbons.

Maggie and I had the same doctor. He had a machine in his office that did the readings. He drew a little bit of blood and put it into a little receptacle on the machine. It looked like a big laser printer, smooth white plastic and blinking, green lights. In a few minutes, the machine hummed and something inside it spun and the humming grew louder and shook the floor a little. He smiled at us, arms folded. The machine printed out the certificates on special paper, the same pinkish color as those new five-dollar bills. He put them face-down on a tray and handed them to us. Maggie and I sat down on the examination table, butcher paper crinkling and creasing under us, bunching between us as Maggie scooted closer. The doctor left us alone.

Maggie asked me if I was feeling nervous. I told her no, even though that was a lie and she could see it in my face.

"I can tell when you're nervous," she said. "You look like you're reading small print when you're nervous."

"I am now," I said. "Thanks."

"Oh, it's all right," she said, and put her hand on my leg. She was always misreading my sarcasm. If there were a chance I was nervous, she took it seriously. I was joking this time. I told her so. She nodded and held my hand.

"We can wait," she said. "We'll just sit here. We don't have to turn it over at all. Nobody will ever know."

We sat in silence for a long time. I told her later that I wanted to stay there forever, our futures vibrating in the midpoint between knowing and not knowing, the moment stretched to fill a lifetime. Would that have been a state of order? Knowing either way is a switch flipped to either side. But what if you refuse to touch it? Is that order or chaos?

History has turning points, moments around which pivot the events that follow. I sometimes imagine it to be a railroad switch that shunts a train from one path to another. Sometimes it's just a big pop, a whack of a stick and the piñata shatters and the candy pours out.

I don't know when this moment happened. It might be when Maggie and I looked at our certificates together and she started crying and I put my arm around her. That's when my life changed, because instead of warmth of closeness, I wanted to crawl away, the click of a cog, the next step. It sank into me, a realization made suddenly clear, a contrast from the moments that filled up our lives before. We weren't kids anymore, and we weren't going to be together forever. A teenager's mind isn't ready for that.

I pulled HEAT DEATH OF THE UNIVERSE. I already knew what that was, but I had to explain it to Maggie. I started to explain it to her to distract her from what she had pulled, because it was also pretty unique. My valiant efforts didn't work. Three days later and we were sitting on her bed with her parents downstairs worrying and worrying, filling the house with the sickly smell of anxiety. After all these years of having the blood readings, people were still slaves to it. Stephen Hawking would say that we're slaves to order, but it seemed pretty chaotic at Maggie's house.

Maggie was worried and weepy. I couldn't blame her. CANCER or PLANE CRASH or HEART ATTACK were what you expected to pull, and those are things you can deal with. They seem distant and unreal, like life was before we had the machine and its holograms and red-dyed paper and you knew that because your grandparents both died of heart attacks that you were prone to that, too. The machine gave us more order, but it didn't really take away the chaos.

"It means I'm going to live for a really long time," I said. "I don't think anybody else has pulled that. At least nobody I know of. I guess it's kind of a big deal."

"I've never heard of it," she said.

I shrugged. "It's when all the heat in the universe dies, right? Atoms stop spinning. It'll be really cold. It's all kind of theoretical, though. Well, it was."

"How long will you live?"

I was embarrassed—she was envious of me. I expected a lot of people would be. I didn't see what the big deal was, though. The woman I loved had pulled NUCLEAR BOMB.

"It's about ten centillion years away," I said. "I looked it up."

"Is that a real number?"

"Yeah. It's ten with about three hundred zeroes behind it."

"How could somebody live that long?"

I shook my head and stared at my feet. "I can't even imagine."

Her hands were trembling. She ran her fingers through her hair and clutched her stomach. She was crying again.

"Other people will pull NUCLEAR BOMB," she said. "They have to. A nuclear bomb doesn't kill just one person."

"You have to stop obsessing about it," I said, quietly. "It's not helping anything."

"How can I not think about it?" she said. I couldn't believe she still had enough water in her to cry again, but she did. She cupped her hands over her face. I hated seeing her so sad.

"You can't do this, Maggie," I said. "You just can't."

"We have to tell somebody about it," she said. "This is something everybody needs to know."

"I don't think that's a good idea," I said.

"But what if—"

"You can't think about what-ifs. You have to think about school and graduating, okay? If it's a problem, somebody else will pull it.

You know that's true. If there's going to be a nuclear bomb, then other people will get it. Just like September 11."

"That happened because people didn't talk about what they got!"

"Do you think that would have helped? If they had told people what they got, then how do you know it wouldn't have happened anyway? It had to happen, Maggie. That's what they pulled."

"Don't you think it's weird that nobody told anybody else what they got?" She was starting to raise her voice. I didn't want that to be our first argument.

I put my hand on her knee.

"Don't tell me you believe that stuff," I said. "Just because some guys on YouTube say it's a conspiracy doesn't mean it is."

"Have you watched it?"

"No," I said. "But I read about it. Look, Maggie, that's silly. There were thousands of people there. How would the government get them all to work at the same building? Or to fly on the same plane?"

"The people in the Pentagon pulled MISSILE," she said. "It's true."

"That's just a rumor. It's an urban legend. Stop it, Maggie."

"I'm scared," she said, her anger melting into convulsing sobs.

I put my arm over her shoulder and hugged her close to me.

After September 11, Stephen Hawking didn't comment on the conspiracy, because nobody had really thought about it. In a letter to the New York Times, he said that order was winning, even though it seemed like it wasn't. War and terrorism are agents of chaos, he said, but the Western world was the bastion of order, and that we would win. Bringing peace and democracy was just another way of bringing order. We were more powerful. We would win, and the Middle East would be quiet and peaceful, eventually. The American military was the ice cube. I thought about that a lot.

—‡—

It was all over the news within a few days. Other people had pulled NUCLEAR BOMB and went public with it, but not Maggie. Her parents were pretty down on the government, and went to war protests and things, and they were worried about what they would do with the information. They didn't want their daughter to be put through the wringer of the Patriot Act, which is what a lot of people were expecting.

Since it was illegal to get your blood read before you were 18, and nobody older than that had pulled the nuke, everybody just assumed it was going to happen much later, decades down the road, when all fifteen people who had pulled the nuke just happened to be in the same place at the same time where a nuclear bomb would go off.

I didn't talk much about what I had pulled because it was so strange. It seemed so weird that somebody would live so long. It was crazy to even consider, but I was thinking about that a lot at the time, and thinking about how if you pull something it's pretty likely to happen.

Within a few weeks, the FBI was all over our town. They were all over other towns, too, like spiders, building webs between the Nuclear Kids, as the NUCLEAR BOMB pullers were being called by the press. The FBI interviewed me, and asked me politely to see my cert, which I did, because I didn't want to cause trouble. There were two agents, a man and a woman. They seemed young, too young to be carrying guns around. The man saw my cert and scrunched his nose up and showed the woman, and she shook her head.

"What does that mean?" she said, to me. I shrugged.

"I'm not sure," I said. It was kind of a lie.

"Have you told anybody else?"

"Just my girlfriend. My parents don't know."

"Why didn't you tell your parents?"

"I didn't want them to worry."

"Then you *do* know what this means," she said, pointing to the cert in her hand.

"I sort of do," I said. "It's when all the heat in the universe dies. It's sort of the end of the universe, I guess."

"That can't be real," she said, to me, as if I were lying to her.

"That's what it says," I said. "It's never wrong, is it?"

"No," she said, shaking her head. "No, it isn't."

"Hey, this kid's a genius," said the man, who was looking at the trophy on my shelf. The trophy wasn't for Being a Genius, it was for a Whiz Kids competition a few years earlier.

The woman looked over his shoulder at the trophy. "A lot of kids win those."

"No, he invented something. Right?"

"Sort of," I said.

"An immortality machine," said the woman.

"I discovered a new kind of algae," I said.

"That's it," said the man. "With holistic properties."

"No," I said. "It's just algae."

"I thought I read that somewhere," he said. "It kills cancer or something."

"I haven't heard that," I said.

"Oh. I must have made it up. Sorry to bother you."

"It's OK," I said, relieved that they would be going.

"Hey, one more thing," he said. His partner put my cert back on the desk. She hovered over it for a few moments, shaking her head, as if she still couldn't believe what it said. "What did your girlfriend pull?"

"She wouldn't tell me," I lied. "She says it's private."

"But you told her yours," he said.

"Yeah," I said.

"You don't think it's private?"

"It can be, I guess."

"But not to the kid who's going to live to the end of the universe, right?"

"Yeah," I said. "I guess so. I really didn't think about it much."

"Hey, if you find a cure for cancer, let me know, okay?" he said, smirking.

"Yeah, sure," I said. "Does it matter, though? If you pulled CANCER, right?"

He looked at the woman, who shrugged and walked out of the room. He looked back at me.

"I didn't pull CANCER," he said. "But you never know."

"Yeah," I said. "I guess it wouldn't matter if you did."

He chuckled and put his hands in his pockets. "Cancer can cause a lot more than death. A cert is just how it ends, right? It's not the whole story."

Sometimes you can feel the changes coming. You can't sleep right the night before, and you're tired and not dealing with your feelings very well, and you're not prepared for it when it happens. Maybe it's order asserting itself, freezing the top layers while the stew roils and boils underneath, like when my mom puts chicken soup in the fridge so the fat rises to the top and hardens and she can ladle it out.

I had a lot of nasty dreams about car accidents and jigsaw puzzles and big, long scars on Maggie's face and her teeth falling out.

The next day was the first day of school after the big New Year's break. There were police cars all over the parking lot, and some government cars. I walked to homeroom, and the man from the FBI was there. He nodded to me as I sat down at my desk. My homeroom teacher looked nervous, and told me to have a seat. I wondered how Maggie was.

"You've probably heard on the news," she said. I hadn't, and a few other kids hadn't, either, so she started to explain. She was having trouble finding the right words.

"There are a few other people who have pulled...something that might not be good for the rest of us. And Agent Williams here is—"

Agent Williams, the FBI guy who looked too young to carry a gun, put his hand on her shoulder and stepped forward.

"No need to get excited, kids," he said, because some of the others were starting to raise their hands. "This is just a routine investigation. We got permission from the school board to have you all tested, in some cases for the second time." He looked right at me and smirked a little. "It's all going to be very smooth and organized, so I don't want anybody freaking out, okay?"

Nobody freaked out. They converted the gym to a big laboratory, with beds and curtains everywhere and the blood-reading machines set up in the corners. Some of the younger kids cried when they got their blood taken, but that was all. Doctors and nurses and other people in blue scrubs and lab coats were all over the place, carrying racks of samples to the machines.

They put us in our homerooms and told us not to wander off, but the force of that authority was fading. The teachers looked more worried than the kids, and weren't really paying attention. I didn't have the nerve to get up and find Maggie, but she would try to find me. I decided it was best to stay put.

I sat on the gym floor with a few of the other kids, nerds like me, except while I had found a place all by myself in the wide, deep strata of high school culture, they had stuck together and taken the chess club and the computer club stratum as their own, as the previous nerds and geeks had graduated after initiating them. Now they were on top, the smartest kids in school. Well, except for me.

"Hey, Brian," said one of the nerds, a kid whose name I couldn't remember. I think it was Jake, but I never really cared to learn it. He was a junior. "What did you pull?"

"That's a personal question," I said, not taking my eyes away from the book I was reading, Stephen Hawking's book, the one that had gotten me thinking so much. I had to read it again, and was reading it a lot. I was back at the part where he was describing the machine's inner workings. He thinks the machine hangs on a cosmic string, tied like a noose around our necks.

"You don't have to tell me," he said. "I was just curious."

"I didn't pull the nuke," I said.

"I hope I do," said the Junior, proudly. He had obviously been thinking about it.

"That's stupid," I said.

"No it isn't," he said, but not just to me. The other nerds were shaking their heads and rolling their eyes. This kid was probably the one with all the stupid theories. Every friend group has one. "Do you know how a nuke kills you? You're incinerated. You probably won't even know it's coming. That's a lot better than EMPHYSEMA or something. Do you know how EMPHYSEMA kills you? You drown in your own mucous."

"You're crazy," I said.

"Oh really? Why? What, did you pull EMPHYSEMA? Or AIDS?"

"Shut up," I said.

"I'm telling you, the nuke is the way to go."

"There are lots of ways a nuke can kill you," I said. "Not just in the first blast, either. Do you know how radiation poisoning kills you? Say you take about a thousand rads or so. For the first few days, you're fine. You don't even know anything's wrong. You might even feel great, like you just got laid, but that's a bad example because you don't know what that's like."

A couple of the other nerds giggled.

"But then you start getting diarrhea, as the cell walls in your intestines break down and die. It's not just 'I ate too many M&Ms'

diarrhea, either. It's bloody and chunky. That lasts for a few days, and then you go crazy from the pain and the diarrhea and the radiation scrambling your circulatory system, and you start bleeding out of every hole in your body."

I had the nerds squirming. A couple of them stood up and walked away. The Junior stared at me with the same expression he probably had when his mom told him there was no such thing as Santa Claus.

"But you're right," I said. "I hope you pull the nuke, too. It's a better way to die, right?"

I didn't care about the rules anymore, and I wanted to make a good exit. I went over to the bleachers. I still didn't see Maggie anywhere. I asked one of her friends where she was, but her friend didn't know. She said her parents had come to take her out of school after homeroom. She wasn't the only one, either.

"I heard you pulled OLD AGE," said her friend, after a few awkward moments of standing around, like teenagers do.

"Where did you hear that?"

"I dunno. Just a rumor I guess. People were asking me like I should know."

"I didn't pull OLD AGE. Nobody does."

"That's not true," she said. "My mom's first boyfriend did."

"Did you actually see his cert?"

"No," she said. "Why would my mom lie about it?"

"I don't know," I said. "It just seems kind of implausible."

"Why?" I got that question a lot.

I shrugged. "It's really ambiguous."

"So? Lots of certs are ambiguous."

"Don't mistake the exception for the rule," I said.

"What?" She was getting annoyed. I got that a lot, too.

"Just because somebody gets a weird, ambiguous cert doesn't mean they all are. Or even most of them."

She shrugged and looked away.

"I was wondering," she said. "Did you and Maggie do it?"

"That's private," I said. She didn't see me blush.

"Yeah," she said. "You know what you said about ambiguous stuff? I was thinking. I think that's what it's all about, you know? It's ambiguous for a reason. That's why nobody pulls YOUTH."

"That's silly," I said. "Nobody pulls OLD AGE, either."

"Whatever," she said, and shrugged and walked away.

People were always walking away from me. I started to think that if I was going to live forever, I was going to be pretty lonely.

I tried to call Maggie, but her parents weren't answering the phone. I went to bed sad and worried, so I snuck one of my mom's Tylenol PMs to help me sleep.

That stuff gives me weird dreams. I dreamed I was standing on a charred ball of dirt, like a chunk of hamburger that sticks to the grill, all wrinkled and black and ashy. I watched the sun gutter and spit and go out, like a wick on a dead candle. It was cold. My breath came out and crystallized in front of me, a growing cloud of spiky ice.

Some dreams are like an emotion magnified into a wide, flat layer and wrapped around your whole brain, so everything that happens in the dream is stained with it. I woke up in the middle of the night, convinced that I was the only person left on earth, in the universe. Reality filtered in slowly, muffled and grey. I heard my dad snoring in the next room, and pulled the blankets close. I got myself back to sleep by imagining Maggie next to me. I missed her warmth.

It was happening all over the country. By the next day, the number of kids who had pulled the nuke was over a thousand. A lot of people were starting to get worried. I stopped watching the news with my parents because I couldn't stop thinking about Maggie and what was going to happen to her, or what was going to happen to all the other people who had pulled it. Everybody was comparing it to 9/11. Now that we know that these people are going to die from a nuke, maybe we can do something about it. Maybe we can avoid another one.

A lot of parents didn't want their kids to get their blood drawn, and kept their kids home. The FBI was using the Patriot Act to get their blood by force. I started to think that Stephen Hawking was wrong, that chaos was going to win. A nuclear bomb is pretty much the definition of chaos, after all.

I walked to Maggie's house after school. She was anxious, but I think seeing me made her feel better. We hugged in her kitchen, and her mom and dad left the room to leave us alone. Her parents didn't mind. The boy genius who would live forever could go console the Nuclear Kid.

I had only been there for a few minutes when they came to test her. Her parents were furious but powerless, which made them even more furious. They looked at me when the FBI agents came to the door, as if I could do anything. Agent Williams was there with some cops and an ambulance that the government was renting out. It had a machine in the back, humming as it warmed up.

I sat on Maggie's bed, waiting. I listened to her iPod. She was listening to a lot of Tori Amos lately, songs about rape and wrath.

Williams came into the room and sat down on the bed. I muted the iPod, Tori's pounding piano ringing echoes in my ears.

He looked concerned, and then looked away, pretending to scrutinize the posters on Maggie's wall.

"It's scary, I know," he said.

I didn't respond, hoping my stare would drive him away.

"I guess you've got it made, though. A couple of trillion years, right?"

"I guess so," I said.

"There will be a lot of girls to love," he said, suddenly, like he couldn't keep it in anymore, in that fragile moment where small talk cracks and shatters under the weight of Bigger Issues. "My high school girlfriends are distant memories. I hardly ever think about them."

"Thanks," I said.

He chuckled, and said "I'm glad they're still teaching sarcasm."

"What are you going to do to them?"

"I'm not going to do anything," he said.

"Until they tell you to."

"Don't make more of this than it is. Nothing like this has ever happened before. If we can see something coming, don't you think we should do something about it?"

"What does it matter? If I'm not going to die in a nuke, what if I stayed right by her? Moved in, worked from home, holed up in a bunker? I'm still not going to die of a nuke."

Williams sighed and rubbed his eyes with his palms, then sat back on the bed, resting his shoulders on Maggie's *The Nightmare Before Christmas* poster. Jack Skellington loomed over his shoulder, grinning.

He reached into his wallet and pulled out a yellow, crumpled cert. The stamp had been worn away, and the corners were soft and blunt.

"It's only fair," he said.

I tried to act disinterested, I tried to be disinterested, but curiosity moved my hand.

It was his cert, and the cause of death was OLD AGE. I stared at him, ready to accuse him of faking it.

He shook his head and took it out of my hand. He pushed play on the iPod, and left me to myself.

Tori sang about earthquakes.

The universe began as a wad of crumpled paper. Since then, invisible hands have been smoothing it out. Stephen Hawking thinks the machine makes those hands human, and makes them move faster.

Nobody pulls YOUTH because there's no ambiguity. The exception is the rule. There is so much irony that it has lost its meaning. A metaphor can kill, a homonym can predict. Nobody pulls YOUTH because there's no joke in it.

Hawking is wrong because the order is imposed, it's an ice cube made of human thought. We believe the cube freezes the lava, but it's just as hot as it was before.

I poked around on the Internet for a little while. The numbers were up. Three thousand, now. Rumors of camps being set up in the desert. Tent cities for children. The government won't comment. The ambulance in front of Maggie's house says enough.

The ambulance pulled away with Williams in the passenger seat. He saw me at the window and waved.

Did he know what I was planning to do? He planted the seed, after all. I took it as a blessing.

Maggie came back to her room and sat down mechanically on her bed next to me.

"You're nervous," she said. Maggie. Always worried about me, not worried enough about herself. I would have to worry for her.

"There are three heavy-metal bands called 'Heat Death of the Universe.' There are twelve books by that title and one independent movie. There are a hundred thousand Google hits with those words."

"I don't know what you're saying," she said.

"That FBI guy showed me his cert. He pulled OLD AGE, Maggie. It's true. It does happen."

I held her hand.

"I've figured it out. The exception is the rule. People pull OLD AGE but they don't pull YOUTH. Ambiguity is built into it. The machine doesn't tell us how we're going to die, it picks a word to describe it. It's unspecific for a reason."

"For what reason? You're scaring me."

"I don't know," I said. "A joke, maybe. Or a test. You can't die of youth but you can be shot by a young person. You can die of old age but you can also be killed by an old person. What you pull is what you're going to die of, but it's just language. It's just words. It doesn't define anything until you start acting on it. Until you force it. We make the order out of the chaos, but the chaos is still there if we want it. That's how people deal with the certs and the machine and knowing how you're going to die. They just don't think about it. They don't act on it. They just live their lives."

She didn't like my enthusiasm.

"It's not a joke," she said. "There's nothing funny about nuclear war."

"Your cert doesn't say NUCLEAR WAR. It says NUCLEAR BOMB. That can mean a thousand things, and only one of those is nuclear war."

"Then why is everybody so worried?"

"September 11. Hiroshima. Chernobyl. Governments can't take the risk, or don't want to. I can't really blame them. Last year, a hundred thousand people died of INFLUENZA. I looked that up too. What if they put all those people in one place? What if they rounded them up and put them in camps?"

"I don't know," she said, watching me talk, watching me gesture. She looked worried, maybe a little scared. I squeezed her hand.

"That would make something happen, Maggie. That's what takes the chaos away. That's what forces the order. It's not the certs that crystallizes the order into something sharp, it's us. It's what we do with them."

"What does that have to do with the flu?"

"Because if you force everybody together, then they won't just all get the flu randomly at once. That's not how it works. It would be bad, Maggie. The universe or order or God or whatever would have to impose a way on those people for them all to die of the same thing. Like bird flu, or something worse. It would be an outbreak, probably. It would be bad."

"But if nobody else pulled flu, it wouldn't matter."

"Not everybody dies of the bird flu. The cert isn't the whole story, it's just the end. It's just the last couple of words in your story. If there's a big flu outbreak, lots of other bad things will happen. Rioting and violence and food shortages. Now all those people who pulled STARVATION or GUNSHOT will have the order crystallized for them, too. It's going to be really bad, Maggie. But we're not talking about the flu, it's even worse. It's a nuclear bomb. I can't even imagine what's going to happen."

I took a deep breath and held her other hand. "I pulled HEAT DEATH OF THE UNIVERSE, but that doesn't mean I'm going to die in a centillion years. It can mean anything. It's just words. It's just the end of the story. That's what your cert can be, too. The end of the story, not the whole thing. We have to go, Maggie."

"What are you—"

"Don't argue, OK? We have to go. Far away. Into the wilderness somewhere."

"We don't know anything about the wilderness!"

"We'll learn. There are lots of places to hide out there."

"I don't want to," she said. She was starting to cry again.

"They're building camps in the desert. You know that, right?"

"Yes," she said, quietly.

"To put you all there, away from the rest of us. They're taking away the ambiguity. They're crystallizing the causality. They're going to make a nuke go off there, Maggie."

"They wouldn't do that! Would they?"

"Oh, I don't know. I don't think so. But they won't have to. Hawking is right, but for the wrong reasons. Order is taking over because we're imposing it. The chaos is still there, but the machine lets us choose not to take it. A nuke is going to go off there because that's what all the people pulled. If you put a lot of people together with that reading, it's the only way it can happen."

"Oh God," she said. She was silent for a long time, and I was out of breath. Finally, she looked at me, red rims around her eyes.

"We have to go," she said.

I'm not sure where we'll end up. Maggie suggested finding her uncle, the one out in the woods somewhere. She doesn't know exactly where he is, but he'll know more about surviving out there than we do. She has a few ideas of where he is, so we'll start there.

Maggie might still be worried, but she isn't showing it. I've given her some hope, and she's given me some, too. Hawking might be right, but I don't think he is.

I feel better about my own cert, too. I'm leaving the ambiguity on the table, next to this document. Mom, Dad, I'm sorry for taking the car and taking some money. I think you know it's for the best. Maggie and I aren't going to be slaves to order like everybody else. I understand why the government is going to put people in those camps. I don't think they have a choice. All those people who pulled PLANE CRASH and FALLING and BURNED ALIVE in September 11 didn't tell anyone what they got. There wasn't a database tracking them. That didn't happen because it was inevitable, it happened because a bunch of terrorists made it happen. Nobody who died on September 11 pulled TERRORISM. There's no joke in it.

My certificate, my reading, isn't the whole story. I'm writing it as I go, day after day, with Maggie next to me. I don't know how things will go, or how we're going to survive.

I only know how it ends.

Story by James Foreman
Illustration by Ramón Pérez

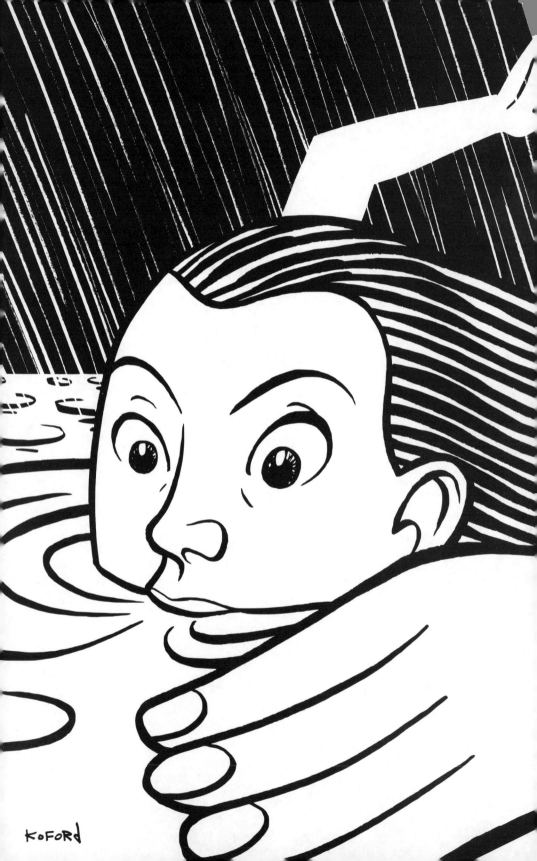

DROWNING

I saw the first ads in March. A week or two later it was all over the news, and then for the next few months you could not get away from it. Still, none of us expected it to have the impact it did. It was a killer. By November I had only had eight or nine dreams when I used to have three or four a week. This is how I make my living. I have a dream and then I wait. Eventually they come to the office or sometimes I run into them somewhere else, we talk about it, and they give me money. At least, that is how it had been working.

Right then I was down to my last week's worth of savings. I had sold my car in August and my stereo and most of my office equipment in September and every day I was looking around thinking about what to cannibalize next. I was getting more and more pessimistic.

Then I had a dream that I thought was a paying one and I woke up that morning feeling pretty good, not a hundred percent but maybe sixty-five. In the dream I was painting a room with a small bunch of lilies. Specifically, I was back working for Denny Mankino.

I had worked for Denny for two miserable years before I started this new line of work. Denny was a nice enough guy most of the time but maybe two days a week he was a nightmare. He always apologized afterwards, and always paid on time, but I was still thinking about going to work for someone else. I had my first dream around then.

The dream was about our client. She was a nice person I did not know a thing about, other than she always said hi and once she brought me a coffee. In the dream, she was swimming in a pool filled with milk, trying to empty it by drinking as she swam. At the end of each lap the pool would be maybe half-full. The problem was that the whole time she was swimming it was raining milk. Not hard, but enough to keep filling the pool. Now the strange part, as opposed to the weird part, was that in a barn maybe thirty yards away, a farmer was spinning a millstone. It was a huge, regular millstone-type millstone, but he spun it like it weighed nothing, like it was a lazy Susan on your kitchen counter. This is what was making it rain. Like I said, strange. But it was just a dream and when I woke up I forgot about it.

That afternoon while Denny was out doing whatever he did, the client came home, walked up to me and started pouring out a dream she had had in which I was holding an invoice she had to pay. She did not even take off her coat, just walked right up to me and started talking.

I had no idea what was happening and thought maybe she was not a nice person but a maniac and I was about to find out how wrong I had been, but then I noticed that she was drinking from a big carton of milk and my dream came back to me like a bolt of shimmery cloth unfurling across the floor.

We went into the kitchen, sat down, and I told her all about it. When I got to the part about the guy, the farmer, she started paying close attention.

"He had a medium-sized freckle above his right eye, half in the eyebrow." She slowly nodded her head as though she knew what I would say next, and then got up and went over to the sink. I waited. When she finally turned around she said, "Can I give you some money?" She looked like a huge weight had been lifted off her. I was glad she was feeling better, but the notion of taking money kind of creeped me out.

"I beg your pardon?"

"You've just helped me. A lot."

I gave her a moment to tell me how but she did not. Instead she found her checkbook and wrote out a check. She handed it to me. It was for five thousand dollars, payable to 'cash.'

As you can imagine, I was dumbfounded, and I guess since I was not saying anything, she felt the need to. "The guy in your dream is my brother. At least, it makes perfect sense if he is. He died, nine years ago tomorrow."

"Oh. I'm sorry." I had no idea what I was supposed to do.

She wasn't finished. "And now, finally, I think I understand. I'm sorry, but I'm kind of freaked out by all this and I'd rather not talk about it. We don't have to talk about this anymore, do we?"

I didn't want to jinx either of us, and now that I had a great big check from nowhere, I didn't want to jinx it either, but I had no idea what we were supposed to do.

"I don't know. Let's see. If you have to tell me, I guess you can come find me. Are you sure you want to give me this? It seems like a lot."

She sat down and looked very calm and smiled a really nice smile. "Yes."

I waited, but she wasn't saying anything else. "Okay then."

She went back to the sink and poured out the milk, and I went back to work.

She never got back in touch with me so I never found out what it was all about, but her check was good. So there was that.

Within about six months the clients were coming pretty steadily. I quit working for Denny and got the office, and for maybe four or five years I made a nice living. It was kind of like I was just walking around, delivering things, but with no real time pressure, and at almost every stop people gave me money. Though it was kind of aimless, there was a weird logic to it all.

Then the machine came along.

I was not convinced that my new dream about Denny was a paying one. Who was supposed to be my client? Myself? That was creepy. The dream just did not make sense the way others had. So I sat in my office, waiting to see what was going to happen next. And then Mr. Watson came in, which I was absolutely not expecting at all.

Mr. Watson was the shop steward of my local, Local 111 of the S.S.C.W.I. For a long time I kind of thought the union was a scam, a way of conniving me out of 5% of my earnings, until they helped me out of a legal scrape that otherwise would have sunk me. That, and they offered a pretty good medical package that included dental, and of course a pension.

For a moment, just long enough to see that he was not my client, I looked at him without saying anything. He sat down on the corner of my desk and looked back at me. I had no idea what he was up to so I kept my yap shut. It must have looked pretty silly, both of us staring at each other, blank-faced, as though we were having some kind of conversation but without actually speaking.

He did not look good. He was in his late fifties and cultivated a Columbo look anyway: rumpled trench coat, cigarette, bad hair-cut and if you got close enough a deep, almost subliminal smell of smoke, but still. He was close enough that I smelled the smoke. That was his day job. He was an investigator for the fire depart-ment; the rumor was that he had a perfect record. I do not think this had anything to do with his side job, though; he was just a tenacious and thorough guy. He once explained that he was really only a witness anyway. "If you pay close enough attention," he'd said, "ninety-nine percent of the time it's obvious how it all burned down."

"Okay," he finally said, then got off the corner of my desk, walked over to the window, looked down at the street and then came back and sat in my client's chair, the one people used to sit in and then give me money from.

"You do any other work in here? A side job of some kind?" he said, taking in my steadily-emptying office.

"I was a house painter before this."

"That's right. That's not such bad work."

"I didn't mind it, but my boss had some real problems."

He looked around some more, nodding his head. "You don't even have a coffee machine?"

"Sold it. I can call down to the diner, they'll send one right up."

"The Brazilian place?"

"No, the other one."

"Oh. Yeah, sure."

I made the call. When I hung up he didn't say anything. He

seemed distracted, maybe even morose, which was not like him at all. He was generally a pretty light-hearted guy.

For laughs I started my spiel. I thought he might get a kick out of it. I sat on the edge of my chair, leaned comfortably forward onto the desk, looked him in the eye, and said in my most neutral voice, "So, I had this dream."

He gave me a very stern look. "This is no laughing matter," he said. He was really in a sour mood.

"But I did have a dream."

"Seriously now?"

"Well, kind of. I mean, I have one I'm working on but I don't know who the, uh, client is yet."

"Oh." He looked away, annoyed. "That's what we thought. Look, it's also why I'm here. We're having some problems down at the hall. As you might have heard, we got no orders coming in. You're maybe one of ten people who've had anything in the last six months or so. Ever since that fucking machine came along. So, I just came to tell you, and luckily you don't have any medical stuff going on, but we're going to have to cut back on medical coverage, substantially, and no more dental."

I had a dentist appointment next week. I was finally going to take advantage of the dental plan. This really was no joke.

I first met Mr. Watson maybe a month after I got my office. He walked into my waiting room one morning and said, "What kind of a waiting room is this if you got no magazines?"

I got up to see who it was and didn't recognize him. "I beg your pardon?"

"If this is your waiting room, where're the magazines?"

"I guess not many people actually wait there. Can I help you?"

He gave me a slightly surprised look. "Oh. I'm Jerry Watson, I'm the shop steward of Local 111 of the S.S.C.W.I."

I gave him a blank look.

"The Sub and Supra Consciousness Workers International. We call it the S.S.C.W.I., though, to keep from freaking people out."

He stuck out his hand and I took it. He had a firm, comfortable handshake and an open, honest face. Immediately, for no good reason at all, I liked him.

"I came by to take your application."

"My application?"

"To join the union. If you want. There's no pressure, honestly, but we do offer a pretty good health and benefits package, and we watch your back if things get out of control."

"Out of control?"

"Like that guy last month who didn't want to admit he was cheating on his wife? If that had gotten out of hand, we could step in for you. But, really, it's your choice. I have the form for the application here, and if you're accepted we'll mail you the medical and all the rest of that crap, so you can look it over at your leisure."

I was pretty surprised, as you might expect. Of all the big changes my life had been going through, I did not foresee this. I had not even belonged to the Painter and Plasterer's Union. There was something about Mr. Watson I trusted though. He reminded me of an uncle who would bail you out and keep it quiet. So when I got over my surprise I asked him the one thing that had really been nagging at me, figuring if anyone knew he would. Namely, what the hell was going on?

"Oh. Right. Well, it's like a swimming pool, a big swimming pool everyone swims in every day. Some for longer than others, but no one for too long because the water is too cold. The only ones who stay in for a long time are some coma victims, and a lot of them are kind of only half in, half out.

"Sometimes there're fewer people in the pool, and sometimes there're lots more, and when there're lots and lots more, we go out and get new hires."

"Like me?"

"I guess. I dunno, you ever have these dreams before?"

"I dunno."

"There you go. There're a lot more we don't know than we do."

The other workers in the local were, for the most part, just like me. Regular, boring people: accountants, lawyers, teachers, maintenance workers, actors. Most all of them kept their day jobs and no one made a big deal about this sideline. I suspect most would have even denied it if asked; it was all pretty far-fetched. The "union hall" was actually just the backroom of a diner where we met periodically, or if you had something come up, Mr. Watson or one of the other officers would meet you there.

"The problem is this new machine has been giving a lot of people the idea that they don't need to swim in the pool anymore. And that, as you might have guessed, has seriously screwed with the natural order of things."

"Huh. Is there anything we can do about it?"

"We're working on that."

We were both quiet for a moment. The coffee came, and after the guy left, I thought I might as well ask him. "You do it yet?"

He looked at me with a deeply annoyed look. I half expected him to tell me to blow it out my ass. I was not just giving him a hard time though, I really was curious about whether he had checked it out. These machines were scabbing our work and I wanted to know he was on top of it.

"You mind if I smoke?" he finally asked. I got the ashtray from the windowsill and put it on the desk, close to him.

He lit up, offered me one. I put up my hand. He leaned forward in his seat, took a sip of his coffee, and made a surprised face. "Wow, that's good coffee."

"Isn't it though? You'd never guess."

He put the cup back on the edge of my desk. "I did do it. Not just out of a sense of professional responsibility."

"So you were curious?"

"About what? How I'm going to die? Who gives a shit how they die? I'll die when I die and after I die I'll be dead, so what do I get from knowing 'how' I die? No, I had to know how it felt."

He squinted and looked past me out my window, made a small grimace like he had sciatica, then back.

"And it was weird. It wasn't what I expected. I was hoping it would be something big, you know, but it wasn't. I mean, all right, you suddenly know how you're gonna die and that's something I had to sleep on for a couple of nights to really get a handle on. But on a deeper level, on the level where we earn our living, well, let's just say I can see how it's polluting the waters.

"For about half an hour after I found out, I felt like I was catching a wave, like, you know when a car goes over a hump and you get that 'Whoa!' feeling? It was like that, and then on the other side of that I felt very calm, and at that moment I knew it was bullshit."

"Bullshit? But it works. It tells you how you're going to die."

"Well yeah, but that's not what it's selling. And they better not because it's fucking expensive so they sell it as the be-all and end-all. Which is the bullshit part, because they're selling peace of mind, and we all know peace of mind is a racket." He finished his cigarette and stubbed it out in the ashtray. "What did you think of it?"

I tried to give at least half a smile. I wanted to tell him what I thought he wanted to hear, but I could not. Ever since third grade when Sister Anne-Marie found out I was lying about eating the choc-olate eggs in the Easter display and wailed for a solid half-hour, I just do not have it in me. Call it coercive but I loved Sister Anne-Marie, and every time I'm faced with the opportunity to lie I see her sweet-ness and know lying will once again break her heart and I cannot do it. Surprisingly, this has brought me far less trouble than you might think.

"I haven't done it."

He seemed taken aback. I didn't think he would be so surprised. I almost wished I could un-say it.

"You what? This is your vocation."

"I know and you're right. But it just smells of really bad luck and I can't bring myself to do it."

"Bad luck?" He suddenly looked like he'd never thought of it that way, and wasn't sure if it was worth the effort. "Bad luck," he said again, and then suddenly started to lighten up.

His phone rang and he dug it out of a pocket, bringing his pack of cigarettes up with it. He lit one up as he answered. He made a couple of grunting noises and stood up, then put his phone away. "I gotta go. Work."

The office suddenly felt very small and hot and I had to leave too. I had to. I stood up with him and grabbed my jacket. "Let me walk down with you."

He seemed to have let go of any misgivings he had about my choice. In fact, he seemed happy now.

In the stairwell he turned back to look up at me. "I'm gonna die by drowning." He gave a little "would you get a load of that" eyebrow bump as he said it.

"Really?"

"Yeah. So I just bought a boat."

"What if you pass out in the tub?"

"Exactly! Those fucking assholes. I wish I could get the Teamsters on their asses."

We got out to the street. It was cold. It was supposed to be warm today. At least, that's what the weatherman had said this morning.

Mr. Watson stopped at his Fire Department car, which was parked at a hydrant. He had a ticket under the windshield wiper.

"Sorry about the bad news, kid. Maybe things will turn around, and in six months we'll all be back at work."

He stuck out his hand and I shook it. It was strong but not overbearing, like he could pick me up and put me on his shoulders if he felt like it. Like he was going to do that at any instant. I instantly felt a huge surge of confidence. "Yeah, maybe so."

"I think it will. Sit tight. Hey, I hear that diner around the corner —the one run by the Brazilian couple—has a great lunch deal."

That was a great idea. I didn't want to go back inside and it was close enough to lunchtime. I was hungry, wasn't I? I was. "Yeah, I think I'll go by there."

"Good idea. You do that. Take care of yourself, kid," he said, and for a moment he sounded almost sad. He got into his city car, plucking the ticket off the windshield, and disappeared into the traffic.

I'd been to the Brazilian place a couple of times, and as soon as I passed through the front door I remembered their meat dishes were pretty good, but not much else was. I thought about turning around but what the hell, I was already there. I took a seat at the counter and my neighbor looked at me and then jumped. "Holy crap! Nick! I was just thinking about you!"

It was Denny. I could not believe it and then I did.

For a solid two seconds, maybe even three—which is a long time for this kind of mistake—I was confident he was my client. Mr. Watson was right, it was all going to turn around. I relaxed, sat back and got ready for the moment when I would tell him about my dream.

Denny did not notice. He was still all enthused to see me. "You were a great worker, you know that? I don't think I ever told you, and I never realized it until later, but you were one of the best workers I ever had. I owe you an apology for all the shit you must have put up with."

Despite myself I laughed. He seemed really, genuinely happy

to see me. Which was nothing like the scowling, surly bastard he'd been. He looked better, too; his skin was clearer, and he looked me in the eye with nothing but pleasure at seeing me.

"That's nice of you, Denny. How're things?"

"Oh, pretty good. Pretty great, actually. I met this girl, Lucky, and I got sober. I don't think you knew that. I'm an alcoholic."

He looked at me candidly, with a touch of sad self-deprecation. I did not know this about him, and was surprised.

"I'm sober now two years and almost seven months."

"Wow. Denny that's great. Really. I'm really happy for you."

Denny looked at his watch. The plate in front of him was empty. I suddenly realized he wasn't in his painter's whites.

"You're not painting anymore?"

"Oh, I still have the business but no, I got people to do the work. Hey, I'm sure you're not interested, but if you want work I got a spot for you. Your own truck. If it works out, maybe a crew. Lucky is setting up a health package and stuff and maybe I could offer that soon."

Denny was like a different person, it was all kind of hard to believe. I suddenly thought that must have been some kind of woman he met.

He was holding his card out to me. It was crisp and expensive-looking. He used to peel them off a paint-soaked stack that lived in the bottom of a bag. He would hand you this dirty, half-ripped piece of crap with a faded rainbow logo and you just knew he was a loser. This card was the exact opposite.

I looked at the card without reaching for it. Denny got a softer look, as though he suddenly realized maybe he was being too hard for the circumstances, like he often used to be. I noticed this and smiled. He wasn't sure what to do with that and proffered the card again.

I'm not the kind that believes we are faced with the inevitable every day, but at times the future is, genuinely, unavoidable, and you have to be a fool to try to get out of its way.

The pool expands, the pool contracts.

I took the card.

Story by C. E. Guimont
Illustration by Adam Koford

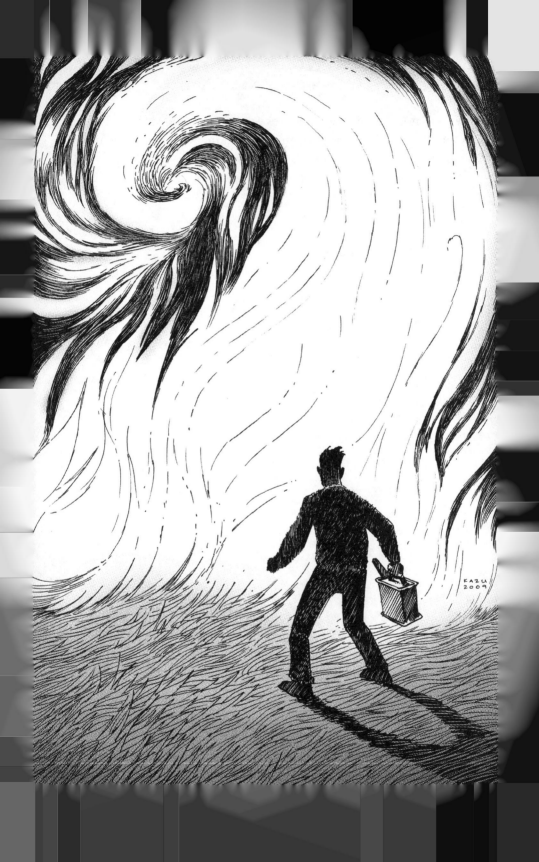

?

HE HAD NOT READ HIS SLIP OF PAPER. It was folded in an envelope in his left pocket. In his right pocket were several books of matches, and he was wearing a backpack. He pushed his way through the scrubby pine trees on the west border of the barrens.

"This isn't how it works, you know. The machine is playing word games."

He hopped across a clear stream, feet sinking into the sandy bank on the other side, wetness seeping over the soles of his sneakers. Water was bad. He needed dry brush.

"The universe doesn't work by word games. You have to think with words to play word games."

He kicked at a snake, daring it to bite, but it disappeared into the undergrowth.

"You can't just say what's going to happen ahead of time. That's not how physical law works. That's narrative. And when reality is twisted to fit narrative, that's not natural. That's someone making stories happen."

A few strands of spiderweb brushed his cheek and eyelash, and he swatted at the air around his face. He was climbing higher. He spotted a cluster of dry-looking bushes in the fading light, and took one of the kerosene bottles from his backpack.

"We have tales about this. The Oracle makes a prediction, and it comes true in an ironic way. Every legend has them. But that's how you tell the legends apart from reality. In reality, the magic doesn't work."

He unscrewed the cap on the kerosene bottle and started splashing the liquid over the dead leaves. He continued until the bottle was empty and the brush was thoroughly soaked.

"There are paradoxes, too. Playing word games only frees you from them for so long. You're messing with things, somehow, keeping people dying the right way no matter what we do. If we watch long enough we'll see your hand move. I'm not stupid. You can't just change things like this."

The breeze was strong and westerly, and there was plenty of brush downwind. He struck a match, stared for a moment, and then dropped it among the fuel-soaked leaves.

"Physics works by saying that if you set things up like so, this is what will happen. Curses say that no matter how you set things up, this is what will happen. And curses don't work. They never have. That's not how our universe goes. They're in all of our stories, but that's 'cause we're people, and we can figure out a way to make them adapt to each new situation. It takes a mind to do that."

The grove was ablaze. He turned from the heat and walked away.

"It takes a mind," he repeated as he went, "and yet those people are all dead, just as their papers predicted. So where does that leave us?"

There was no answer. He reached the car. It was a Chevy Nova with no glass in the back window. He had bought it for $300, cash.

"I never expected an answer. I never thought the priest or the rabbi or the monk knew any more than I did. I was at peace with an uncaring universe. So what the hell is this all about? For the first time, a chance at some answers, and you're playing games?"

He pulled out onto the freeway, and settled the speedometer at seventy. Any faster and he might get pulled over. In any event, the car wouldn't go any faster.

"Are you even paying attention? Am I just talking to myself? Maybe you're on autopilot. Maybe you haven't noticed me yet."

He drove silently for an hour, then got off at a random exit.

"You can't just announce that it's all been a game and then expect me to keep playing. I spend my life waiting for some fucking answers and then you wave this in front of me. I'm not going to sit around and passively watch how it all plays out and laugh at your cleverness. I want to talk to you. I want to know who the hell you are."

He passed an all-night Wal-Mart parking lot, drove on for half a mile, and turned right onto a dirt road. He followed it for a bit, then turned off the road and maneuvered the car between the trees down into a small ravine, where the wheels stuck in the mud. He turned off the car, took his backpack, and walked toward the Wal-Mart.

"So who are you, anyway? Are you what waits on the other side, with the papers guiding us to you? Or are you a petty, stupid animal like us, a level above but just as lost, playing games? Do you know your own destiny, your own end? Does the same reaper who collects our souls wait, somewhere, for you? What does it say on YOUR piece of paper?"

He reached the parking lot, and walked down the rows of cars. He found an old Reliant K with a cold hood—good, its owners probably wouldn't return for a while—took a crowbar from his backpack, broke the window, opened the door, and climbed inside. He fumbled around with the wires under the steering wheel, hoping that there would be an obvious pair of wires labeled "CONNECT THESE TO HOTWIRE CAR" but in the end he had to pry the ignition apart and turn the rotator switch to start the car. He pulled out onto the street and headed back toward the freeway, wind buffeting his face through the shattered window. Maybe someone had seen him at the

barrens, but they'd be looking for a Chevy Nova. Keep changing
cars. Can't get caught by a roadblock once they notice the pattern.
Have to do this right.

"I'm not afraid anymore. But I'm angry. This isn't right. This
isn't natural. We're being pushed around, and I want to know who
you are. Who the hell are you? What am I doing out here? I have a
mother, and a father, and brothers, and I'm on a highway in a stolen
car hundreds of miles from home, and I could die anywhere, and
it's all to play games with you so you'd better fucking come out and
talk to me!" He felt a tightness in his chest and a sudden lump in his
throat. He blinked away tears. "I'm not crazy. There are hundreds
of bodies buried with their little pieces of paper, and it's not natural,
and I want to know WHO THE FUCK YOU ARE." The words hurt
his own ears.

He drove for another hour, a Google Maps printout in his lap,
the location of the next fire marked with a red teardrop-shaped icon.

"In elementary school," he said, after a time, "kids would come
up to you and ask the question, 'Are you P.T.?' It was a trick question, of course. If you said yes, they called you a pregnant teenager.
If you said no, they'd say you weren't potty-trained. All you could do
was reject the question. You could even," he added conversationally,
"punch the kid in the mouth when he asked."

They'd probably see the pattern by morning. The local police
would be alerted, waiting near the locations of the last few fires.
He'd have to be careful.

"When the question doesn't make sense, you can reject it. But
this is much worse. Here, there's only one way out. And you're standing there next to it, grinning. Well, fine. You win. I can't quit. I'm
in your stupid game." He shifted in the seat and heard the envelope
crinkle in his pocket. He stared up at the stars through the glass.
"But I'm not reading your paper until you give me some answers."

—‡—

Morning drew near. Spot fires burned across the Ohio valley, forming a curious pattern. Perhaps someone out there would glance at the Earth, would see the great question mark he had burned into its skin. Perhaps the mind behind the Machine was deaf to his ramblings, but it had to notice the hundred-mile-tall message drawn in fire. It was the Machine's move now.

He sat on a flat stone in a Kentucky field, far from any roads. The police wouldn't find him here, not for a long time. He'd starve to death first.

"I don't know what you know, but I know I'm done searching half-heartedly for answers. I have your attention, across whatever space and time separates us. Whatever is going to happen to me can happen here. I'm not moving to eat or drink. If that's the way you've decided it will happen, then I guess that's the way it will happen. But it's your decision, not mine. You can't pretend you're ignoring this."

He lay back on the rock.

"So maybe I'll die here. Maybe this is how it ends, with my questions unanswered."

The setting moon hung over the horizon. People claimed it bore a face, but he had never been able to see it.

"But if you have even a bit of honesty in you, the paper in my pocket doesn't say 'SUICIDE.' It says 'MURDER.'"

There was no reply.

Story by Randall Munroe
Illustration by Kazu Kibuishi

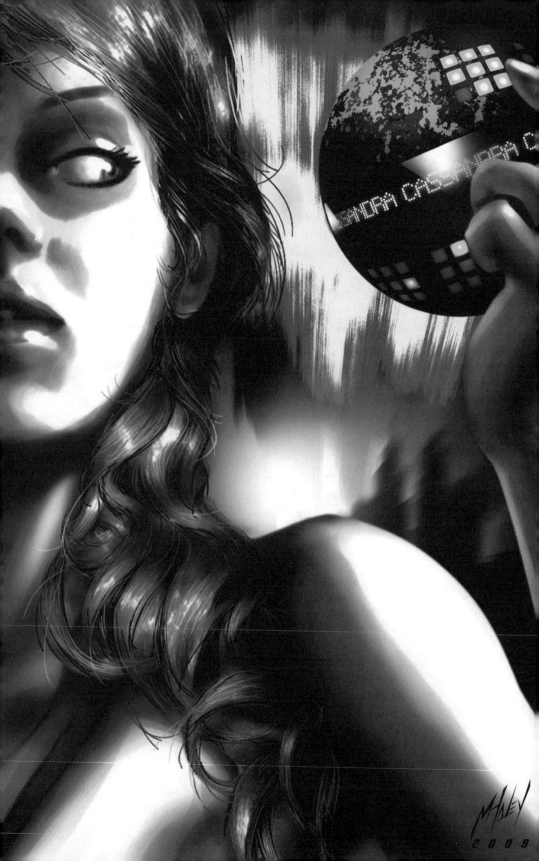

CASSANDRA

It was like that movie, back in the day, where the machine asks the kid, "How about a nice game of chess?"

"No," he types back. "Let's play Global Thermonuclear War."

That's what the slip of paper in my hand read. "Global Thermonuclear War."

I was sixteen years old. A girl, just about a woman.

You may have heard about the Delvice, which is what the marketing droids decided to call it back in the day when they thought it was going to change the world. The "Delphi Device." Clever, huh? Stick your finger in, feel a little prick, find out how you're going to die. There were jokes about some unfortunate early ad copy: "I'm just sorry for the guy who has everybody feeling his little prick." But it was really that simple, if anyone could figure out what it all meant.

Where did the words come from? The internals were simple: A few cells of your blood were vaporized by a laser, and the optical spectrum was fed into your basic quad-core PC running a huge neural net.

It had some limitations. The result was always in English. And while the machines never made an error when they were calibrated properly, like any other device, they could go wrong. Then they just produced plausible nonsense. People got predictions like "Colorless Green Ideas," which was meaningful enough to kill Chomsky's theory of language, but not much else.

The rest of the time the words had meaning, but not always the obvious meaning. Words are ambiguous. It has something to do with being a tool for thought.

Whatever the machine said, you usually lacked the context to interpret it properly. "Hit by car" might as easily refer to an amusement park ride as a highway mishap. "Crushed by a pig" might mean a block of iron or an angry sow. "Gunshot" covered the bases from artillery to BBs.

So despite the early predictions that it was going to change everything, it really didn't. I mean, what use is a prediction that seems tuned up to mislead? And who really wants to know? People had been ignoring doctors' advice for years. It was that much easier to ignore the output of a machine that you couldn't even ask for a second opinion.

It became a novelty for a generation: a "you-tell-me-yours-and-I'll-tell-you-mine" topic of conversation on a first date, and then faded into obscurity like any of a dozen other inventions whose time never quite came.

Did you know there was once a guy who built flying cars? Really. They worked, too. They just didn't work well enough to be popular enough to change anything. It's easy to build a novelty. It's hard to make the world reorganize itself so that what used to be a novelty becomes a necessity. Bill Gates managed it with personal computers. Henry Ford with automobiles. Edison with electricity. Bell with telephony, and RCA with radio and television, even if they had to "borrow" the latter from Farnsworth. But not many others.

The Delvice never became a necessity, and novelties don't last. Some folks had fun with it, though. When I was doing research after getting my own prediction I found out about one guy who, for a while, ran a successful Web site that would generate a list of possible interpretations for any cause of death. The lists usually ran into the tens, sometimes the hundreds.

But it soon became obvious that a few short words just weren't enough to encode the kind of information people care about. Most of the time.

I never told anyone about the prediction I got. It hardly seemed to mean anything, especially once I'd read a few accounts of radical ambiguity. Words on paper from some ancient toy in a back-country mall that hadn't been maintained for decades. Maybe mine was a nonsense phrase that happened to look meaningful. Might as well ask the once-popular Magic 8-Ball something. It got "Outlook not so good" right. I don't know if anyone ever asked it about Internet Explorer.

The next few years of my life were full of the usual girly things: boys, toys, sports, and school. Despite dire predictions in the early years of the new millennium, things were shaping up not too badly, and by mid-century anyone with a brain could get along pretty well.

I completed a double-major in business and math, and found myself working in New York as a second assistant actuary. The Chief Actuary was a wizened old man with a gentle smile and an old-fashioned manner that hid a timid and conventional mind. There's something about being in the business of predicting death that attracts the mediocre. But a job is a job, and with student loans to pay off it was good money and a convenient place to start what at that time I liked to think of as the long climb over the bodies of my enemies, all the way to the top.

The Chief, as we called him, made a point of taking new associates out to lunch in the few weeks after their arrival at the firm, and

I took that opportunity to ask him about the Delvice. Having moved to the big city, I was thinking again about that strange prediction from years ago, wondering what it really meant, and imagining the tall smoky men nodding their broad-brimmed hats over the skyscrapers while pedestrians screamed through the streets like badly-inked extras in an old comic book.

I didn't feel comfortable approaching the issue directly, but got him talking about the old days, before gene-mapping and other death-prediction technologies were routine. He had some good stories to tell, mostly about the changes in courtship and marriage that resulted from routine paternity testing, but when I asked, "What about the Delvice? Isn't it a little surprising that it never caught on?" he looked like he'd swallowed a frog.

"Hardly surprising at all," he snapped. "It's a toy."

"Gene mapping was a toy once, too."

"Gene mapping was a tool, even when it was too cumbersome to use. It was clear from the beginning that we could create meaningful probability distribution functions based on people's genetic proclivities, even before routine measurement became possible. With gene mapping we could associate a given haplotype with a dozen possible causes of natural death, and sub-divide the population into risk categories accordingly. If someone had DFN-8 they were going to go deaf and have poor balance, and we knew what the odds were of them dying because of it.

"The Delphi Device was too well named. It never produced anything susceptible to statistical analysis. Two people might die of cancer at the age of seventy-five and one of them would be told 'Cancer' and the other 'Old Age'. Two people might die in the same car crash and one would be told 'Drunk Driver' and the other 'Blunt Force Trauma.' And the odds are that the one who had been drinking would get the drunk driver prediction.

"Actuarial art is not just about numbers, it's about categories, and we carefully choose categories of causes that matter to us. Diseases we can cure, accidents we can prevent, chronic conditions we can treat. Those are what matter. The Delvice used some *other* kind of categorization scheme, and it was too capricious to offer any statistical guidance, much less individual assurance."

I nodded and tried to look intelligently interested, although so far he hadn't said anything I didn't know. And nothing that explained his apparent hostility toward the machine.

"Then there was the time element. Suppose you knew you were going to die of heart failure. At what age? Without that little bit of information you really don't know anything that you didn't know before, even in the old days when we just had things like family history and lifestyle to go on.

"Finally, and most famously, there was the interpretation issue. I recall one case where a man was predicted to die from a falling meteorite. Astrophysicists spent a fortune following him around, waiting to get the rock still hot from its descent through the atmosphere. And of course he wound up dying in a museum during the making of a documentary about his predicament when one of the exhibits fell on him. So even in cases where there seemed to be no room for ambiguity there were too many possibilities."

"And no one ever tried to get past those issues?"

"Oh, we tried. I myself once headed up a division of the company that was tasked with finding a way to aggregate sufficient data to make statistically valid inferences from Delvice forecasts. It was very nearly the demise of my career." He grimaced at the painful memory. "At first it looked straightforward. There are techniques for dealing with imperfect data, but as someone once said, 'data' is not the plural of 'anecdote.' To perform any sort of statistical inference we must have some sort of homogeneity. And there wasn't any way of imposing that on the Delvitic results. In the end, my team was able to prove mathematically that there was a kind of maximum entropy

principle behind the predictive mechanism: prediction was only possible if the sum total of knowledge in the world remained constant.
Anything else would have violated the second law of thermodynamics, which even a poor statistician like me knows isn't going to
happen. So in a sense the feeling of knowledge that the Delvice predictions created was just that: a feeling. The simple fact of knowing
how you were going to die necessarily changed the world in such a
way that the knowledge couldn't do you any good. It didn't create
any new information—it just collected little bits of information from
a million places and concentrated them in one place.

"We called it the Ignorance Theorem. It was quite a significant
result from a purely theoretical perspective, and in fact the mathematician responsible later went on to win the Fields Medal for his
work on extended probability measures over non-Borel subsets.
He was obsessed with finding a loophole in his original result, possibly because his own Delvitic prediction involved something that
appeared both equally unlikely and unpleasant. To do with sex and
horses, as I recall."

I opened my eyes wide with slightly salacious girly curiosity at
this, and his pale skin took on a genteel flush, but he didn't fill me
in on either the details of the prediction or the actual fate of the
mathematician in question. (My later research showed it was every
bit as unlikely, and far more unpleasant, than even those fleeting
scenes that had spattered my imagination initially.)

"The board of directors, as you might imagine, wasn't much interested in theoretical results, regardless of how interesting they might
have been to academics. They didn't even allow us to publish what
we had, hoping rival firms would continue to invest in something we
knew to be a dead end. It took me several years to make up for that
failure, and I was fortunate to salvage my career at all. No matter
what anyone tells you, they always shoot the messenger. If he's very
lucky, as I was, it's only a flesh wound."

"So even if someone had an unambiguous prediction, they wouldn't be able to do anything about it?"

"That is correct. It's a bit like these oddball quantum phenomena we used to hear so much about, that some people thought were going to allow faster-than-light communication. A fellow I knew in college got stuck with that one as his first job out of school. Apparently everyone who understood anything about the problem knew it could never be used to send signals, but someone in senior management at his employer decided it 'just made sense,' to use the catch-phrase of the arrogant and ignorant." He shook his head sadly in memoriam to a career cut short. "Poor man. He was an absolute genius, a true prodigy in quantum information theory. I hired him as a consultant on the Delvice project, and his own contribution to the work was critical.

"It was taking quite a risk on my part, what with corporate chairs being the only secure university employment these days, and him having been blacklisted. The motto of the modern corporation is: 'If at first you don't succeed, hide any evidence you ever tried.' If that means ruining a few careers here and there it's just too bad. That was the last intellectual work he was able to secure, although I understand he has continued his own theoretical research, despite turning his hand to plumbing for a living. Which I suppose has its remuneration—financially, if in no other way.

"In any case, his experience was a cautionary tale for me, and with his advice I was able to present the final result to the board without quite falling on my own sword."

I almost smiled at the sudden image of him dressed in ramshackle armor like a knight, but had the sense to restrict myself to a weak smile. He was clearly touchy on the subject of careers ruined by the ignorant asking for the impossible. But I could hardly help asking, "But how does that work? If someone had a clear prediction, say, 'Death by hurricane,' wouldn't they be able to know that a hurricane was going to hit?"

"Yes, but when? And where? And will they be in more than one hurricane? We had great hopes for such people, but unfortunately the general principle meant that only a few unambiguous predictions could exist, and even when we could find people who had them, it gave us nothing useful. A dozen people in Los Angeles were found with 'Earthquake' predictions, but that's hardly new information. All it told us was that there would be people killed in California by earthquakes. 'Film at eleven,' as we used to say."

I let the obscure reference go. Film?

"So even in the case where someone knew they were going to die in a singular global catastrophe—a war or famine or plague—they couldn't do a thing to prevent it?"

"Not unless they can also violate the second law of thermodynamics. It would be the equivalent of building a perpetual motion machine. Strictly impossible. Even if they published their prediction, no one would believe them, or the act of publishing it would cause the event to occur. Like a central banker warning of a panic and causing a run on the banks.

"As I said, the marketing people did a better job than they could possibly have dreamed when they named the Delphi Device. The Greeks understood the vagaries of prediction. They knew that knowledge can't be created out of nothing, and in this case the price of knowing one thing is the inability to do anything about it. I would have thought that someone with your name would appreciate that, Cassandra, but I suppose hope really does spring eternal among the young."

I've spent many years since then pondering what he told me, and learning far more math and physics than I ever dreamed existed in those days as a lowly actuarial assistant. I even broke into the company's archives and verified that the theoretical work the Chief's group did decades ago is sound. I've worked through the proofs myself, and I can't see any way around it.

By concentrating the knowledge of how one is going to die into a few simple words, the same information is lost from a million other places that might prevent that occurrence from actually coming to pass. The Ignorance Theorem might be summed up as: "To know what is going to happen to an individual, there must be a loss of information about the group." And by removing information from that dynamic context, we remove the possibility of change.

I hooked up with the Chief's quantum-mechanic friend a few years ago and found he had indeed continued to work on the Ignorance Theorem. He had been able to prove that it is the act of measurement that actually fixes the individual's fate. Free will is a collective phenomenon—individuals only have it when they are an ignorant atom within a larger group. It is in the dynamics, the ebb and flow of information passing freely between individuals in a billion small ways, that makes the process of choice possible. The group can be in a mixture of a million "information eigenstates" at once, each representing a possible future, all evolving as an uncertain whole.

The Delvice picks out one possible future from that mix and collapses the collective wavefunction into a single state relative to the fate of that individual. Which suggests there is one desperate way to reverse the process.

I am not taking this course lightly. I went back to that old back-country mall where I got my prediction so many years ago and bought their machine, certainly one of the last in existence. It was cheap. I've been testing people ever since—my job, now in the upper echelons of the insurance business, has given me access to a lot of blood samples. It isn't exactly ethical, but I have never been at risk of being caught.

I can't tell anything from the data. I wondered if there would be an increase in "Fire" predictions for younger people who were more likely to live until the bombs fell. But the Ignorance Theorem holds.

There is nothing in the data that unambiguously pointed to a sudden increase in violent death. There can't be.

It was only a matter of time before the final thought occurred to me. I am the only person who knows of my prediction. Perhaps I am the only one who got it. The "meteorite man" was certainly unique in his fate. Maybe I am, too.

Suicide won't work. People tried that back in the day—terminally depressed souls who were told by the Delvice they were going to die of cancer and tried to shoot themselves or poison themselves or drown themselves. It never worked. They either failed entirely— the gun misfired, or the "poison" turned out to be candy—or they floated back to the surface and lived out their days as institutionalized vegetables until they died, as predicted, of cancer.

What I need to do is not destroy my life, but rather disperse the knowledge of how it is going to end. If I do that, then perhaps it won't happen. It is the only thing I can think of in my increasingly desperate quest. But I must not reveal to anyone what my prediction is, or they would have to share my fate.

Fate. There's another fine Greek concept.

I've lived well these past years, knowing that tomorrow we all might die. I've never married, never had children. I regret that, if I regret anything. But I've been able to enjoy myself in ways that others, trapped in more conventional lives, might not. Known pleasures and adventures that were made all the more intense by the growing certainty that in the end I must forget them all.

I've destroyed my machine. I really hope it is the last one in existence. I've not been able to find any others. I've done a bit of other destruction, too. Archives, records. It would be hard, though not impossible, for anyone to build a new one. And if they do, I've arranged things so that they will eventually be sent all the information I have on the Ignorance Theorem and the collective nature of free will.

Penultimately, I have murdered my quantum collaborator. His body won't be found. His prediction read simply, "Cassandra." Death by me. When he first heard my name he gave a small start, and then a slow smile spread across his features and he nodded. He was a very old man, even for these long-lived times. His first words were, "I'm happy to say I've been waiting for you for a very, very long time. And I think I am indeed ready to meet you at last." He was a good friend, and helped me to understand the nature of the problem and the only possible solution. But he knew too much. If he didn't know the exact nature of my prediction he guessed the general sense of it. He had to die. And the machine said I had to kill him.

As for me, administering electro-shock therapy to yourself isn't easy, but I'm pretty sure my set-up will work. It's amazing what you can find on iBay. Complete with manuals, even. This old Russian gear is supposed to be the best.

I have it wired so there is a program of shocks that will be administered until I am unable to speak the pass-phrase, which is, as you might expect, "Global Thermonuclear War." As soon as I say it I'll be shocked again. Once an hour has passed with no shocks an automated email will alert the building super. Just one line: "Emergency. Send paramedics to Unit 10-C." If that doesn't work, my rent is due tomorrow, which will certainly bring him to the door soon enough.

I don't know why I'm writing this, even. Before I shock myself the first time I'll scrub the drive and burn this machine.

But I guess I wanted to review in my own mind what brought this to pass. Decades of knowing, or at least suspecting that I knew, how the world was going to end. With tensions rising again in Micronesia over thermo-electric rights to the Western Pacific Basin it is time to act. If I can disperse the knowledge in my mind, turn it back into a million random acts of a million anonymous human beings, put the world back into a superposition of possible futures, it might just be enough to prevent the end.

The paramedics who are called to my side will be changed, however slightly, by responding to that call instead of some other. The doctors and nurses will have the course of their lives deflected. Perhaps I'll even make the news, changing in some small way the minds of many thousands of people who will see a story about me instead of something else. In these things I still have a choice. If not in the manner of my passing, then at least in the manner of my living.

There is no certainty I will succeed. Perhaps I am committing mental suicide for nothing. But I have to try.

I have read a great deal on the effects of electro-shock, and there is a good chance I'll be rehabilitated. I've given much thought to what I might do with the rest of my life, and concluded that the only way to avoid future disasters of this kind is for humanity to expand beyond just one world. We have been to Mars and back. It is time to go there and stay.

The note beside my bed read simply: "Only one Earth is not enough." I'm afraid to say anything more, afraid I will give in to some subconscious temptation that would eventually lead me right back to this point.

I have done what I can. If it works, I will have saved humanity. And no one, not even I, will ever know.

Goodbye.

Story by T. J. Radcliffe
Illustration by Matt Haley

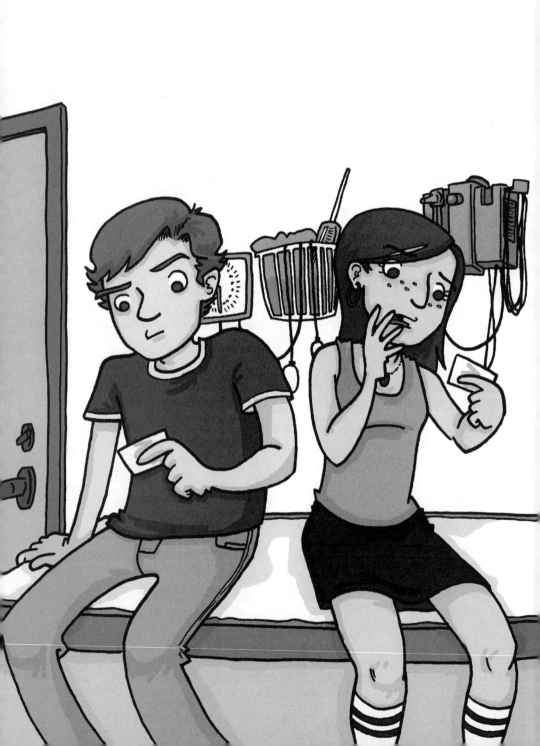

Contributors

Camille Alexa lives with fossils, dried branches, pressed flowers, and other dead things in ¼ of an Edwardian house in the Pacific Northwest. She's fond of big dogs, warm bread, post-apocalyptic love stories, and the serial comma. Her short fiction collection, *Push of the Sky,* earned a starred review from Publishers Weekly and has been nominated for the Endeavour Award. More at CAMILLEALEXA.COM.

John Allison lives near Manchester, UK and intends to keep positive despite all the evidence suggesting that he do otherwise. See his comics and his upbeat attitude at SCARYGOROUND.COM.

Kate Beaton draws men in fancy hats for a living. On an exciting day she'll draw a character with epaulets. Her website is HARKAVAGRANT.COM.

Matthew Bennardo has lived in Cleveland, Ohio, for the past twenty years. His stories have previously been published in Asimov's Science Fiction and Strange Horizons, among other markets. He can be contacted at: MATTHEW.BENNARDO@GMAIL.COM.

Brandon Bolt draws cartoon pictures in order to eat, and has made a variety of other unclever life decisions. Perhaps you will be affected by one of them one day. To start, read the cartoon he draws at NOBODYSCORES.COM. There is also a portfolio site at LOOSENUTSTUDIO.COM if perhaps you are interested in having some pictures drawn, which experts concede is possible.

Vera Brosgol spends her days drawing storyboards for animation in Portland, Oregon. At night she produces illustrations and comics, and her first book, *Anya's Ghost,* will be published by First Second in Spring 2011. Her website is VERABEE.COM.

Jeffrey Brown is the author of numerous autobiographical graphic novels such as *Clumsy* and *Funny Misshapen Body* as well as humorous work including *Incredible Change-Bots* and *Cats Are Weird.* WWW.JEFFREYBROWNCOMICS.COM

Scott C. is Scott Campbell, art director for *Psychonauts* and *Brütal Legend* at Double Fine Productions. Scott has done numerous comics that have appeared in such anthologies as *Hickee, Flight, Beasts!,* and *Project: Superior.* He has also painted many clever little paintings that have shown in such places as San Francisco, Los Angeles, Portland, Montreal, and Japan. SCOTT-C.BLOGSPOT.COM

Mitch Clem has made a ton of comics, including *My Stupid Life* (published by New Reliable Press) and *Nothing Nice to Say* (published by Dark Horse Comics). Everything about him lives at MITCHCLEM.COM.

Daliso Chaponda is a writer & comedian who writes fiction on trains as he travels to stand-up gigs. His fiction is often dark and depressing to compensate for the vacuousness of his night-job. He has been shortlisted for the Carl Brandon Society Award, Northwest Breakthrough Comedian Award, and so on. He likes strawberries. WWW.DALISO.COM

John Chernega lives in southern Minnesota with his wife and sons. Aside from a few corporate catalogs, "Almond" is his first published work. You can read his blog at CHERNEY.VOX.COM. He keeps a nondescript business card on his nightstand that says "Clumsy Hippopotamus", but he refuses to divulge whether it's from a machine of death, or if he's been moonlighting as a clumsy hippopotamus.

Danielle Corsetto is the creator of the webcomic "Girls With Slingshots," the comedic story about two girls, a bar, and a talking cactus, which can be found at GIRLSWITHSLINGSHOTS.COM. She lives with two cats and a 9-year-old goldfish in Shepherdstown, West Virginia in a very old house. These days she spends most of her time drinking alone and talking to herself.

Chris Cox is a deranged, one-eyed hunchback wandering by night through the wastelands of Pawtucket. His age isn't known, but sightings go back three hundred years and he's generally believed to be a cannibal. Author of one and a half phenomalous black comedy novels, he's represented by ParkEast Literary Agency, with whom he only communicates via cryptic notes written on apples injected with larvae. Needless to say, he's a tricky one. EVERWAKE_@HOTMAIL.COM

Ben "Yahtzee" Croshaw was born and raised in England but now lives in Australia. Primarily a gaming writer, he is responsible for the "Zero Punctuation" video reviews at The Escapist online magazine. His first novel, *Mogworld*, has been published by Dark Horse Books. He can be reached through his personal site at FULLYRAMBLOMATIC.COM.

Alexander Danner writes and teaches comics. His most recent series is "Gingerbread Houses," a retelling of Hansel and Gretel illustrated by Edward J. Grug III. "Gingerbread Houses" and other fairy tales can be found at PICTURESTORYTHEATER. COM. More of Danner's stories and experiments can also be found at TWENTYSEVENLETTERS.COM. He is co-author of the textbook *Character Design for Graphic Novels,* and he teaches Writing the Graphic Novel at Emerson College.

Aaron Diaz gave up a life of professional science to draw comics on the internet. He shares a name with a Mexican pop star. DRESDENCODAK.COM

Rene Engström is a cartoonist and illustrator living and working out of Östersund and Malmö, Sweden. She has just wrapped up the 300-page online graphic novel *Anders Loves Maria.* RENEENGSTROM.COM

Jess Fink is the author of *We Can Fix It: A Time Travel Memoir,* published by Top Shelf. She has seen the all-knowing Space Rainbow and eaten its gummy heart. She also makes T-shirts. Her erotic webcomic about a Victorian robot is at: JESSFINK.COM/ CHESTER5000XYV

James Foreman lives in Pittsburgh and is probably drinking coffee. He blogs about his life's esoterica at: JAMESFOREMAN.COM.

Tom Francis is a writer and editor for PC Gamer magazine and PCGamer.com. He keeps a pet blog called James at PENTADACT.COM, and you can e-mail him at PENTADACT@GMAIL.COM.

Rafa Franco was born on a wee town in Argentina 27 years ago. Graphic designer by trade, he has had some art and a couple of articles published where you will never find them, and has managed to unwillingly produce some small-time freelance graphic design work. Like an idiot savant, he roams the muddy slime of mediocrity and has the common sense to let the occasional spark of creativity out to the world. If you feel like traveling fifteen thousand miles south to the city of La Plata near Buenos Aires, you may catch him starring in a play as a 70-year-old backwater whore. Or you can reach him at RFRANCO81@YAHOO.COM. It's okay.

Dorothy Gambrell is the last living American to enjoy listening to the radio. She draws unfortunate cartoons on a regular basis at CATANDGIRL.COM.

Shaenon K. Garrity is the creator of the daily webstrips "Narbonic" and "Skin Horse" (the latter co-written with fellow contributor Jeffrey Wells), as well as many other comics both on- and offline. She occasionally writes scripts for Marvel Comics, a disproportionate number of which involve department-store Santas. She also works as a freelance manga editor for VIZ Media and teaches at the Academy of Art in San Francisco. She lives in Berkeley with her husband, Andrew Farago, and their neurotic cat Tesla.

KC Green does comics online and off. He did some comics for Nickelodeon magazine and then they closed their doors. He blames himself every day. Currently he
does the webcomic "Gunshow" at GUNSHOWCOMIC.COM, but for how long until his
unfocused, child-like mind wanders on to something else? You can try to find more
of his work, old and new, at his unfinished website KCGREENDOTCOM.COM.

William Grallo is the son of Lou. He was the winner of the Will Inman Award for
Poetry and a runner-up for the Ursula K. LeGuin Award for Imaginative Fiction.
He has had fiction published in Rosebud magazine and online at ALWAYSBLACK.COM.

C. E. Guimont lives in Berlin, Germany. His previous two novels, *The Ten Lies She
Told Me and The One or Two I Told Her* and *That Business With the Rabbit* are in Staten
Island's Fresh Kills dark archive.

Matt Haley is best known as a comic-book illustrator for DC, Dark Horse and
Marvel. Currently drawing the sequel to *Badass* (Harper), he directs film and
watches Japanese kids' shows when sober. MATTHALEY.COM

Christopher Hastings is the creator of *The Adventures of Dr. McNinja*. He lives in
Brooklyn with his fiancée, Carly, and their dog, Commissioner Gordon. You can
read his comic for free at DRMCNINJA.COM, and you can email him for free at
CHRIS@DRMCNINJA.COM.

Paul Horn is an infographics journalist, illustrator and man-about-town. His comic
"Cool Jerk" is found in finer comics shops and at COOLJERK.COM. He and his wife
Darlene live in San Diego and enjoy writing blurbs in the third person.

Sherri Jacobsen writes copy for movie marketing by day, and rewrites copy for
finicky movie marketing executives by night. This is her first appearance in a
publication not bound by staples.

John Keogh is an itinerant rambler with fists of steel and a nose for trouble,
currently roughhousing his way through New England. You can see him try to
do right by his kin on LUCID-TV.COM.

Karl Kerschl has been drawing comics professionally for 15 years. He has worked on
Superman, The Flash, Robin and *The Teen Titans*, among other heroic things, and is the
author of the Eisner-nominated webcomic "The Abominable Charles Christopher."
More of his work can be found at KARLKERSCHL.COM.

Kazu Kibuishi is the creator of the *Amulet* graphic novel series for Scholastic Graphix and the *Flight* comics anthology for Villard Books. He lives and works in Alhambra, California. BOLTCITY.COM

Adam Koford is the creator of a book called *The Laugh-Out-Loud Cats Sell Out.* During the day he works for a video game company making secret things he's not allowed to talk about unless there's an official public relations envoy present. ADAMKOFORD.COM

Douglas J Lane's narrative weirdness has appeared in T*ales of the Unanticipated* and *Pure Francis*, and can be found in the forthcoming anthology *Seasons In The Abyss*. He currently juggles his day job with his work on a novel and a flaming chainsaw. He can be reached—and might even reply—at DJ.DOUGIEJ@GMAIL.COM.

Roger Langridge is currently the cartoonist behind the Eisner- and Harvey-nominated *Muppet Show Comic Book* and writer of Marvel's all-ages superhero book, *Thor: The Mighty Avenger*, putting in occasional bursts of activity on a web strip, "Mugwhump the Great", whenever he gets a spare moment. His past credits include his multi-award-nominated self-published comic, *Fred the Clown*, and being co-writer and artist of Marvel's *Fin Fang Four*.

K M Lawrence may be writing in Ireland, or may be writing in England. Either way, he can be contacted at KLUDGECO.COM.

David Malki ! is the author of the Eisner-, Harvey- and Ignatz-nominated comic strip "Wondermark." His latest collection is *Dapper Caps & Pedal-Copters*, published by Dark Horse Books. He lives in Los Angeles and he likes to fly airplanes. Read comics, contact him, etc. at WONDERMARK.COM.

Erin McKean is a lexicographer (look it up). She lexicogs as the founder of Wordnik. com, and blogs about dresses at DRESSADAY.COM. She has written one novel, four books about wacky words, and enough email to cover the entire moon with a layer of alphanumeric characters five ems deep.

Brian McLachlan makes two webcomics: "The Princess Planet" and "Smooth N Natural." He does a lot of work for kids, including stuff for Owl magazine, Nickelodeon magazine, Nelson Textbooks and the graphic novel *Ticket To Space* for Scholastic Canada. Basically, a lot of children have probably added moustaches to his illustrations. He's also worked for Vice, YM, Dragon, The Toronto Star, Oni Press and other incongruous publishers.

Kevin McShane is a cartoonist, designer, actor, filmmaker, writer, photographer, and a dozen other things that won't impress you either. He can be found digitally at KEVINMCSHANE.ORG.

Dylan Meconis is the creator of *Bite Me!* and *Family Man*. Should one come across her tricorner hat (lost in a pheasant shoot), please send it home to DYLANMECONIS.COM.

Camron Miller is an amateur writer and classics student. A graduate of St Bees School and the Lawrenceville School, he divides his time between the University of London, the Surrey Hills, and a seaside village near the Lake District National Park. He can be reached at CAMRONMILLER@HOTMAIL.COM.

Carly Monardo lives and draws in Brooklyn, NY with her fiancé and their ridiculous dog. A graduate of the School of Visual Arts Animation Program, Carly has worked on such shows as *Sunday Pants, SuperNormal,* and *Venture Bros.* She also works as a free-lance illustrator. You can find more of her work at WHIRRINGBLENDER.COM.

Randall Munroe, a cartoonist from southern Virginia, is the creator of the webcomic "xkcd" (XKCD.COM), one of the most popular comics on the Internet. Formerly a roboticist at NASA, he now makes a living writing comics. He spends his time drawing, traveling, and training computers to beat humans at Rock-Paper-Scissors. He lives in Somerville, Massachusetts.

Nation of Amanda enjoys using swear words and painting and drawing comics, not in that order. She currently lives with, is engaged to, and frequently collaborates with Mitch Clem who cannot even believe how awesome she is. Her blog lives at NATIONOFAMANDA.LIVEJOURNAL.COM.

Ryan North is an author who lives in Toronto, which is in Canada. He writes a comic strip called "Dinosaur Comics" which you can pick up in book form at your local bookstore, or which you can just read for free at QWANTZ.COM. They're pretty okay! You can reach him through his website.

Pelotard has worked at Microsoft in Dublin, at the European Space Agency in Noordwijk-an-Zee in the Netherlands, and has found his degree in theoretical physics completely useless in his current career at a translation agency. He lives outside Stockholm, Sweden, with his family, and can be reached at PELOTARD@PELOTARD.COM.

Ramón Pérez is an overcaffeinated Canadian who likes to draw picture books for the likes of Marvel and DC Comics, while at the same time indulging his own peculiar muse by regaling the world with tales such as "Kukuburi" and quirky comedies the likes of "ButterNutSquash." For a deeper foray into his mind and meanderings visit RAMONPEREZ.COM.

Brian Quinlan recently earned a degree in English with a concentration in Creative Writing at Virginia Tech. He has yet to decide what the hell he'll do next. Brian can be contacted at: BDPQUINLAN@GMAIL.COM.

T. J. Radcliffe is a mercenary scientist and poet living in Kingston, Ontario, Canada. When not sailing or hiking he writes poetry to go with the whimsical and beautiful images created by Hilary Farmer at GREENTEADOODLES.WORDPRESS.COM, with whom he has a graphic-novel/epic-poem/web-comic in development. He is also working on a self-referential novel about the nature of stories called *Metastory*, helps mentor a FIRST Robotics team, is an adjunct professor at Queen's University working on cancer genetics, pretends to keep a day job, and has serious plans to get some sleep in the late fall of 2037. He can be reached via his website: TJRADCLIFFE.COM

Jesse Reklaw has been drawing the weekly comic strip "Slow Wave" since 1995, and has two collections published: *Dreamtoons* and *The Night of Your Life*. Find more online at SLOWWAVE.COM.

Katie Sekelsky lives in Pennsylvania. She has had illustrations published with the Harvard University Press and featured in Cooper-Hewitt's National Design Triennial. Her work can be seen on her mother's refrigerator (by appointment only) and at KSEKELSKY.COM.

Gord Sellar is a graduate of Clarion West 2006, and has lived in South Korea since 2002. His writing has appeared in Asimov's Science Fiction, Clarkesworld, Interzone, and Jetse de Vries' *Shine* anthology, as well as in *The Year's Best Science Fiction Vol. 26*, edited by Gardner Dozois. He was a finalist for the John W. Campbell Award for Best New Writer in 2009. Visit his website at GORDSELLAR.COM.

Kean Soo is the author and illustrator of the *Jellaby* series of graphic novels. He spends a distressing amount of time on the Internet, and not enough on his website, SECRETFRIENDSOCIETY.COM.

Jeff Stautz lives in Vancouver, Canada. He is the Fiction Editor of *PRISM international*, is a former Fishtrap Fellow, and was a writer-in-residence at the Montana Artists' Refuge. His work has appeared most recently in *The First Line* and is forthcoming in *Event*.

Cameron Stewart is the multiple-award nominated illustrator of *Batman & Robin*, *Seaguy*, *Catwoman*, and *The Other Side*. His serialized online graphic novel *Sin Titulo* won the 2010 Eisner Award for Best Digital Comic, and can be found at SINTITULOCOMIC.COM.

Kris Straub is the cartoonist behind the webcomic "Chainsawsuit" and the sci-fi humor saga *Starslip*. He's also co-author of the Harvey Award-nominated *How To Make Webcomics*, published by Image. Kris has lived in every city in America for at least one second.

James Lafond Sutter is the Fiction Editor for Paizo Publishing, creators of the Pathfinder Roleplaying Game. He is the award-winning author of numerous game products and short stories, and his fiction has appeared in such venues as *Black Gate*, *Catastrophia*, and *Apex Magazine*, as well as been translated into several languages. His anthology *Before They Were Giants* pairs the first stories of SF greats from William Gibson to China Mieville with new interviews and writing advice from the authors themselves. For more information, visit JAMESLSUTTER.COM.

Marcus Thiele (familiarly known as *Marcus Parcus)* disappeared under mysterious circumstances at the age of 27 and was hastily replaced with a life-like replica. The pretense of his continued existence and artistic output is maintained through the silence, exile and cunning of the skilled estate representatives at THEMONKEYMIND.LIVEJOURNAL.COM.

Kelly Tindall is Canadian, and his drawings can be found all over a bunch of Image comic books. Go say "hi": KELLYTINDALL.BLOGSPOT.COM.

Dean Trippe is an alien robot ninja wizard (from the future) who makes comics. He is a former comic shop manager, a lifelong superhero fan, and has an actual degree in comics. For more of his work, visit DEANTRIPPE.COM.

J Jack Unrau is a freelance writer and vagabond librarian whose work has appeared on Wired.com, CBC Radio and in Broken Pencil. Living in China taught him valuable lessons about taking pictures of riot police. J's online home is THEDUBIOUSMONK.NET.

Bartholomew von Klick lives beneath a bridge in Missouri, emerging only to collect a toll from passers-by. He sometimes mutters about all the things he would like to eat, but has not yet been able to kill. He has thirty-six cats, and a beautiful wife who rises from the grave every night to hunt and bring him snacks from the orphanage.

Julia Wainwright lives in Suffolk, England, where she writes stuff, makes things, and grows 0.1 percent of her own food. She's just happy to be here. Julia can be reached at JULIACW@NTLWORLD.COM.

Jeffrey C. Wells is the co-creator of the award-winning webcomic "Skin Horse", found online at SKIN-HORSE.COM. He himself has also won awards, but they were for things like "Worst Opening Line of a Science Fiction Story", so if you want to award him with things so he no longer feels inferior to his own webcomic, that would be great. He lives in the wilds of rural Wisconsin with a wonderful spouse, a dial-up modem, and more pets than you can shake a stick at. Watch him do his thing at JEFFREYCWELLS.LIVEJOURNAL.COM.

David Michael Wharton (INHETET@GMAIL.COM) is a freelance writer and journalist from Texas. When not sweating in the trenches as an editor for Creative Screen-writing Magazine, he hammers out screenplays and short fiction and swears one of these days he's going to get around to that novel, damn it.

Shannon Wheeler is the Eisner-winning creator of the comics *Too Much Coffee Man*, *Postage Stamp Funnies* and *How To Be Happy*. His cartoons appear regularly in the New Yorker. TMCM.COM

Living deep in the savage lands known as the 'Dirty Jerz,' Kit Yona runs an auto salvage yard, adds income via poker whenever possible and plays rugby with an enthusiasm that far outstrips any athleticism he might believe he possesses. In his lack of spare time Kit edits and writes for the fantasy book review site The Griffin or the Agate (THEGRIFFIN.COM) to justify the time spent getting his Masters degree in English. He blames his appearance in this tome on his beautiful muse of a wife, Laura. He can be tormented/harassed/contacted at JYDOG1@GMAIL.COM.

Copyright

thank you for reading our book